Point of Care Medicine

A Concise Guide to the Care of the Hospitalized Patient

Point of Care Medicine

A Concise Guide to the Care of the Hospitalized Patient

Anthony D. Slonim, MD, DrPH
Executive Vice President/Chief Medical Officer
Barnabas Health
West Orange, New Jersey
Professor, Medicine, Pediatrics, Community and Public Health
University of Medicine and Dentistry of New Jersey
New Jersey Medical School
Newark, New Jersey

Alexander B. Levitov, MD, FCCP, FCCM, RDCS
Professor of Medicine
Eastern Virginia Medical School
Department of Internal Medicine
Division of Pulmonary and Critical Care Medicine
Norfolk, Virginia

Paul Marik, MD
Professor, Internal Medicine
Eastern Virginia Medical School
Norfolk, Virginia

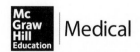

New York   Chicago   San Francisco   Lisbon   London   Madrid   Mexico City
Milan   New Delhi   San Juan   Seoul   Singapore   Sydney   Toronto

Point of Care Medicine: A Concise Guide to the Care of the Hospitalized Patient

1 2 3 4 5 6 7 8 9 0 DSS/DSS 18 17 16 15 14 13

ISBN 978-0-07-176298-4
MHID 0-07-176298-1

This book was set in ITC New Baskerville by Aptara, Inc.
The editors were James F. Shanahan and Kim J. Davis.
The production supervisor was Richard Ruzycka.
Project management was provided by Indu Jawwad of Aptara, Inc.
Shenzhen Donnelley was printer and binder.

This book is printed on acid-free paper.

Library of Congress Cataloging-in-Publication Data

Point of care medicine / [edited by] Anthony D. Slonim, Alexander B. Levitov, Paul Marik.
   p. ; cm.
  Includes bibliographical references and index.
  ISBN 978-0-07-176298-4 (hardcover : alk. paper) – ISBN 0-07-176298-1 (hardcover : alk. paper)
  I. Slonim, Anthony D.   II. Levitov, Alexander.   III. Marik, Paul Ellis.
  [DNLM: 1. Hospitalization–Outlines.   2. Evidence-Based Medicine–Outlines. WX 18.2]

362.11–dc23   2012040996

Contents

Section 3: Special Populations

Contributors

Shrirang Ajvalia
Intern, Medical Affairs
Barnabas Health
West Orange, New Jersey

Shilpa Amara, PharmD
Medical Communications Specialist
Barnabas Health
South Plainfield, New Jersey

David P. Bahner, MD, RDMS,
FACEP, FAIUM, FAAEM
Associate Professor
Director of Ultrasound
Ohio State University
Department of Emergency Medicine
Columbus, Ohio

Jody P. Boggs, MD
Chief Resident, Internal Medicine
Eastern Virginia Medical School
Norfolk, Virginia

Christian H. Butcher, MD, FCCP
Carilion Medical Center
Roanoke, Virginia

James S. Cain, MD, FACP
Clinical Assistant Professor of
Medicine
University of Virginia and Edward Via
School of Medicine, Virginia Tech
Chief of Medicine and Medical
Director, Dialysis
Carilion Medical Center
Roanoke, Virginia

David J. Castaldo, MD
Program Director, Internal Medicine
Eastern Virginia Medical School
Norfolk, Virginia

Ronald S. Chamberlain, MD,
MPA, FACS
Chairman and Surgeon-in-Chief,
*   Department of Surgery*
Saint Barnabas Medical Center
Professor of Surgery
University of Medicine and Dentistry
*   of New Jersey (UMDNJ)*
Livingston, New Jersey

Catherine J. Derber, MD
Assistant Professor, Division of
*   Infectious Diseases, Department of*
*   Internal Medicine*
Eastern Virginia Medical School
Norfolk, Virginia

Himanshu Desai, MD
Assistant Professor, Department of
*   Medicine*
Division of Pulmonary and Critical
*   Care Medicine*
Eastern Virginia Medical School
Norfolk, Virginia

Allison R. Durica, MD
Section Chief, Maternal Fetal Medicine
Assistant Professor, Obstetrics and
*   Gynecology*
Virginia Tech Carilion School of
*   Medicine and Research Institute*
Roanoke, Virginia

Ronald W. Flenner, MD
Associate Professor, Division of
*   Infectious Diseases, Department of*
*   Internal Medicine*
Associate Dean for Medical Education
Eastern Virginia Medical School
Norfolk, Virginia

L. Beth Gadkowski, MD, MPH, MS

*Assistant Professor, Division of
    Infectious Diseases, Department of
    Internal Medicine*
Eastern Virginia Medical School
Norfolk, Virginia

B. Mitchell Goodman, III, MD

*Assistant Professor, Department of
    Internal Medicine*
Eastern Virginia Medical School
Norfolk, Virginia

Hannah L. Hays, MD Fellow

*Medical Toxicology, Department of
    Emergency Medicine*
Ohio State University
*Central Ohio Poison Center at
    Nationwide Children's Hospital*
Columbus, Ohio

Michael Hooper, MD

*Assistant Professor, Department of
    Medicine*
*Division of Pulmonary and Critical
    Care Medicine*
Eastern Virginia Medical School
Norfolk, Virginia

**Colin G. Kaide, MD, FACEP,
FAAEM, UHM**

*Associate Professor of Emergency
    Medicine*
*Board-Certified Specialist in
    Hyperbaric Medicine*
Specialist in Wound Care
*Ohio State University Department of
    Emergency Medicine*
Columbus, Ohio

Nina Khachiyants, MD

Assistant Professor of Medicine,
*Virginia Tech Carilion School of
    Medicine and Research Institute*
Roanoke, Virginia

Joan K. Kowalec, MD

Department of Medicine
Newark Beth Israel Medical Center
Assistant Professor, Internal Medicine
*New Jersey Medical School, University
    of Medicine and Dentistry*
Newark, New Jersey

Robert G. Lahita, MD, PhD

Chairman, Department of Medicine
Newark Beth Israel Medical Center
*Professor, Internal Medicine, New
    Jersey Medical School*
University of Medicine and Dentistry
Newark, New Jersey

**Alexander B. Levitov, MD, FCCP,
FCCM, RDCS**

Professor of Medicine
Eastern Virginia Medical School
Department of Internal Medicine
*Division of Pulmonary and Critical
    Care Medicine*
Norfolk, Virginia

Paul Marik, MD

Professor, Internal Medicine
Eastern Virginia Medical School
Norfolk, Virginia

Amanda B. Murchison, MD

*Clerkship Director-Assistant Residency
    Program Director*
*Assistant Professor, Obstetrics and
    Gynecology*
*Virginia Tech Carilion School of
    Medicine and Research Institute*
Roanoke, Virginia

**Vijayashree Murthy, MS, DNB,
MCh**

Department of Surgery
Saint Barnabas Medical Center
Livingston, New Jersey

Edward C. Oldfield, III, MD
*Professor and Chief, Division of
    Infectious Diseases, Department of
    Internal Medicine*
Eastern Virginia Medical School
Norfolk, Virginia

Armin Rashidi, MD
Division of Internal Medicine
Eastern Virginia Medical School
Norfolk, Virginia

Jeffrey Schnader, MD
Professor of Medicine
Eastern Virginia Medical School
Hampton, Virginia

Anthony D. Slonim, MD, DrPH
*Executive Vice President/Chief
    Medical Officer*
Barnabas Health
West Orange, New Jersey
*Professor, Medicine, Pediatrics,
    Community and Public Health*
*University of Medicine and Dentistry
    of New Jersey*
New Jersey Medical School
Newark, New Jersey

Lauren S. Sparber, MD, MS
Department of Surgery
*University of Medicine and Dentistry
    of New Jersey*
Newark, New Jersey

Prasanna Sridharan, MD
*Saint George's University School of
    Medicine*
Grenada, West Indies

Sami G. Tahhan, MD
Division of Internal Medicine
Eastern Virginia Medical School
Norfolk, Virginia

Stephanie B. Troy, MD
Assistant Professor
*Division of Infectious Diseases,
    Department of Medicine*
Eastern Virginia Medical School
Norfolk, Virginia

Patrice M. Weiss, MD
*Chair, Department of OB/GYN,
    Professor*
*Carilion Clinic/ Virginia Tech
    Carilion School of Medicine and
    Research Institute*
Roanoke, Virginia

Dedicated to the memory of my Grandma Betty
who taught me everything I needed to know by age 5.
Anthony D. Slonim

Dedicated to Irina and Alexandra.
Alexander B. Levitov

Dedicated to my wife Susan and my pugs, Molly
and Ernie, the source of all my inspiration.
Paul Marik

Preface

We are pleased to introduce *Point of Care Medicine: A Concise Guide to the Care of the Hospitalized Patient,* which was conceptualized as a concise and "ready reference" for the physician providing hospital-based care for adult patients. We are hopeful that the book's organization will be helpful for both the intern and experienced hospitalist. In a volume of this size, decisions need to be made about what content to include or exclude. This book is not intended to replace major textbooks of medicine, but to provide evidence-based information to assist with on-call problem solving and treatment. The aim of this work was to prioritize the common problems encountered during hospitalization and provide supplemental information in easy-to-access websites and reference materials.

We are grateful to the chapter authors who worked diligently to provide us with chapters that were robust in content, but where every word mattered. We would like to add a special note of thanks to Maria Levitov for her assistance. As a first edition, there will clearly be things that we missed or wish we had done better. Please feel free to contact and inform us of ways to improve this volume's use for its intended purpose. We hope that you find this book useful in your care of patients.

Anthony D. Slonim, MD, DrPH
Alexander B. Levitov, MD, FCCP, FCCM, RDCS
Paul Marik, MD

Section 1: General Medical Issues

CHAPTER 1

Bedside Procedures

Christian H. Butcher

INTRODUCTION

Procedures are an essential component of health care delivery, and competence assures the best possible outcome. Beyond technical expertise and skill, components of competency include a thorough understanding of the indications, contraindications, and risk-to-benefit ratios for each procedure. In addition, the ability to recognize and manage procedural complications should be considered a fundamental part of any procedure-related curriculum.

AIRWAY MANAGEMENT

Patients who are unable to adequately ventilate or protect their airway from foreign material, such as food, oral secretions, and blood, must be managed both expeditiously and skillfully to optimize outcomes.

Head Tilt and Jaw Thrust

Indications

- Relief of soft tissue airway obstruction (tongue, posterior oropharyngeal crowding)
- Often used in conjunction with bag-mask ventilation

Contraindications

- Cervical spine injury or previous cervical fixation (head tilt)
- Severe rheumatoid arthritis or ankylosing spondylitis (head tilt)
- Down syndrome (head tilt)
- Trauma to the lower face or mandible (jaw thrust)
- Jaw thrust may be poorly tolerated in awake patients

Mechanism

- Brings tongue forward away from posterior oropharynx
- Straightens upper airway, thereby creating a more direct line from the mouth to the trachea

Technique: Head Tilt

- Place patient in supine position.
- Place one hand on the forehead and the other hand below the chin.
- Without flexing or extending the neck, tilt the head back by applying downward pressure on the forehead while lifting the chin.
- The mouth should remain closed.

Technique: Jaw Thrust

- Place patient in supine position.
- Standing at the head of the bed, slightly open the mouth.
- Place fingers under the angle of the mandible on both sides.
- Lift the mandible up and out, attempting to lift the lower teeth (or gum) over the upper teeth.

Advantages

- No need for anesthesia
- May act as a respiratory stimulus in sedated patients

Disadvantages

- May cause discomfort (jaw thrust)
- Jaw dislocation
- Does not prevent aspiration

Complications
- Ineffective airway
- Damage to the spine in susceptible patients (rheumatoid arthritis, ankylosing spondylitis)

Oral and Nasal Airways (see http://www.healthsystem.virginia.edu/Internet/Anesthesiology-Elective/airway/equipment.cfm)

Indications
- Relief of upper airway obstruction, usually from soft tissues (tongue)
- Used as an adjunct for bag-mask ventilation
- Acts as a bite block after orotracheal intubation or for procedures such as bronchoscopy to protect the scope

Contraindications
- Severe oropharyngeal or nasal trauma or occlusion.
- Basilar skull fracture or previous skull base or posterior pharyngeal surgery (nasal airway).
- Coagulopathy or late-stage pregnancy can complicate nasal airway insertion by causing potentially life-threatening epistaxis.

Mechanism
- Oral airways act to both lift the tongue forward and away from the posterior oropharynx, and to create a patent pathway through the oropharynx by depressing the tongue away from the palate.
- Nasal airways work by creating a channel that bypasses the oropharynx.

Technique (Oral Airway)
- Select an oral airway of appropriate length. An acceptable length would extend from the patient's earlobe to the corner of the mouth.
- Open the mouth and depress the tongue with either a tongue blade or your finger (or thumb depending on your position).
- Consider anesthetizing the oropharynx with a topical anesthetic spray.
- Insert the airway so that the concave side is against the tongue.
- Initially, the tip should point toward the posterior oropharynx.
- Insert the airway slowly, attempting to follow the contour of the tongue with the tip of the airway.
- If done correctly, at the end of insertion your wrist will be flexed and your hand will resemble the head and neck of a swan.

Technique (Nasal Airway)
- Use a long cotton-tipped swab covered with lidocaine jelly to both anesthetize the tract and to help assess patency. Insert the swab all the way to the posterior nasopharynx.
- Compare both sides for ease of insertion of the swab, then remove swab.
- Choose the side that will accommodate the largest airway, based on the ease of swab insertion.
- Consider instilling a 10% phenylephrine solution or spraying oxymetazoline into the nare of choice.
- Have soft, flexible nasal airways of several different sizes set aside.
- Based on visual inspection and swab insertion, choose the largest airway likely to be successfully inserted into the nare, then insert slowly and advance straight back to the posterior nasopharynx, taking care to maintain position under the inferior turbinate (the floor of the nose).
- If the airway is curved, insert it with the curved side down.
- If the airway will not pass, use a smaller airway. *Do not force a nasal airway.*
- The airway should reflect off the posterior nasopharynx and begin to travel toward the glottis. If this does not occur, take the tube out and bend it slightly at the tip, then reinsert.

Advantages
- Oral airway: can be used in cases of nasal trauma or fracture and skull base injury, causes less bleeding in the coagulopathic patient, and may act as a respiratory stimulus in the sedated patient

- Nasal airway: can be used in cases of oral trauma, has less gag response than oral airway, works well in patients with poor mouth opening or in seizing patients, and may act as a respiratory stimulus in the sedated patient

Disadvantages and Complications

- May require topical anesthesia.
- Cannot be used in cases of facial or nasal trauma.
- May cause bleeding.
- May cause nasal or pharyngeal mucosal trauma and lacerations.
- Must only be used in spontaneously ventilating patients or in conjunction with bag-mask ventilation.
- An improperly selected oral airway can worsen upper airway obstruction by forcing the tongue posteriorly.

Bag-Mask Ventilation (see http://www.acep.org/content.aspx?Id=40992)

Indications

- Any condition resulting in a lack of adequate spontaneous ventilation
- Often used after sedating for either laryngeal mask airway (LMA) insertion or endotracheal intubation

Contraindications

- Airway, breathing, and circulation supersede all other concerns in a patient who succumbs to respiratory arrest; bag-mask ventilation may be the best option until a definitive airway can be established.
- If the situation is more elective, the following have been described as relative contraindications:
  - Vomiting
  - Full stomach
  - Hiatal hernia
  - Trauma to face or trachea
  - Tracheoesophageal fistula
  - Cervical spine injury or disease

Mechanism

- Positive pressure either augments ventilation in spontaneously breathing patients or provides ventilation in apneic patients.
- Provides supplemental oxygen to the conducting airways.

Technique

- Obtain the necessary equipment: Yankauer suction catheter, face mask, Ambu bag, oxygen, positive end-expiratory pressure (PEEP) valve.
- Place the patient in supine position, with the neck extended slightly forward (anatomic sniff position, similar to that used for intubation).
- Place either an oral or nasal airway.
- Two-person technique is superior: One person stands at the head of the bed and places the mask over the mouth and nose. A seal is made by pressing down with the thumb and thenar eminence of both hands while the fingers, placed under the mandible and chin, lift the mandible up. The second person delivers positive pressure by squeezing the Ambu bag.
- One person technique is occasionally unavoidable: Stand at the head of the bed and place the mask over the mouth and nose. Cup the mask with the thumb and index finger, while placing the remaining fingers under the mandible and chin (C-grip). Apply downward pressure with the thumb and index finger, and upward pressure with the remaining fingers.
- A perfect seal is unnecessary; an air leak is acceptable as long as ventilation is adequate.
- Delivered breaths should be synchronized to the patients respiratory efforts, if present.
- Be careful not to cause breath stacking (important in chronic obstructive pulmonary disease and asthma patients).
- Use a PEEP valve or squeeze and hold the Ambu bag (inspiratory pause) in difficult to oxygenate patients (pulmonary edema, acute respiratory distress syndrome).
- Consider cricoid pressure to constrict the upper esophagus thereby preventing inadvertent gastric insufflation.

Advantages

- Provides positive pressure, which either provides ventilation to the apneic patient or augments inadequate ventilation in the spontaneously breathing patient
- Noninvasive technique ideal for patients requiring temporary ventilatory assistance

Disadvantages and Complications

- May cause severe gastric distention.
- May cause hemodynamic compromise either reflexively from gastric distention (vagal response) or from air trapping and elevated intrathoracic pressure with resultant decreased venous return. Cricoid pressure and lower respiratory rates reduce these risks.
- May cause vomiting.

Laryngeal Mask Airway (LMA) Insertion (see video: www.youtube.com/watch?V=tgoyjzsunk0)

Standard LMA

- An LMA is a type of supraglottic airway that does not traverse the vocal cords, but instead rests upon and makes a seal with the glottic structures.
- The components of the tube include an aperture that rests on the supraglottic structures, an inflatable cuff that surrounds the aperture and facilitates the seal, an inflation line connected to a pilot balloon similar to standard adult endotracheal tubes, and a long flexible airway tube that protrudes from the mouth after placement.
- Although this type of airway is a relatively recent addition to the airway armamentarium, it has been widely accepted and integrated into airway management algorithms.

Intubating LMA

- Similar in most respects to a standard LMA.
- The inner diameter of the tube is large enough to accept up to a size 8.0 endotracheal tube.
- The airway tube is usually shorter and more rigid than a standard LMA to facilitate correct positioning of the endotracheal tube.
- The aperture contains an epiglottis elevating bar that forces the epiglottis forward (anteriorly) to allow passage of the endotracheal tube.
- Because of the rigid design, the intubating LMA is a cross between an LMA and a rigid laryngoscope, being easily manipulated outside the mouth.

Indications

- An alternative for situations when bag-mask ventilation or endotracheal intubation are difficult.
- Often used in the operating room for relatively short surgical procedures.
- Can be used to support ventilation during bronchoscopy.
- Intubating LMA facilitates endotracheal intubation while allowing for simultaneous ventilation.

Contraindications

- Orofacial trauma
- Upper airway or pharyngeal obstruction from tumor or abscess
- Need for high-pressure mechanical ventilation (air leaks)
- Full stomach

Technique

- Select a tube of the correct size. LMAs come in sizes from 1 to 5, with most adults requiring either size 4 (women, small men) or size 5.
- Inflate the cuff to ensure there are no leaks.
- Deflate the cuff all the way.
- Lubricate the sides and back of the LMA with water-soluble lubricant.
- Place patient in anatomic "sniff" position.
- Open the mouth, ensuring visualization of the posterior oropharynx.
- Grasp the LMA like a pencil at the junction of the tube and mask; the aperture faces forward.
- Place the back of the LMA against the upper teeth.
- Use the index finger of the grasping hand to push the LMA up against the hard palate while inserting in order to avoid the tongue.

- Once the tip of the mask reaches the posterior oropharyngeal wall, use the index finger to push both posteriorly and inferiorly toward the glottis until the LMA is seated.
- Remove the index finger while applying pressure to the tube with the other hand.
- Inflate the cuff and test the seal by connecting and delivering a breath with an Ambu bag. Auscultate the chest and epigastrium as with standard endotracheal intubation.
- If a large air leak is present, deflate the cuff and insert the LMA further or reinflate with less air.
- If airway resistance appears too high during bag ventilation, the tip of the mask may have folded upon itself or the epiglottis may be causing mechanical obstruction. In that case, reposition the tube.

Advantages

- Allows for positive pressure ventilation
- Does not traverse the vocal cords, which reduces risk of vocal cord trauma and tracheal damage
- Can be placed without laryngoscopy
- Can be used as a backup in case of unsuccessful endotracheal intubation

Disadvantages and Complications

- Requires experience
- Requires sedation
- Occasionally associated with unacceptably large air leaks
- Does not prevent aspiration

Rapid Sequence Endotracheal Intubation (for overview, see https://ezcompetency.com/modules/4.php)

Endotracheal intubation can be performed emergently or electively. The technique is similar regardless of the acuity, however, the goal of rapid sequence intubation (RSI) as performed in emergent situations is to induce anesthesia quickly enough to avoid use of bag-mask ventilation. RSI is usually performed in nonfasting individuals who are at high risk of aspiration; bag-mask ventilation further increases aspiration risk.

Although intubation of the trachea can be achieved through the oral or nasal route, the oral route is preferred because of a lower risk of complications such as bleeding from nasal or oropharyngeal trauma, as well as reduced incidence of paranasal sinus infection. However, if intubation is necessary and the oral route is not an option, or if the patient cannot be sedated for laryngoscopy, the nasal route is preferred. Nasotracheal tubes should be removed and replaced by orotracheal tubes as early as possible.

Indications

- Inability to protect airway from foreign substances (blood, oral secretions, gastric contents, tracheobronchial secretions)
- Altered mentation resulting in apnea
- Acute respiratory failure, either hypercapnic, hypoxic, or mixed
- Anticipated multisystem failure such as severe trauma or severe sepsis
- Electively for operative procedures or bronchoscopy

Contraindications

- Orofacial trauma that either obstructs the upper airway or distorts landmarks.
- Penetrating neck trauma is NOT a contraindication to intubation, but may dictate the technique used and the desired position of the endotracheal tube.
- Pregnancy, coagulopathy, nasal trauma or occlusion, basilar skull fracture or nasal cerebral spinal fluid (CSF) leak, and previous skull base surgery or repair of craniofacial defects are contraindications to nasal intubation.
- Cardiac arrest: these patients can often be intubated without the use of induction agents, sedatives, or neuromuscular blockers. No need for RSI.

Technique

- Notify the most experienced clinician available that you are about to intubate a patient.
- Perform a rapid airway assessment using a validated assessment tool, such as **Look** externally. **Evaluate** using the 3:3:2 rule. **Mallampati** classification. **Obstruction**. **Neck** mobility (LEMON) assessment method (see http://www.acep.org/content.aspx?Id=33992)

- Mallampati score (see table at http://www.mymedal.org/index.php?n=Military.310501)
- Measurements:
  - Thyromental distance (3 fingerbreadths)
  - Mouth opening (3 fingerbreadths)
  - Jaw protrusion (1 fingerbreadth)
- Atlanto-occipital extension
- Pathology in the airway causing occlusion or distortion of landmarks
- If the results of the LEMON American College of Emergency Physicians (ACEP 1C) assessment predict a difficult airway, alternative airway strategies should be considered (videolaryngoscopy, bronchoscopic intubation, surgical airway) and consultation with an experienced clinician, if possible, should be done.
- Obtain the necessary equipment
  - Ambu bag
  - Rigid laryngoscope (check to ensure proper function)
  - Oxygen source
  - Suction apparatus and Yankauer
  - Size 6.0 to 8.0 cuffed endotracheal tubes are adequate for most adults (check the cuff)
  - 10 cc air-filled syringe
  - Stylette
  - Anesthesia:
    - Induction agent: etomidate, ketamine, or thiopental
    - A rapid onset sedative: midazolam
    - Neuromuscular blocker: succinylcholine, vecuronium, cisatracurium
  - Resuscitation medications
    - Vasopressors and cardiac stimulants such as atropine, dopamine, epinephrine, phenylephrine
    - Intravenous (IV) fluids
  - Additional personnel to monitor and record vital signs and obtain additional medications and equipment
- Position the patient appropriately in the sniff position.
  - This position results in alignment of the oropharyngeal airway with the vocal cords, facilitating direct vision of the cords.
  - The position is achieved by placing pillows under the head and slightly extending the neck. *Avoid hyperextending the neck.*
  - In the awake patient experiencing respiratory distress, it is advisable to begin induction prior to placing the patient supine; this helps avoid unnecessary agitation.
- Ensure adequate cardiopulmonary monitoring devices are attached and working properly (where applicable).
  - Blood pressure should be cycled every 2 to 3 minutes.
  - Continuously monitor heart rate and rhythm.
  - Continuously monitor oxygen saturation.
- Induce anesthesia.
  - There is no high-quality supportive evidence for premedication prior to RSI (atropine, lidocaine, etc.).
  - Administer induction agent and sedative, followed by neuromuscular blocking agent in rapid succession.
  - Ensure adequate induction and the ability to ventilate the patient before administering neuromuscular blocker.
- Preoxygenation and ventilatory assistance during the procedure may be necessary, especially in patients with limited cardiopulmonary reserve.
- If preintubation ventilatory assistance is used (bag-mask ventilation) consider using gentle cricoid pressure (ACEP 1C) to reduce the risk of esophageal insufflation.
- Open the mouth by using the thumb and index finger of the intubating hand.
  - Place the thumb on the lower teeth (or gumline) while placing the index finger on the upper teeth.

- Apply pressure by extending the thumb against the lower teeth and flexing the index finger against the upper teeth, which results in a scissors-like motion resulting in mouth opening.
- Insert the laryngoscope (MacIntosh or Miller blade) and follow the contour of the tongue with the blade tip.
- If a MacIntosh blade is used, attempt to wedge the tip of the blade between the tongue and the epiglottis (the epiglottis will be included in the view).
- If a Miller blade is used, insert until the tip of the blade covers both the tongue and the epiglottis (the epiglottis will be excluded from view).
- Once the laryngoscope is in satisfactory position, lift the handle up and over the chest at approximately a 45-degree angle to the floor, without changing the angle of the wrist (angling the wrist, and thus the laryngoscope, increases the risk of damaging the teeth).
- Suction all secretions.
- Visualize as much of the vocal cords as possible, but visualization of the posterior commissure is usually adequate.
- Once the cords are visualized, insert the lubricated endotracheal tube (ETT) (with cuff deflated) in such a manner as not to obstruct your view and direct the tip toward the vocal cords.
- Slight upward angulation of the ETT tip may facilitate insertion.
- If significant resistance is met, consider using a smaller tube.
- If the glottic opening is anterior, and the tube cannot be manipulated through the vocal cords, consider intubating first with an angled-tip bougie (Coude tip), then insert the ETT over the bougie.
- Confirm satisfactory position of the tube with end-tidal carbon dioxide monitoring (deliver at least 5–6 breaths to ensure carbon dioxide is from a pulmonary source), auscultation of the chest, auscultation over the stomach, and by monitoring pulse oximetry and vital signs. Confirm ETT position with a chest x-ray.
- Remember that there is a delay in pulse oximetry of up to 30 to 45 seconds.
- If unsuccessful, continue efforts unless hemodynamic compromise, desaturation, or airway trauma occurs, then immediately stop, clear the airway, and resort to bag-mask ventilation or, if bag-mask ventilation is not possible, proceed to emergent surgical airway (see Complications [Difficult Airway] section p. 9)

Advantages

- Bypasses soft tissue upper airway obstruction
- Provides an effective, secure airway
- Less air leak than either bag-mask ventilation or LMA
- Allows for ventilation with higher pressures than LMA
- Reduces, but does not eliminate, risk of aspiration when compared to bag-mask or LMA

Disadvantages and Complications

- Requires experience.
- Requires anesthesia.
- Can result in trauma to the oropharynx, vocal cords, glottic structures, and trachea (mucosal or vocal cord laceration).
- Improper technique or difficult anatomy predispose to dental damage.
- Esophageal intubation is a frequent occurrence; early recognition is essential.
- Right mainstem intubation is common; suspect if peak pressures are high, asymmetric chest expansion or unequal breath sounds are observed, or if unilateral lung sliding is seen on transthoracic ultrasound.
- Pneumothorax is relatively rare (0.1% in one series), but potentially serious.

Management of Epistaxis (see http://emedicine.medscape.com/article/863220-overview)

Initial Management

- Assess vital signs and respiratory status; epistaxis can quickly lead to both hemorrhagic shock and respiratory compromise.
- Obtain appropriate equipment:
  - Light source

- Suction apparatus
- Cotton-tipped swabs
- Water-soluble lubricant
- Vasoconstrictor, such as 1:1000 epinephrine or oxymetazoline
- Silver nitrate sticks
- Lubricated nasal packing (ribbon gauze)
- Nasal speculum
- Inspect the nose and posterior pharynx closely and note the side involved, whether the bleed is anterior or posterior (if possible), and the rate of bleeding.

Anterior Epistaxis (90%)

- Most commonly originate from the Kiesselbach plexus
- Usually occurs in younger patients
- Usually seen as obvious unilateral low-volume bleed
- Management:
  - Apply ice to bridge of nose.
  - Instill vasoconstrictor into affected nostril and apply pressure to that side of the nose, occluding the nostril on that side.
  - Wait 10 minutes.
  - Inspect nose; if no further bleeding, no further intervention is necessary.
  - If bleeding continues, inspect thoroughly, removing clots if necessary to localize the bleeding site.
  - If a bleeding site is found, instill 2% lidocaine solution into the nare and use silver nitrate to cauterize the bleeding site.
  - If bleeding continues, anterior nasal packing will be necessary.
  - Commercially available nasal tampons are better tolerated than traditional ribbon gauze nasal packs.
    - Cut nasal tampon to the appropriate size.
    - Lubricate with water-soluble lubricant.
    - Insert along the floor of the nasal cavity, advancing as far posterior as possible.
  - If nasal tampons are not immediately available, traditional ribbon gauze packing should be used.
    - With your finger, anchor one end of the lubricated ribbon gauze on the upper lip just below the affected nostril.
    - Use a lubricated cotton-tipped swab to introduce folds into the nasal cavity, advancing the gauze along the floor of the nose as far posteriorly as possible.
    - Continue to introduce folds of gauze into the nose until the entire cavity is full.
    - Trim any gauze protruding from the nose.
  - Prescribe prophylactic antibiotics to cover typical nasopharyngeal organisms (staphylococcus).
  - Arrange for removal of the packing after 48 to 72 hours.

Posterior Epistaxis (10%)

- Associated with larger volume blood loss than anterior epistaxis
- Occurs in older patients in the setting of medical illness (vascular disease, anticoagulation)
- Can be more rapidly fatal because of hemorrhagic shock or respiratory compromise
- Should be treated as a true medical emergency
- Management:
  - Assess airway, breathing, circulation.
  - Consider sending blood for immediate type and crossmatch.
  - Place IV and start volume replacement, if necessary.
  - Obtain 2 Foley catheters and topical antibiotic ointment.
  - Anesthetize the affected side with 2% lidocaine.
  - Insert Foley catheter into the nostril and advance posteriorly.
  - Visualize the Foley catheter protruding down the posterior oropharynx.
  - Inflate the balloon with 10 cc water and apply gentle traction on the catheter until it seats.

- Tape to nose in a similar fashion as an nasogastric (NG) tube.
- Place anterior nasal pack as described above.
- Consider placing bilateral packs.
- Admit the patient for observation and obtain ear, nose, and throat consultation.
- Both anterior and posterior nasal packs can cause necrosis.
- Sinusitis is possible.
- If antibiotic therapy is not administered, toxic shock syndrome can ensue.

Complications (Difficult Airway)

- With a difficult airway, consider marking patient and consulting anesthesia.
- Airway management is a high-risk endeavor; failure to secure an adequate airway in a critically ill or sedated patient will result in serious morbidity or death.
- Scores designed to predict difficult airway or difficult intubation are, unfortunately, poorly predictive.
- It takes years to accumulate the skills necessary to effectively combat difficult airway situations, as these situations are relatively infrequent.
- The definition of "difficult airway" according to the American Society of Anesthesiologists is a situation where a trained anesthesiologist has difficulty with mask ventilation or with endotracheal intubation.
- Difficult mask ventilation
  - Incidence between 2% and 8%
  - Failure to maintain saturation (< 92%) despite proper technique
  - Inability of the anesthesiologist to provide adequate face mask ventilation because of one or more of the following:
    - Inadequate mask seal
    - Excessive gas leak
    - Excessive resistance to the ingress or egress of gas
  - Signs of inadequate face mask ventilation include:
    - Absent or inadequate chest movement
    - Absent or inadequate breath sounds
    - Auscultatory signs of severe obstruction
    - Cyanosis
    - Gastric air entry or dilatation
    - Decreasing or inadequate oxygen saturation
    - Absent or inadequate exhaled carbon dioxide
    - Absent or inadequate spirometric measures of exhaled gas flow
    - Hemodynamic changes associated with hypoxemia or hypercarbia
      - For example, hypertension, tachycardia, and arrhythmia
- Difficult tracheal intubation
  - Incidence between 1.5% and 8%
  - Intubation requiring multiple attempts in the presence or absence of pathology
  - Failed intubation
- Difficult laryngoscopy also qualifies as a difficult airway
  - Cannot visualize any part of the vocal cords
  - May or may not lead to difficult intubation
- Factors associated with increased risk of difficult tracheal intubation include morbid obesity, pregnancy, patients undergoing cervical spine surgery, and laryngeal pathology.
- Always notify the most experienced clinician available in the event that a difficult airway situation arises de novo or if a patient has risk factors.
- If a patient has a history of difficult intubation, notify the difficult airway team or the most experienced clinician available when making decisions regarding management of the airway (tube changes, extubation, etc.).
- Do not attempt to handle a difficult airway situation unless either you are adequately prepared or there is no alternative.
- For more information, see the article entitled "Practice Guidelines for Management of the Difficult Airway" (*Anesthesiology*. 2003;98:1269–77).

CARDIOVASCULAR

For all vascular cannulation procedures ultrasound guidance should be considered (see http://www.asecho.org/files/VC.pdf).

IV Catheter

Indications

- IV fluids, antibiotics, sedatives

Contraindications

- No true contraindications
- Avoid sites of active infection
- Avoid extremities with disrupted venous return
- Avoid extremities that are edematous
- Avoid sites of trauma or burns

Equipment

- Most IV catheters are between 1 inch and 1.25 inches.
- Longer catheters are more stable and can be left in place for longer periods of time.
- Larger bore catheters are the gold standard for infusing blood or fluids rapidly.
- Resistance to flow is proportional to catheter length and inversely proportional to diameter, so a short large-bore catheter has the less resistance than a longer catheter with a smaller diameter.
- Most insertion sets include skin prep, catheter, retractable safety needle, and sterile dressing

Technique

- Perform a rapid survey of the anatomy, inspecting for areas or trauma, erythema, and edema.
- Note the medical history regarding previous lymphadenectomy, peripheral arteriovenous (AV) fistula placement (Brescia-Cimino fistula, etc.).
- Identify the most peripheral vein that will likely accept cannulation.
- Adhere to universal precautions.
- Apply tourniquet above the proposed site and palpate the target vein.
- Note the location and course of the vessel.
- Cleanse the skin and your gloved finger with the skin prep solution.
- Stabilize the vein between your thumb and index finger by applying counter tension to the overlying skin.
- Puncture the vessel at a 45-degree angle to the skin along its course.
- A flash of blood in the catheter indicates successful cannulation.
- Slowly slide the catheter over the needle into the target vessel.
- Secure with a clear bio-occlusive dressing.
- If unsuccessful, change to a more proximal site and reattempt
- If still unsuccessful, consider using ultrasound to identify candidate veins, assess patency, and to mark an insertion site.
  - Ultrasound is associated with up to a 91% success rate in cases of failed peripheral IV placement.

Advantages

- Easy to learn.
- Does not require anesthesia.
- Can handle large volume infusions depending on the gauge of the catheter and the size of the vein.
- Serious complications are rare.

Disadvantages and Complications

- Must be exchanged after 72 hours.
- Subcutaneous leaks are common.
- Thrombophlebitis.
- Cannot administer vasopressors or high osmolar solutions through a peripheral vein.

Arterial Blood Gas Sampling

Indications

- Assess blood oxygen, carbon dioxide, and acid-base status.
- Assess for dyshemoglobinemias, such as methemoglobinemia and carboxyhemoglobinemia.

Contraindications

- Abnormal Allen test.
- Avoid sites with evidence of active infection.
- Avoid AV fistulas (Brescia-Cimino fistula).
- Avoid areas with known anatomic distortion from surgery, burns, and so forth.

Technique

- Perform a rapid survey of the anatomy, inspecting for areas or trauma, erythema, and edema.
- Note the medical history regarding previous lymphadenectomy, peripheral AV fistula placement (Brescia-Cimino fistula, etc.).
- Select an appropriate site, preferably the most peripheral site available.
- Alert the patient that he or she may experience some discomfort.
- For radial artery sampling, position the arm on a stationary surface with the palm facing up.
- Perform the Allen test (see http://www.youtube.com/watch?V=jq0ai5uxx68).
  - There is some debate as to the value of the Allen test in predicting who is at risk of hand ischemia; however, the test continues to be performed on a routine basis, especially in the setting of radial artery harvesting for coronary bypass grafting.
  - Occlude both the ulnar and radial artery simultaneously.
  - Ask the patient to clench the fist (if applicable), then open the hand.
  - Release the ulnar artery and observe for reperfusion of the palmar skin.
  - If reperfusion does not occur with release of the ulnar artery, the patient may have a rudimentary ulnar circulation; another site should be chosen.
- Consider performing a sonographic Allen test:
  - Use a high-frequency vascular (linear array 7–12 MHz) probe with color Doppler to localize the palmar arch.
  - Occlude the radial artery and observe for continued circulation in the palmar arch or digital arteries (you may see a reversal of flow as the radial artery is occluded).
  - The Allen test suggests that radial artery cannulation or harvesting is safe.
  - Using either static guidance to mark a suitable site for cannulation, or cannulation under dynamic guidance has been shown to reduce the number of unsuccessful attempts.
  - If a hematoma occurs while using ultrasound, arterial flow is still readily apparent with the application of Doppler or color Doppler to the two-dimensional (2D) image, enabling subsequent attempts.
- Palpate the artery using landmarks: medial to the styloid process of the radius, and proximal to the scaphoid tubercle.
- If the artery is poorly or completely nonpalpable because of hemodynamic compromise or adipose tissue, consider using ultrasound.
  - High-frequency linear-array transducer with color-flow Doppler
- Mark or note the location of the artery.
- No need to anesthetize; injection of local anesthesia is just as painful as the procedure itself.
- Using a standard blood gas analysis kit, cleanse the skin with alcohol or commercially available skin prep solution.
- Puncture the skin over the artery at a 30- to 45-degree angle to the axis of the forearm.
- Advance no more than 1 to 1.5 cm.
- Arterial blood will flash back into the syringe fairly rapidly.
- If no blood is obtained, *slowly* pull the needle out; if a through-and-through puncture occurred (through the posterior wall of the artery), there should be a flash of blood when the needle tip reenters the lumen.
- If no blood is obtained, consider repeating at a more proximal site.
- If no blood is obtained at all from the radial site, consider either switching to the other radial artery, or consider a brachial or femoral stick.

Advantages

- Arterial blood gas analysis gives invaluable information regarding the acid-base and oxygenation and ventilation status of a patient.
- Radial artery sampling is safe and easy to perform, because of its superficial location.
- In the setting of shock, the femoral artery is typically easily palpable, or at least makes for a larger sonographic target than the radial artery.

Disadvantages and Complications

- The radial artery is difficult to palpate in the setting of shock or peripheral vascular disease.
- Rare instances of hand ischemia have occurred following arterial blood sampling.
- Hematoma formation that may impinge on arterial supply to the hand.
- Vasovagal response is possible.
- Vessel laceration requiring surgical repair is possible.

Arterial Catheterization

Indications

- Useful for patients in whom noninvasive blood pressure measurement is unreliable:
  - Patients with diabetes
  - Patients with peripheral vascular disease
  - Patients with morbid obesity
  - Patients with severe lymphedema
- Allows for continuous, beat-to-beat hemodynamic monitoring
  - Assess fluid responsiveness in critically ill patients based on:
    - Respiratory variation in peak arterial pressures
    - Pulse contour analysis
  - Allows titration of vasopressors and cardiac inotropes
- Enables frequent blood gas analysis
- Radial artery cardiac catheterization (similar technique, different equipment)

Contraindications

- Abnormal Allen test (radial artery)
- Known or suspected arterial compromise of a given extremity

Technique

- Role of ultrasound:
  - The radial artery is a small target.
  - Patients requiring arterial line placement are usually hypotensive with diminished palpable pulses.
  - Significant anatomic variation exists in up to 2.6% of patients (radial).
  - Techniques of ultrasound guidance for central venous catheter insertion are easily adapted to arterial catheters, because from an ultrasound guidance perspective, the procedures are very similar.
- The most commonly cannulated arteries are the radial, axillary, and femoral, with the radial approach being the most common.
- Advantages of the radial artery are:
  - The wrist is easily accessible.
  - Dual circulation is present in the hand (in most patients).
  - The wrist is a relatively clean site (compared to the femoral artery).
  - It is important to understand, however, that radial artery catheterization is not risk free.
- Long-term catheterization of the brachial artery may be associated with catastrophic limb ischemia because of the relatively small caliber of the vessel and the absence of dual blood supply to the distal upper extremity.
- The femoral approach is commonly used, usually in the setting of failed radial placement (or predicted failure).
- Femoral pressures and waveform are more accurate and reliable.
- The axillary artery is a larger target and is associated with less of a risk of limb ischemia than the brachial, but catheterization is cumbersome to perform.

- Other sites of cannulation include ulnar, dorsalis pedis, tibialis posterior, and temporal arteries.
- Insertion kits can vary depending on the intended site of insertion:
  - Radial arterial lines are typically inserted with an all-inclusive needle-catheter-guidewire apparatus.
  - Femoral arterial lines are usually similar to central venous catheters, in that insertion is through a modified Seldinger technique using a needle, guidewire, dilator, and separate catheter.
- Radial artery catheterization (for femoral artery catheterization, see Central Venous Catheter Placement, Femoral section below):
  - Obtain informed consent after discussing specific risks such as limb ischemia, need for surgical embolectomy, repair of pseudoaneurysm, infection, bleeding, and scar.
  - Obtain the necessary equipment:
    - Angiocatheter (20- or 22-gauge) *or* commercially available radial artery cannulation kit
    - Alcohol swab
    - Skin prep solution
    - Sterile gauze
    - 1% lidocaine
    - 25-gauge needle
    - 3- to 5-cc syringe
    - Skin suture or commercially available nonsuture catheter securing device (reduces catheter-related bloodstream infection rates)
    - Sterile towels and/or fenestrated drape
    - Pressure tubing
    - Pressure transducer
    - Pressure bag
    - 1 L normal saline
    - Monitor or display
    - Ultrasound
    - Marking pen
  - Position the patient appropriately with the arm extended, the ventral aspect of the forearm exposed, and the hand resting on a bedside procedure table.
  - Place a towel roll under the wrist, which should result in slight dorsiflexion of the wrist.
  - Secure the hand and towel roll to the underlying procedure table.
  - Use palpation or ultrasonography to locate the artery and to select an insertion site; mark an appropriate site.
  - Cleanse the area with alcohol.
  - Infiltrate the skin and subcutaneous tissue with 1 to 2 cc lidocaine.
  - Prep and drape the area in usual sterile fashion.
  - Reidentify the radial artery by palpation, confirming the site; palpation and localization may be more sensitive and accurate if the palpating finger is along the axis of the vessel, rather than at a 90-degree angle to the vessel.
  - Using the angiocatheter or the commercially available cannulation apparatus, puncture the skin at a 30- to 45-degree angle and advance toward the pulse or directly under your skin mark until a flash of blood is seen.
  - If blood is not seen, slowly remove the catheter; through-and-through sticks, which will be revealed on catheter withdrawal, are not uncommon.
  - If there is still no blood, withdraw the catheter almost to the skin surface, then systematically redirect if unsuccessful, remove the catheter and reevaluate the site.
  - Select a more proximal site if vasospasm or hematoma formation obscures the artery from palpation (if ultrasonography is used, neither of these problems preclude further attempts at the same site, as long as blood flow is maintained).
  - When changing sites, apply pressure for 5 minutes to the original site to prevent hematoma formation.
  - Assuming blood is returned, advance either the catheter, or in the case of the all-in-one kits, advance the guidewire followed by the catheter.

- If the guidewire does not advance easily, withdraw it and decrease the angle of the catheter (keeping the tip in the vessel, lay the catheter down closer to the patients' hand), then readvance the wire.
- Remove either the needle or the guidewire-needle apparatus and observe for pulsatile blood flow.
- If no flow is seen, the catheter is not in the vessel lumen; start again.
- *Do not reintroduce the needle or guidewire into a catheter that is not intraluminal,* or you will damage or cut the catheter.
- Ask the assistant or nurse to connect the transducer circuit to the catheter; observe the waveform to ensure an arterial source.
- Secure the catheter with nylon skin suture or a commercially available catheter securing device.
- Place a sterile dressing.
- Troubleshooting
  - The transducer must be zeroed and at the appropriate height to give an accurate pressure reading:
    - If the transducer is too high, the pressure will be underestimated.
    - If the transducer is too low, the pressure will be overestimated.
  - Dampened waveforms may be caused by:
    - Air in the circuit
    - Kinked or partially occluded catheter
    - Pressure bag problems
  - Exaggerated waveforms are usually from catheter "whipping," seen more often in larger vessels and result from vigorous blood flow.

Advantages

- Obtains more accurate blood pressure in a beat-to-beat fashion when compared to noninvasive blood pressure monitoring.
- Femoral artery waveform provides a very accurate representation of central arterial pressures, and therefore is reliable (more than the radial artery) for calculating cardiac output.
- The femoral artery may be accessed more quickly than the radial artery.

Disadvantages and Complications

- Arterial line complications are rare, but potentially catastrophic.
- Venous puncture.
- Multiple arterial punctures.
- Hematoma formation.
- Failed placement.
- Limb ischemia.
- The radial arterial waveform, because of its distal location, is an inaccurate representation of more central arterial pressures, especially in the setting of vasopressor use; this can lead to poorly informed treatment decisions.

Central Venous Catheter Placement (Femoral, Subclavian, Internal Jugular)

Central venous catheter (CVC) placement is one of the most common invasive procedures performed in the hospital setting. Consequently, although vascular access procedures are associated with a relatively low rate of serious complications, the large number of these procedures performed annually translates into a large absolute number of complications. Therefore, it is imperative that the operator fully understand the risks, benefits, indications, and contraindications to the placement of these catheters, and take every precaution to reduce the risk of complications. For the purposes of this discussion, central line placement refers to both standard multilumen catheters, and nontunneled catheters used as introducers and for dialysis access.

Indications

- Central access for administration of high-osmolality infusions such as total parenteral nutrition
- Short-term central access for administration of IV antibiotics
- Vasopressor administration
- Hemodialysis access

- Apheresis, plasmapheresis
- Access for chemotherapeutics
- Monitoring central venous pressure
- Poor peripheral access

Contraindications

- Venous occlusion from stenosis or thrombosis.
- Severe coagulopathy or thrombocytopenia (relative; case dependent).
- Superior vena cava syndrome.
- Infection at proposed insertion site.
- Internal jugular (IJ) should be avoided in setting of contralateral IJ thrombosis or stenosis.
- Subclavian should be avoided in patients requiring hemodialysis because of incidence of stenosis.
- Femoral should be avoided in cases of deep vein thrombosis (DVT) or in patients at high risk of DVT.

Technique

- All clinicians tasked with placing CVCs should undergo formal training designed to allow familiarization with local equipment and procedures and to provide education on measures proven to reduce complications such as central line-associated bloodstream infections (CLABSIs).
- Lines placed emergently or under conditions where all policies were not strictly adhered to should be removed as early as possible, preferably within 48 hours.
- Lines placed at outside institutions should be immediately surveyed for evidence of infection; if there are clinical signs of infection, consider immediate replacement using a de novo cannulation (no wire changes).
- A vascular access team, whose responsibilities include insertion, maintenance (tubing changes, declotting, dressing changes), data collection in regard to CVCs, and assessing ongoing need for CVCs in each patient may be appropriate.
- Nurses and other staff should, with the help and cooperation of whomever is placing the line, complete a procedure checklist focused on:
  - Ensuring that informed consent was obtained
  - Identification of the patient and procedure ("time out")
  - Ensuring compliance with infection control practices
  - Adherence to other safety practices (appropriate patient position, sedation, monitoring, disposal of biohazardous materials, proper handling of sharps)

Central venous Cannulation Site Selection Criteria

- The subclavian site is generally preferred for a long-term cannulation, total parenteral nutrition, and caustic medications.
- The femoral site should be avoided, but can be used for less than 72 hours if no site is available or if emergency renal replacement therapy is provided.
  - The IJ vein provides the easiest access to central vein under the ultrasound guidance.
  - The frequency of complications associated with particular site should be considered (Table 1-1).
  - Role of ultrasound

TABLE 1-1. RISK OF COMPLICATIONS ACCORDING TO CENTRAL VENOUS CANNULATION SITE

	Internal Jugular (%)	Subclavian (%)	Femoral (%)
Pneumothorax	0–1	2–3	N/A
Hemothorax	0	<1	N/A
Arterial puncture	5–10	3–5	5–15
Failed attempt	15–20	5–15	15–40

- Complications occur in up to 5.4% of CVC insertions in experienced hands.
- Several meta-analyses, multiple review articles, and numerous standardized procedure guidelines investigating or advocating the use of ultrasound for CVC placement have been published, including a position paper from the American Society of Echocardiography and the Society of Cardiovascular Anesthesiologists (see http://www. asecho.org/files/VC.pdf).
- These and other studies demonstrate that the use of 2D ultrasound during CVC insertion is associated with:
  - Fewer complications (risk reduction [RR] 57%)
  - Fewer attempts before successful cannulation (RR 41%)
  - Fewer failed procedures when compared to a landmark-based approach (RR 86%)
  - Shorter procedure times
- As a result, the Agency for Healthcare Research and Quality in the United States and the National Institute of Clinical Excellence in the United Kingdom have issued statements advocating ultrasound guidance in central venous access procedures (see http://www. nice.org.uk/guidance/TA49).
- Despite these evidence-based guidelines, some providers continue to resist and do not use ultrasound at all, or use it only in potentially "difficult to cannulate" patients such as the morbidly obese or in cases of failed cannulation.
  - Predicting which patients will be difficult to cannulate is difficult and inaccurate.
- The recognition of a failed attempt, as may arise from an occluded vessel, can only be viewed retrospectively after the failure has occurred.
- Therefore, using ultrasound in all central venous access procedures is recommended, in an effort to improve safety.
- Step-by-step guide
  - Obtain the proper equipment and personnel:
    - Ideally a kit containing all essential equipment and components, standardized throughout all the units of a given hospital or health system, should be used to prevent complications caused by unfamiliarity with equipment
    - Central line kit
      - CVC
      - Lidocaine
      - Chlorhexidine skin prep solution
      - Gauze
      - Several needles (18-, 22-, 25-gauge)
      - Several syringes
      - Sterile saline flushes
      - Cannulation needle and catheter
      - Guidewire
      - Dilator(s)
      - Needleless caps
      - Suture or commercially available catheter-securing device
      - Clear sterile dressing
      - Consider ultrasound-friendly needles
      - Ultrasound with high-frequency linear-array transducer (with or without color flow or Doppler)
      - Sterile sheath for the ultrasound transducer
  - Set up a sterile field on a rolling procedure table

Internal Jugular Vein

- The first step in successfully cannulating the internal jugular vein is proper positioning of the patient.
- Rotate the head slightly contralaterally, with the neck extended.
- Excessive rotation of the neck and head may lead to significant distortion of the anatomy and may increase the amount of overlap of the carotid artery and jugular vein.
- Place the bed in Trendelenburg position.
- The ultrasound machine should be placed by the ipsilateral side of the bed, at about the level of the patients' waist.

- Establish a sterile field on a bedside table and place within easy reach.
- Perform an initial examination of the landmarks without ultrasound and select an insertion site.
- The site should then be confirmed with ultrasound. There are two reasons for this:
  - Immediate feedback regarding landmark-based site selection
  - Facilitates teaching both the landmark-based approach and ultrasound-guided approach
- If ultrasound is used, the target vessel and surrounding structures should be identified, and the patency of the vessel should be confirmed and documented in the procedure note.
- Be sure to scan the entire length of the vessel, including the junction of the internal jugular and subclavian vein, looking for evidence of thrombosis (Figure 1-1A):
  - Lack of compressibility
  - Lack of color-flow signal or Doppler signal
- Once a satisfactory insertion site is identified, notify the assistants and nursing staff about the plan.
- Using proper technique, dress with mask, cap, gown, and sterile gloves.
- The patient's skin can now be prepped and full barrier precautions used to maintain sterility and reduce the incidence of catheter-related infections.
- Before cannulation, a second ultrasound examination should be performed to ensure that the original insertion site is still viable.
- Open the sterile ultrasound sheath.
- Have the assistant hold the transducer, with ultrasound gel applied to the transducer surface (can be nonsterile gel), in a position such that the operator and the assistant can both acquire the transducer, and place it in the sterile sheath in one motion.
- Note that instead of using an assistant, the transducer can be "picked up" by the operator, whose hand is inside the sterile sheath (like a puppet; Figure 1-1B). The sheath can then be extended to cover the transducer cord.
- Apply sterile rubber bands to secure the sheath in place.
- Orientation needs to be acquired any time the probe is removed from the patient and set down:
  - Orient by touching the transducer surface and noting the resulting image; ensure that you are not looking at a backward image.
- After the site is confirmed with ultrasound, set up the catheter as per normal routine:
  - Set aside all needed equipment in the order that it will be used.
  - Flush the catheter and attach the needless hubs to all but the middle port.
  - Open local anesthetic and draw into syringe with 19-gauge needle.
  - Discard 19-gauge needle into an approved sharps device and apply a 25- or 22-gauge needle to syringe.
  - Anesthetize the skin over the proposed cannulation site.
  - Attach the cannulation needle to a syringe.
- During cannulation, always use the same insertion site and needle trajectory that you would if you were using the landmark-based approach (lateral, medial, etc.).
  - Do not disregard proper needle trajectory by not paying attention to the needle while looking at the ultrasound image.
  - Center the vessel lumen on the screen (when visualizing in the transverse plane); remember that when the vessel is centered on the screen, it is directly underneath the middle of the transducer head.
  - Perform a "mock poke" to confirm your proposed insertion site relative to the underlying vessel. This is done by laying the cannulation needle on the skin surface, then applying the transducer over it (Figure 1-1C). If the needle is in the right place, the acoustic shadow produced by the needle should be directly over, or be superimposed on, the target vessel (Figure 1-1D).
  - Puncture the skin approximately 0.5 to 1 cm proximal to the transducer and aim the needle toward the target vessel, usually at about a 30- to 45-degree angle to the skin.
  - For IJ cannulation, the target is toward the ipsilateral nipple.
  - If the needle tip cannot be visualized indenting either the subcutaneous tissue overlying the vessel or the vessel itself, move the probe along the axis of the vessel while slightly "agitating" the needle; this will accentuate the image of the needle and tip.
  - The point of the V caused by indenting the subcutaneous tissue above the vein with the needle tip should be directly over the vessel.

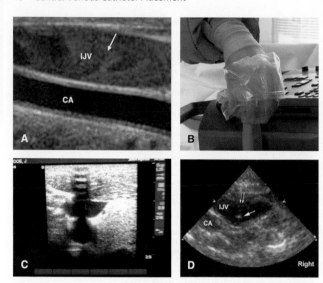

Figure 1-1   Placement of the internal jugular line. **A.** Prescreening. There is a clot in the internal jugular vein marked by the arrow. **B.** Proper placement of the sterile sheath over the linear array ultrasound transducer. **C.** "Mock poke" technique with the needle under the transducer and the needle ultrasound "shadow" overlying the image of internal jugular vein. **D.** cannulated internal jugular vein (IJV). CA, carotid artery. Arrow points at the line within the lumen in the short-axis view.

- Be sure to visualize the tip of the needle at all times; it is very easy to misinterpret the shaft of the needle as the tip; be sure to move the probe axially along the vessel frequently to keep the tip in view.
- If done properly, the needle tip should be seen entering the lumen at approximately the same time as the flash of blood is obtained in the syringe.
- Once the vessel has been successfully cannulated, the transducer can be set aside.
- Anchor the needle to the skin *carefully*; minimize movement of the needle once it is inside the vessel.
- Detach syringe; nonpulsatile blood should emanate from the needle hub.
- Insert the guidewire into the needle.
- Slowly advance the guidewire; inserting the wire too quickly negates the flow-directed characteristics of the flexible wire and predisposes to malposition.
- Insert the wire no more than 20 cm (hash marks on the wire are length measurements).
- The wire should advance smoothly and without significant resistance.
- Remove the needle without altering the position of the wire (do not pull it out).
- Make a small skin stab with the pointed end of the scalpel, just at the point where the wire enters the skin. Do not cut the wire.
- Advance the dilator over the wire.
- Grasp the dilator near the tip and advance through the dermis; continue to grip the dilator approximately 1 to 2 cm from the tip and advance in stages into the vessel.
- Grasping the dilator near the hub while inserting predisposes to wire kinking.
- Remove the dilator and apply pressure to the newly dilated tract with gauze.
- Advance the catheter over the wire, taking care to back the wire out through the central port before advancing into the skin.
- Do not let go of the wire at any time during the procedure (until it is removed).

- Advance to 15 to 16 cm for the right IJ; 17 to 20 cm for left IJ.
- Intravascular position of the needle can be confirmed with ultrasound (see Figure 1-1D); save a picture for documentation in the medical record.
- Secure the line with suture or a commercially available line-securing device.
- Once the line is in place, consider agitated normal saline solution contrast to confirm intraluminal position and a quick ultrasound examination of the anterior chest to evaluate for a pneumothorax by looking for bilateral "sliding pleura"; this should be included in the procedure note.

Subclavian Vein

- Differences in ultrasound localization (compared to IJ)
  - The subclavian vein is more difficult to visualize ultrasonographically than either the internal jugular, axillary, or femoral veins because of its position under the clavicle.
  - Proper imaging requires significant angulation and manipulation of the transducer.
  - Using a small footprint 5-MHz curvilinear probe facilitates imaging the subclavian vein.
  - The subclavian can be imaged from either a supraclavicular or infraclavicular approach, but the infraclavicular approach may be difficult in obese patients.
  - Once the vein is identified, assess its patency with color-flow Doppler; inability to compress the vein with the transducer makes it difficult to assess the vein for clot by compression alone.
  - In my experience, it is usually easier to visualize the subclavian with a longitudinal, supraclavicular view in obese patients and a subclavicular view in thin patients.
  - Cannulating the subclavian under dynamic guidance is associated with a longer learning curve because of transducer manipulation and the use of the longitudinal view; however, the procedure itself is largely the same as that outlined under the IJ Vein cannulation section.
- Differences in technique (compared to IJ)
  - Stand at the patient's side.
  - Set up ultrasound on the contralateral side.
  - The rule of thumb is to palpate the infraclavicular depression at the junction of the deltoid and pectoralis muscle (deltopectoral groove); the deepest point of this depression, which is usually approximately 1 cm below the clavicle, is the ideal insertion site.
  - Palpate the sternal notch: once inserted in the skin, the needle will be advanced straight toward this landmark.
  - Insert the cannulation needle into the skin to a depth of approximately 1 cm.
  - Place the middle finger of the noncannulating hand on the sternal notch.
  - Orient the thumb of the noncannulating hand straight down (pointed right toward the floor), just under the clavicle along the expected trajectory of the advancing needle.
  - While keeping the needle parallel to the floor (do not angle under the clavicle; move both hands simultaneously to keep the needle parallel to the floor), press down with the thumb and direct the needle under the clavicle.
  - Aspirate while advancing.
  - If you advance the needle to the hub without obtaining a flash of blood, withdraw the needle by all but 1 cm, then redirect slightly cephalad.
  - All other steps are identical to IJ cannulation.

Axillary Vein

- Using the axillary vein for central venous access has many unique advantages over other sites:
- Because the insertion site is on the anterior chest, the axillary approach likely shares a low incidence of catheter-related infections with the subclavian approach.
  - Unlike the subclavian vein, axillary vein cannulation may be associated with fewer complications, such as pneumothorax, hemothorax, and chylothorax.
  - The axillary vein is easier to compress than the subclavian vein, which allows easier recognition of clots.
- Unlike the standard subclavian approach, axillary cannulation could potentially cause a brachial plexus injury, particularly if a far lateral puncture is performed.
- One distinct disadvantage of the axillary approach is the unique dependence on ultrasound to ensure localization and subsequent cannulation; landmark techniques are not as effective as with the other common sites used to access the central venous system.

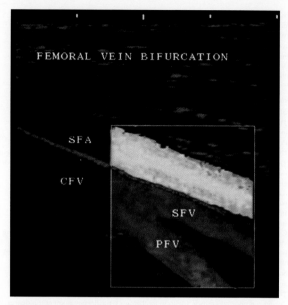

Figure 1-2   Ultrasound anatomy of the superficial femoral artery and the bifurcation of the common femoral vein. Note colored Doppler direction. BART, blue away from, red toward (the transducer). See color insert.

Femoral Vein

- Differences in ultrasound localization (compared to IJ)
- The ultrasound machine should be placed on the contralateral side of the patient, directly across from the operator.
- The entire area should be scanned, with identification of all vascular structures, including the femoral artery, common femoral vein, and saphenous or profunda femoris vessels if possible (Figure 1-2).
- Once the vein is identified, it should be evaluated for the presence of clot.
- Additionally, a longitudinal view of the vein should be obtained as it dives under the inguinal ligament, and the ligament itself should be marked on the skin. This ensures that an intraperitoneal puncture will not occur.
- The patient is placed in reverse Trendelenburg position.
- Palpate the femoral artery; the femoral vein usually lies medial to this (nerve, artery, vein, empty space, lymphatics).
- Palpate the inguinal ligament, which traverses the straight line between the anterior superior iliac spine and the pubic tubercle.
- Examine the leg for evidence of DVT or ischemia; if suspicious, consider an alternative location.
- Several clinically important complications may occur that lead to significant morbidity:
  - Accidental (or intentional) femoral arterial cannulation, especially in coagulopathic patients, may cause life-threatening retroperitoneal hemorrhage and hematoma.
  - Puncturing the artery in an already ischemic leg can lead to worsening ischemia either by clot formation or plaque embolism.
  - Inadvertent puncture of the femoral nerve during needle cannulation can cause severe pain.
  - A puncture site that is too proximal can result in inadvertent puncture of intraperitoneal structures (bowel).

- Once a cannulation site has been selected, set up the equipment as directed under IJ cannulation above.
- When cannulating the femoral vein, insert the needle at a 30- to 35-degree angle and direct toward the umbilicus.
- All other steps are similar to IJ or subclavian puncture.

Advantages over Other IV Access

- Allows infusion of hyperosmolar solutions and vasopressors
- Stable IV access
- Does not have to be changed every 72 hours
- When properly cared for, can last up to 7 to 10 days before needing replacement

Disadvantages and Complications

- Table 1-1 shows the risk of Complications According to Central Venous Cannulation Site.
- Requires skilled and educated clinicians.
- Requires labor-intensive education and surveillance programs designed to maximize safety and to ensure compliance with best practices.
- Although vascular access procedures are associated with a relatively low rate of serious complications, the large number of these procedures performed per annum translates into a large absolute number of complications.
- An improved understanding of complications and why they occur may assist the physician in reducing their risk.
- Complications of central venous catheterization have been well described and may be categorized in several different ways:
  - Immediate complications are those that occur as a consequence of the procedure itself (also known as mechanical complications):
    - Multiple venous punctures
    - Arterial puncture or cannulation
    - Hematoma
    - Hemothorax
    - Pneumothorax
    - Thoracic duct injury with or without chylothorax
    - Catheter tip malposition
  - Delayed complications occur later in the hospital course:
    - CLABSI
    - Thrombosis
    - Vessel or heart chamber perforation (especially with left-sided catheters)
  - Risk of CLABSI is substantially decreased by:
    - Full barrier precautions
    - Hand hygiene prior to the procedure
    - Keeping the number of hubs to the absolute minimum
    - Accessing the line as infrequently as possible
    - Scrubbing ports with an alcohol swab or commercially available port cleansing device before accessing
    - Strict adherence to the drying times recommended by skin prep manufacturers
  - Thrombosis may be reduced by assuring that the catheter tip position is in a high-flow area (distal third of the superior vena cava), and is not in direct contact with a vessel wall.
  - Patient-related factors that increase the risk of complications:
    - Large body habitus
    - Presence of coagulopathy
    - Prior surgery with distortion of the superficial or deep anatomy
    - Vascular anatomic variation
  - Operator factors include:
    - Level of experience
    - Presence of fatigue
    - Use (or nonuse) of ultrasound for guidance

- Complications from these procedures are likely to be associated with excess direct costs derived from prolonged hospital and intensive care unit lengths of stay and additional procedures, such as chest tube insertion or hematoma evacuation, to treat the complications.
- A single episode of iatrogenic pneumothorax has an attributable length of stay of 3 to 4 days.
- Indirect costs such as additional provider time and patient suffering are also important issues to consider.

Peripherally Inserted Central Catheter (PICC) Lines and Midlines

A PICC line is a long catheter (up to 60 cm long) that is inserted through a peripheral vein, but whose tip lies within the central circulation. In contrast, a midline is a long peripherally inserted catheter that does not reach the central circulation, usually about 20 cm in length.

Indications

- Midlines are for the infusion of fluids, antibiotics, and other medications over a prolonged period of time, up to 6 weeks.
- PICC lines have the same indications as midlines, with the addition of high osmolal solutions and solutions with nonphysiologic pH, as well as vasopressors.
- An institutional algorithm that governs IV access taking into consideration indications, patient factors, and alternatives when deciding on the type of vascular access device may avoid excessive and inappropriate PICC line use. The algorithm used at our institution is shown in Figure 1-3.
- One of the most common reasons cited for placing PICC and midline devices is difficulty obtaining adequate peripheral access. This can, in part, be avoided by providing nursing and support personnel with ultrasound guidance principles for peripheral IV access.

Contraindications

- Venous thrombosis of the extremity
- Air embolism
- Catheter fracture
- Infection

Technique

- Matching the catheter to the specific need of the patient is the first step.
- Always use the smallest diameter catheter possible.
  - Thrombosis risk is increased from the following: large catheter diameter, cephalic vein placement, "peripheral" placement (outside of the vena cava, so-called midclavicular catheters), long duration of catheterization, and presence of underlying solid-tumor malignancy or hypercoagulation disorders.
- PICC line and midline insertion requires the same degree of sterility as a central line.
  - The risk of catheter-related infection with midlines and PICC lines is substantially lower than that of CVCs, but is still a significant problem.
  - Factors associated with higher infection rates are:
    - Use of any skin prep other than 2% chlorhexidine
    - Lack of full barrier precautions (cap, mask, gown, and large drape)
    - The use of catheters with more than a single lumen (the more lumens, the higher the risk)
- There are several midline and PICC line kits on the market. It is important to review the needs of your particular patient when selecting a catheter.
  - A PICC that is capable of handling high-pressure infusions, such as may be used with IV contrast agents may be indicated.
  - PICC lines come with one, two, or three lumens and range in size from 4 to 6 French.
  - Midlines are typically single lumen, but also may be dual lumen. Typical sizes are 2 to 5 French.
- Obtain all necessary equipment:
  - PICC or midline insertion kit
  - Full-length drape
  - Cap, mask, gown, sterile gloves
  - Ultrasound

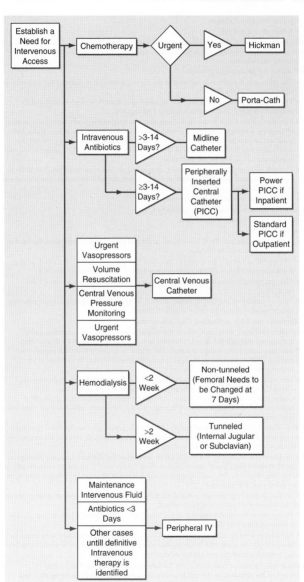

Figure 1-3 Intravenous Access Algorithm.

- Sterile transducer sheath
- Sterile ultrasound gel
- Examine the target arm and compare to the contralateral arm, paying particular attention to areas of skin infection and cellulitis, and comparing arm circumference (evidence of existing thrombosis).
- Position the patient appropriately.
  - The right arm is preferable because of the higher incidence of catheter-tip malposition when inserted in the left arm.
  - The patient is positioned supine, the shoulder is abducted 90 degrees and slightly externally rotated, and the elbow is flexed 90 degrees.
  - This allows easy access to the basilic vein and may help reduce catheter tip malposition by forming a straight line from the insertion site to central venous system. If the arm is left at the patient's side, the catheter tip must negotiate a turn when entering the subclavian; this increases the risk of the catheter either entering the ipsilateral internal jugular vein or coiling in the subclavian.
  - The risk of air embolization with PICC or midline placement is unknown, but likely to be negligible and roughly the same as that with peripheral IV insertion. Trendelenburg position, therefore, is probably not necessary.
  - The arm is secured with tape or restraints.
- Measure the arm circumference and record.
- Scan the target arm with ultrasound.
- Role of ultrasound:
  - For both midline and PICC line insertion, 2D and color Doppler ultrasound is used to "map" the extremity of interest.
  - All superficial vascular structures of the distal brachium should be identified, paying particular attention to differentiating artery from vein and assessing vein size.
  - After mapping is complete, a candidate vein is selected for insertion and then marked.
  - Patency should be assessed by noting normal venous flow characteristics and ensuring compressibility along the entire length of the vessel.
- There are two basic methods of PICC placement:
  - First, a Seldinger technique, where the vessel is cannulated with a needle, a wire is threaded through the needle followed by needle withdrawal, and a dilator and tear-away introducer is then inserted. The dilator is removed from the introducer, and the PICC is inserted to the appropriate position, followed by removal of the introducer.
  - The second method requires cannulation with a device similar to an Angiocath, where the vessel is cannulated by a needle-angiocatheter combination. The angiocatheter acts as the introducer; once cannulation is achieved, the needle is removed and the PICC is inserted through the angiocatheter, which is then "torn away" and removed.
- The desired PICC kit is opened and the line itself is prepared. Usually, these lines have a long metallic obturator that provides stiffness during insertion; this should be partially withdrawn to allow for catheter trimming.
- The desired catheter length is estimated by measuring the distance from the proposed insertion site to the glenohumeral joint, adding the distance from the glenohumeral joint to the sternal notch, then adding approximately 6 cm to allow for proper positioning in the distal superior vena cava.
- The best catheter tip position is the distal third of the superior vena cava, at the junction of the superior vena cava and right atrium.
  - This position causes the catheter tip to "float" within the lumen, which is associated with a lower incidence of thrombus formation.
  - The superior vena cava has a higher flow rate compared to the axillary, subclavian, or brachiocephalic veins, which has implications for thrombus formation and damage to the vessel from infusion of caustic substances.
- Once this distance is determined, the catheter should be trimmed to length.
  Do not cut the obturator, as this will produce a sharp point capable of puncturing the vessel.
- Prep and drape the patient.
- Rescan the area and confirm the position of the target vein.

- Cannulate the vessel under dynamic guidance as described in the Central Venous Catheter section above.
- When access to the vein is obtained, remove any dilators that may be present, leaving the introducer in place.
- Insert the midline or PICC and advance slowly to the hub.
- Quickly advancing the catheter increases the risk of catheter tip malposition. By slowing the rate of advancement, the catheter becomes more "flow directed" and follows the flow into the correct position.
- Remember, the catheter was trimmed to an appropriate length already, so advancing the hub will ensure correct tip position.
- When the catheter is fully advanced, remove the inner stylette or obturator, attach a syringe, and aspirate blood to confirm an intravascular position.
- Ultrasound can also be used to evaluate for catheter tip malposition by scanning the ipsilateral internal jugular vein and contralateral subclavian, if possible.
- The line can then be secured by a suture, or one of several commercially available adhesive devices and dressed appropriately. When placing a PICC, a portable chest radiograph should be obtained to confirm correct placement.
- The lines should be cared for in an identical fashion as central lines.

Advantages

- Relative longevity.
- Ease of insertion.
- Low rate of serious complications.
- Less phlebitis than peripheral IVs.
- Midlines do not require chest radiography to confirm position.

Disadvantages and Complications

- Hematoma.
- Arterial insertion.
- Catheter tip malposition into the ipsilateral internal jugular vein.
- Coiling in the subclavian vein or a thoracic branch such as the thoracodorsal vein.
- Cardiac arrhythmia.
- Nerve injury.
- Thrombosis.
- Air embolism.
- Catheter fracture.
- Infection.
- Pressure measurements are less reliable when obtained with a PICC.

Insertion of Pulmonary Artery Catheter

The perceived utility of pulmonary artery catheterization has declined significantly over the last decade.

Indications

- Diagnosis and management of patients with pulmonary hypertension
- Diagnosis of intracardiac shunting
- Diagnosis of cardiac tamponade
- Evaluation of cardiac filling pressures in the absence of significant valvular pathology or external applied pressures (such as mechanical ventilation)
- Preoperative assessment of cardiac transplant candidates
- Postoperative monitoring of cardiac function in cardiac surgical patients
- Aspiration of air emboli

Contraindications

- Venous occlusion from stenosis or thrombosis
- Severe coagulopathy
- Recent pulmonary surgery (pneumonectomy, lobectomy, surgical pulmonary arterial embolectomy)
- Tricuspid or pulmonic valve stenosis, thrombosis, or endocarditis

Technique (see http://www.youtube.com/watch?v=HdlCH_h_hao)

Pericardiocentesis (see http://www.wonderhowto.com/how-to-perform-pericardiocentesis-195377/)

The pericardial space usually contains less than 1 cc/kg of pericardial fluid, which acts as a lubricant between the visceral and parietal pericardium. The parietal pericardium is a dense fibrous structure that is poorly distensible. As such, the pericardial space cannot accommodate the rapid accumulation of fluid without compromising cardiac performance, quickly leading to shock and death. Therefore, early recognition and drainage of impending or actual tamponade is a critically important skill.

Indications

• Life-threatening hemodynamic collapse resulting from cardiac tamponade

Contraindications

• None, if done for the appropriate reason

Technique

• Obtain the necessary equipment:
  • Pericardial drain kit with long (spinal) needle, guidewire, dilator, and drainage catheter
  • Sterile prep (chlorhexidine)
  • Sterile towels
  • Two 10-cc syringes
  • Needles: 25- and 19-gauge
  • Scalpel
  • Local anesthetic (1% or 2% lidocaine)
  • Ultrasound machine with sterile transducer sheath
  • Alligator clip and electrocardiograph machine
• The patient should be placed in mild reverse Trendelenburg.
• Place an NG tube to decompress the stomach.
• Ensure adequate cardiac monitoring and support (fluids, oxygen, etc.) if time permits.
• Using the cardiac transducer (3–5 MHz phased array), obtain a 4-chamber subcostal view and confirm the presence of fluid.
• Pericardial fluid will appear as an anechoic to slightly echoic fluid collection anterior to the right ventricle (transudative fluid will be anechoic; infected fluid may be highly echoic and complex appearing).
• Measure the distance from the skin to the fluid.
• Prep and drape the patient.
• Infiltrate the skin in the subxiphoid region with 5 to 10 cc lidocaine.
• Using ultrasound, reacquire a subcostal 4-chamber view.
• Using dynamic guidance, insert the needle (with alligator clip attached to lead V_1 of a standard electrocardiograph machine) at a 45-degree angle, aiming cephalad and toward the left nipple, toward the fluid collection.
• Keep the needle tip in the ultrasonographic view at all times.
• Once fluid is obtained, remove the syringe and advance a guidewire into the pericardial space.
• Remove the needle, leaving the guidewire in place.
• Make a small skin incision at the insertion site.
• Dilate with the small-bore dilator included in the kit.
• Insert the drainage catheter over the wire into the pericardial space.
• Remove the wire.
• Secure the catheter and place to gravity drainage bag or to bulb suction.
• Place a sterile dressing.
• If just an emergent pericardiocentesis is performed and a pericardial drain is not placed (not recommended because of high risk of reaccumulation), remove enough fluid to stabilize the patient then obtain cardiology or cardiothoracic surgery consultation for definitive drainage.

Advantages

- Quickly lifesaving
- If ultrasound is used, it can be performed safely at the bedside with small risk of major complications.

Disadvantages and Complications

- Risk of complications is very high with blind approach.
  - Laceration of the myocardium
  - Laceration of coronary arteries
  - Liver puncture
  - Pneumothorax or hemothorax
  - Pneumopericardium
  - Air embolism
  - Gastric or colonic perforation
- Pericardial infection: risk increases with catheter dwell time.

THORACIC

Pneumothorax (Needle Decompression)

Indications

- Decompression of hemodynamically significant pneumothorax

Contraindications

- None, if performed for the correct indication

Technique

- Equipment
  - Percutaneous pleural drain or 16-gauge Angiocath (any catheter device will work)
  - Chlorhexidine skin prep solution
  - Sterile towels
  - Lidocaine
  - Stopcock
  - Bulb suction or self-contained chest drainage system
  - Wall suction (optional)
- Confirm tension pneumothorax by assessing for the following: absent breath sounds, tracheal deviation to the contralateral side (from the absent breath sounds), elevated jugular venous distention, hypotension, and tachycardia.
- Place patient in semirecumbent position.
- Cleanse the skin overlying the second intercostal space in the midclavicular line.
- Remove any flash chamber or obturator from the needle.
- Insert the Angiocath into the second intercostal space, above the third rib, at a 90-degree angle to the chest wall.
- Listen for a rush of air.
- Remove the needle, leaving the catheter in place.
- Secure the catheter with tape.
- Consider applying bulb suction, a stopcock that can be opened for intermittent decompression, or connection to a chest drainage chamber.
- Assess the patient for improvement; if no improvement, investigate for other causes of hemodynamic compromise.

Advantages

- Quick, lifesaving technique
- Buys time to arrange or perform a definitive procedure

Disadvantages and Complications

- Hemothorax
- Cardiac perforation
- Tamponade
- Intercostal artery or nerve transaction

Thoracentesis (Figure 1-4; see www.youtube.com/watch?v=xIXR4Aoi8qo and www.youtube.com/watch?v=UBY3cQiQ6Ko)

Indications

- Diagnostic thoracentesis allows a determination of the etiology of pleural fluid.
- Therapeutic thoracentesis improves symptoms of dyspnea.
- Therapeutic thoracentesis almost never improves oxygenation unless the patient already has significant pulmonary disease, but may help improve the mechanics of breathing, relieving dyspnea and improving ventilation.

Contraindications

- Severe coagulopathy (relative; assess risk-to-benefit ratio)
  - Studies indicate that increased INR is not associated with a higher risk of bleeding complications when ultrasound is used.
- Agitated patient
- Very small effusions unless the operator is experienced and ultrasound is used

Technique

- Ultrasound should be considered for guidance:
  - Prospective studies have shown a significant reduction in risk of pneumothorax and hemothorax when ultrasound is used.
  - Allows for identification of small effusions.
  - Differentiates between pleural fluid and atelectasis or infiltrate.
  - Allows characterization of pleural fluid (anechoic collections are much more likely to be transudative, complex collections are more likely to be exudative).
- Consider pleural manometry to help identify unexpandable lung.
- Thoracentesis may be performed in the upright or supine position.
- May be performed either posteriorly or laterally.
- A posterior approach in an upright position is appropriate if the patient is able to cooperate.
- Mechanically ventilated patients may be leaned forward to facilitate a posterior approach; alternatively, a supine mechanically ventilated patient may be approached laterally.
- Equipment
  - Standard thoracentesis kit.
  - Sterile towels.
  - Lidocaine.

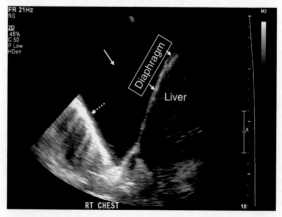

Figure 1-4   Ultrasound guidance for thoracentesis (image of the thorax and the pleural effusion).

- Skin prep solution (chlorhexidine).
- Vacuum bottles or gravity drainage bag.
- Containers for diagnostic studies (red top blood tube for chemistry, purple top for cell count and differential, sterile specimen jar or tube with no additive for cytology, blood culture tubes for pleural fluid culture).
- Ultrasound machine with 5-MHz curvilinear probe (smallest footprint available to image better through the ribs).
- Pleural manometer setup.
- If the above-mentioned thoracentesis kit is not available, a long 18-gauge angiocatheter and 60-cc syringe with a one-way valve or stopcock is acceptable.
- Sterile gauze and tape.
- Position the patient appropriately for the procedure.
- If the patient is upright, ensure stabilization with a table and an assistant.
- If the patient is supine, position the patient at the edge of the bed, so that the lateral chest wall extends beyond the side of the bed by a few inches. This allows insonation of the posterolateral chest wall with ultrasound and ensures an adequate window for needle insertion.
- Use ultrasound to localize and quantitate the fluid collection.
- Note the echo consistency of the fluid: anechoic versus echoic versus complex appearing.
- Note any adhesions present.
- Note the depth of the fluid from the skin surface.
- Note the angle of insonation; this will be the same angle and trajectory used for needle insertion.
- Once an adequate insertion site has been identified, mark the skin.
- Prep and drape in sterile fashion.
- Anesthetize the skin, subcutaneous tissues, and chest wall with 5- to 10-cc 1% lidocaine.
- Using the angle and trajectory obtained during the ultrasound examination, insert the thoracentesis catheter or angiocatheter into the skin and subcutaneous tissues.
- Apply gentle suction and slowly advance into the pleural space.
- If ultrasound is used for dynamic guidance (recommended for small effusions), keep the needle tip in view at all times and guide into the fluid collection.
- If ultrasound was not used for identification and localization of fluid, and no fluid was obtained after a reasonable depth of needle insertion, consider radiographic guidance of some sort (computed tomography [CT], ultrasound).
- Once fluid is obtained, aspirate into a 60-cc syringe and hand off to an assistant for further processing (into blood tubes, culture bottles).
- Connect gravity drainage bag or vacuum bottles.
- If pleural manometry is used, connect to the transducer circuit and have the assistant calibrate and zero the transducer; note the pressure during drainage.
- Pleural pressure that drops below 15 to 20 cm H_2O during drainage is indicative of poorly expandable lung, and increases the risk of reexpansion pulmonary edema and pneumothorax.
- Upper limits on the amount of fluid that can be safely removed are not well supported in the literature; large fluid collections drained rapidly may cause unsafe pressure fluctuations in the chest and may cause fluid shifts.
- Remove the needle and apply a bandage.
- Once the fluid is drained, a postprocedure ultrasound can be performed to identify pneumothorax.
- Routine postprocedure chest radiography is controversial; data supports an individualized approach based on operator experience and skill, whether or not ultrasound was used, and signs or symptoms of complications during the procedure (chest pain, dyspnea, aspirated blood).

Advantages

- Allows for rapid drainage of pleural fluid
- Relatively noninvasive
- Can be repeated if necessary

Disadvantages and Complications

- Cannot effectively drain highly viscous fluid collections (empyema).
- Loculations often prevent complete chest drainage and lung expansion.
- Pneumothorax (1.5% to 30%).
- Hemothorax.
- Nerve damage.
- Cardiac puncture.
- Liver, spleen, or kidney puncture.
- Can cause empyema.
- May need to be repeated.

ABDOMINAL AND GASTROINTESTINAL
(see http://www.youtube.com/watch?V=r7maXwlCFw)

Abdominal Paracentesis

Indications

- Diagnosis of intraabdominal pathology
  - New onset ascites
  - Spontaneous bacterial peritonitis
- Therapeutic paracentesis
  - Recurrent ascites in setting of hepatic disease
  - Relieve pressure in abdominal compartment syndrome (if fluid is a contributor)

Contraindications (All Relative and Must Be Individualized)

- Severe coagulopathy (INR greater than 2 in elective cases) or thrombocytopenia less than 20,000
- Gastric or bowel distention
- Bladder distention
- Pregnancy
- Abdominal wall infection
- Acute abdomen

Technique

- Obtain necessary equipment:
  - Paracentesis or thoracentesis tray
  - 18-gauge angiocatheter (at least 1.75 in if possible)
  - Sterile skin prep solution (chlorhexidine)
  - Sterile towels and drape
  - Lidocaine
  - Needles: 19- and 25-gauge
  - Scalpel
  - Two 10-cc syringes
  - One 60-cc syringe
  - Red top tube for chemistry, purple top tube for cell count and differential, blood culture bottles
  - Sterile gloves
  - Drainage apparatus (gravity drainage bag or vacuum bottles)
  - Gauze
  - Tape
  - Ultrasound machine with 5-MHz curvilinear transducer (optional but highly recommended)
  - Sterile transducer sleeve
- Position the patient in the supine or semirecumbent position.
- Consider decompressing the stomach with an NG tube; decompress the bladder with a Foley catheter.
- Use ultrasound to identify the fluid collection (Figure 1-5).

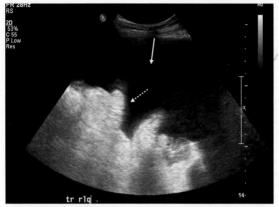

Figure 1-5   Ultrasound guidance for paracentesis (image of the abdominal cavity and the ascites).

- Note the amount, echogenicity (anechoic, complex), and best window for needle insertion.
  - Make sure to identify all abdominal viscera, including the liver, kidneys, spleen, bladder, and bowel.
  - Mark an appropriate insertion site on the skin, noting the depth and angle of insonation (which will be duplicated with the needle if dynamic guidance is not used).
- Prep and drape the area.
- Anesthetize the skin with 5 to 10 cc 1% or 2% lidocaine in the usual manner (raising an intradermal skin wheal, then injecting deeper while intermittently aspirating to prevent injection into a vessel).
- When fluid is obtained with the anesthesia needle, withdraw without injecting further.
- Make a small skin nick with the scalpel.
- Insert the needle-catheter device into the skin nick and advance slowly toward the fluid collection while aspirating.
- There is no conclusive evidence that a zigzag insertion technique reduces the risk of persistent fluid leak on needle removal.
- Once fluid is obtained, advance the needle another 0.5 to 1 cm then stop; remove the needle, leaving the catheter in place.
- Advance the catheter to the hub.
- Connect the 60-cc syringe and aspirate fluid for samples; hand off to an assistant for further processing.
- Connect gravity drainage bag or vacuum bottles.
- Large-volume paracentesis should be performed with caution, especially in patients who have not had large amounts of fluid removed.
- There is some evidence that intravascular volume expansion with albumin prevents hemodynamic complications of large-volume paracentesis, but this remains controversial.
- If the fluid ceases in a stuttering manner, slowly withdraw the catheter until flow improves.
- If the flow does not improve, or if blood is suddenly aspirated, kink the tubing to stop suction and remove the catheter.
- Apply pressure for several minutes, then apply a bandage.
- If large-volume paracentesis was performed, monitor for hemodynamic complications, which are often silent; instruct the patient to monitor urine output and assess for symptoms of presyncope.

Advantages

- Allows for relatively noninvasive diagnosis of intraabdominal pathology
- Safe and effective
- Minimal training required

Disadvantages and Complications

- Persistent fluid leak from puncture site
- Perforation of gastrointestinal (GI) tract
- Secondary peritonitis
- Hepatic, splenic, or renal laceration
- Hemoperitoneum
- Hematoma formation
- Hepatorenal syndrome (in cirrhotic patients following large-volume paracentesis)
  - Consider volume expansion with albumin.

NG Intubation

Indications

- Enteral nutrition
- Diagnosis of upper GI bleeding
- Relief of acute gastric distention (following bag-mask ventilation for example)
- Decompress proximal GI tract in setting of distal obstruction (small bowel obstruction, gastric outlet obstruction)
- Prevention of aerophagia in the setting of bowel obstruction, ileus, or pseudoobstruction

Contraindications

- Facial or nasal trauma precluding insertion.
- Skull base fracture, CSF leak.
- Recent esophageal or gastric surgery.
- Esophageal varices are not an absolute contraindication, but passing an NG tube in the setting of recent banding of varices should be approached with caution.

Technique

- Obtain the appropriate equipment.
  - Viscous lidocaine
  - Water-soluble lubricant
  - NG tube
  - One 60-cc syringe
  - Stethoscope
- Place the patient in a comfortable position.
- Measure the tube from the nose to the earlobe, then add the distance from the earlobe to the epigastrium.
- Ask the patient to sniff viscous lidocaine.
- Lubricate the tube with water-soluble lubricant.
- Flex the neck.
- Insert the tube in the nose, pass along the floor of the nasal cavity.
- Resistance will be met when the tube encounters the posterior nasopharyngeal wall; continue advancing several centimeters, then begin asking the patient to swallow.
- Continue advancing the tube slowly until in place.
- Connect the 60-cc syringe filled with air to the tube.
- Auscultate the epigastrium while injecting the air and listen for gastric sounds.
- Ask the patient to speak (if applicable) to ensure that the tube has not passed through the vocal cords (cough alone is unreliable as many patient with correctly placed tubes experience cough during insertion).
- Secure the tube to the nose with tape.
- Strongly consider obtaining a chest radiograph prior to initiating enteral feeding.

Advantages

- Allows access to the upper GI tract for feeding, identification of upper GI bleeding, administration of enteral medications, decompression of the stomach, prevention of aerophagia

Disadvantages and Complications

- Insertion into the lower respiratory tract
- Epistaxis
- Discomfort
- Paranasal sinus disease (consider orogastric tube in intubated mechanically ventilated patients)
- Ulceration of the nares
- GI bleed from gastric mucosal erosion, more likely when the tube is placed to high suction

GENITOURINARY

Bladder Catheterization

Indications

- To relieve urinary retention
- To better assess urine output in nonambulatory or incontinent patients
- To lavage the bladder in cases of bleeding
- Antibiotic bladder washes
- Collection of clean urine for microbiologic or cytologic examination

Contraindications

- Suspected urethral rupture (pelvic trauma, pelvic fracture)
- History of urethral stricture or deformity or congenital abnormality
- Acute prostatitis

Technique

- Obtain equipment:
  - Bladder catheterization kits include a catheter (Foley), skin cleanser, lubricant, 10-cc syringe, fenestrated drape, gloves, and a gravity drainage bag
- Have the opened kit within arms' reach.
- Coat the catheter with a liberal amount of lubricant.
- Position the patient appropriately: supine for men, and frog-legged for women.
- Place sterile towels or the fenestrated drape around the penis or the vulva.
- Cleanse the area thoroughly.
  - Grasp the penis with one hand, apply skin cleanser liberally around the entire glans with the other hand.
  - Open the labia minora and identify the urethral meatus; cleanse the entire area.
- Grasp the catheter and insert into the urethra.
- Advance until the hub of the catheter reaches the urethral meatus, or until urine is returned (will not require advancement to the hub in women).
- If urine is not returned, irrigate the catheter with saline to confirm position.
- Inflate the balloon with 10 cc normal saline.
- Connect gravity drainage bag.
- If difficulty ensues during insertion, most commonly in men with prostate hyperplasia, note the location of the obstruction.
- If the obstruction seems distal along the course of the urethra (toward the meatus), a smaller catheter may be helpful.
- If the obstruction is more proximal along the urethra (toward the prostate), the problem may be stricture at the bulbomembranous junction (urethra has an angle at this location) or prostatic hyperplasia.
  - In either case, a coude-tipped catheter inserted with the tip pointing at the 12 o'clock position (assuming the patient is supine) may help negotiate the angle.
  - Palpation of the perineum and digital pressure from outside may help the catheter negotiate the angle.

- If still unsuccessful, never attempt to force the catheter through an area of resistance; the urethra is particularly susceptible to development of "false passages" that often require cystoscopy to both identify the problem and to pass a catheter.
- Have a low threshold for obtaining urology consultation to help with difficult cases.

Advantages

- As above (indications)

Disadvantages and Complications

- Creation of false passages
- Hematuria: common, usually self-limited, but may be severe in coagulopathic patients
  - Must irrigate the bladder to prevent clot formation
- Cystitis
- Epididymitis
- Urethral stricture
- Bladder perforation
- Urethral perforation (if the balloon is inflated while in the urethra)

Bladder Pressure Assessment

Indications

- Diagnosis of intraabdominal hypertension and abdominal compartment syndrome

Contraindications

- None

Technique

- Equipment: an in-line pressure manometer (column manometer, or more commonly a pressure transducer system)
- Ensure that the bladder is relatively empty (less than 50 cc)
  - Full bladders may overestimate bladder pressure.
- Zero the transducer or ensure that the bottom of the column is at midbladder height in the supine patient (4–5 cm below the pubic symphysis).
- Open the stopcock and allow the pressure to equilibrate.
- Pressure 12 mm Hg or more is abnormal.
- Pressure 25 mm Hg or more indicates abdominal compartment syndrome (in the right clinical context).

Advantages

- Easy, reproducible method for ascertaining intraabdominal pressure

Disadvantages and Complications

- Accuracy has been debated.
- Subject to misinterpretation or errors in measurement.

MUSCULOSKELETAL

Knee Injection and Aspiration

Indications

- Diagnosis of septic arthritis
- Diagnosis of inflammatory arthropathies
- Allows for examination of crystals and cell counts
- Injection of corticosteroids

Contraindications

- Overlying skin infection
- Severe coagulopathy or bleeding disorders
- Presence of prosthetic joints
- Bacteremia without systemic antibiotics on board

Technique

- Equipment

- Local anesthesia (1% lidocaine)
- Skin prep solution
- Sterile towels
- Needle: 18- or 19-gauge
- Needle: 25-gauge for anesthetic
- Appropriate tubes for samples
- Two 10-cc syringes
- Sterile gloves
- Ultrasound machine with linear array transducer (optional)
- Position the patient supine with the leg fully extended at the knee.
- Palpate the knee, specifically noting the presence of fluid.
- If ultrasound is available, use the high-frequency linear array transducer in a longitudinal orientation to locate the quadriceps tendon (fibrous structure attaching to the superior pole of the patella).
  - Fluid often collects below the quadriceps tendon in the suprapatellar fossa.
  - Note the location and depth of the fluid.
- Prep and drape the area.
- Anesthetize the skin overlying either the medial or lateral suprapatellar recess (to either side of the quadriceps tendon).
- Insert the needle and aim for the center of the patella, taking care to advance the needle under the patella.
- Once fluid is obtained, aspirate the joint completely.
- Debris may obstruct the needle; periodically rotate the needle or clear the needle intermittently by injecting a small amount of the aspirated synovial fluid.
- Place fluid into correct containers for laboratory analysis.
- If injection is to be performed, disconnect the syringe used for aspiration and connect the syringe containing corticosteroid, and so forth.
- Inject slowly; there should be no resistance to injection.
- Remove the needle and place a sterile bandage.

Advantages

- Allows diagnosis of articular pathology
- May be therapeutic if debris is removed or corticosteroids are injected

Disadvantages and Complications

- Infection
- Bleeding
- Failure

Bone Marrow Aspiration and Biopsy

Aspiration is used to assess cell morphology; biopsy is used to assess for architecture and cellularity of the bone marrow.

Indications

- Unexplained anemia (assess bone marrow cellularity)
- Unexplained leucopenia
- Unexplained thrombocytopenia
- Pancytopenia
- Suspected hematologic malignancy (special histochemical stains required)
- Suspected lymphoma
- Suspected storage disease
- Suspected infiltrative disease (ie, amyloidosis)
- Fever of unknown origin (obtain bone marrow cultures at bed side)

Contraindications

- Hemophilia and other inherited clotting disorders
- Severe disseminated intravascular coagulopathy
- Sternal bone marrow aspiration should be avoided in all patients

- Infection at insertion site
- Previous radiation at proposed site

Technique

- Equipment
  - Alcohol prep pads, double-ply, large
  - Povidone iodine (Betadine) swab sticks (packets of 3)
  - Ear speculums
  - Gauge sponges 3 × 4 in (7.5 × 10 cm)
  - Plastic isolation gowns
  - Isopropyl alcohol swab sticks (packets of 3)
  - Latex gloves, examination, nonsterile
  - Latex gloves, sterile
  - Lidocaine HCL, injection, 1%, 10 mg/mL, 20 mL vials
  - Needles, 22-gauge, 1–1/2 in
  - Small fenestrated sheet, sterile, 30 × 30 in with 1½ × 2-in fenestration
  - Sodium bicarbonate solution, 8.4% (1 mEq/mL), 50 mL vials
  - Sodium heparin, 100 USP Units/mL, 2 mL vials
  - Spinal needles, 3½ in (Quincke type point)
  - Subcutaneous needles, 26-gauge, 5/8 in
  - Blank labels
  - Bone marrow aspiration needle, 15-gauge, 4 in
  - Bone marrow biopsy needle, J-type, 11-gauge, 6 in (15 cm)
  - Contoured Jamshidi bone marrow biopsy-aspiration needle (11-gauge, 4 in)
  - Disposable plastic syringes, sterile, 10 cc
  - Disposable plastic syringes, sterile U 20 cc
  - Disposable scalpel (γ radiation sterilized: 2.5 mrad, 25 KGy)
  - Illinois sternal-iliac aspiration needle, 16-gauge, adjustable length (3/16 to 1–7/8 in)

Procedures

- Place patient on the side with knees flexed with the head averted to one side.
- Palpate the patient's back for landmarks and identify the center of the posterior superior iliac spine.
- If not readily palpable, consider ultrasound.
- Prep in the sterile manner and place sterile drapes.
- With steady twisting motion, advance biopsy (Jamshidi) needle to the center of the posterior superior iliac crest.
- Unlock and remove the obturator.
- Advance needle approximately one-half to 1 cm farther into the marrow cavity. The needle should remain stationery when not manipulated.
- Rotate the needle clockwise and counterclockwise 6 times to free the specimen of the cortical bone.
- Remove specimen and place into container.
- In case of aspiration, either biopsy or aspiration needle can be used.
- Remove obturator only when the needle is stationary in the bone.
- Aspirate the necessary volume of bone marrow.

Complications

- Broken needle
- Hemorrhage
- Infection at aspiration site
- Perforation of iliac bone

Punch Biopsy of the Skin

Indications

- Conditions requiring a full-thickness biopsy
- Small lesions (usually > 8 mm)

Contraindications

- Suspected malignant lesions requiring a large-margin (melanoma)
- Large lesions (> 8 mm)
- Severe coagulopathy (relative)
- Infection at the site of biopsy
- Allergy to topical antibiotics or local anesthetics

Technique

- Measure the size of the lesion to be removed, or if a general condition (rash) is to be biopsied, locate an area that has both affected and nonaffected skin.
- Select an appropriate size skin punch (2–8 mm) and place on sterile tray along with 4-0 nylon skin suture, small sterile scissors, and a needle driver or clamp.
- Mark the area to be biopsied.
- Cleanse the skin with alcohol.
- Infiltrate the area with 1% or 2% lidocaine solution.
- Prep and drape the area.
- Using an appropriate-sized punch, apply the punch to the skin at a 90-degree angle.
- Apply gentle pressure and rotate the punch until it has cut to the desired depth (approximately 3 mm).
- Remove the punch and ensure that the lesion is now free floating.
- Grasp the lesion with the clamp (gently to prevent crush artifact) and use the scissors to remove any subcutaneous connective tissue.
- Place the specimen in fixative.
- Close the skin incision with interrupted 4-0 nylon skin sutures.
- Do not close the skin too tightly, as swelling will occur which may cause the skin to become necrotic.
- Apply antibiotic ointment and a sterile bandage.
- Remove sutures in 7 to 10 days (7 for low-tension areas, 10 days for high-tension areas such as around joints).

Advantages

- Easy to perform.
- Most punches are disposable, precluding the need for autoclaving.
- No specialized training is necessary.

Disadvantages and Complications

- Can remove only small lesions.
- Damage to underlying structures may occur.
- Skin infection.
- Bleeding.
- Bruising.

NEUROLOGIC

Diagnostic Lumbar Puncture

Indications

- Evaluate the central nervous system for evidence of infection, hemorrhage, or malignancy.
- CT is falsely negative in up to 7% of cases of subarachnoid hemorrhage (SAH), therefore SAH cannot be ruled out without lumbar puncture (LP).
- Measure central nervous system pressure.
- Injection of medications (anesthesia, chemotherapeutics).

Contraindications

- Increased intracranial pressure, which may lead to herniation (controversial)
- Severe coagulopathy or thrombocytopenia less than 50,000 per microliter
- Evidence of infection over the planned insertion site
- Anatomic abnormalities of the spine that would interfere with needle insertion

Role of Imaging in Decision Making

- *Routine CT screening prior to LP is not supported in the literature.*
- CT should be considered in the following conditions, all of which are associated with increased risk of increased intracranial pressure:
- Focal neurologic findings on examination:
  - Gaze palsy
  - Arm or leg drift
  - Abnormal visual fields
  - Abnormal language
- Age older than 60 years.
- Immunocompromised status.
- Known intracranial mass or space occupying lesion.
- Recent seizure (within 1 week).
- Altered consciousness:
  - Inability to follow 2 commands
  - Inability to answer 2 consecutive questions correctly
- Papilledema.
- CT findings of unequal intracranial compartment pressures, and therefore increased risk of herniation include:
  - Lateral shift of midline structures
  - Loss of the suprachiasmatic and basilar cisterns
  - Obliteration of the fourth ventricle
  - Obliteration of the superior cerebellar and quadrigeminal
  - Plate cisterns with sparing of the ambient cisterns
- In patients found to have physical examination findings consistent with elevated intracranial pressure, the focus should shift away from LP and toward diagnosis of the underlying cause and subsequent management of increased intracranial pressure.

Technique

- Obtain the appropriate equipment:
  - Lidocaine for topical anesthesia
  - Fenestrated drape or sterile towels
  - Spinal needle with obturator
  - Needles for anesthesia: 25- and 22-gauge
  - One 10-cc syringe
  - Collection tubes
  - A clear graded column manometer and stopcock for CSF pressure measurement
  - Ultrasound machine with either 5-MHz curvilinear probe or 6- to 13-MHz linear-array probe (if landmarks are difficult to palpate)
- Position the patient either in the lateral decubitus position or seated upright.
- Ensure patient comfort by placing a pillow under the head, or if seated upright have a table available for the patient to rest on (pressure cannot be accurately measured in an upright patient).
- Have the patient flex the hips and neck as much as possible; if the patient is not cooperative, administer incremental doses of sedative and have an assistant maintain correct position of the patient (do not sedate a patient seated upright).
- Select an insertion site:
  - Draw an imaginary straight line connecting the highest palpable part of the iliac crests.
  - The L4 to L5 interspace is typically where the line intersects the spine.
- Clean the skin over the proposed insertion site, then drape.
- Anesthetize the skin and subcutaneous tissues; follow the proposed spinal needle track and anesthetize the entire track (stop if you meet resistance).
- Insert the spinal needle and aim cranially by approximately 20 degrees, taking care to follow a midline trajectory.
- A slight increased resistance, followed by a sudden loss of resistance ("pop") will be felt when the needle penetrates the ligamentum flavum.

- Remove the obturator and observe for fluid return.
- If no fluid is obtained, reinsert the obturator and advance the needle by increments, removing the obturator after every stage of advancement until fluid is obtained.
- Take care not to insert the needle too far (may be "hubbed" in overweight patients).
- If bone is encountered, pull the needle back to the subcutaneous tissues and redirect.
- *Tip: Do not redirect a deeply buried needle,* as this may cause damage and is generally ineffective.
- *Tip:* Use a systematic approach to redirection, do not blindly "jab," but rather aim slightly more cranially or caudally with each successive attempt.
- *Tip:* ensure that the patients hips are not leaning toward or away from you, otherwise you will not be advancing the needle in a true midline trajectory.
- If blood is obtained:
  - Wait to see if it clears (traumatic tap).
  - Wait to see if it clots (traumatic tap).
  - If it does not clot or clear, the patient may have an SAH.
- If CSF is obtained, place a 3-way stopcock on the end of the needle, then attach a graded column in the upright position. Open the stopcock and allow CSF to fill the column and come to rest, then record pressure:
  - Normal is less than 15 cm H_2O.
  - Abnormal is greater than 20 cm H_2O.
  - Borderline is 15 to 20 cm H_2O.
- Empty the column into collection tubes. Send for:
  - Cell count and differential
  - CSF protein and glucose
  - Gram stain and culture, bacterial antigens
  - Special tests: India ink, fungal or viral studies, and so forth
- Remove the stopcock and obtain additional CSF straight from the spinal needle for cell counts.
- Withdraw needle and place sterile bandage over the insertion site.
- Be sure to observe for changes in neurologic examination.
- No need for routine bed rest following LP.

Ultrasound-Guided Lumbar Puncture

- Use either a 5-MHz curvilinear probe (overweight patients) or a high-frequency linear-array probe (nonobese patients).
- Position patient for LP.
- Scan the spine along its axis (longitudinally) and identify the L4 and L5 spinal processes.
- Align the spinal processes so that the intervening space is centered on the screen.
- Mark the skin under the center of the probe, which corresponds to the space between L4 and L5.
- Turn the probe 90 degrees and again identify either the L4 or L5 spinal process; align in the center of the screen.
- Mark the skin under the center of the probe.
- There will be two skin marks, one longitudinal and one transverse; the intersection of the two should be the insertion site.

Disadvantages and Complications

- Postprocedure headache ("spinal headache")
  - Onset is usually 24 to 48 hours after LP.
  - Analgesics and fluids relieve symptoms in most patients.
  - Caffeine may be helpful.
- Episodes of paresthesia, which are usually self-limited
- CSF leak from the insertion site. This can be treated with an epidural blood patch.
- Herniation, which is a rare but often fatal complication, requires emergent management including neurosurgical consult.

CHAPTER 2

Environmental Emergencies

Colin G. Kaide, Hannah L. Hays, and David P. Bahner

ENVIRONMENTAL EMERGENCIES

Hypothermia

Statistics

- There are 20 to 100,000 environmental emergencies per year worldwide.
- Environmental emergencies cause approximately 700 deaths per year in the United States.
- Most cases occur in an urban setting and are related to exposure attributed to alcoholism, illicit drug use, mental illness or homelessness.
- Other affected groups include people in an outdoor setting for work or pleasure.

Definition

- Accidental or intentional drop of body core temperature to 35°C (95°F) or below (Table 2-1)

TABLE 2-1. ETIOLOGY OF AND FACTORS CONTRIBUTING TO HYPOTHERMIA

Decreased Heat Production	Increased Heat Loss	Impaired Thermoregulation
Endocrine Failure	**Environmental**	**Peripheral Failure**
Hypopituitarism	Immersion (conduction heat loss)	Neuropathies
Hypoadrenalism	Wet clothing (conduction/evaporative heat loss)	Acute cord transection
Lactic acidosis		Spinal cord injuries
DKA/Alcoholic ketoacidosis	**Induced Vasodilatation**	**Central Failure/Neurologic**
Insufficient Fuel	Pharmacologic/Toxicologic	SAH or CVA
Hypoglycemia	Vasodilators	CNS trauma
Malnutrition	Beta-blockers	Hypothalamic dysfunction
Extreme exertion	Hypoglycemic agents	Parkinson's disease
Neuromuscular Physical Exertion	Depressors of consciousness	Cerebellar lesion
Age extremes	**Erythrodermas**	Neoplasm
Impaired shivering	Burns	Multiple Sclerosis
Inactivity	Psoriasis	
Lack of adaptation	**Iatrogenics**	
	Cold infusion	
	Heatstroke treatment	
	Induced hypothermia (post arrest)	

CNS, central nervous system; CVA, cerebrovascular accident; DKA, diabetic ketoacidosis; SAH, subarachnoid hemorrhage.

Severity and Expected Changes (Table 2-2)

TABLE 2-2. PATHOLOGICAL CHANGES IN HYPOTHERMIA

	Core Temp		Characteristics
	°C	°F	
Mild	37.6	99.6	Normal rectal temperature
	37.0	98.6	Normal oral temperature
	36.0	96.8	Increase in metabolic rate and blood pressure and preshivering muscle tone
	35.0	95.0	Urine temperature 34.8°C (94.6°F); maximum shivering thermogenesis
	34.0	93.2	Amnesia, dysarthria, and poor judgment develop; maladaptive behavior; normal blood pressure; maximum respiratory stimulation; tachycardia, then progressive bradycardia
	33.0	91.4	Ataxia and apathy develop; linear depression of cerebral metabolism; tachypnea, then progressive decrease in respiratory minute volume; cold diuresis
Moderate	32.0	89.6	Stupor; 25% decrease in oxygen consumption
	31.0	87.8	Extinguished shivering thermogenesis
	30.0	86.0	Atrial fibrillation and other arrhythmias develop; poikilothermia; cardiac output two-thirds of normal: insulin ineffective
	29.0	85.2	Progressive decrease in level of consciousness, pulse, and respiration; pupils dilated; paradoxical undressing
	28.0	82.4	Decreased ventricular fibrillation threshold; 50% decrease in oxygen consumption and pulse; hypoventilation
	27.0	80.6	Loss of reflexes and voluntary motion
Severe	26.0	78.8	Major acid-base disturbances; no reflexes or response to pain
	25.0	77.0	Cerebral blood now one-third of normal; loss of cerebrovascular autoregulation; cardiac output 45% of normal; pulmonary edema may develop
	24.0	75.2	Significant hypotension and bradycardia
	23.0	73.4	No corneal or oculocephalic reflexes; areflexia
	22.0	71.6	Maximum risk of ventricular fibrillation; 75% decrease in oxygen consumption
	20.0	68.0	Lowest resumption of cardiac electromechanical activity; pulse 20% of normal
	19.0	66.2	Electroencephalographic silencing
	18.0	64.4	Asystole
	16.0	60.8	Lowest adult accidental hypothermia survival
	15.2	59.2	Lowest infant accidental hypothermia survival
	10.0	50.0	92% decrease in oxygen consumption
	9.0	48.2	Lowest therapeutic hypothermia survival

Multiple System Involvement

- Central nervous system (CNS)
  - CNS progressively deteriorates from confusion to coma.
  - Areflexia below 28°C (82.4°F): Patellar reflex is last to disappear.
  - Electroencephalogram appears flat at 19°C (66.2°F).
  - Less than 5% of patients have focal symptoms; if focal findings appear on examination, use computed tomography to look for intracranial pathology.
  - Antidiuretic hormone inhibition may cause a "cold diuresis" with fluid and electrolyte shifts.
  - If not a primary exposure, look for CNS pathology.
- Cardiovascular
  - Bradycardia.
  - Dysrhythmias: Initially, slow atrial fibrillation is common below 30°C (86°F).
  - Decreased cardiac output.
  - Hypotension.
  - Risk of ventricular fibrillation is greatest when temperature is lower than 22°C (71.6°F).
  - J wave or Osborn wave is seen on electrocardiogram.
  - Third spacing and cold diuresis cause hypovolemia.
- Respiratory
  - Initial stimulation of respiratory drive
  - Progressive decline in minute ventilation
  - Bronchorrhea
  - Cough impaired; aspiration common
  - Pulmonary edema
- Hematopoietic
  - Hemoconcentration.
  - White blood cells initially increase but then decrease because of sequestration and bone marrow depression.
  - Cold coagulopathy:
    - Cold induces thrombocytopenia.
    - Clotting factors become less active when cold.
  - Oxyhemoglobin curve shifts to the left (decrease in available oxygen).
- Other systems:
  - Gastrointestinal (GI) motility is decreased.
  - Insulin is inactivated.

Diagnostic Evaluation

- Complete blood count, coagulation studies
- Urinalysis, blood urea nitrogen, creatinine
- Electrolytes, glucose
- Chest x-ray
- Electroencephalogram
- Arterial blood gas (*do not correct for temperature*) (Table 2-3)

Treatment

- Handle all victims carefully: Rough handling has been known to precipitate ventricular fibrillation.
- Prevent further heat loss.
- Anticipate an irritable myocardium and hypovolemia.
- Treat hypothermia before treating frostbite.
- ABCDEs
  - **A**irway with cervical spine immobilization if any question of trauma, intubate if necessary; be ready for dysrhythmias.
  - **B**reathing—provide oxygen.
  - **C**irculation—intravenous (IV) normal saline; initially avoid lactated Ringer solution.
  - **D**isability—record quick neurologic examination.
  - **E**xposure—remove wet clothes, look for injuries.

TABLE 2-3. CORRECTED AND UNCORRECTED BLOOD GAS ANALYSES

Which has a higher measured pH: boiling water or near-freezing water? They both will have a *measured* pH of 6.8. The blood gas machine will warm or cool the test sample to be measured, to the temperature of 37°C (98.6°F) and then read the pH. Likewise, blood sent to the lab at any temperature will have the pH measured at 37°C (98.6°F). Let us take the example of a patient whose core temperature is 25°C (77°F) and who is maintaining an adequate respiratory rate for his or her temperature (probably by artificial means at this temperature!). If these givens are true, the patient would be ventilating slower than a person at 37°C (98.6°F). For sake of argument, let us say the rate is appropriate for the quantity of carbon dioxide produced at this subnormal temperature (ie, the patient should be in acid-base balance). If the laboratory is told that the patient's core temperature is 25°C (77°F), the laboratory will use an artificial correction factor (ΔpH/C° = 0.015) derived from laboratory data and correct the pH to the given temperature. The laboratory would report a corrected pH of 7.58. This "corrected pH" represents what the pH probe would read if it were stuck into the patient and allowed to read the actual pH at the patient's temperature, instead of at 37°C (98.6°F) (the way the machine usually does). This pH of 7.58 is appropriately high.

If the same case is replayed without informing the laboratory that the patient's temperature is 25°C (77°F), the laboratory machine will heat the blood to 37°C (98.6°F), a reading will be taken, and an uncorrected value will be reported. If the patient is in true acid-base balance (if the ventilator is set properly or the patient is spontaneously breathing at the correct rate), the uncorrected number from the laboratory will be 7.4. (Note: If you stuck a probe into the patient and used the actual body temperature to measure the pH without warming the blood to 37°C [98.6°F], the pH would read 7.58, which is the same as that corrected for temperature.) The pH (uncorrected) of 7.4 indicates that the patient is in perfect acid-base balance.

Bottom Line: If you obtain an uncorrected pH of 7.4, the patient is in perfect acid-base balance at *any temperature*. If you obtain an uncorrected pH of 7.28, you will automatically know that at any temperature, this patient is not in acid-base balance and his or her pH should be brought back close to 7.4 (uncorrected). In some cases this may require intubation and relative hyperventilation (possibly a rate of 12 breaths per minute instead of what we usually think of as hyperventilation at 16–20 breaths per minute).

- Measure temperature with low-reading esophageal, rectal, or bladder thermometer.
- Consider thiamine, 50% dextrose, naloxone.
- Use fluids before vasopressors.
- Look for hidden trauma.
- Look for potential cause.
- Watch for "after-drop."

Rewarming (Table 2-4)

- **Heated humidified oxygen:** The respiratory tract is an effective site for heat exchange with heating of both the pulmonary vasculature and the oxygen itself. The heart is then perfused with warmer blood. Because of the low thermal conductivity of dry air, humidification is required for effective heat transfer. Heat is delivered effectively with a mask but is greatly augmented by an endotracheal tube.

    Another benefit of heating the airway is that it stimulates pulmonary cilia and reduces the amount and viscosity of cold-induced bronchorrhea.

    Although shivering may be reduced with this method of core rewarming, the core temperature is elevated nonetheless.

    The ideal temperature of the air to be delivered is 45°C (113°F). Minor modification of respiratory equipment may be required to achieve this temperature.

- **Expected rate of rewarming:** 1 to 2.5°C (1.8–4.3°F) per hour; rewarming rate is higher with an endotracheal than with a mask.
- **Indications:** All patients with moderate to severe hypothermia.
- **Contraindications:** None.
- **Heated infusions:** Rewarming a hypothermic patient with heated IV fluids *is not* effective. Maximum warming is only 0.33°C (0.66°F) per liter. To increase a patient's temperature from 26°C (80°F) to 32°C (90°F) would require 6 × 3 = 18 L of warmed saline!

TABLE 2-4. REWARMING

Passive External Rewarming (PER)

Discussion: This method is focused on preventing any further loss of heat from a body by providing insulation and removing the patient from the offending environment. No outside heat is added to the patient and peripheral vasoconstriction is maintained. It is appropriate in mild hypothermia or as adjunctive to active rewarming.

Use: *The stable patient with a core temperature > 32°C (89.6°F) is the ideal candidate for this treatment.* PER may be used in any patient as initial treatment in the field, or to prevent further heat loss in the emergency department. For this technique to cause an increase in body temperature, the patient *must be able to generate heat.* The patient will lose this ability at < 32°C (89.6°F).

Rate of Rewarming: 0.5–1°C/h (0.9–1.8°F/h)

Active External Rewarming (AER)

Discussion: This method involves delivery of heat directly to the skin or external surface of the patient. Heat may be applied to the whole patient or selectively to the trunk. Mixed results have been obtained during study of this technique with paradoxically high mortality rates when aggressive AER is applied in severe hypothermia to the whole body. This may be secondary to after-drop and pH changes in arterial blood. In previously healthy patients with mild hypothermia, AER appeared to be safe but offered no advantages over PER and core rewarming. The problem of core after-drop hypothermia and hypotension may be ameliorated by applying AER only to the trunk.

Methods of AER include:

- Radiant heat
- Hot-water bottles
- Plumbed garments
- Electric heating pads and blankets
- Forced circulated hot air
- Immersion in warm water.

Use: The application of AER alone must be done cautiously with close monitoring for adverse thermic and blood pressure changes. Application should be limited to the trunk only. Truncal AER may be used safely in conjunction with active core rewarming.

Rate of Rewarming: Variable

Active Internal/Core Rewarming (AIR)

Discussion: This method involves the delivery of heat to the core. This is done either directly by lavage of core structures with heated irrigation solutions or indirectly via heating the blood or the inspired air. Additionally, microwave radiation can cause direct heating of tissues.

Methods of core rewarming include:

- Heated humidified oxygen
- Heated infusions
- Heated irrigation of hollow viscous (gut, bladder, colon)
- Heated irrigation of body cavities (peritoneal, pleural, mediastinal)
- Bypass with heat exchangers (and/or oxygenators)
- Diathermy

Use: See list of indications for active core rewarming.

Rate of Rewarming: 1–10°C/h (1.8–18°F/h), depending on method used. Effects are usually cumulative.

In the hypothermic patient or in the normothermic patient requiring massive infusions of crystalloid and blood, all infusates should be heated to at least body temperature (37°C [98.6°F]). This is done to prevent iatrogenic hypothermia, or worsening of existing low temperatures.

- **Expected rate of rewarming:** 0.33°C (0.66°F) per liter of fluid warmed to 42°C (107.6°F).
- **Indications:** Any moderate to severe hypothermic patient or any patient receiving massive infusions or transfusions.

- **Contraindications:** None.
- **Heated irrigation of hollow viscous:**
  - Heated irrigation of virtually every orifice has been tried as a method of rewarming hypothermic patients.
  - Although irrigation of the stomach, colon, and bladder have the ability to raise core temperature, they are limited by the available surface area.
  - Further, prolonged irrigation of these surfaces will induce electrolyte fluxes.
  - To address this problem, intragastric and intracolonic balloons filled with warm water have been used effectively in lieu of direct irrigation.
  - Warmed fluids used for direct irrigation should have a dwell time of several to 15 minutes.
  - The patient should be intubated before gastric lavage is performed as airway protection.
  - **Expected rate of rewarming:** 1 to 1.5°C (1.8–2.7°F) per hour
  - **Indications:** Moderate to severely hypothermic patients as an adjunct to other methods of rewarming.
  - **Contraindications:** GI tract injury. This should not be the only method of rewarming.
- **Heated irrigation of body cavities:**
  - The peritoneal, thoracic and mediastinal cavities, through diagnostic peritoneal lavage (DPL), tube thoracostomy, and thoracotomy respectively, can all be irrigated with warmed solutions.
  - In ascending order, these methods have progressively greater ability to raise core temperature rapidly.
  - They are, however, more invasive than previously described methods.
  - Through a DPL catheter, normal saline, lactated Ringer solution or 1.5% dextrose dialysate heated to 40 to 45°C (104–113°F), may be instilled into the peritoneum 2 liters at a time.
  - The fluid is left to dwell for 20 to 30 minutes and then exchanged.
  - Using dialysate, effective detoxification of certain substances and manipulation of certain electrolytes can be attained.
  - The thoracic cavity can be irrigated with saline heated to 40 to 42°C (104–107.5°F) through anterior and posterior chest tubes (at the second or third intercostal space of the anterior midclavicular line and at the fifth or sixth intercostal space of the post-posterior axillary line).
  - Irrigation with this inflow/outflow system can be done using a Level 1 pressure infuser (180–550 mL min) or by hanging heated IV bags.
  - Care must be taken so as to not cause a *tension hydrothorax* by not allowing for enough time for adequate drainage of the posterior chest tube.
  - Single chest tube lavage can be done infusing 200 to 300 cc of saline at a time and removing the fluid by suction after each aliquot.
  - The technique of thoracic irrigation has the advantage of allowing for preferential heating of the mediastinal structures.
  - Further, the "thoracic pump model" of cardiopulmonary resuscitation (CPR) is preserved so as to facilitate blood movement in what may be a very hard, noncompliant heart.
  - This technique is best reserved for patients who are not perfusing, unless extracorporeal warming is immediately available.
  - The technique of placing the chest tubes may precipitate a malignant rhythm, especially if a chest tube is banging up against the heart.
  - Right-sided tubes may help to avoid this complication.
  - Irrigation of the mediastinum (heart) can be done through a left-sided thoracotomy (or median sternotomy), and the heart can be directly irrigated with saline warmed to 40 to 42°C (104–107.5°F).
  - The pericardium need not be opened unless tamponade physiology is appreciated.
  - This technique is reserved for patients in cardiac arrest or those who are otherwise not perfusing.
  - Defibrillation can be attempted at 1 to 2°C (1.8–3.6°F) intervals starting above 26°C (78.8°F).
  - Unless a perfusing rhythm is obtained, irrigation can be performed until the heart reaches a temperature of 32°C (89.6°F).
  - By opening the chest, the thoracic pump is lost, and internal cardiac massage may be difficult because of a noncompliant heart.
  - **Expected rate of rewarming:**
    - Peritoneal irrigation: 1 to 3°C (1.8–5.4°F) per hour.

- Thoracic irrigation: Reported in 1 series to be up to 20°C (36°F) per hour but probably not so dramatic in most cases.
- Mediastinal irrigation: Works as well as or better than thoracic lavage.
- **Indications:** Moderate to severe hypothermia. Thoracic or mediastinal irrigation should be reserved for nonperfusing rhythms or severe hypothermia in patients for whom bypass is available.
- **Contraindications:** See above.
- **Extracorporeal blood rewarming:**
  - Extracorporeal blood rewarming (ECR) is a process in which blood is removed from the circulatory system, heated, and subsequently returned to the body.
  - In addition, the blood may be oxygenated before it is returned.
  - The available methods of bypass differ primarily in which side of the circulatory system the blood is removed from and returned to.
  - All of the systems offer the advantage of rapid rewarming at a controllable rate up to 2°C (3.6°F) every 5 minutes.
  - Some of the newer systems do not require the use of heparin and some use heparin-coated circuits.
  - This expands their use to patients with known bleeding sources in whom anticoagulation is contraindicated.
  - The addition of an in-line oxygenator would allow perfusion of tissues with oxygenated, heated blood, despite cardiopulmonary arrest.
  - These methods of ECR are designed to be used in hypothermic patients in full cardiac arrest or in cases in which adequate rates of rewarming are not attained by less invasive methods.
  - **Femoral-femoral bypass:** This technique, which requires a pump, oxygenator, heater and perfusionist is the gold-standard for ECR. The femoral vein is cannulated and a line is placed so that the catheter tip is at the level of the atrium-inferior vena cava junction. Blood is removed, heated, oxygenated, and returned to the femoral artery at the rate of 2 to 3 liters per minute. CPR can be performed during insertion of the catheters to allow for continued perfusion. Although newer, heparinless systems are available, most bypass units will require anticoagulation.

    Disadvantages to this system include limited availability and the risk of anticoagulation. At high flows, rewarming rates of up to 1 to 2°C (1.8–3.6°F) every 3 to 5 min are attainable. The use of concomitant vasodilator therapy may augment flow rates and effectiveness.
  - **Arteriovenous rewarming:** This circuit uses the patient's systolic blood pressure to drive the system. Typically, the femoral artery and vein are cannulated. Arterial blood is run through a countercurrent fluid warmer and returned to the venous side. While this system offers a wider availability and does not require a perfusionist, pump, or anticoagulation, it does need systolic blood pressure of at least 60 mm Hg to run the circuit.
  - **Venovenous rewarming:** This is also possible but it does not provide circulatory support and it needs an active method to remove and replace the warmed blood.
  - **Hemodialysis:** Using either a 2-site cannulation or the simple, single site, 2-way flow catheter, 200 to 250 mL of blood per minute can be dialysed and rewarmed. The great advantage to this system is that the personnel and facilities already exist to do dialysis in most hospitals. Further, any electrolyte abnormalities are easily managed through dialysis. This method, while effective, is slower and provides less heat exchange than 2-vessel cardiopulmonary bypass.
  - **Expected rate of rewarming:** Varies depending on the system used and the maximum attainable flow rate but temperature increases of up to 1 to 2°C (1.8–3.6°F) every 3 to 5 min are attainable.
  - **Indications:** Severe hypothermia with either cardiac arrest or failure of less invasive methods to increase temperature at an acceptable rate.

Management of Specific Emergencies during Rewarming (Table 2-5)

Frostbite

- Phases of injury
  - Prefreeze
    - Secondary to chilling; vasospasticity
  - Freeze-thaw
    - Caused by actual ice crystal formation

TABLE 2-5. SPECIFIC EMERGENCIES

Respiratory Emergencies

Intubation is necessary when:

- Airway protection is needed for lavage or altered mental status.
- Respiratory rate or depth is not adequate to keep the uncorrected pH close to 7.40.
- The patient is not able to adequately oxygenate.
- Airway bronchorrhea interferes with lung function.

Ventilation and Oxygenation

100% oxygen should be used during resuscitations and it should be heated to 45°C (113°F) if possible.

Ventilation rate of the hypothermic patient by bag-valve-mask is usually slower than in normothermic patients but rate should be adequate to keep the uncorrected pH at 7.4.

Remember:

Carbon dioxide production is decreased in hypothermia (decreases by 50% for each 8°C [14.4°F] drop in temperature). Patients may have respiratory rates of 4–10 breaths per minute and still adequately oxygenate and ventilate.

Cardiac Emergencies

CPR is indicated when:

- No signs of life are present.

CPR is contraindicated when:

- Do not resuscitate (DNR) status is established.
- The chest wall is immobile because of decreased compliance.
- Any pulse is present by palpation or Doppler.

Arrhythmias

Atrial arrhythmias

Do not produce a rapid ventricular response. They are common in moderate and severe hypothermia and do not require treatment. They resolve spontaneously as temperature rises to normal.

Bradycardia

Slow heart rate is a normal response in hypothermia. It *is not* responsive to atropine. If the clinical condition requires, symptomatic bradycardia may be treated with external pacing. Internal pacing may trigger a malignant ventricular arrhythmia.

Ventricular arrhythmias

These include ectopy and fibrillation. Most cases of preexisting ectopy (frequent premature ventricular contractions) will disappear with hypothermia. Ventricular fibrillation can be induced by cardiac stimulation, ranging from jolts and bumps to CPR, to Swan-Ganz catheter (or introducer wire) placement. Likewise, it can be spontaneous. Prophylaxis with drugs has not, as of yet been adequately studied in humans.

- Lidocaine is still waiting to be proven effective as prophylaxis. In established hypothermic ventricular fibrillation (VF), lidocaine has been shown to have no effect.
- Bretylium was a good candidate as a prophylactic agent, but human studies showed little effect. Further studies were not done before it was removed from the market. In animal models it seemed to work extremely well.
- Magnesium sulfate at the dose of 100 mg/kg, in one study chemically defibrillated most patients who were on bypass at 30°C (86°F).
- IV amiodarone, another class III antiarrhythmic agent, would be interesting to study for its effects under hypothermic conditions.
- Electrical defibrillation at up to 200 J should be tried one time at the onset of VF at any temperature. Subsequent shocks will not likely restore a perfusing rhythm until the core temperature is above 30°C (86°F). In the thoracic lavage and extracorporeal rewarming protocols, defibrillation can be attempted at 1 to 2°C (1.8–3.6°F) intervals starting above 26°C (78.8°F).

(continued on next page)

TABLE 2-5. SPECIFIC EMERGENCIES *(Continued)*

Asystole

Asystole, especially in the field, may be difficult to differentiate from fine VF. Asystole may actually be the presenting rhythm of a hypothermic patient, completely bypassing VF. Some authors suggest that asystole is more common as a presenting rhythm than VF. It should be treated as per advanced cardiac life support protocols. It is noteworthy that many patients have been successfully resuscitated from hypothermic asystole.

Hypotension

Hypothermia will decrease mean arterial pressure and cardiac index. Cardiac output drops to ~45% of normal at 25°C (77°F). Peripheral vasoconstriction will occur increasing the supraventricular rhythm. Evaluation of what should be a normal blood pressure will be difficult. If the patient is hypotensive despite fluid therapy and rewarming, and blood loss is not considered a possible cause, dopamine infusion may be started and titrated to systolic blood pressure of ~100 mm Hg.

Termination of Efforts

Resuscitation efforts can be terminated if:

· DNR status is documented and verified, or obvious signs of death exist.
· All efforts at resuscitation have failed and the patients T°>32°C/89.6°F
· Studies showing a potassium > 10 an extremely poor prognostic indicator may be confirmed an used as a criteria for termination of resuscitation

- Vascular stasis
  - Changes in the blood vessels, including spasticity and dilation; plasma leakage, stasis coagulation, thrombosis
- Late ischemic
  - Result of thrombosis; tissue necrosis, gangrene
- Degrees of injury
  - Difficult to predict extent of injury on initial evaluation.
  - Classified like burns.
  - Fingers, toes, nose, ears, and genitalia are first to suffer.
  - Clinical presentation:
    - Coldness, numbness, stinging, burning, pain, throbbing
  - First degree:
    - Erythema
    - Numbness
    - White or yellowish plaque
    - Edema
  - Second degree:
    - Erythema
    - Edema
    - Superficial blisters
    - Blisters with clear or milky fluid
  - Third degree:
    - Deeper blisters with hemorrhagic fluid.
    - Injury is deep into the dermis.
  - Fourth degree:
    - Injury is completely through the dermis and involves the subcuticular tissues.
    - Leads to mummification with muscle and bone involvement.
- Treatment
  - Address life-threatening conditions first, especially hypothermia.
  - Do *not* rewarm if there is any chance of refreezing.

- Do *not* rewarm by massaging.
- Treat like a burn.
- Rapid rewarming is treatment of choice:
  - Immerse patient in circulating warm water (40–42°C [104–107.6°F]).
  - Rewarm until skin is pliable and erythematous at the most distal part.
- Narcotics are often needed.
- Blisters: Care of blisters is controversial although most agree to débride clear blisters.
- Tetanus prophylaxis.
- Pad between fingers and toes and all splints.
- Elevate.
- Ibuprofen.
- Aloe vera.
- Observe for necrosis and demarcation.

HEAT-RELATED ILLNESS

Epidemiology

- Approximately 500 people die from heat-related illness each year in the United States.
- It is hard to know the exact number as it is underreported.
- In 1995, there were 800 reported deaths in Chicago.
- In 1999–2003, the Centers for Disease Control and Prevention reported 3442 deaths (688 per year), a 54% increase over preceding years.
- In August 2003, there were 35,000 reported deaths in Europe.
- The elderly are at risk for classic heat stroke.
- There are three risk groups for children: neonates, toddlers, and adolescents.

Mechanisms

- Increased heat production
- Decreased heat dissipation: radiation and evaporation
- Impaired thermoregulation: illness, drugs, and behavior (Table 2-6)

Minor Heat Emergencies

- Heat edema
  - Clinical presentation
    - Peripheral edema developing during the first few days in a hot environment
  - Treatment
    - Usually self-limited, does not require medical therapy.
    - Do not use diuretics.
- Heat syncope

TABLE 2-6. DRUGS THAT CAN CAUSE OR COMPLICATE HYPERTHERMIA

Anticholinergics

Salicylates

Diuretics

Phenothiazines

LSD

Sympathomimetics

   Cocaine

   Amphetamines (including MDMA [Ecstasy])

- Clinical presentation
  - Syncope after prolonged standing in a hot environment. Incidence decreases with acclimatization.
- Treatment
  - Cool the victim and administer oral fluids (gentle rehydration). Heat syncope is usually self-limited. Rule out cardiac syncope.
- Heat cramps
  - Clinical presentation
    - Painful, spasmodic muscle cramps that usually occur in heavily exercised muscles
    - Recurrent cramps that may be precipitated by manipulation of muscle
    - Onset during exercise or after the work effort
  - Treatment
    - Rest in cool environment.
    - Give oral rehydration solution with ¼ tsp salt in 1 Q drinking water.

Major Heat Emergencies

- Heat exhaustion
  - Clinical presentation
    - Flulike symptoms: malaise, headache, weakness, nausea, anorexia, vomiting.
    - Tachycardia, orthostatic hypotension.
    - Sweating is generally present.
    - Temperature is lower than 40°C (104°F).
    - Mental status and neurologic examination are normal.
  - Treatment
    - Place in cool, shaded environment.
    - Orally rehydrate if capable, but patient may need IV fluids because of large amount of volume lost as sweat.
    - Active cooling measures: ice packs to neck, axillae, groin.
    - Spray with tepid water and fan (one of the most effective ways to cool).
    - *Patient must avoid further heat stress for 48 hours.*
- Heat stroke: A true medical emergency with a high mortality rate (up to 80% in some series) (Table 2-7)

TABLE 2-7. CLASSIC HEAT STROKE VERSUS EXERTIONAL HEAT STROKE

There are 2 types of heat stroke, classic and exertional. The major difference is how they develop.

Classic heat stroke happens as the result of chronic dehydration and exposure to high temperatures. The dehydration leads to the inability to sweat, which is the major mechanism by which heat is lost by the body.

- Excess heat gain, impaired loss.
- Occurs during heat waves.
- Most often seen in older adults, the very young, poor, or debilitated.
- With or without inciting medications.
- Sweating is usually impaired.

Exertional heat stroke results from an increased production of heat during exercise, along with an impaired ability to lose heat. It usually is seen in a hot setting, especially when there is high humidity. It can, however, develop in normal temperatures during very hard exercise. Inadequate hydration can play a major role in the development of heat stroke.

- Excess heat production, overwhelmed heat loss mechanism
- Most often seen in young, healthy, athletes, military, etc.
- *More likely to still be sweating*
- Worse systemic involvement
- Rhabdomyolysis, acute renal failure, coagulopathy, hypoglycemia

TABLE 2-8. COOLING METHODS

Evaporative Methods (↓ T°: 0.06°C [0.1°F] per min)

Pros

· Well tolerated by patients

· Effective cooling

Cons

· Constant spray necessary

· Set-ups not readily available

Ice Water Immersion (↓ T°: 0.1°C [0.2°F] per min)

Pros

· Rapid cooling is possible

· Easy to set up (body bag or tub + ice water)

Cons

· Shivering possible (treat with diazepam or chlorpromazine)

· Not comfortable for patients

Strategic Ice Packs (↓ T°: 0.02°C [0.05°F] per min)

Pros

· Easy to do in the field

· Okay for mild exhaustion

Cons

· Not fast enough for heat stroke

- Clinical presentation
  - Temperature is generally higher than 40.5°C (105°F).
  - Skin is usually hot and dry, but sweating may be present in exertional heat stroke.
  - Mental status changes: delirium, seizures, coma.
  - Tachycardia.
  - Orthostatic changes, hypotension.
  - Hyperventilation.
- Treatment
  - Immediate cooling (Table 2-8)
    - Ice packs to neck, axillae, chest well, groin.
    - Spray with tepid water and fan.
    - Immerse in cool water if vitals stable.
    - Stop active cooling at 38.9°C (102°F).
    - Internal cooling rarely needed or used.
    - Avoid and prevent shivering (benzodiazepines may be useful).
  - Airway breathing circulation (ABCs).
  - IV fluid: treat volume depletion.
  - Dantrolene is ineffective.
  - Monitor for complications and treat.
- Prognostic factors
  - Good prognosis
    - Recovery of CNS function during cooling
    - Expected in majority of patients receiving prompt and aggressive treatment
  - Poor prognosis
    - Coagulopathy with liver hepatocyte damage
    - Lactic acidosis in classic form
    - Rectal temperature higher than 42.2°C (108°F)

- Prolonged coma of more than 4 hours
- Acute renal failure
- Hyperkalemia
- Aspartate aminotransferase higher than 1000 U/L

INSECT BITES AND STINGS

Stinging Insects Kill More People Annually than do Snakes

Hymenoptera—Honeybees, Yellow Jackets, Wasps, Hornets, Bumble Bees, and Fire Ants—Account for Majority of Insect-Related Deaths

- They have complex poisons with numerous components, for example, there are nine different antigens in honeybee venom.
- Sensitized patients are at the greatest risk to develop life-threatening reactions.
  - They make up 1% of the general population.
- It takes 300 to 500 stings of a venomous insect to kill an average person.

Reactions

- Local
  - Majority of cases
  - Local redness, pain, swelling
  - May extend more than 6 inches beyond the sting
  - May persist longer than 24 hours
  - Treatment
    - Remove stinger, if present (bees only).
    - Ice and elevate.
    - Local wound care: tetanus prophylaxis.
    - Antihistamines, steroids (perhaps beneficial)
- Mild generalized
  - Symptoms away from the sting site are itching, hives, nausea, and wheezing.
  - Treatment:
    - Antihistamines, steroids
    - Inhaled beta-agonists for wheezing
    - Local wound care: tetanus prophylaxis
    - Observation for 6 to 8 hours
    - Consider epinephrine if wheezing:
      - Use 0.3 cc epinephrine.
      - Intramuscular (IM) is the best route to use; subcutaneous is no longer recommended.
- Severe generalized
  - It is classically immunoglobulin E-antibody mediated.
  - Clinical presentation:
    - Anaphylaxis, laryngoedema, circulatory collapse, loss of consciousness.
    - Most deaths occur within first hour.
    - Usually the more rapid the onset, the worse the reaction.
  - Risk factors are previous reactions, reexposure, and atopy.
  - Histamine:
    - Pain, irritation, itching
    - Capillary membrane leak: edema, third space loss, increased secretions, hives
    - Vasodilatation: decrease in peripheral vascular resistance, hypotension
    - Smooth muscle irritability and spasm: laryngospasm, bronchospasm, GI cramping
    - Theoretical direct cardiac and CNS irritability
  - Treatment:
    - ABCs: intubate *early*
    - IV fluids: support blood pressure

TABLE 2-9. IV EPINEPHRINE USE

In refractory patients who are not improving with IM epinephrine, IV epinephrine is indicated. IV epinephrine must be given very slowly.

Inject 1 mg of epinephrine into a 1 L bag of normal saline. Use either of the following concentrations:

· 1 mg in 1 cc (1:1000 dilution) OR
· 1 mg in 10 cc (1:10,000 dilution) (This is crash cart epinephrine.)

Start drip at 1 cc/min, which is 1 mcg/min. Piggyback this slow drip into a high-flow IV to allow rapid delivery to the patient. Titrate to the patient's response.

Do not push undiluted epinephrine: This may cause fatal arrhythmia.

- Epinephrine is the drug of choice: initially may be given IM, but may need IV drip (Table 2-9)
- Steroids
- Inhaled beta-agonists for bronchospasm
- H$_1$ and H$_2$ blockers
- Admit all.
- Send patient home with EpiPen.
- Refer for desensitization treatment.

CHAPTER 3

Toxicology

Colin G. Kaide, Hannah L. Hays, and David P. Bahner

INTRODUCTION

- Twenty-four-hour per day consultation is available at regional poison centers throughout the United States for assistance with management of poisoned patients.
- At each regional poison center, 24-hour medical backup is provided by a medical toxicologist.
- Help can be obtained by calling the national toll-free number, 1–800–222–1222.
- Aside from providing recommendations regarding acute ingestion, assistance in management of other conditions is available and includes: chronic overdose, envenomations, chemical burns, and assistance in excluding poisoning as a possible etiology of patient presentation.

GENERAL APPROACH TO THE POISONED PATIENT

- Stabilize all instabilities:
  - ABCs (air\way, breathing, circulation) need to be managed and stabilized
- Comatose patients:
  - Consider naloxone:
    - The triad of opioid-induced coma is respiratory depression (respiratory rate ≤8 breaths per minute), altered mental status, and miosis.
    - Dose:
      - For patients in cardiac arrest or who are unstable (periarrest) give 0.4 to 2 mg intravenously (IV), intramuscularly (IM), or by intraosseous infusion (IO).
        - Repeat every few minutes until a response is seen.
      - For patients suspected of having underlying opioid dependence, smaller doses are recommended. Doses as low as 0.04 mg IV/IM/IO have been used.
        - *Caution: Naloxone can precipitate acute withdrawal.*
      - For pediatric patients use 0.1 mg/kg IV/IM/IO, maximum 2 mg.
      - Larger doses may be needed in patients with overdoses of buprenorphine, fentanyl, diphenoxylate and atropine, pentazocine, propoxyphene, or clonidine.
      - If no response is seen after a dose of 10 to 15 mg IV/IM/IO, consider other diagnoses.
      - *Warning: The duration of action of naloxone is often less than the offending opioid:* Repeated dosing or IV infusion may be needed.
      - Other routes are nebulized, intranasal, subcutaneous, or endotracheal tube.
  - Flumazenil:
    - It has no place in the standard coma cocktail.
    - Its use is only recommended by some experts under certain, selective circumstances.
    - The use of flumazenil may precipitate seizures in patients with overdose of cyclic antidepressants, medications with proconvulsant effects, or in patients with underlying benzodiazepine dependence.
  - Glucose:
    - As an alternative obtain a rapid fingerstick blood glucose level to exclude glucose derangements as an etiology of coma.
    - Dose:
      - Adults:
        - Give 50 to 100 mL of a 50% dextrose solution slow intravenous push (IVP).

- Children:
  - Do not use a 50% dextrose solution.
  - Use 2 to 4 mL/kg of a 25% dextrose solution slow IVP.
  - Ensure that the patient has a secure IV.
- Thiamine:
  - Thiamine is indicated to prevent and treat Wernicke-Korsakoff syndrome.
  - Cause of Wernicke-Korsakoff syndrome:
    - Malnourishment (including chronic alcoholism)
  - Symptoms of Wernicke encephalopathy:
    - Altered mental status
      - Confusion, confabulation, hallucinations, amnesia
    - Ataxia
    - Ocular findings
      - Nystagmus, ophthalmoplegia, anisocoria, sluggish pupillary responses
  - Dose:
    - Adults: 100 mg slow IVP
    - Can also be given IM or orally
  - Should be given concurrently with glucose
    - *Caution:* There is no literature to support definitive need for thiamine *before* administration of glucose.
- Consider and exclude nontoxicologic causes.
- History
  - Patient
    - Although an accurate history is of paramount importance in the evaluation of poisoned patients, the clinician should be wary of overreliance on the information provided by suicidal patients given the tendency for emotional factors to hinder accurate recall and reporting of details.
  - Family and friends
    - They can be valuable sources for determining the time of onset, motive for overdose (confirm suicidality in patient who is denying), and substances involved.
    - Many patients will text message or post on social media during time of distress or suicidal overdose.
  - Paramedics
    - They can relay valuable information regarding the scene:
      - Identity of and number of bottles at the scene
      - Other substances available in the home
    - Ask them to stay until initial patient stabilization.
  - Information to obtain:
    - What was ingested? (or possibly ingested)
    - When did the ingestion occur?
      - What is the exact time of overdose?
      - Is ingestion acute or chronic?
    - Why did the patient take the overdose?
    - How was it ingested?
      - By what route was it ingested: oral, inhalation, injection (IV, IM, subcutaneous), rectal, or intravaginal?
    - How much was ingested?
- Physical examination
  - Take vital signs: temperature, blood pressure, heart rate, respiratory rate (Tables 3-1 through 3-4).
  - General appearance
    - Level of consciousness
      - Use of the Glasgow Coma Scale (GCS) is controversial in toxicology.
        - Not validated for assessment of airway protective reflexes in poisoned patients.

TABLE 3-1. DRUGS AFFECTING TEMPERATURE

Hyperthermia	Hypothermia
Bath salts	Ethanol[a] (and other alcohols)
Sympathomimetics[b]	Barbiturates
MAOIs	Opioids
PCP	Vasodilators
Neuroleptic malignant syndrome	Hypoglycemics
Serotonin syndrome	Sedative-hypnotics
Salicylates	Beta-blockers
Withdrawal	
Anticholinergics	

MAOI, monoamine oxidase inhibitor; PCP, phencyclidine hydrochloride.

[a]Ethanol causes a vasodilatory response leading to poikilothermia. In essence, heat transfer will occur between the patient and the environment such that the patient's body temperature approaches the temperature of the environment. Clinically, this means that ethanol intoxication can lead to hypothermia, hyperthermia, or normothermia, depending on the surrounding environment. Because the ambient temperature is generally cooler than the core temperature, hypothermia is the more common clinical manifestation seen.

[b]Sympathomimetics include cocaine, amphetamines, and amphetamine derivatives (MDMA [Ecstasy]).

- Application of the GCS hinges on fact that patients are giving their "best response."
  - This patient population is often not giving best response.
- The mantra, "GCS less than 8, think intubate" does not necessarily apply.
  - Some poisoned patients with GCS less than 8 maintain airway protective reflexes (eg, γ-hydroxybutyrate [GHB] poisoning)
  - Some poisoned patients with normal GCS may need intubation (eg, cyclic antidepressant poisoning)
- Level of distress
- Signs of trauma
  - Poisoned patients are more likely to sustain physical injury.

TABLE 3-2. DRUGS AFFECTING BLOOD PRESSURE

Hypertension	Hypotension
Sympathomimetics[a]	Beta-blockers/Calcium channel blockers
Anticholinergics	Cyanide
Ergot derivatives	Cyclic antidepressants
Phenylpropanolamine	Iron
MAOIs	Opiates and opioids
Ketamine	Theophylline
Withdrawal	Phenothiazines
Black widow spider envenomation	Sedative-hypnotics

MAOI, monoamine oxidase inhibitor.

[a]Sympathomimetics include cocaine, amphetamines, and amphetamine derivatives (MDMA [Ecstasy]).

TABLE 3-3. DRUGS AFFECTING HEART RATE

Tachycardia	Bradycardia
Anticholinergics	β-blockers
Cyclic antidepressants	Cyclic antidepressants
PCP	Calcium channel blockers
Sympathomimetics[a]	Cardiac glycosides (digitalis)
Theophylline	Cholinergics
Withdrawal	Cyanide
Ephedrine	Opioids
Carbon monoxide and cyanide	Clonidine

PCP, phencyclidine hydrochloride.
[a]Sympathomimetics include cocaine, amphetamines, amphetamine derivatives (MDMA [Ecstasy]).

- Perform HEENT (head, ears, eyes, nose, throat) examination.
  - Eyes (Table 3-5)
    - Pupil reactivity
    - Nystagmus
    - Scleral or conjunctival injection
    - Scleral icterus
  - Mucous membranes
    - Dry (anticholinergic)
    - Moist (sympathomimetic)
- Skin
  - Color change: pallor, erythema, cyanosis
  - Presence or absence of sweating
  - Heat production: warm, cool
  - Track marks, skin popping
    - Be sure to check in between fingers and toes.
- Abdomen
  - Bowel sounds
  - Tenderness
  - Palpable bladder
  - Organomegaly
  - Stool guaiac

TABLE 3-4. DRUGS AFFECTING RESPIRATORY RATE

Increased	Decreased
Carbon Monoxide	Alcohols
Cyanide	Barbiturates
Drug-induced metabolic acidosis	Benzodiazepines
Drug-induced hepatic failure	Opioids
Drug-induced methemoglobinemia	
Salicylates	

TABLE 3-5. DRUGS AFFECTING PUPIL SIZE

Miosis (small pupils)	Mydriasis (large pupils)
Cholinergics	Anticholinergics
Opiates/opioids[a]	Sympathomimetics[b]
Clonidine	
Nicotine	LSD
Phenothiazines	MAOIs
PCP	Withdrawal

LSD, lysergic acid diethylamide; MAOI, monoamine oxidase inhibitor; PCP, phencyclidine hydrochloride.
[a]Meperidine is unique among opioids in that pupillary response is variable.
[b]Sympathomimetics include cocaine, amphetamines, amphetamine derivatives (MDMA [Ecstasy]).

- Genitourinary
  - Patient may need rectal or vaginal inspection if concealment of drugs is suspected.
- Neurologic
  - Level of consciousness
  - Strength and sensation
  - Cerebellar function
  - Gait examination
  - Abnormal movements
    - Choreoathetoid movements
    - Akathisia
    - Dystonia
    - Tremor
  - Clonus
  - Reflexes
  - Seizures (Table 3-6)
- Odor (Table 3-7)
  - Odor of ethanol does not rule out other etiologies of coma (trauma, head injury).

TABLE 3-6. DRUGS THAT CAN CAUSE SEIZURES (PLASTIC)

P	PCP, pesticides, phenothiazines, propoxyphene
L	Lead, lithium, local anesthetics (lidocaine), lindane
A	Anticholinergics, antibiotics (penicillin, imipenem, chloroquine, dapsone, fluoroquinolone)
S	Salicylates, sympathomimetics (amphetamines), strychnine, selective serotonin reuptake inhibitors (SSRIs)
T	Theophylline, toxic inhalants (toluene, hydrogen sulfide, cyanide)
I	Isoniazid (INH), insulin, propranolol (Inderal), industrial acid (hydrofluoric acid)
C	Cyclic antidepressants, cocaine, carbon monoxide, camphor, caffeine, carbamazepine

PCP, phencyclidine hydrochloride.

TABLE 3-7. ODORS CAUSED BY PARTICULAR INTOXICANTS

Odor	Possible Intoxicant
Bitter almonds	Cyanide
Carrots	Water hemlock (cicutoxin)
Fishy	Zinc or aluminum phosphide
Fruity	Ethanol, acetone, isopropyl alcohol, chlorinated hydrocarbons (chloroform)
Garlic	Arsenic, DMSO, organophosphates, yellow phosphorous, selenium, tellurium
Glue	Toluene, other solvents
Pears	Chloral hydrate, paraldehyde
Rotten Eggs	Hydrogen sulfide, N-acetylcysteine, disulfiram, stibine, mercaptans
Shoe Polish	Nitrobenzene
Wintergreen	Methyl salicylate

DMSO, dimethylsulfoxide.

- Laboratory evaluation
- "Suicide Panel"
  - Given the paucity of signs and symptoms associated with some suicidal ingestions and the understanding that the history given by the suicidal patient is sometimes inaccurate, the ollowing battery of tests is generally recommended in all suicidal patients presenting after confirmed or suspected overdose:
- Serum acetaminophen level
  - Acetaminophen is a very common constituent in over-the-counter medications.
  - Patients may not know they have taken it.
  - Signs and symptoms may not appear until 12 to 24 hours post-ingestion.
- Serum salicylate level
  - This is controversial as routine screening test.
  - It is a very common constituent in over-the-counter medications.
  - The classic triad of tinnitus, gastrointestinal (GI) upset, and hyperventilation are reproducible at specific serum concentrations and should be readily detectable by an experienced, mindful clinician; however, symptoms often evolve over time and might not be present on initial evaluation.
- Electrolyte panel, including sodium (Na^+), potassium (K^+), chloride (Cl^-), and carbon dioxide (CO_2)
  - This panel allows calculation of the anion gap (AG).
  - A normal AG accounts for unmeasured anions present in a normal human (anionic proteins including albumin, sulfate, and phosphate).
  - $AG = Na^+ + [Cl^- + CO_2]$
    - Normal AG is 8 to 12 mEq/L.
  - The most common cause of an elevated AG metabolic acidosis (AGMA) is lactic acidosis (Tables 3-8 and 3-9); however, presence of this metabolic derangement in your patient should prompt a thorough evaluation for other possible causes.
    - Refer to the toxic alcohol section below.
    - If it is determined that lactic acidosis is the cause of the AGMA, then the etiology of the lactic acidosis should also be determined.
  - Test renal function (blood urea nitrogen [BUN], creatinine).

TABLE 3-8.   DRUGS THAT CAN CAUSE AN ELEVATED ANION GAP
             METABOLIC ACIDOSIS

C	Cyanide, carbon monoxide
A	Alcoholic ketoacidosis[a], acetaminophen[b]
T	Toluene
M	Methanol, metformin[c]
U	Uremia
D	Diabetic ketoacidosis (DKA)
P	Phenformin[c], paraldehyde[d]
I	Iron, isoniazid, ibuprofen
L	Lactic acid
E	Ethylene glycol
S	Salicylates, starvation

[a]NOTE: acute ethanol use does not cause an elevated anion gap (AG).
[b]In rare circumstances, severe acetaminophen poisoning can cause an elevated AG by increasing production of 5-oxoproline via the γ-glutamyl cycle; however, presence of an elevated AG metabolic acidosis should first prompt investigation of other causes.
[c]Phenformin (no longer Food and Drug Administration approved) and metformin can cause an elevated AG by way of lactic acidosis.
[d]Paraldehyde is a prebenzodiazepine sedative hypnotic that is no longer used clinically but was left on this table for historical purposes.

- Perform a urine pregnancy test in all female patients of child-bearing age.
- Electrocardiogram (ECG)
  - An ECG is controversial as a routine component of testing for the overdose patient.
  - Many (hundreds) of drugs have effects on cardiac rhythm, rate, and intervals.
    - Even poisons not typically thought of as altering cardiac function (eg, cocaine, diphenhydramine) can do so.
  - Check for arrhythmia, prolonged intervals (QRS, QTc), and other abnormalities (Figure 3-1).
  - Consider continuous cardiac monitoring and continuous pulse oximetry if there is:
    - A high risk of overdose (based on the characteristics of patient presentation or substance[s] involved)
    - An abnormal initial ECG
    - Abnormal vital signs
- Radiography: using plain films (Table 3-10)
  - Can be useful to guide whole bowel irrigation (WBI) and possibly confirm exposure of a large amount of a radiopaque drug
  - Cannot be used to rule out significant ingestion
- Specific drug levels
  - Determining specific levels can guide management and disposition decisions in both acute and chronic poisoning.

TABLE 3-9.   DRUGS THAT CAN CAUSE A LOW ANION GAP

Bromide	Lithium

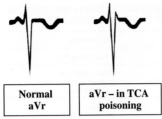

<table>
<tr><td>**Normal
aVr**</td><td>**aVr – in TCA
poisoning**</td></tr>
</table>

Figure 3-1   TCA, tricyclic antidepressant.

- The National Academy of Clinical Biochemistry, in collaboration with clinical biochemists, medical toxicologists, forensic toxicologists, and emergency physicians, has recommendations regarding what toxicology tests should be routinely available in the toxicology laboratory (Table 3-11).
  - This does not mean that this is a panel of tests that should be routinely ordered on all poisoned patients.
- Screening for drugs of abuse
- Most centers offer testing for a handful of commonly abused drugs.
  - Generally, this screen is a radioimmunoassay performed on the patient's urine.
    - This screen does not give a quantitative level, rather it gives a "positive" or "negative" result depending on whether the drug or its metabolites are present in sufficient quantity to register a result.
    - Substances commonly screened for include cocaine, opiates, amphetamines, benzodiazepines, phencyclidine hydrochloride (PCP), and δ-9-tetrahydrocannabinol (THC).
  - *This screen does not indicate intoxication.*
  - This screen is not generally helpful for or aid in clinical decision making.
    - This screen is often required for admission to psychiatric facilities.
  - *False-positive results are common.*
    - The type and frequency of false-positive results varies from laboratory to laboratory.
    - The best approach to determine what types of substances can cause a false-positive result on a urine drug screen is to call the toxicology laboratory that ran the test and speak with an experienced individual.
    - Many laboratories have a readily available list of what agents can cause a false-positive result.
- Comprehensive drug screens
  - Comprehensive tests can screen for the presence of hundreds of drugs and drug metabolites.
    - This number is small when compared to the number of available drugs (thousands).

TABLE 3-10. SUBSTANCES THAT MIGHT BE VISIBLE ON X-RAY

C hloral hydrate
H eavy metals
I odine
P henothiazines, packets (eg, cocaine and heroin body stuffers)
E nteric-coated products
S olvents

TABLE 3-11. TOXICOLOGY LABORATORY STUDIES RECOMMENDED TO BE ROUTINELY AVAILABLE

Qualitative	Quantitative
Amphetamines	Acetaminophen
Barbiturates	Carbamazepine
Cocaine	Cooximetry
Opiates[a]	Digoxin
Propoxyphene[b]	Ethanol
Phencyclidine	Iron
Tricyclic antidepressants[c]	Lithium
	Phenobarbital
	Salicylate
	Theophylline
	Valproic acid

[a]Specific opiates and opioids detected varies depending on the characteristics of the machine, but usually detects natural opiates (morphine, codeine, heroin) with or without varying synthetic and semisynthetic opioids. Discussion with laboratory personnel regarding which opioid you are concerned with is the best way to choose the appropriate test.
[b]May change given its current status.
[c]Often subjected to numerous false-positive results secondary to its chemical structure. Discussion with laboratory personnel should reveal which drugs are known to cause false-positive tricyclic antidepressant results in a particular laboratory.

- The best approach is to call the toxicology laboratory and discuss your concerns to determine the best test for a given scenario.
- Screens can be performed on serum or urine.
  - Urine is generally preferred as results remain positive for longer periods of time.
- Screens generally use gas or liquid chromatography and mass spectrometry.
- More accurate than radioimmunoassay
  - Fewer false-positive results
- *Positive result does not necessarily indicate intoxication.*
- Can be useful and alter management if:
  - Patient is very ill.
  - History is unobtainable or limited.
- Osmolar gap
  - A normal osmolar gap accounts for unmeasured osmotically active particles present in a normal human.
  - The osmolar gap is pertinent to the evaluation of toxic alcohol exposure.
  - An elevated AG acidosis accompanied by an elevated osmolar gap should raise concern for toxic alcohol poisoning.
    - Other conditions where this metabolic derangement can be seen are:
      - Alcoholic ketoacidosis
      - Diabetic ketoacidosis
  - Osmolar gap = measured osmolarity − calculated osmolarity
  - Normal osmolar gap is −14 to +10 mmol/L.
  - Calculated osmolarity = $2[Na^+]$ + BUN/2.8 + glucose/18
    - There are many different formulas, although the above formula is the most common.

TABLE 3-12. CAUSES OF ELEVATED OSMOLAR GAP

Ethylene glycol	Methanol
Isopropyl alcohol	Acetone
Mannitol	Lactic acidosis
Magnesium	Dimethyl sulfoxide (DMSO)
Renal failure	Osmotic contrast dyes

- Measured osmolarity is determined by the laboratory.
  - *Measured osmolarity must be specifically ordered.*
  - This is not the same osmolarity listed along with a routine chemistry panel, which instead is simply a calculated value obtained by applying one of several formulas.
- An accurate osmolar gap can only be obtained if the specimen used for the measured osmolarity is drawn at the same time as the specimen used to measure serum chemistries (and thus supply the values for calculation of the osmolarity).
  - Most experts recognize that a measured osmolarity is not initially ordered on all patients presenting with possible overdose and is instead added after recognition of an elevated AG.
  - Because certain toxic alcohols can volatilize over time, it is recommended that a fresh specimen be drawn after the AGMA is identified, to prevent a falsely low osmolar gap.
    - The clinician should keep in mind; however, that after ingestion of toxic alcohols, osmols are being metabolized over time.
- Pitfalls:
  - Overreliance on the osmolar gap
    - The osmolar gap is a helpful diagnostic tool when elevated (Table 3-12).
    - Normal value does not definitively rule out poisoning by toxic alcohols as the toxic alcohol is metabolized over time, generating toxic metabolites that are not osmotically active, but do cause metabolic acidosis.
  - Not ensuring that the measured serum osmolarity is obtained by the *freezing point depression* method
    - Boiling point elevation is the other possible method for measuring serum osmolarity.
      - It is faster, *but*
      - It is problematic in the toxic alcohol-poisoned patient because boiling the specimen can allow some of the toxic alcohol to evaporate off, giving a falsely low measured osmolarity.
  - Failing to order a chemistry panel (to calculate osmolarity) *and* a measured serum osmolarity at *the same time*
    - Waiting until *after* the chemistry panel is back and an elevated AG is noted and *then* ordering measured osmolarity will invalidate results.
    - The proper action is to order a serum osmolarity from a *fresh* specimen *and* a repeat chemistry panel.
  - Assuming that the serum osmolarity listed along with the chemistry panel is a measured osmolarity
    - This represents a laboratory *calculation* using one of various formulas and is not a measured value.
  - Conversion factors
    - Table 3-13 provides the conversion factors traditionally used to estimate the serum level of the osmol of interest.
      - Less useful when more than one is ingested

TABLE 3-13. CONVERSION FACTORS FOR SUBSTANCES COMMONLY
CONTRIBUTING TO AN ELEVATED OSMOLAR GAP[a]

Ethanol	4.6
Methanol	3.2
Ethylene glycol	6.2
Isopropyl alcohol	6
Acetone	5.8

[a]Estimated serum level of a given osmotically active substance listed above = osmolar gap × conversion factor.

- Cooximetry
  - Certain arterial blood gas analyzers can provide direct measurement of the percent of carboxyhemoglobin, methemoglobin, and oxyhemoglobin.
  - Cooximetry cannot differentiate sulfhemoglobin from methemoglobin.

ENHANCED ELIMINATION

- GI decontamination
- Ipecac
  - It is a mixture of chemicals derived from plants that induce emesis by direct irritation of the GI mucosa as well as stimulation of the chemoreceptor trigger zone in the cerebral medulla.
  - It is no longer recommended for home, prehospital, or in-hospital use because risk outweighs benefit.
  - Parents should be discouraged from storing ipecac and other emetics in the home.
- Gastric lavage
  - It is used very infrequently.
  - Classic teaching states that it can remove approximately one-third of toxin from the stomach.
  - Indications (all should be met):
    - Protected airway
    - Life-threatening ingestion of a noncharcoal-responsive poison that has no antidote, the removal of one-third of which might have a significant effect on outcome
    - Ingestion occurred recently enough so as to allow initiation of orogastric lavage within 1 hour from overdose
    - The substance of interest should fit through the lavage tube:
      - Some products are too large to fit through the tube and therefore are likely not amenable to removal by this method.
  - Recent review of all cases reported to the Central Ohio Poison Center in Columbus, revealed that use of orogastric lavage was *recommended* in a total of 2 cases during 2010.
  - Methods
  - Ensure protected airway.
  - Use a 36 to 40 French (Ewald) orogastric or nasogastric (NG) tube (smaller tube may work for liquids).
  - Place patient in left lateral decubitus position.
  - Aspirate orogastric tube once in position to remove poison.
  - Instill 200 mL aliquot of tepid water or saline and then remove by aspirating back up through the tube.
    - Use saline and avoid excessive amounts of lavage fluid in children to prevent electrolyte shifts.
    - Repeat until lavage fluid is clear.

- Risks
  - Can promote vomiting, which puts the patient at risk for aspiration (even in intubated patients)
  - Can cause esophageal and gastric perforation
  - Accidental placement into the respiratory tract
- Whole Bowel Irrigation (WBI)
  - Uses polyethylene glycol electrolyte lavage solution (PEG-ELS), given at high flow rates via NG tube, to force poisons through the GI tract
  - Indications
    - Large ingestions of drugs that are not (well) adsorbed to charcoal
    - Large ingestions of sustained-release products that are dangerous in overdose
    - Patients ingesting drug-filled packets, bags, or condoms
  - Contraindications
    - Bowel obstruction and ileus
  - Methods
    - Ensure protected airway.
    - Place NG tube.
    - Start at a low (200 mL/h) rate and increase as tolerated to goal rate of 2000 mL/h.
      - Patients cannot drink this much PEG-ELS on their own, and the only way to do this properly is with use of an NG tube.
      - Children should receive 35 mL/kg/h or 500 mL/h.
    - Many sources state to continue WBI until rectal effluent is clear; however, the true end point is expulsion of all the poison (can follow abdominal x-ray if radiopaque poison).
      - *Clear rectal effluent might happen in 1 hour without significant expulsion of poison.*
    - Stop WBI if no stool output after 8 to 10 L in adults or 150 to 200 mL/kg in children.
- Activated charcoal
  - It has an incredible surface area in which substances are "caught" in the "holes" of the carbon and are held there by weak van der Waal forces for the duration of transit through the GI tract.
  - It adsorbs most toxins (see Table 3-14 for exceptions).
    - Although it is commonly used, there are no studies to support a positive effect on patient-oriented outcomes.
  - It should not be given to patients without a protected airway:
    - "Cheeseburger test": if your patient cannot sit up in bed and eat a cheeseburger, then he or she cannot have activated charcoal.
  - Usual dose is 1 g/kg body weight (50–100 g in adults).
  - Alternative dose is 10× the amount of poison ingested.
- Dialysis
  - Characteristics of drugs that make them amenable to removal by hemodialysis (Table 3-15)
    - Small volume of distribution
    - High molecular weight
    - Low protein binding

TABLE 3-14. POISONS NOT REMOVED (WELL) BY ACTIVATED CHARCOAL

C	Caustics[a] (acids and alkali)
H	Heavy metals (potassium, iron, lithium), hydrocarbons
A	Alcohols (ethanol, methanol, ethylene glycol, isopropanol)
R	Rapidly absorbed substances
C	Cyanide

[a]Absolute contraindication to activated charcoal use.

TABLE 3-15. SUBSTANCES REMOVED BY HEMODIALYSIS

Ethylene glycol	Methanol
Salicylates	Theophylline
Lithium	Phenytoin

- Other methods of enhanced elimination are beyond the scope of this chapter but might include:
  - Multidose activated charcoal
  - Bile acid-binding resins
  - Urinary and serum alkalinization
  - Charcoal hemoperfusion
  - Continuous arteriovenous hemodialysis and continuous venovenous hemodialysis

SPECIFIC TOXIDROMES

- A toxidrome is a set of expected, frequently encountered copathologies that can help to identify a particular known ingestion.
- Sympathomimetic syndrome
  - See Table 3-16:
    - α_1/α_2 and β_1/β_2
    - Alpha- or beta-blockade
    - Mixed
  - Examples, cocaine, bath salts, amphetamines
- Cholinergic syndrome
  - The prototype agent is *acetylcholine.*
  - See "Chol" in Table 3-16.
  - Causes:

TABLE 3-16. SYMPATHETIC/PARASYMPATHETIC SYNDROMES

	α_1	β_1	$\alpha\beta$	Lytics	Cholinergics	Anti-cholinergics
Blood pressure	↑↑↑	↓	↑↑↑	↓	↑/↓	↑
Heart Rate	↓	↑	+/−	↓	↑/↓	↑
Temperature	+/−	+/−	↑	↓	↔	↑
Respiratory Rate	+/−	↔	+/−	↓	↓	↔
Level of Consciousness	Agitated	↔	Agitated	↓	↔	↓/Agitated
Pupils	Dilated	↔	Dilated	Pinpoint	Pinpoint	Dilated
Skin	Wet	↔	Wet	↔	Wet	Dry
Mucus Membranes	Dry	↔	Dry	↔	Wet	Dry
Bowel	+/−	↔	+/−	↔	↑↑	↓

Alpha$_2$ causes decreased release of norepinephrine (causes decreased blood pressure).
Beta$_2$ stimulation causes dilation of vascular beds in muscles.

TABLE 3-17. "WET" SYMPTOMS

S	Salivation
L	Lacrimation
U	Urination
D	Diarrhea
G	Gastric emptying (vomiting, diarrhea)
E	Emesis
BBB	Bronchorrhea, bronchospasm, bradycardia
Other	Miosis

- Organophosphates
- Carbamates
- Nerve agents
  - Sarin, soman, VX
- Muscarine-containing mushrooms
  - Clitocybe
- Oximes
  - Pralidoxime
- Effects are primarily muscarinic
- Symptoms (Table 3-17)
  - *Patients do not die from SLUDGE*: They die from bronchorrhea and bronchospasm.
    - They also die of nicotinic receptor agonist mechanism, which can occur and is manifested by muscle fasciculations and weakness.
  - SLUDGE can lead to seizures, coma, and respiratory failure.
- Treatment
  - Supportive care
  - Atropine
    - The treatment end point is resolution of bronchorrhea and bronchospasm.
    - Very large amounts might be needed in organophosphate exposures (>50 mg or more).
      - *Remember to use preservative-free atropine if using large amounts.*
  - Pralidoxime (2-PAM)
    - The only oxime approved for use in the United States
    - Traditional antidote for organophosphate and carbamate poisoning
    - Must be given soon after exposure to derive any benefit
- Anticholinergic syndrome
  - The prototype agent is *atropine.*
  - See "AC" in Table 3-16.
  - Causes:
    - Scopolamine
    - Antihistamines
    - Jimson weed
  - Effects are primarily muscarinic.
  - Symptoms:
    - "The anti-SLUDGE"
    - Red as a beet
    - Hot as a hare
    - Dry as a bone

- Mad as a hatter
- Blind as a bat
- Tachy as a leisure suit
- Seizing like a squirrel
- Opioid syndrome
  - Respiratory depression (respiratory rate ≤8 breaths per minute)
  - Miosis
  - Depressed mental status

SPECIFIC POISONS (Table 3-18)

- Acetaminophen
  - One of most common hospital calls to poison centers is for acetaminophen poisoning.
  - It is one of the most common coingestants.
  - With therapeutic use, nontoxic pathways (sulfation and glucuronidation) account for 96% of acetaminophen metabolism.
    - In acetaminophen metabolism, 4% is metabolized to a toxic metabolite, N-acetyl-para-benzoquinoneimine (NAPQI).
      - Under normal circumstances, this toxic metabolite is rapidly detoxified by glutathione.
      - In overdose situations, glutathione stores are depleted, and NAPQI accumulates.
  - NAPQI causes direct hepatic damage:
    - The low end of the toxic range (ingested dose) is 150 mg/kg.
  - Risk of hepatotoxicity can be predicted by the Rumack-Matthew nomogram:
    - It can only be used for single acute ingestions, defined as one in which the entire ingestion occurs within an 8-hour period.
    - Detectable acetaminophen levels obtained prior to 4 hours post-ingestion cannot be plotted on the nomogram, and therefore, cannot be used to determine risk of hepatotoxicity.
      - Undetectable acetaminophen levels obtained between 1 and 4 hours post-ingestion can be used to exclude ingestion.
  - Levels identified as potentially hepatotoxic based on the Rumack-Matthew nomogram indicate that the patient should be treated with the antidote, N-acetylcysteine (NAC).
    - NAC works by multiple mechanisms to prevent hepatotoxicity, the most well-known of which is that it replenishes glutathione stores.
    - NAC is available for oral and IV administration.
    - There is no point in the course of acetaminophen overdose that would be "too late" to start NAC unless the patient is dead; however, if started within 8 hours, no benefit is lost.
      - Therefore, no benefit of NAC is lost while waiting for a 4-hour level, and presumptive treatment of early presenting patients (patients presenting prior to 8 hours) is not recommended.
    - IV and oral NAC are equally efficacious in treating acetaminophen overdose.
      - The IV form is preferred in patients with fulminant hepatic failure, pregnancy, and intractable vomiting (after brief, aggressive trial of antiemetics).
      - The oral form tastes horrible.
        - Affects compliance
        - Causes an approximately 50% incidence of nausea and vomiting
- Salicylates
  - Aspirin is the most common.
    - Other:
      - Methyl salicylate (oil of wintergreen)
      - Bismuth subsalicylate (Pepto-Bismol)
  - The classic triad is most commonly seen in acute overdose and early presenters:
    - Tinnitus
    - GI upset (nausea, vomiting, abdominal pain)
    - Hyperventilation (tachypnea, hyperpnea, or both)

TABLE 3-18. POISONS AND ANTIDOTES

Poison	Antidote/Classic Treatment
Acetaminophen	N-acetylcysteine (Acetadote)
Anticholinergics (atropine, plants)	Physostigmine[a]
Benzodiazepines	Flumazenil[a]
Beta-blockers	Glucagon, diazoxide[a], high-dose insulin/ euglycemia, intralipid
Botulism	Botulism antitoxin
Black widow spider	Latrodectus antivenin
Calcium channel antagonists	Calcium, glucagon, high-dose insulin/ euglycemia, intralipid
Carbon monoxide	Oxygen
Cholinergics (organophosphates, carbamates, nerve agents, mushrooms, hemlock)	Atropine, glycopyrrolate, pralidoxime[a]
Coumarin and warfarin	Phytonadione (vitamin K)
Crotalids and elapids	Crotalid antivenin FAB; Micrurus antivenin
Cyanide	Nitrites, sodium thiosulfate, hydroxycobalamin
Digoxin, cardioactive steroids	Digoxin FAB
Enterohepatic circulation drugs	Multidose activated charcoal
Ethylene glycol	Fomepizole, ethanol, thiamine, pyridoxine
Fluoride	Calcium salts
Heavy metals	
Arsenic and arsine gas	Dimercaprol (BAL), succimer, dimerval
Iron	Deferoxamine
Lead	Dimercaprol, succimer, dimerval, Ca-EDTA, penicillamine-D
Mercury	DMSA succimer, dimercaprol, dimerval, penicillamine-D
Thallium	Prussian blue
Hydrofluoric acid	Calcium gel
Isoniazid (INH)	Pyridoxine (vitamin B_6)
Methanol	Ethanol, fomepizole, folic acid (vitamin B_9)
Methemoglobinemia	Methylene blue
Niacin (vitamin B_3)	Aspirin
Opiates, opioids	Naloxone

(continued on next page)

TABLE 3-18. POISONS AND ANTIDOTES *(Continued)*

Poison	Antidote/Classic Treatment
Radioactive agents	
Americium	DTPA-Ca or DTPA-Zn
Cesium and thallium	Prussian blue (ferric hexacyanoferrate), sodium polystyrene sulfonate (Kayexalate)
Iodine	Saturated solution of potassium iodide (SSKI)
Plutonium	DTPA-Ca or DTPA-Zn
Sulfonylureas	Dextrose[b], octreotide, glucagon[a], diazoxide[a]
Torsades and increased QT drugs	Magnesium
Tricyclic antidepressants, sodium channel blockers, weak acids	Sodium bicarbonate

Ca-EDTA, calcium disodium edetate; DMSA, dimercaptosuccinic acid; DTPA-Ca, diethylenetriamine pentaacetic acid calcium; DTPA-Zn, diethylenetriamine pentaacetic acid zinc.
[a]Routine use is not recommended. Discussion with a medical toxicologist or physician experienced in the management of the specific poisoning and indications for the antidote is strongly encouraged prior to use.
[b]Initial treatment of choice for hypoglycemia, but should not be given prophylactically as it can stimulate insulin release, worsening hypoglycemia.
(Courtesy of Mark L. DeBard, MD, FACEP.)

- Three phases:
  - Primary respiratory alkalosis
    - Aspirin enters the central nervous system (CNS) and causes stimulation of the cerebral medulla.
  - Respiratory alkalosis with metabolic acidosis
    - Aspirin becomes incorporated into intracellular cytochrome complexes, inhibiting oxidative phosphorylation.
    - Aerobic metabolism is halted and adenosine triphosphate generation becomes increasingly dependent on anaerobic metabolism, leading to lactic acidosis and hyperthermia.
    - In addition to the primary derangement, the respiratory alkalosis becomes a true compensatory mechanism.
  - Overwhelming metabolic acidosis
    - The body's ability to adequately compensate for the metabolic acidosis is overwhelmed.
    - Signs and symptoms are hypoglycemia, neuroglycopenia, noncardiogenic pulmonary edema, altered mental status, and seizure.
- Treatment
  - Follow the ABCs, provide supportive care, and consider activated charcoal.
    - *Warning: Intubation of the salicylate patient can cause rapid, severe worsening of metabolic acidosis that can be fatal.* Consultation with a medical toxicologist or physician experienced in the management of salicylate poisoned patients is strongly encouraged.
  - Aspirin is enterohepatically recirculated, and therefore, patients may benefit from multidose activated charcoal.
  - Urinary alkalinization
    - The recipe is 5% dextrose in water plus 3 ampoules of sodium bicarbonate to run at 1.5 times maintenance.
      - Add potassium chloride supplementation to prevent severe hypokalemia secondary to intracellular shift caused by bicarbonate administration.
      - A dose of 20 mEq in adults should suffice.
      - Ensure that the patient is not in renal failure.

- Goal urine output is 1 to 2 mL/kg/h.
- Check the following hourly until stable or improving, then decrease frequency as indicated by clinical scenario:
  - Urine pH (goal ≥7.5)
    - Blood pH (venous okay, goal 7.45–7.5)
      - Avoid severe alkalemia (pH >7.55) as this shifts hemoglobin-oxygen dissociation curve to the left.
    - Serum potassium
      - Hypokalemia may prevent adequate urinary alkalinization.
    - Serum salicylate level
- Hemodialysis
  - Clinical deterioration despite aggressive maximal therapy
  - Respiratory failure necessitating intubation
  - Coingestion of CNS depressants that prevent the patient from achieving adequate, compensatory respiratory alkalosis
  - Renal failure preventing adequate urinary alkalinization secondary to patient inability to tolerate fluid load
  - Heart failure preventing adequate urinary alkalinization secondary to patient inability to tolerate fluid load
  - Serum salicylate level greater than 40 to 60 mg/dL in chronic salicylism
  - Serum salicylate level greater than 80 to 100 mg/dL in acute salicylism

Section 2: Medical Specialties

CHAPTER 4

Cardiology

Alexander B. Levitov

GATHERING DATA

Common Cardiovascular Signs and Symptoms

Chest Pain (Angina is typical.)

Angina

- Grading:
  - **1 point** for retrosternal pain radiating to the left arm 30 min or less. (Using the characteristic of 'pressure' for chest pain is an unreliable method of differentiating cardiac from non cardiac chest pain.)
  - **1 point** for pain provoked by exertion
  - **1 point** for pain relieved by rest or nitroglycerin at home (not the emergency department)
  - **Score: 3** = typical angina, **2** = atypical angina, **0–1** = nonanginal chest pain
  - If angina lasts longer than 30 minutes, consider acute myocardial infarction (MI).

Pleuritic Chest Pain

- Sharp, increased by deep inspiration and cough and possibly local pressure, relieved by leaning forward.
- Consider myocarditis, pericarditis, or pulmonary embolism.

Tearing Chest Pain

- Midscapular, posterior sudden and onset with maximal intensity
- Consider dissecting thoracic aortic aneurysm

Cardiac Syncope

- Sudden, no prodrome, short duration

Shortness of Breath (dyspnea)

- Occurs with pulmonary or cardiac problems
- Associated with angina or second and third *angina* grading points above (**angina equivalent**).

Paroxysmal nocturnal dyspnea

- Sudden, onset of dyspnea at night is a sign of congestive heart failure (CHF)

Pedal Edema

- May be a sign of right ventricular (RV) failure

Palpitations

- Often a symptom of tachycardia or arrhythmia

Claudication

- Pains or cramps (caused by ischemia) provoked by exercise and relieved by rest

Weight gain

- May be sign of CHF **or unsuccessful** cardiac and CHF therapy.

Cardiovascular Review of Systems

- **Coronary artery disease risk factors:** age, weight, male gender, previous MI or atherosclerotic disease elsewhere
- **Cardiac interventions:** pacemaker; implantable cardioverter-defibrillator (ICD); left ventricular assist device (LVAD); valve illness, repair, or replacement; coronary artery bypass grafting; any cardiac surgery as a child; percutaneous coronary intervention (PCI)
- **Drugs of abuse:** including delivery (eg, intravenous [IV]); tobacco, alcohol, cocaine, methamphetamines, other drugs

- **Family history** coronary artery disease, sudden death
- **Medications:** Antiarrhythmics, antipsychotic, anticonvulsives, statins, warfarin and other anticoagulants
- **Illnesses:** Diabetes, dyslipidemia, hypertension, stroke, aortic aneurysm, deep venous thrombosis, pulmonary embolism
- **Socioeconomic status:** level of education, use of Internet, income (eg, Can the patient afford medications?)

Physical Examination of the Heart Great and Large Vessels

Formulating a clinical diagnosis depends heavily on an understanding of the relevant anatomy and the examination of the normal and abnormal signs of the cardiovascular system.

- To review cardiac anatomy see the Atlas of Human Cardiac Anatomy at http://www.vhlab.umn.edu/atlas/index.shtml (accessed July 5, 2011).
- To review a tutorial on the cardiac physical examination see Heart Sounds and Cardiac Arrhythmias at http://www.blaufuss.org (accessed July 5, 20115).

General Considerations

Figure 4-1 demonstrates the correlation of the left ventricular cycle with heart sounds from the cardiac physical examination, the electrocardiogram, and cardiac pressures and volumes.

Increased end diastolic volume in association with low left ventricular ejection fraction (EF) usually identifies the presence of systolic heart failure, whereas low end diastolic volume can be a sign of hypovolemia (when associated with high EF) or diastolic heart failure (if EF is low).

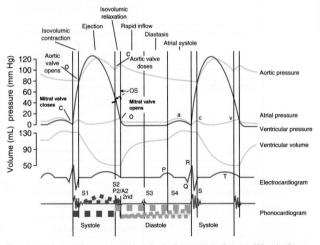

Figure 4-1 Cardiac cycle demonstrating mechanical and auditory properties: Interrupted blue triangle indicates aortic and pulmonary stenosis murmur; interrupted blue line indicates mitral and tricuspid valve regurgitation murmur; interrupted red triangle indicates mitral and tricuspid valve murmur; interrupted red line indicates aortic and pulmonary regurgitation murmur. Valves follow close-open ("COCO") pattern; on the chart, the aortic valve is on top (high pressure) and the mitral is on the bottom (low pressure). The difference in pressures (ie, pressure gradient) between the heart chambers results in blood flow with the velocity being proportionate to the gradient: end systolic volume (ESV), 120–130 mL; end diastolic volume (EDV), 50–60 mL; stroke volume (SV) = EDV − ESV (70–80 mL). Ejection fraction (EF) measured in percent is SV/EDV = (EDV − ESV)/EDV (65–70%). The right ventricle cycle is with the same volume but lower; the average is one-quarter of the ventricular pressure because of higher right ventricle compliance.

Heart Sounds and Murmurs

Heart Sounds

Heart sounds are created by cardiac structures during the cardiac cycle:

- S_1 Closure of atrioventricular valves
- S_2 Closure of the semilunar valves

TABLE 4-1. CARDIAC MURMUR CLASSIFICATION

Murmur Type	Description	Special Characteristics
Stenotic Murmurs	• Occur during flow phases when ventricular volumes change • Shorter than regurgitant murmurs (by isovolemic phase)	Vary with flow and are crescendo/decrescendo or crescendo/decrescendo (diamond shape)
Regurgitant Murmurs	• Occupy the entire phase of the cycle (described as holo (systolic/diastolic) or pan (systolic/diastolic) • Right-sided murmurs (eg, tricuspid or pulmonic valve) vary with respiration	
Systolic Murmurs		5 maneuvers altering systolic murmurs: (Valsalva, Amyl Nitrate, Leg Raising, Squatting, Hand Grips = phenylephrine [VALSH])
	Aortic/pulmonic stenosis	Aortic stenosis murmurs increase with leg raising and amyl nitrate, whereas Valsalva, squatting and hand grips reduce these murmurs. (↑LA ↓SVH)
	Hypertrophic obstructive cardiomyopathy (HOCM)	Valsalva test and amyl nitrate increase HOCM murmurs whereas leg raising, squatting, and hand grips reduce these murmurs.(↑VA ↓LSH)
	Mitral/tricuspid regurgitation	Leg raising and hand grips increase mitral valve regurgitation murmurs whereas Valsalva test and amyl nitrate reduce these murmurs. Squatting does not affect these murmurs(↑LH ↓VA)
	Ventricular septal defect	
	Mitral valve prolapse	Late systolic with midsystolic click Longer and higher pitched Mid to late and lower pitched Varies with patient position
Continuous Murmurs	Patent ductus arteriosus Coarctation of the aorta Arterial-venous fistula	
	Ruptured sinus of Valsalva test aneurysm	May be associated with a left superior vena cava syndrome

↑LA, increased with leg raising and amyl nitrate; ↓SVH, decreased with squatting, valsalva and hand grips; ↑VA, increased with valsalva and amyl nitrate; ↓LSH, decreased with leg raising, squatting and hand grips; ↑LH, increased with leg raising and hand grips; ↓VA decreased with valsalva and amyl nitrate.

- **Split S$_2$** Normal with inspiration
  - Abnormal in bundle-branch block (BBB)
  - Paradoxical split: left bundle-branch block (LBBB)
  - Fixed: atrial septal defect (ASD)
- **S$_3$** Occurs at the termination of the rapid left ventricular (LV) filling phase (70% passive)
- **S$_4$** Represents atrial contraction (and therefore absent in atrial fibrillation)

Murmurs and Bruits

Murmurs are created by abnormal flow patterns in and around the heart and often signify pathology of heart valves or great vessels (Table 4-1). Bruits are created by abnormal flow (usually increased flow velocity) in great and large vessels.

Pulses, Pressures, and Waveforms (Table 4-2)

TABLE 4-2. VITAL SIGN CHARACTERISTICS

Arterial Pulses	Description	Indicates
Pulsus tardus et parvus	Weak delayed upstroke	AS, LV failure, hypovolemia
Bisferiens	Bounding, (double-beating)	AI, PDA, vasodilatory shock
Blood Pressures	Check both arms Check arm and leg Measure pulse pressure (systolic-diastolic normal ≈ 50–60 mm Hg)	If different, consider aortic dissection If BP in arms > BP in legs, consider coarctation of the aorta *Increased:* AI, vasodilatory shock *Decreased:* Cardiac tamponade/obstructive shock
Jugular pressure (JP) Waveform examination Jugular venous distension (JVD)	The A wave corresponds to atrial systole. The C wave occurs at the beginning of the ventricular systole when AV valves bulge toward the atria. The X descent is caused by atrial diastole and rapid atrial filling. The V occurs because of pressure increase in the atrium, when tricuspid valve is closed. The Y descent is caused by rapid emptying of the atrium following the opening of the tricuspid valve.	JP
	Large A wave	TS, PS, AV dissociation
	Large V wave	ASD, MVR
	Exaggerated pulsation + large V wave	TR
	Rise in JVD during inspiration (Kussmaul sign) + steep Y-descent	Constrictive pericarditis, less commonly in pericardial tamponade

AI, aortic insufficiency; AS, aortic stenosis; ASD, atrial septal defect; AV, atrioventricular; BP, blood pressure; LV, left ventricular; MVR, mitral valve regurgitation; PDA, patent ductus arteriosus; PS, pulmonary stenosis; TR, tricuspid regurgitation; TS, tricuspid stenosis.

MEDICAL SPECIALTIES

TABLE 4-3. CARDIAC BIOMARKERS

Test	Indicates	Timeframe
Cardiac Troponins (T and I)	Indicates myonecrosis if positive (exceeds 99th percentile for reference group) on one occasion in 24-h period (ACC/AHA class IA)	Detectable in 6 h; elevated up to 12 days
CKMB	CK total >2.5 suggest myonecrosis	Elevated in MI, myocarditis, and cardioversion; increase 4–8 h, peak at 24 h (8 h after reperfusion) returns to normal in 24–48 h
Myoglobin	Frequently used in ED	Single elevated *myoglobin* (>110 µg/L) in 3–6 h after onset of symptoms improves early detection of MI (NPV 89%) and is associated with increased 6-mo mortality risk (TIMI class IB)
Glycogen Phosphorylase Isoenzyme BB (GPBB)	"New marker"	Rapid increase in blood levels can be seen in MI ACS. Elevated in 1–3 h after onset of ischemia

ACC/AHA, American College of Cardiology and American Heart Association; CK, creatinine kinase; CKMB, creatinine kinase myocardial band; ED, emergency department; MI ACS; myocardial infarction acute coronary syndrome; NPV, negative predictive value; TIMI, Thrombolysis in Myocardial Infarction risk score.

Diagnostic Testing

- Laboratory (Table 4-3)
- Chest Radiography
    - **Cardiac findings:** Cardiomegaly (enlargement of the cardiac silhouette) structures in Figure 4-2A and B can be used to define specific components such as enlarged cardiac chambers and dilated great vessels.

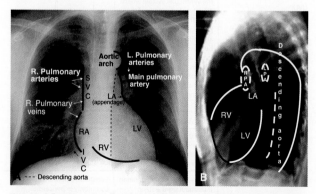

Figure 4-2 **A.** Posterior-anterior radiograph of the chest demonstrating normal landmarks. IVC, inferior vena cava; L, left; LA, left atrium; LV, left ventricle; R, right; RA, right atrium; RV, right ventricle; SVC, superior vena cava. **B.** A lateral radiograph of the chest demonstrating normal landmarks. LA, left atrium; LPA, left pulmonary artery; LV, left ventricle; RPA, right pulmonary artery; RV, right ventricle.

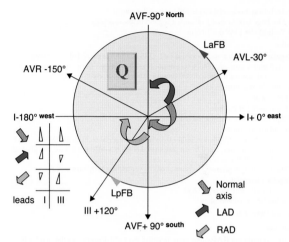

Figure 4-3 Provides determinants for QRS axis. Leads are aVF, aVL, and aVR. LAD, left axis deviation (northeast); LaFB, left anterior fascicular block; LpFB, left posterior fascicular block; RAD, right axis deviation (southwest).

- **Pulmonary findings related to cardiac disease:** Pulmonary vascular redistribution (increased diameter of the vessels to the upper lobes of the lungs) of more than one-half may be associated with cardiomegaly and pleural effusion(s).
- Regional lung hypoperfusion caused by pulmonary embolism (PE) (**Westermark sign**).
- **Other findings:** Calcifications of aorta and coronary arteries, presence of bioprosthetic or mechanical valves, repair rings, cardiac hardware (pacemakers, ICDs, ventricular assist devices etc.)
- Figure 4-2A and B demonstrate posterior-anterior and lateral radiographs of the chest demonstrating the normal landmarks and structures. Also see Heart Sounds and Cardiac Arrhythmias at http://www.blaufuss.org (accessed July 5, 2011).
- Special Tests
  - **Electrocardiogram (ECG) basics** (Figures 4-3 and 4-4)
    - **Rate in beats per minute (bpm)**
    - **Number of large horizontal boxes between consecutive QRS complexes is 300** (see Figure 4-4)
  - Differentiated ECG paper speed is 25 mm/s
  - Each small horizontal box is 40 msec (0.04 seconds)

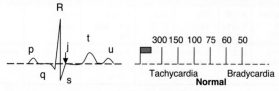

Figure 4-4 Electrocardiogram (ECG) complexes and determining heart rate.

- Each large horizontal box is 200 msec (0.2 seconds)
- Five large boxes equal 1 second; it is good to assess pauses
- Vertical box 1 mV per 10 mm

Rhythm

- **Regular** sinus rhythm is indicated if each QRS complex is preceded by a P wave:
  - Atrial flutter with fixed block is commonly misinterpreted by the automated reader; suspect if rate is a fraction of 300 bpm (ie, 150, 100, 75, etc.)
  - Third-degree heart block
  - Junctional
  - Idioventricular rhythm
  - Supraventricular tachycardia (SVT)
- **Irregularly irregular**
  - Most likely atrial fibrillation rather than multifocal atrial tachycardia (MAT) (MAT is commonly misinterpreted by the automated reader; 3 different P-wave morphologies and PR intervals).
  - May be multiple premature contractions or ventricular tachycardia (VT).
- **Regularly irregular**
  - Atrial flutter with variable block
  - Second-degree heart block

Axis (see Figure 4-3)

Definitions

- **Left axis deviation (LAD):** axis more negative than –30 degrees (northeast), S > R in II.
- **Right axis deviation (RAD):** axis more positive than +90 degrees (southwest), S > R in lead I.
- Quick assessment: look at leads I and III in QRS complexes point in the opposite directions, same in LAD as in RAD (mnemonic is "right reaches, left leaves")

Intervals and Complexes Duration and Voltage (Table 4-4; see Figure 4-4, for intervals and complexes)

Bundle-Branch Blocks

- Figure 4-5 patterns P and R show right bundle-branch block (RBBB) and LBBB respectively, which are common patterns. Beware if seen in the setting of myocardial ischemia particularly in right coronary artery (RCA) territory, which could indicate an inferior MI.
- QRS longer than 120 msec (QRS duration)
- **Right** (RBBB) mnemonic is "**RBBB** Large **R** in **Right**-sided V lead (V_1)" (Figure 4-6 and see Figure 4-5, pattern P)
- **Left** (LBBB) mnemonic is "LBBB Large R in **Left**-sided V leads (V_5-V_6)" (see Figure 4-5, pattern R)
- **Hemiblocks:** QRS shorter than 120 msec (see Figure 4-3)
  - Left anterior hemiblock (LAH) (a.k.a. left anterior fascicular block) axis more negative than –45 degrees: qR-I, rS-III/F

TABLE 4-4. NORMAL INTERVALS AND COMPLEXES DURATION AND VOLTAGE (SEE FIGURE 4-4)

	P	PR	Q	QRS	Q(S)T(c)	T
Duration/ lead (msec)	II <120 V_1 <40	>120 <200	<40	60–100 No or small RV_1	<1/2 RR (<440)	
Voltage h/d (mm)	II <2.5 V_1 <1.5	Depression <1 mm	<1/4 R in same complex	See LVH/RVH R + S > 5-limb >10 Vs	Elevation >1 Depression <1	3-limb 7-V

LVH, left ventricular hypertrophy; RVH, right ventricular hypertrophy.

Atrial rate / Ventric rate   Rhythm & rate disturbances

A. Ectopic atrial contraction

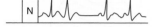

N

B. Sinus tachycardia

100+ | 100+

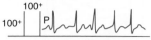

P

C. Paroxysmal supraventricular tachycardia

160 | 160

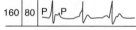

P

D. Atrial tachycardia with block (2:1)

160 | 80

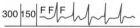

P   P

E. Atrial flutter (2:1 block)

300 | 150

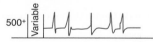

F F F

F. Atrial fibrillation

500+ | Variable

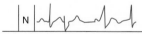

G. Ectopic ventricular contractions

N

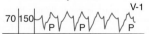

H. Ventricular tachycardia

70 | 150

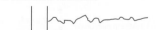

V-1
P   P   P

I. Ventricular fibrillation

Atrial rate / Ventric rate   Conduction disturbances

J. First degree heart block

70 | 70

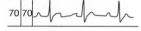

K. Second degree heart block

80 | 40

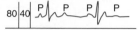

P   P   P   P

L. Third degree heart block (complete H. B.)

80 | 40

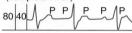

P P   P   P   P

M. Wenckebach

80 | 50

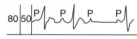

P   P   P   P

N. Wolff-Parkinson-White with delta waves

70 | 70

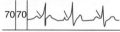

O. Wolff-Parkinson-White without delta waves

70 | 70

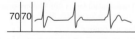

P. Right bundle branch block

70 | 70

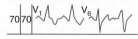

V_1 V_6

R. Left bundle branch block

70 | 70

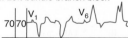

V_1 V_6

Figure 4-5   A summary of the electrocardiogram (ECG) patterns of cardiac arrhythmias and conduction abnormalities: patterns A through R.

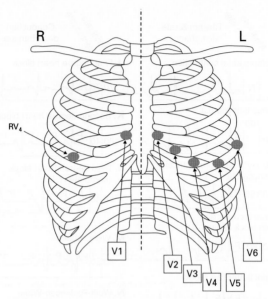

Figure 4-6   Precordial lead placement ᵣV₁-ᵣV₆ are right precordial leads used in the diagnosis of right ventricular myocardial infarction. (Image recreated by Maria Levitov.)

- Left posterior hemiblock (LPH) (a.k.a. left posterior fascicular block) axis more positive than +110 degrees: r**S**-I q**R**-III (mnemonic is "reverse previous")
- **Bifascicular blocks:** LAH plus RBBB, LPH plus RBBB
- **Trifascicular block:** LBBB plus first-degree atrioventricular (AV) block or bifascicular blocks plus first-degree AV block

Abnormal Patterns

- P wave (Figure 4-7; left atrial enlargement [LAE], right atrial enlargement [RAE])
- **PR**-Short: Less than 120 msec PR; for preexcitation syndrome, expect delta wave, slurred QRS upstroke. Long (PR duration) greater than 200 msec indicates first-degree AV block; PR depression indicates pericarditis.
- **Q** wave: depth more than one-quarter R height in same complex, or duration longer than 40 msec indicates MI, preexcitation syndrome, LBBB, pneumothorax, pulmonary embolism (PE) (SI QIII, TIII), hypertrophy (see hypertrophic cardiomyopathy [HCMP]

II   LAE = "p mitrale"   II   RAE= "p pulmonale" > 2.5 mm

V1 >1 mm   V1 >1.5 mm

>120 msec.

Figure 4-7   Electrocardiogram (ECG) criteria for left atrial enlargement (LAE) and right atrial enlargement (RAE).

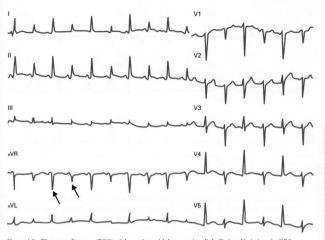

Figure 4-8   Electrocardiogram (ECG) of the patient with large pericardial effusion. Variations in QRS morphology from beat to beat (arrows) is an "electrical alternans."

and hypertrophic obstructive cardiomyopathy [HOCM]) or infiltrative cardiomyopathy (see restrictive cardiomyopathy [RCMP])) (septal Qs)

- **QRS:** see Table 4-4 for normal duration and voltage.
- **Low voltage:** hypothyroidism, pericardial may be with "electrical alternans" (Figure 4-8) or pleural effusion, infiltrative cardiomyopathy (RCMP)
- **RV$_1$:** consider lead misplacement (common), *posterior MI,* RVH (see below), RBBB, preexcitation syndrome, rarely dextrocardia, Duchenne muscular dystrophy, constrictive pericarditis
- **Poor R-wave progression:** R wave is less than 2 to 4 mm in leads V$_3$ or V$_4$ or reversed R-wave progression, R in V$_4$ less than R in V$_3$ or R in V$_3$ less than R in V$_2$ or R in V$_2$ lead misplacement; old anteroseptal (LAD distribution) MI; right ventricular hypertrophy (RVH); left ventricular hypertrophy (LVH); LBBB; preexcitation syndrome (see arrhythmias)
- **Ventricular hypertrophy (VH):** ECG criteria have poor predictive value (requires echocardiographic diagnosis):
  - **RVH:** RAD R > S in V$_1$ + RV$_1$ >5 mm, S in V$_6$ >7 mm
  - **LVH:** SV$_1$ + RV$_5$ or V$_6$ >35 mm or R in RVL >11 mm
- **Widened QRS** (QRS duration)
  - BBB, premature ventricular contractions, aberrantly conducted premature atrial contractions, quinidine, flecainide, severe hyperkalemia
- **QT** (QTc = QT/√ RR NL < 440 msec) **prolongation** (QT duration)
  - Drugs: antiarrhythmics class IA and III antipsychotics (ie, haloperidol); tricyclics; lithium; antimicrobials, commonly fluoroquinolones and macrolides, less commonly antimalarials and antivirals; methadone; for complete list, see Arizona Center for Education and Research on Therapeutics at http://www.azcert.org/medical-pros/drug-lists/CLQTS.cfm (accessed July 5, 2011).
  - Electrolyte abnormalities and endocrine disorders: hypokalemia (pseudoprolongation), hypocalcemia (true prolongation), hypomagnesemia, hypothyroidism, **hypothermia** (Osborn waves) (Figure 4-9)
  - Intracerebral hemorrhage, carotid hypersensitivity or surgery (or neck dissection)

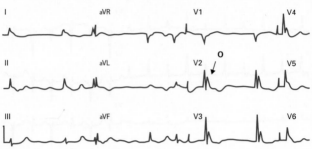

Figure 4-9 Electrocardiogram (ECG) of the patient with severe accidental hypothermia demonstrating Osborn wave arrow –O.

- Congenital (Romano-Ward syndrome autosomal dominant without deafness, Jervell and Lange-Nielsen syndrome autosomal recessive, associated with congenital deafness)
- **ST elevation** (STE) (Figures 4-10A and B; Figure 4-11)
  - STE plus acute MI (AMI) is **STEMI** (convex upward, see Figure 4-10A) in the leads corresponding to coronary territory (see Figure 4-10A) often with T-wave inversion, left ventricular aneurysm persistent STEMI changes "frozen ST elevation"
  - Coronary spasm: variant or Prinzmetal angina shorter duration than AMI corresponding to coronary territory
  - Pericarditis (concave upward) in all leads except aVR and V_1; longer duration, followed later by T-wave inversion (when ST returns to normal limits)
  - LBBB, LVH, Brugada syndrome, (downsloping STE in V_1-V_2) (see Figure 4-11)
  - Normal variant (concave upward) interrupted line (Figure 4-12), common in young J-point elevation 1 to 4 mm V_2 to V_5
- **ST depression**
  - Non-ST-segment elevation myocardial infarction (non-STE + MI = **NSTEMI**)
    - Positive stress (test) intentional or unintentional because of myocardial ischemia in the leads corresponding to coronary territory

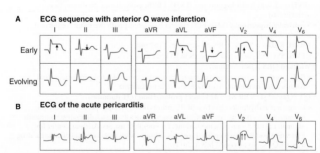

Figure 4-10 A. Electrocardiogram (ECG) of the ST-segment elevation myocardial infarction: Notice ST-segment elevation corresponds to the coronary anatomy. Notice "reciprocal" ST-segment depression. **B**. ECG of the acute pericarditis. Note PR interval depression (single arrow) and S T-segment elevation in multiple leads (double arrows). Notice ST-segment elevation does not correspond to the coronary anatomy.

Brugada syndrome

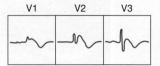

V1	V2	V3

Figure 4-11 Electrocardiogram (ECG) consistent with Brugada syndrome.

- STEMI "reciprocal" changes (see Figure 4-10A)
- LVH "strain" pattern, LBBB (I, aVL, V$_5$,V$_6$)
- Digitalis, hypokalemia (plus U waves)
- **Peaked T waves** AMI "hyperacute phase" **indicates hyperkalemia**
- **T-wave inversion** (see Figure 4-10A): evolving anterior leads I, aVL V$_2$-V$_6$
  - NSTEMI in the leads corresponds to coronary territory LVH, RVH ("strain" pattern)
  - **Hypothermia** (see Figure 4-12): in combination with Osborn waves
  - Increased intracranial pressure (deep symmetrical, "cerebral T")
  - Drugs (digoxin), acid-base disorders, rate related; may be normal or nonspecific
- U waves: hypokalemia (with flat T wave indicates "pseudo-prolongation" of QT interval [QU]), hypocalcaemia
  - **ECG libraries**
    - ECG library at the University of Wales, http://www.ecglibrary.com/ecghome.html (accessed July 5, 2011)
    - ECG Learning Center, University of Utah, http://library.med.utah.edu/kw/ecg/image_index/index.html (accessed July 5, 2011)

Bedside Echocardiography (Echo), Transthoracic Echocardiography (TTE) and Transesophageal Echocardiography (TEE)

- Usually performed in standard views (Figures 4-13 through 4-16)
- May identify reversible causes of cardiac arrest or shock (American College of Cardiology [ACC]/American Heart Association [AHA] class IA).

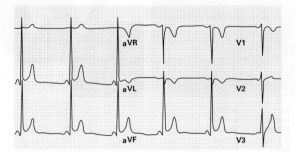

Figure 4-12 Normal variant J point elevation. Notice concave ST-segment elevation does not correspond to the coronary anatomy. (Image recreated by Maria Levitov.)

Parasternal long axis PLAX

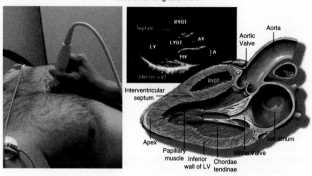

Figure 4-13 Bedside echocardiography. Transducer position indicates expected image and cardiac anatomy in parasternal long axis view. AV, aortic valve; LA, left atrium; LV, left ventricle; LVOT, left ventricular outflow tract; MV, mitral valve; RVOT, right ventricular outflow tract.

- In acute MI (ACC/AHA class IA) used to assess LV function and presence of regional wall motion abnormality (RWMA), which suggests ischemia (in parasternal short axis [PSAX] views, all walls are able to be visualized [see Figures 4-13 and 4-14])
- For RV MI (inferior wall) and mechanical complications (acute ventricular septal defect [VSD], which is more common in septal and anterior wall MI), papillary muscle rupture (more common in inferior wall MI) and perforation
- To assess valvular integrity and function, cardiac source of emboli, aortic root
- TEE preferred if dissection suspected
  - ACC/AHA echo guidelines, *Appropriate Use Criteria for Echocardiography*, available at http://content.onlinejacc.org/cgi/content (accessed July 5, 2011)
- **Arterial and venous**, including Doppler ultrasound evaluation of the peripheral vessels (see also peripheral vascular disease)

Parasternal short axis PSAX

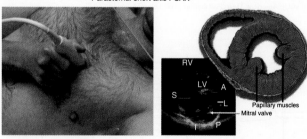

All	Anterior
Ladies	Lateral
Purchase	Posterior
In	Inferior
Sears	Septum (intraventricular)

Figure 4-14 Bedside echocardiography. Transducer position indicates expected image and cardiac anatomy in parasternal short axis view. Cardiac segments are marked with initial letters and corresponding mnemonic.

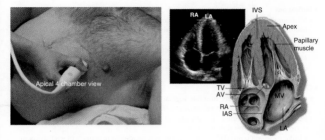

Figure 4-15   Bedside echocardiography. Transducer position indicates expected image and cardiac anatomy in apical 4-chamber view. IVS, interventricular septum; LA, left atrium; RA, right atrium. IAS, iteratrial septum; TV, tricuspid valve; AV, aortic valve.

- For arterial study, see the American College of Radiology guidelines at http://www.guidelines.gov/content.aspx?id=32533 (accessed July 5, 2011)
- For venous study, see http://www.guidelines.gov/content.aspx?id=32534 (accessed July 5, 2011)

Exercise Tolerance Test (ETT) (a.k.a. "stress test")

- Treadmill protocol in the order of decreasing exercise level:
  - **Bruce protocol**
    - 1-minute Bruce
    - 2-minute Bruce
    - 3-minute Bruce (most common; 3-minute workloads increase in 3 metabolic equivalent [MET] increments)
    - Modified Bruce
  - **Naughton** (3-minute increases in 1 MET increments)
- Maximal load if target heart rate (HR) is 220 bpm minus patient's age) or double product = HR × SBP > 30,000 is achieved, where SBP is systolic blood pressure.
- If submaximal with known coronary artery disease (CAD) (ie, post-MI evaluation) consider pharmacologic:
  - Pharmacologic if unable to exercise
    - **Dobutamine** is used with asthma (or severe chronic obstructive pulmonary disease) reversed by administering a beta-blocker
    - **Adenosine or dipyridamole** in patient with poorly controlled hypertension, glaucoma, or BBB; reversed by administering theophylline

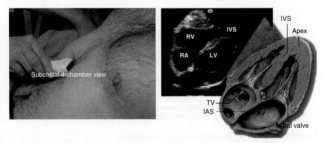

Figure 4-16   Bedside echocardiography. Transducer position indicates expected image and cardiac anatomy in subcostal 4-chamber view. IVS, interventricular septum; RV, right ventricle. IAS, iteratrial septum; TV, tricuspid valve; AV, aortic valve; LV, left ventricle; RA, right atrium.

MEDICAL SPECIALTIES

- **Indications**
  - Medium risk of coronary heart disease according to risk factors of smoking, family history of CAD, hypertension, diabetes and high cholesterol (ACC/AHA class IA) nearly always combined with imaging
  - Follow up for CAD when clinically indicated (ACC/AHA class IIB): ischemia localization (AHA/ACC class IA) and assessment of myocardial viability (usually pharmacologic), evaluation of exercise tolerance, differential diagnosis of chest pain (symptom reproduction with exercise)
- **Contraindications**
  - Acute MI within 48 hours, unstable angina, uncontrolled cardiac arrhythmia (eg, VT), severe symptomatic aortic stenosis, aortic dissection, PE, pericarditis
  - **Positive ECG:** Horizontal ST depression or STE (highly positive) in the leads corresponding to coronary territory
  - Duke treadmill score (DTS) = maximum exercise time in minutes − (5 × ST segment deviation in mm) − (4 × angina index), where 0 = no angina, 1 = nonlimiting angina, 2 = exercise limiting angina
  - DTS 5 = low risk (4-year survival 99%)
  - DTS between 4 and −10 = intermediate risk
  - DTS less than −10 = high risk (4-year survival 79%)
- **Imaging**
  - Echo TTE in parasternal long axis (PLAX), PSAX (apical 4-chamber and apical 2-chamber views in Figures 4-13 through 4-16)
  - Radiotracer (Figure 4-17), such as technetium 99m (^{99m}Tc) sestamibi or thallium 201 single-photon emission computed tomography (SPECT) (perfusion scintigraphy), rubidium 82-positron emission tomography (PET) (possibly better images) or double tracers (gated to assess LV function)
  - Reversible defect: ischemia, particularly if corresponding to coronary territory
  - Fixed: scar indicates previous infarct
  - May be false negative in left main and 3-vessel disease
- **Summary of ETT recommendations:** see ACA/AHA Guidelines for Exercise Testing: Executive Summary at http://circ.ahajournals.org/cgi/content/full/96/1/345 (accessed July 5, 2011)
  - Patient able to exercise
    - ST-T normal during ETT
- In women, echocardiography possibly better
  - Patient able to exercise
    - ST-T abnormal indicates LBBB, LVH, medication effect
- Consider ETT plus SPECT, PET, or echocardiography
  - Patient unable to exercise
    - Pharmacologic protocol plus SPECT, PET, or echocardiography
  - Patient unable to complete ETT
    - Consider ambulatory ECG or event monitor

Cardiac Magnetic Resonance Imaging (MRI) and Computed Tomography (CT)

- **Indications**
  - Constrictive pericarditis, assessment of myocardial viability, cardiac masses, cardiomyopathies
  - For high-grade coronary stenosis, consider computed tomography angiography (CTA), magnetic resonance angiography (MRA)
  - For all clinical indications and appropriateness criteria see *Appropriateness Criteria for Cardiac Computed Tomography and Cardiac Magnetic Resonance Imaging* at http://www.asnc.org/imageuploads/CCT-CMRApprop080706.pdf (accessed July 5, 2011)

Cardiac Catheterization and Coronary Angiography

- **Indications**
  - High-risk noninvasive assessment; AMI with intent of revascularization (ACC/AHA class IA)

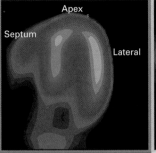

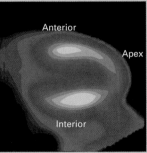

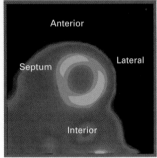

Figure 4-17 Correlation of coronary anatomy and imaging segments (positron emission tomography, single-photon emission computed tomography, etc.). (Images recreated by Maria Levitov.) See color insert.

- Cardiac care system class III to IV angina. Status post successful resuscitation or VT. Suspected failure of revascularization (ie, stent closure). AMI with carcinogenic shock or heart failure. Before valve surgery or repair (ACC/AHA class IB).
- Worsening noninvasive assessment. Unclear chest pain. Unexplained LV systolic dysfunction (ACC/AHA class IC).
- For *ACC/AHA Guidelines for Cardiac Catheterization and Cardiac Catheterization Laboratories*, see http://circ.ahajournals.org/content/84/5/2213.full.pdf+html (accessed February 13, 2011)
- **Risks of the coronary angiography**
  - AMI 5:10,000 doubles in high-risk patients
  - Allergic reaction to contrast or medications
  - Contrast-induced nephropathy
    - To calculate risk use web calculator, A Risk Score to Predict Contrast-Induced Nephropathy after Percutaneous Coronary Angioplasty, at http://www.zunis.org/Contrast-Induced%20Nephropathy%20Calculator.htm (accessed February 16, 2011)
    - Higher in patients with diabetes and patients with chronic renal disease
    - Vessel injury
    - Bleeding, including retroperitoneal
    - Arrhythmias
    - Stroke
- **Consider the following prior to cardiac catheterization:**
  - Question patient about reaction to contrast or seafood (iodine)
  - Perform bedside ultrasound assessment of femoral arteries and veins.

- Get complete blood count (CBC), prothrombin time, partial prothrombin time, serum creatinine (clearance in elderly and if muscle mass is diminished)
- Contrast nephropathy prevention
  - Acetylcysteine 600 mg BID PO × 72 h
- IV fluids possibly 150 mEq sodium bicarbonate in 1000 cc of 5% dextrose in water over 8 hours, on call to the catheterization laboratory

SPECIFIC CONDITIONS

Coronary Artery Disease (CAD)

- Evaluate chest pain for asymptomatic or minimally symptomatic atherosclerotic CAD in the emergency department.
- *Probability analysis and regional nature* (corresponding to coronary territory) is key to evaluating CAD (Figure 4-18; see Figures 4-10A and B).
  - **Probability analysis** is based on the combination of symptoms and CAD risk factors.
- Probability of CAD is based on symptoms and Framingham study risk categories (Table 4-5):
  - Diabetes, smoking, recommendations of the Fifth Joint National Committee on Prevention, Detection, Evaluation, and Treatment of High Blood Pressure (JNC5), LVH, and National Cholesterol Education Program total and low-density lipoprotein cholesterol categories

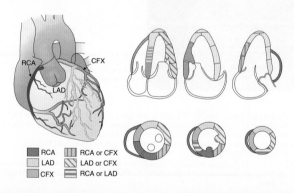

Coronary Artery	Area	Leads	Imaging: Echo, PET, SPECT
LAD	Antero-septal	V_1-V_4	Antero-Septal
RCA>>Cfx.	Inferior/right ventricle	II, III, AVF	Inferior +/− Right Ventricle
Cfx.	Lateral +/− apex	I, AVL +/−V_5, V_6	Lateral wall +/− Apex
LAD, >CFX, >RCA	Apical	V_5, V_6	Apex
LAD/1st SP	IVS	V_1-V_2	Interventricular Septum
RCA>CFX	Posterior	RV_1, ST V_1, V_2	Posterior / Inferior wall

Figure 4-18 Coronary anatomy and echocardiogram segments in apical 2-, 4-, and parasternal short axis views. CFX, circumflex coronary artery; LAD, left anterior descending artery; RCA, right coronary artery.

TABLE 4-5. PROBABILITY OF CORONARY ARTERY DISEASE AS
RELATED TO ANGINA SCORE

| Age | Angina Score | | | | | |
	1 (%)		2 (%)		3 (%)	
30–39	1	5	4	22	26	70
40–49	3	14	13	46	55	87
50–59	8	22	32	59	80	92
60–69	19	28	54	67	91	94+
Sex	♀	♂	♀	♂	♀	♂

- To calculate risk, use the web calculator, General Cardiovascular Risk Profile for Use in Primary Care: 8491 Patients in the Framingham Heart Study, at http://www.zunis.org/FHS_CVD_Risk_Calc_2008.htm (accessed July 5, 2011)
- Probability assessment Tables for 2- and 10-year risks are available at Framingham Heart Study, http://www.framinghamheartstudy.org/risk/coronary2.html (accessed July 5, 2011) and http://www.framinghamheartstudy.org/risk/coronary.html (accessed July 5, 2011)
- For overall probability analysis consider using the calculator, Duke Clinical Score: Prediction of Coronary Heart Disease in a Patient with Chest Pain at http://www.zunis.org/Duke%20Chest%20Pain%20-%20CAD%20Predictor.htm (accessed July 5, 2011)
- **Regional changes** corresponding to coronary territory no matter how unimpressive are more important then nonregional, no matter how dramatic. (For coronary artery territories, see Figure 4-18). Regional changes for ECG are defined as *abnormal Q waves* or any *ST-T segment abnormalities*, corresponding to coronary vessels territories (see Figures 4-10A and B, 4-18). For echo as RWMA, see Figures 4-13–4-18. For radioisotope studies as *perfusion defects*, see Figures 4-17, 4-18).

Acute Coronary Syndromes (unstable angina and NSTEMI)

- **Etiology:** most atherosclerotic coronary disease
- **Presentation:** New angina, rest angina, increase in angina symptoms if myonecrosis present (ie, with biomarkers per Table 4-2)
- **Physical examination:** S₃, S₄ (see Figure 4-1 and Table 4-2); diaphoresis, hypotension
  - **ECG:** ST depression, T inversion
  - **Laboratory results:** NSTEMI with elevated biomarkers
  - Measurement of brain natriuretic peptide (BNP) or N-terminal (NT)-proBNP may be considered to assess global risk (ACC/AHA class IIA, level B).
  - **Echo:** RWMAs corresponding to coronary territory (see Figures 4-13, 4-14, 4-15, 4-16, 4-18)
  - **Resting SPECT/PET:** regional perfusion defect, corresponding to coronary territory (see Figure 4-17, 4-18)
- **Triage:** evaluate probability of death, MI (urgent revascularization), extent of myocardium in jeopardy. **Admit the patient to the intensive care unit/cardiac care unit (ICU/CCU).** Establish Thrombolysis in Myocardial Infarction (TIMI) **risk score** (Tables 4-6A and B).
  - To calculate, use the web calculator, TIMI Risk Score for Acute Coronary Syndrome (UA/NSTEMI), at http://www.zunis.org/TIMI%20UA-NSTEMI%20Risk%20Score.htm (accessed July 5, 2011).
  - For more information, see TIMI Study Group at http://www.timi.org (accessed July 5, 2011).
- **Treatment** (Figure 4-19)
- Antithrombotic agents
  - Aspirin (ASA) 162 to 325 mg (crushed or chewed), 75 to 325 mg/24 h PO (ASA allergy substitute: clopidogrel)
  - ASA plus clopidogrel 300 to 600 mg PO, 75 mg/d (unless imminent coronary artery bypass graft [CABG])

TABLE 4-6A. TIMI RISK SCORE

Historical Characteristics	Points
Age ≥65 years	1
≥3 Risk factors	1
Known CAD	1
ASA use within a week	1
Presentation characteristics	1
≥2 angina episodes over 24 h	1
ST↑ ≥0.5 mm	1
+ Biomarkers	1
Risk score total point	0–7

ASA, acetylsalicylic acid (aspirin); CAD, coronary artery disease; ST↑, ST-segment elevation; TIMI, Thrombolysis in Myocardial Infarction.

- Unfractionated heparin (UFH) 60 U/kg IV bolus (IVB) (maximum 4000 U), 12 U/kg/h (maximum 1000 U/h). Adjust to achieve activated partial thromboplastin time (APTT) 1.5 to 2.5 × control (50–70 sec). *Check CBC every 72 hours: If platelet count is decreased by one-half, then consider heparin-induced thrombocytopenia (HIT) and change to direct thrombin inhibitors (DTIs).* If more than 35,000 U/24 h is needed to achieve APTT, heparin resistance is present (may be caused by concomitant use of nitroglycerin [NTG]; switch to DTI).
- Low-molecular-weight heparin (LMWH) and factor Xa (FXa) inhibitors: enoxaparin 1 mg/kg subcutaneously every 12 h (use caution in renal failure: glomerular filtration rate [GFR] <30 mL/min; monitoring of FXa may be used, if available)
- Fondaparinux 2.5 mg/24 h subcutaneously (caution if GFR <30 mL/min; monitoring of FXa should be used, if available)
- DTIs: bivalirudin 0.1 mg/kg IVB, 0.25 mg/kg/h; in HIT or if PCI is planned, add 05 mg/kg IVB. If already on bivalirudin, increase to 1.75 mg/kg/h.
- Glycoprotein IIb (GPIIb) and GPIIIa inhibitors: in high-risk patients or if PCI is planned, use tirofiban 0.4 μg/kg IV over 30 min, 0.1 μg/kg/min IV × 48 to 96 h

TABLE 4-6B. TIMI RISK SCORE AND PROBABILITY OF DEATH AND REVASCULARIZATION

TIMI Risk Score	Death or MI in 14 Days Plus Urgent Revascularization (%)	
0–1	3	5
2	3	8
3	5	13
4	7	20
5	12	26
6–7	19	41

MI, myocardial infarction; TIMI, Thrombolysis in Myocardial Infarction.
Entry criteria into TIMI 11B: acute coronary syndrome as ischemic pain within 24 hours plus coronary artery disease evidence.

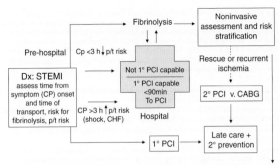

Figure 4-19 Assessment, triage, and therapy of patients with ST-segment elevation myocardial infarction (STEMI). CABG, coronary artery bypass surgery; CHF, congestive heart failure; Dx, diagnosis; PCI, percutaneous coronary intervention; p/, patient; CP, chest pain.

or eptifibatide 180 µg/kg IVB, 2 µg/kg/min IV × 72 to 96 h; if PCI is planned, use abciximab 0.25 mg/kg IVB, 0.125 µg/kg/min.

- *Do not administer fibrinolytic therapy.*
- To calculate bleeding risk, use the Crusade Bleeding Score calculator at http://www.crusadebleedingscore.org/ (accessed July 5, 2011).
- Antiischemic
  - NTG 0.3 to 06 mg sublingual or buccal spray; after 3 doses 5 min apart, consider IV 5 to 10 µg/min, increase by 10 µg/min every 3 to 5 min until symptoms or systolic blood pressure (SBP) is less than 100 mm Hg (no mortality benefit; *do not use if recent use of phosphodiesterase inhibitors,* ie, sildenafil, tadalafil; caution in RV dysfunction)
  - Beta-blockers
  - Metoprolol 5 mg IVB every 5 min × 3 doses (*beta-blocker IV may not improve survival*), 25 mg PO every 6 h, titrate to HR 60 bpm. If the HR is less than 55 bpm, SBP is less than 100 mm Hg, second or third degree heart blocks, bronchospasm, uncontrolled CHF, do not start the medication. If the patient is on the medication already, it should be held or stop if these events occur.
  - Calcium channel blockers (CCBs): diltiazem, verapamil (no mortality benefit) may be tried if beta-blockers are contraindicated.
  - Morphine: consider for those with pulmonary edema and retractable symptoms.
- PCI
  - In centers with a high volume of PCIs with experienced (>75 PCIs performed per year) operators and door-to-balloon time of 90 minutes or less, consider PCI within 24 and up to 80 hours after hospitalization for those with very high predicted mortality (ACC/AHA class II). See the following special considerations:
  - Prinzmetal angina: treat with CCB, NTG
  - Cocaine coronary spasm: Patients with cocaine-associated myocardial ischemia should receive initial treatment with benzodiazepines. *Avoid beta blockers if possible* (may enhance coronary vasoconstriction); give ASA, NTG, and low doses of verapamil to reverse coronary vasoconstriction. For reperfusion, use PCI or thrombolytic therapy.
  - Antiphospholipid antibody syndrome: treat with UFH plus steroids (poor prognosis)
  - Prognosis and discharge triage see STEMI below.
- **ST Elevation Myocardial Infarction (STEMI)**
  - **Etiology:** atherosclerotic
  - **Presentation:** Similar to acute coronary syndrome (ACS), *approximately 25% asymptomatic*
  - **Physical examination:** S_3, S_4 (see Figure 4-1 and Tables 4-1, 4-2); rales, jugular venous distension (JVD) may indicate RV involvement

- **ECG:** ST-segment elevation 1 mm or more and T-wave inversion followed in hours by pathologic Q waves in the leads corresponding to coronary territory but at least 2 leads (see Figures 4-10A and B) plus myonecrosis is present (ie elevated biomarkers [see Table 4-3]) to indicate STEMI "reciprocal" changes (ST-segment depression in other leads). New LBBB (see Figure 4-5, pattern R) same meaning as ST-segment elevation
  - *With preexistent LBBB:* Q in V_5V_6, STE 1 mm or more in leads concordant with QRS, or 5 mm or more STE in leads discordant with QRS; ST-segment depression 1 mm or more in V_1 to V_3
  - *Diagnosis of STEMI with permanent ventricular pacemaker:* QRS or 5 mm or more STE in leads discordant with QRS Sgarbossa criteria.
- **Echo criteria for STEMI:** RWMA (see Figure 4-14) and it is useful to assess LV function and RV involvement but cannot discriminate old from new.
- *Do not use gastrointestinal cocktail or pain reproduction with chest palpation to rule out MI in the emergency department.*
- **Triage:** Admit patient to ICU/CCU, similar mortality and probability analysis as in NSTEMI. Identify candidates for reperfusion. Prevent and treat complications.
- **Therapy**
  - *Immediate adjunct (to reperfusion) therapy*
    - Establish IV line.
    - O_2 to achieve SO_2 over 90%
    - Antithrombotic
    - *Beta-blocker IV may not improve survival;* oral likely beneficial (http://download.thelancet.com/pdfs/journals/lancet/PIIS0140673606692350.pdf [accessed July 5, 2011]), consider ([accessed July 5, 2011]), consider oral metoprolol (ACC/AHA class IA, IV, and IIB).
    - ASA as soon as possible
    - If tissue plasminogen activator (TPA), give recombinant plasminogen activator (rPA) with UFH to a partial prothrombin time of 1.5, 2 × control × 48 h or LMWH 7 days
    - *No GPIIb/IIIa inhibitors after fibrinolysis*
    - Antiischemic, see NSTEMI
    - Morphine, see NSTEMI
    - Consider mild sedation (diazepam 5 mg PO 24 h)
    - Angiotensin-converting enzyme inhibitor (ACEI): *Do not use IV ACEIs.* (captopril 6.25 mg PO TID, increase as tolerated).
    - Angiotensin receptor blocker (ARB) benefit approximately equal to ACEI
    - Consider IV insulin infusion for 48 hours
    - Consider K^+ and Mg^{++}; check and keep normal for at least 48 hours.
    - Hydroxymethylglutaryl-coenzyme A (HMG-CoA) reductase inhibitors (a.k.a. statins, eg, lovastatin PO 20–80 mg/d prior to discharge)
  - Reperfusion strategy
    - Should be implemented if less than 12 hours since presentation.
    - Selection criteria: anginal character pain longer than 30-min duration, with ECG for STEMI (with or without developed new Q waves in involved leads)
    - Time from the onset of symptoms less than 6 hours confers greatest benefit, but effective up to 12 to 16 hours.
- Primary PCI
  - In centers with a high volume of PCIs (>75 PCIs performed per year) with experienced operators and door-to-balloon time of 90 minutes or less (ACC/AHA class IB), consider PCI for those with high predicted mortality if 1 or more significant lesions in 1 or more (see angiography guidelines) coronary arteries and large area of viable myocardium (ACC/AHA class IB), or multiple graft stenosis (ACC/AHA IIC). In other patients and those with contraindications to fibrinolysis, benefits of PCI are unclear.
  - PCI types
    - Balloon angioplasty (percutaneous transluminal coronary angioplasty) because restenosis is a relatively benign disease

- For more information, see *Primary PCI for Myocardial Infarction with ST-Segment Elevation* at http://www.nejm.org/doi/full/10.1056/NEJMct063503 (accessed July 5, 2011)
  - Stents decrease the rate of restenosis, but if restenosis occurs, stent closure can be catastrophic; ASA for life, clopidogrel 4 weeks or more.
  - Drug-eluting stent use is controversial; ASA for life, clopidogrel 1 year or more.
  - For more information, see *Drug-Eluting Coronary Stents—Promise and Uncertainty* at http://www.nejm.org/doi/full/10.1056/NEJMe068306 (accessed July 5, 2011)
- Nonprimary PCI
  - Rescue, recurrent ischemia during hospitalization and ETT prior to discharge.
  - Early routine: 24 hours or less after fibrinolysis (ACC class IIB)
  - Late routine: (later than day 7) *not beneficial*
  - For PCI national guidelines see U.S. Department of Health and Human Services at http://www.guideline.gov/content.aspx?id=34980&search=pci
- PCI complications
  - Bleeding overall rate 2.0%; for those treated with manual compression only, 2.8%; vascular closure device, 2.1%; bivalirudin, 1.6%; vascular closure device and bivalirudin, 0.9%. May be retroperitoneal heart block; decrease requires retroperitoneal ultrasound or CT. Resuscitation, transfusion, surgical consultation (possibly vascular or interventional radiology), but evacuation is seldom necessary.
  - Pseudoaneurysm: pulsatile mass, bruit bedside or formal ultrasound is diagnostic and may guide therapy (compression) (Figure 4-20)
  - AV fistula: for bruit, bedside or formal ultrasound is diagnostic; vascular surgery consultation (Figure 4-21)
  - Cholesterol emboli: (poor 6 months prognosis) eosinophilia, livedo reticularis (Figure 4-22), renal failure
  - Stent stenosis or thrombosis
  - Contrast nephropathy assessment and prevention
  - Reperfusion arrhythmias: (generally benign)

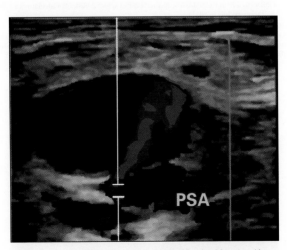

Figure 4-20   Two-dimensional arterial ultrasound and colored Doppler of the patient with femoral artery pseudoaneurysm. PSA, posterior spinal artery. (Image recreated by Maria Levitov.) See color insert.

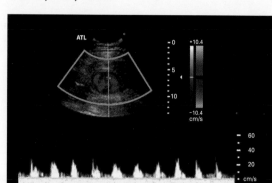

Figure 4-21   Two-dimensional arterial ultrasound continuous wave and colored Doppler of the patient with femoral artery arteriovenous fistula. See color insert.

- Overall PCI:
  - See the web risk calculator, Mayo Clinic Risk Scores to Predict In-Hospital Death and Adverse Events for Coronary Angioplasty, at http://www.zunis.org/Mayo%20Clinic%20 -%20Death%20and%20MACE%20After%20PCI%20-%20Risk%20Calculator%202007. htm (accessed July 5, 2011)
- Cardiothoracic surgery
  - Consider a cardiothoracic surgery consult to evaluate for CABG in refractory angina not amendable to PCI or disabling angina; for patients with diabetes with 2- or more vessel disease; for patients with left main or left main equivalent, that is significant (≥70%)

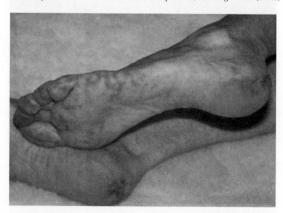

Figure 4-22   Livedo reticularis in patient with atheroemboli. See color insert.

stenosis of proximal LAD and proximal left circumflex artery or 3-vessel disease with impaired LV function (ACC/AHA class I); and for failed PCI.
- To determine overall CABG risk, use the web calculator, A Risk Score to Predict In-Hospital Mortality for Coronary Artery Bypass Graft Surgery at http://www.zunis.org/CABG%20Risk%20Calculator.htm (accessed July 5, 2011)
- Fibrinolysis
- Indications for reperfusion
- Door to needle 30 minutes or less (consider prehospital, emergency department-guided administration by emergency medical services)
- With absence of contraindications:
  - Any history of intracranial hemorrhage, aneurysm, AV malformation or neoplasia
  - Ischemic cerebrovascular accident (CVA) or head trauma within 3 months
  - Aortic dissection *(Stanford type A may cause STEMI because of coronary artery dissection.)*
  - Active bleeding or hemorrhagic retinopathy
  - Known bleeding diathesis INR ≥ 2.0
  - Marked hypertension greater than 180/110 mm Hg
- **Fibrinolytic drugs**
  - TPA 15 mg IVB, 50 mg over 30 min, 35 mg over 60 min
  - rPA 10 unit IVB × 2 with 30-min interval
  - Streptokinase *(no repeated use)* 1.5 million units IVB over 1 h
  - Figure 4-19 summarizes a decision algorithm for PCI versus fibrinolysis.
- **Complications and special considerations**
  Right ventricular MI
- In the setting of RCA distribution (inferior wall myocardial infarction [IWMI]), hypotension, JVD with clear lungs, and Kussmaul sign, bedside echo is diagnostic and can be used to assess right atrial pressure (RAP) (>10 mm Hg) and right ventricular systolic pressure (RVSP), which is usually higher than 30 mm Hg. See the web calculator, Echocardiographic Assessment of Hemodynamics, at http://www.zunis.org/Echocardiographic%20hemodynamics.htm (accessed February 13, 2011)
- RV ECG changes Symmetrical to V leads on the right chest (see Figure 4-6) RV_4 STE more than 1 mm
- Treat with IV fluids; goal 15 more than a RAP that is higher than 10 mm Hg, avoid NTG and diuretics.
- Consider pulmonary vasodilators (inhaled nitric oxide [NO]), intraaortic balloon pump (IABP) or RV assist device)
  Heart block (see Figure 4-5, patterns J, K, L, M)
- Common RCA: AV nodal artery (AV node ischemia), atropine to bedside, tape to bed for transport, temporal transcutaneous or transvenous pacemaker. Heart block in LAD distribution MI equates with poor prognosis.
  Hemodynamic complications
- *Acute pump failure (LV failure), cardiogenic shock* (Figure 4-23)
  - Acute pulmonary edema
  - LAD distribution likely
  - Consider noninvasive therapy (echo, transpulmonary thermo-dilution, pulmonary artery catheter monitoring, and intraarterial blood pressure monitoring).
  - Consider mechanical ventilation (noninvasive positive pressure ventilation or intubation), rescue reperfusion or revascularization, IABP counterpulsation.
  - IABP, LVAD, NTG
  - Inotropes (dobutamine, dopamine, milrinone) and pressors (phenylephrine [Neo-Synephrine], norepinephrine to keep mean arterial pressure [MAP] >60 mm Hg)
  - Diuresis
  - If renal failure supervenes may require continuous renal replacement therapy instead of diuresis.
- *Arrhythmias (see Figure 4-5; see arrhythmias section below)*
  - *No prophylactic antiarrhythmic therapy*

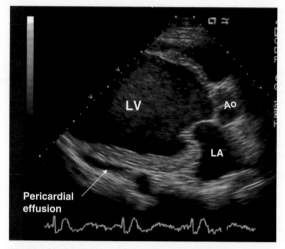

Figure 4-23   Echocardiogram in parasternal long axis view of the patient with severe dilative cardiomyopathy. Ao, aorta; LA, left atrium; LV, left ventricle. See color insert.

- For loss of pulse or consciousness, cardiac arrest, ventricular fibrillation, initiate advanced cardiac life support
- If hemodynamically unstable, use defibrillation and cardioversion
- Otherwise, assure K^+ Mg^{++} are normal; consider beta-blocker (amiodarone).
- UFH for atrial fibrillation consider digoxin (monitor levels in reduced GFR; check for decrease)
- Tolerate reperfusion arrhythmias
- Heart blocks (see Figure 4-5, patterns K and L)
- Second-degree type 1 atrioventricular block (AVB), BBB: atropine to bedside, tape to bed for transport, temporal transcutaneous pacemaker backup
- Second-degree type 2 or third-degree AVB, 2:1 block with QRS longer than 120 msec, consider bifascicular or trifascicular block
- New BBB (Figure 4-5 patterns P and R): transcutaneous pacemaker backup, transvenous pacemaker
- *Mechanical complications*
  - Typically day 3–5 post STEMI, but *may occur sooner (day 1–2)* after revascularization.
  - Acquired VSD (Figure 4-24). Is more common with LAD, but more difficult to repair with RCA infarct. Shock or CHF with new harsh holosystolic murmur. Echo (TTE, TEE) is diagnostic. Temporize with therapy for shock; surgical (or percutaneous) closure offers best outcome. Surgical mortality approximately 20%.
  - Free wall perforation (a.k.a. cardiac rupture) (Figure 4-25): Spontaneous or *may be the result of RV perforation by pacemaker wire* (Figure 4-26). Patient presents with vomiting and chest pain; progressive or recurrent STE echo (TTE, TEE) is diagnostic. Temporize with therapy of shock; tamponade requires emergency surgery. Surgical mortality approximately 50%.
  - Pseudoaneurysm (a.k.a. false aneurysm) (Figure 4-27A): a free wall perforation contained by adherent pericardium and/or scar tissue. Echo (TTE, TEE) is diagnostic. Free rupture likely and requires emergency surgery.
  - Acute mitral valve regurgitation (MVR) (Figure 4-28) is caused by posterior medial papillary muscle (PMPM) from RCA territory (eg, MI) rupture or ischemic dysfunction, which is more common because of singular blood supply of PMPM from

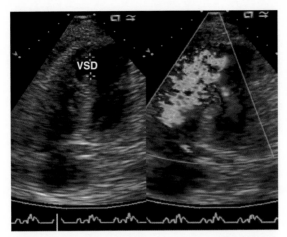

Figure 4-24   Echocardiogram in apical 4-chamber view of the acquired ventricular septal defect (VSD) complicating septal (left anterior descending artery distribution) ST-segment elevation myocardial infarction. See color insert.

patent ductus arteriosus (PDA). Poorly tolerated. Shock or severe CHF (worse then in VSD) with new harsh holosystolic murmur, giant V waves (Figure 4-29 , Table 4-2). Echo (TTE, TEE) is diagnostic. Temporize with therapy of shock; PMPM rupture requires surgery. Surgical mortality approximately 50%, but worse outcome when treated medically (mortality 90%) (see Figure 4-28).

- *Ventricular aneurysm (a.k.a. "true" aneurysm)*
  - No danger of rupture unlike pseudoaneurysm. May cause CHF; "frozen ST Elevation" more than 2 weeks; echo is diagnostic (dyskinetic region) (see Figure 4-26). Elective

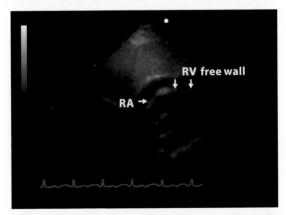

Figure 4-25   Echocardiogram in subcostal short axis view of a right ventricle (RV) free wall ↓↓ perforation with pericardial effusion. RA, right atrium →.

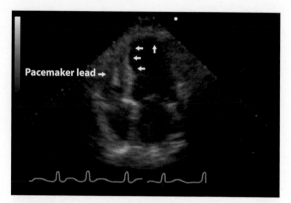

Figure 4-26   Ventricular wall perforation from a pacemaker lead. True apical aneurysm - multiple arrows.

surgery (aneurysmectomy) if malignant arrhythmias, recurrent CHF, or if source of emboli (see Figure 4-27B).

- *LV thrombus*
  - More common with aneurysm
  - Echo is diagnostic (see Figure 4-27B); may need echo contrast if difficult study.
  - Anticoagulation for 3 to 6 months
- *Pericarditis (see pericardial disease)*
  - Pleuritic chest pain. May be occur with pericardial rub; ECG changes are rare except for atrial arrhythmias; no anticoagulation (ASA 650 mg PO 4 times daily).
  - Postcardiac injury syndrome (a.k.a. postpericardiotomy); post-MI syndrome occurred in 4% of patients, but rapidly decreasing with reperfusion strategies. Occurs 1 to 4 weeks or sometimes months after myocardial injury. May reoccur up to 2 years post

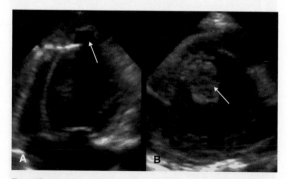

Figure 4-27   Echocardiogram in apical 4-chamber view. **A.** Patient with an apical pseudoaneurysm (white arrow). **B.** Echocardiogram in parasternal short axis view of a patient with apical thrombus (white arrow).

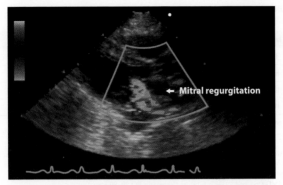

Figure 4-28 Echocardiogram in parasternal long axis view of a patient with acquired mitral valve regurgitation and inferior wall myocardial infarction (right coronary artery distribution). See color insert.

triad: pericarditis, pleuritis, pneumonitis (pulmonary infiltrates) (mnemonic is "3-Ps"). Fever, increased leucocytes, ECG changes, rarely tamponade. No anticoagulation (ASA 650 mg PO 4 times daily); NSAID, may need glucocorticoids.

- Prognosis STEMI, ACS (Table 4-7)
- Global Registry of Acute Coronary Events (GRACE) risk model
  - http://www.outcomes-umassmed.org/grace/acs_risk/acs_risk_content.html (accessed July 5, 2011)
- GRACE calculator
  - http://www.zunis.org/Risk_Calculators/GRACE_Score_and_Risk_Category_Calc.htm (accessed July 5, 2011)
- Triage on discharge
  - Risk-factor assessment (ETT, TTE to assess left ventricular ejection fraction [LVEF]) and lifestyle modification counseling (smoking cessation, control of diabetes [glycated hemoglobin level <7.0], hyperlipidemia)
  - Low-density lipoprotein cholesterol goal less than 70 mg/dL; blood pressure goal 120 to 130/80 mm Hg exercise, weight loss.
  - ASA for 1 year
  - Beta-blocker: indefinitely
  - ACEI/ARB: indefinitely if CHF

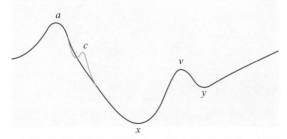

Figure 4-29 Jugular venous pressure and hemodynamic effects of respiration.

TABLE 4-7. KILLIP CLASSIFICATION AND MORTALITY IN ACUTE MYOCARDIAL INFARCTION

Class	Definition	Predicted Mortality (%)
I	No CHF	6
II	S_3 and/or basilar rales	17
III	Pulmonary edema	30–40
IV	Cardiogenic shock	60–80

CHF, congestive heart failure.

- Aldosterone antagonists (spironolactone [Aldactone] 25 mg/d) indefinite if CHF or if LVEF is less than 40%
- Sublingual NTG (for angina as needed)
- HMG-CoA reductase inhibitors (lovastatin PO 20–80 mg/d)

Nonatherosclerotic CAD

- *Can cause the same syndromes as atherosclerotic CAD*
- Etiology
  - Coronaritis (coronary vasculitis), rheumatoid arthritis, systemic lupus erythematosus (SLE), rheumatic, temporal arteritis, cocaine vasculitis, Takayasu arteritis, Kawasaki disease (in children causing coronary artery aneurysms [Figure 4-30]), Churg-Strauss disease.
  - Thrombotic catastrophic antiphospholipid antibody syndrome (a.k.a. Asherson syndrome)
  - Coronary spasm: variant of Prinzmetal angina, cocaine
  - Coronary dissection: Stanford classification type A thoracic aorta dissection, pregnancy
  - Coronary embolism: AV subacute bacterial endocarditis (SBE), mural thrombus, left atrial myxoma

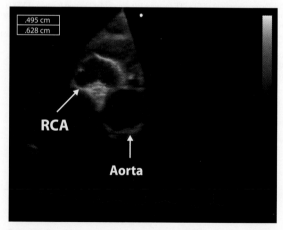

Figure 4-30 Nonatherosclerotic coronary disease. Right coronary artery (RCA) aneurysm in a child with Kawasaki disease. (Compare RCA and aortic diameter.)

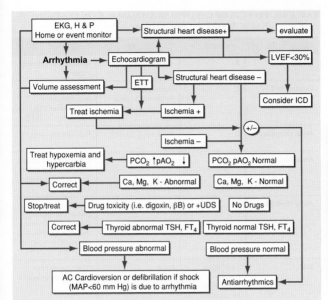

Figure 4-31   Approach to the patient with arrhythmias (in red requires immediate attention). βB, beta-blocker; ECG, electrocardiogram; ETT, exercise tolerance test; FT4, free thyroxine; ICD, implantable cardio defibrillator; LVEF, left ventricular ejection fraction; MAP, mean arterial pressure; PaO₂, partial pressure of arterial oxygen; pCO₂, partial pressure of carbon dioxide; TSH, thyroid-stimulating hormone; UDS, ultrasound Doppler sonography.

Cardiac Arrhythmias

- **Diagnosis**
  - Figure 4-31 summarizes an approach to the patient with acute (or unknown duration) arrhythmias.
  - In hemodynamically unstable or unconscious patients, electrical cardioversion (synchronized) or defibrillation should be considered. The priority should be given to recognizing and correcting conditions that cause or provoke arrhythmias.
  - When arrhythmias are diagnosed, consider obtaining long "rhythm strips" in leads II, aVF and/or V₁. If possible, double the voltage to better identify P waves. A diagnosis of myocardial ischemia can be made simultaneously.
  - Home ECG or event monitoring may be necessary for patients with palpitations but without ECG changes.
  - ETT may be needed to provoke ischemia-related arrhythmias.
  - Consider ECG during carotid sinus massage (CSM) (Table 4-8). (*Do not massage both carotids simultaneously.*)

Tachyarrhythmias

Narrow QRS Complex Tachycardias (see Figure 4-5, Patterns C and D)

- Structural heart disease can be discovered by echo and makes the presence of arrhythmias more significant.
- *Do not attempt antiarrhythmics if sinus tachycardia is present. If patient is hemodynamically unstable or if angina or CHF is present* because of nonsinus tachyarrhythmia, consider

TABLE 4-8. EFFECTS OF CAROTID SINUS MASSAGE ON COMMON NARROW QRS TACHYCARDIAS

Tachycardia	See Figure 4-5	CSM Effects	Treatment
Sinus	B	Gradual rate decrease	Remove precipitating event
Reentry SVT	C	None or abrupt conversion to sinus	CSM ± Valsalva test, adenosine, beta-blocker, CCB, cardioversion (150 J)
Atrial tachycardia	D	Atrial rate 0 Δ, block may ↑	Hold digoxin, correct K⁺
Atrial flutter	E	Block may ↑ VR↓	Beta-blocker, diltiazem, digoxin, cardioversion (start at 50 J) catheter ablation
Atrial fibrillation	F	VR↓	Anticoagulation if chronic, VR control, conversion, if no NSR, then give ibutilide, cardioversion (start at 100 J) (see Figure 4-15)
MAT	≥3 different P-wave morphologies ≥3 PR durations	None	Treat lung disease, amiodarone, verapamil
Preexcitation with antegrade AV nodal conduction	N, O	None or abrupt conversion to sinus	CSM, ± Valsalva test, adenosine, beta-blocker cautious *(cardioversion pads on, defibrillator ready)*

AV, atrioventricular; CCB, calcium channel blocker; CSM, carotid sinus massage; MAT, multifocal atrial tachycardia; NSR, normal sinus rhythm; SVT, supraventricular tachycardia; VR, ventricular response.

immediate cardioversion. Consider pacemaker that detects and terminates arrhythmia (ACC/AHA class IC).

- Caution: if digitalis toxicity is suspected (atrial tachycardia with block, atrial fibrillation with pseudo-regularized ventricular response [VR], atrial flutter with high degree and odd block [3:1, 5:1, 7:1]), withdraw digitalis; consider antidigoxin antibody fragments ("Digibind") if life-threatening digitalis overdose.
- **Atrial fibrillation** (see Figure 4-5, pattern F; Figure 4-32)
  - ACC/AHA management guidelines http://www.zunis.org/AFib%20Management%202007.htm (accessed July 5, 2011)
  - **Paroxysmal** if self-limiting episodes; **chronic** (persistent) if episodes last longer than 7 days; (**permanent**) if episodes last longer than 6 months
  - Evaluate for underlying cause: 50% is caused by thyrotoxicosis, valvular heart disease (mitral valve stenosis [MVS]), pulmonary disease, obstructive sleep apnea, drugs (ethanol [ETOH], cocaine, methamphetamines, theophylline), and ACS.
- **Treatment**
  - **Aimed at rate control and anticoagulation**
  - Anticoagulation with **warfarin** or dabigatran (lower rate of hemorrhagic CVA) (see http://www.nejm.org/doi/full/10.1056/NEJMoa0905561 [accessed July 5, 2011]) 150 mg and 220 mg once daily (coagulation testing not required) to prevent stroke in high- (MVS,

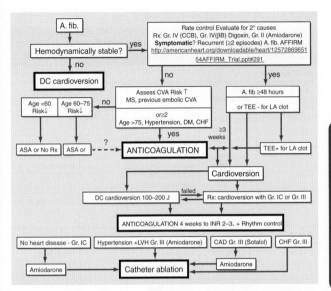

Figure 4-32 Approach to assessment, triage. and treatment of the patient with atrial fibrillation. A. fib., atrial fibrillation; ASA, aspirin; CAD, coronary artery disease; CHF, congestive heart failure; CVA, cerebrovascular accident; DM, diabetes mellitus; Gr., grade; LA, left atrium; LVH, left ventricular hypertrophy; MS, mitral valve stenosis; Rx, drug therapy; TEE, transesophageal echocardiogram. ; ?, indicates uncertainty if anticoagulation should be undertaken.

history of thromboemboli) and moderate- (age ≥75 years, hypertension, diabetes, CHF) risk patients; warfarin to INR 2.0 to 3.0. To assess stroke risk, use the web calculator at http://www.zunis.org/FHS%20Afib%20Risk%20Calculator.htm (accessed July 5, 2011).
- Compare CVA risk to bleeding risk; use of clopidogrel increases bleeding risk (Table 4-9).
- Use **groups II, III, IV drugs for rate control** (see Table 4-10)

TABLE 4-9. HAS-BLED BLEEDING RISK ASSESSMENT TOOL

	Points	Score	Bleeds per 100 Patient-Years
Hypertension	1	Any	1.56
Abnormal renal or liver function	1 each	0	1.13
Stroke	1	1	1.02
Bleeding History	1	2	1.88
Labile INR	1	3	3.74
Elderly (>65 years)	1	4	8.7
Drugs or ETOH	1 each	5	12.5

ETOH, ethanol.

MEDICAL SPECIALTIES

TABLE 4-10. ANTIARRHYTHMIC DRUGS

Group/Drug	Dose (mg, unless noted)	Side Effects	Excretion	Special Comments
IA. QT duration				
Quinidine	Sulfate 200–400 PO Q 6 h Gluconate 324–628 PO Q 8 h	Diarrhea, anemia (Hb↓), thrombocytopenia (Plt↓), hypotension	H	Seldom used
Procainamide	500–1000 IVB, 2–5 mg/min	Nausea, QT duration, lupus-like syndrome, agranulocytosis	H/R	May use in preexcitation (WPW)
Disopyramide	100–300 PO Q 6–8 h	Negative inotrope and chromotrope anticholinergic	H/R	Used in HOCM
IB.				
Lidocaine	1 mg/kg IVB, 1–4 mg/min	Confusion, seizures, respiratory arrest	H	Follow level (*Do not use prophylactically*)
Mexiletine	100–300 PO Q 6–8 h	Nausea, tremor	H	
IC. Nausea, VT, PR duration, QRS duration				
Flecainide	50–100 PO Q 12 h		H/R	
Propafenone	150–300 PO Q 8 h		H	
II. Beta-blocker = Bradycardia Bronchospasm, CHF, AVB				
Metoprolol	2.5–10 IVB Q 5 min × 3, 25–100 PO BID	Beta-blocker	H	Use in ACS, STEMI
Propranolol	0.5–1 Q 5 min (total 0.15 mg/kg, 20–60 PO Q 6 h	Beta-blocker	H / variable	Seldom used IVB
Esmolol	500 µg/kg IVB over 1 min, 50–200 µg/kg/min	Beta-blocker	Hydrolyzed by plasma esterases	Short half-life

TABLE 4-10. ANTIARRHYTHMIC DRUGS *(Continued)*

Group/Drug	Dose (mg, unless noted)	Side Effects	Excretion	Special Comments
III.				
Dronedarone	400 mg BID with meals	Liver injury		Decrease simvastatin dosage Check ALT, AST
Amiodarone	150 over 10 min, 1 mg/min × 6 h, 0.5 mg/min 800–1600 PO Q day × 1–2 weeks, 400–600 × 3 weeks, 200–400 Q day	Thyroid ↓ or ↑, pulmonary fibrosis, QT duration, bluish skin and cornea (microdeposits), complex excretion		Check TFT; pulmonary fibrosis more likely if IV after PO use.
Ibutilide	1 mg over 10 min (may repeat)	TDP, nausea, hypotension	H	
Dofetilide	125–500 µg PO Q 12 h	TDP, headache	R	
Sotalol plus beta-blocker	80–320 PO Q 12 h	Beta-blocker, VT, fatigue	R	
IV. CCB: AV Block, Hypotension, Constipation				
Diltiazem	0.25 mg/kg over 2 min, repeat 0.35 mg/kg after 15 min, 5–15 mg/h 120–360 PO Q day	Above	R/H	VR control in atrial fibrillation; AV block
Verapamil	2.5–10 IVB, 120–480 PO Q day		H	
V. Miscellaneous				
Adenosine	6 IVB, 12 IVB	Hypotension, atrial standstill	R	SVT
Digoxin	0.75–1.5 over 24 h IV or PO 0.25–0.5 PO Q day	AV Block, VT, SVT, nausea , caution in women	R	VR control in atrial fibrillation; level 0.5–0.8 ng/mL

ACS, acute coronary syndrome; ALT, alanine aminotransferase; AST, aspartate aminotransferase; AVB, atrioventricular block; BID, twice daily; CCB, calcium channel blocker; CHF, congestive heart failure; H, hepatic; Hb, hemoglobin; HOCM, hypertrophic obstructive cardiomyopathy; IVB, intravenous bolus; Plt, platelet; Q, every; R, renal; STEMI, ST-segment elevation myocardial infarction; SVT, supraventricular tachycardia; TDP, torsade de pointes; TFT, thrombus formation time; VR, ventricular response; WPW, Wolf-Parkinson-White.

- **Cardioversion:** 100 to 200 J after anticoagulation therapy longer than 3 weeks; may start with addition of UFH or LMWH until INR is greater than 2.0, if no left atrial (LA) thrombus on echo (TEE > TTE) and patient is symptomatic after rate control. Follow by rhythm control strategy (see Figure 4-32).
- **Atrial flutter** (see Figure 4-5, pattern E)
  - Consider if ventricular rate is 150 bpm, 100 bpm, and so forth (2:1 or 3:1); cardioversion with 50 J is usually successful.

Wide QRS Complex Tachycardias (see Figure 4-5, pattern H)

- Differential VT versus aberrantly conducted SVT (*If in doubt assume VT, if hemodynamically unstable direct current [DC] cardioversion.*)
- **SVT** with **aberrant conduction:** typical BBB pattern with rate-related BBB usually RBBB pattern (treat as SVT).

Preexcitation Syndromes (a.k.a. Wolff-Parkinson-White (WPW) syndrome) (see Figure 4-5, patterns N and O): caused by accessory conduction pathway between atria and ventricles (Kent bundle) (see short PR).

- **Narrow complex (SVT)** occurs if conduction is antegrade through the AV node.
- Wide complex (SVT) occurs if antegrade conduction is through an accessory pathway. Often occurs with atrial fibrillation with VR faster than 250 bpm.
- Consider cardioversion (Table 4-10): **grade IA (procainamide),** grade **III (ibutilide),** or if oral, grade **IC (flecainide).** *Do not use CCB, beta-blocker, digoxin, adenosine (may elevate VR).*
- Consider **catheter ablation** if WPW arrhythmias inducible by ETT or **electrophysiologic study (EPS),** particularly if results in unstable hemodynamics.

Ventricular Tachycardia (see Figure 4-5, pattern H)

- *Hemodynamic status has no differential diagnostic value between VT and SVT.*
- **Diagnostic of VT** is presence of capture (within normal limits) or fusion beat (implies bidirectional conduction).
- **EEG criteria favoring VT**
  - AV dissociation
  - QRS duration longer than 140 msec with RBBB configuration (see Figure 4-5, pattern P)
  - QRS duration longer than 160 msec with LBBB configuration (see Figure 4-5, pattern R)
  - QRS-LAD (northeast) with RBBB morphology (see Figure 4-3)
  - QRS-extreme LAD (northwest) with LBBB morphology
  - Concordance of QRS in precordial leads
  - Morphologic patterns of QRS
  - RBBB (see Figure 4-5, pattern R) mono- or biphasic V_1
  - RS (with LAD) or QS in V_6
  - LBBB (see Figure 4-5) RV_1 or RV_2 40 msec or longer
  - Onset of QRS to S nadir duration in V_1 or V_2 70 msec or longer
  - Q in V_6
  - Notched downslope of S in V_1
- **Echo**
  - Can be done in both stable or unstable patient and may be helpful in assessing for ischemia (RWMA), LV function, pericardial disease, and so forth
- **Cardiac MRI:** Consider if infiltrative cardiomyopathy is possible.
- **Cardiac catheterization: EPS**
- **Monomorphic:** Associated with Structural Heart Disease (LV scar, cardiomyopathies, congenital [ie, arrhythmogenic RV dysplasia]) or Primary VT.
- **Therapy**
  - DC cardioversion (100 J) if unstable
  - If stable and acute, **amiodarone** is favored.
  - Chronic: **IA, IB, IC, III** (see Table 4-10)
  - ICD
  - If LVEF is less than 35%, then RV dysplasia, HOCM is indicated (ACC/AHA class IC).
  - **If primary VT:** no heart disease may respond to CCB (verapamil or beta-blocker.)

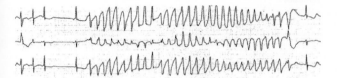

Figure 4-33 Example of polymorphic torsade de pointes ventricular tachycardia.

- **Polymorphic:** increased QT (torsade de pointes) (Figure 4-33) congenital, drug induced, decreased Mg level, ETT induced, Brugada syndrome (see Figure 4-11)
- **Therapy**
  - IV Mg 1 to 2 g IVB; *discontinue all QT during drug therapy.*
  - ICD in congenital QT duration
  - **In both:**
    - **Amiodarone** (see Table 4-10) also if inferior vena cava firing is frequent or disabling.
  - If still disabling, consider catheter ablation.

Ventricular Fibrillation

- See Figure 4-5, pattern I (*It only takes a second to **make sure it is not a monitor artifact.**);* **defibrillate and initiate advanced cardiac life support.**

Bradyarrhythmias

- **Sinus bradycardia**
  - **Causes:** seen in athletes; drugs (CCB, beta-blocker [see Table 4-10]) hypothermia, hypothyroidism, hypoxemia, sepsis
  - **Treatment:** remove primary cause; usually unnecessary, but if symptomatic give atropine 0.6 mg IVB (may repeat 3 times) or transvenous pacemaker.
- **Sick sinus syndrome** (SSS) (a.k.a. tachycardia-bradycardia or "tachy-brady" syndrome): caused by degenerative conduction system disease. Control tachycardia with CCB or beta-blocker; permanent pacemaker is indicated for symptomatic bradycardia component.
- **AVB** (heart block)
  - **First-degree AVB:** PR duration longer than 200 msec; no therapy (see Figure 4-5, pattern J)
  - **Second-degree Mobitz type I:** Wenckebach block (see Figure 4-5, pattern M), narrow QRS (2:1 block with narrow QRS), progressive elevation in PR until QRS (ventricular beat) is dropped, then sequence is repeated. AV nodal conduction abnormality: suspect drugs, AV nodal ischemia with IWMI (RCA distribution [see Figure 4-18]), mitral valve repair or replacement (mitral valve is close to AV node). Worse with CSM; if treatment is needed, give atropine 0.6 mg IVB (may repeat 3 times) or place temporal pacemaker.
  - **Second-degree Mobitz type II** (see Figure 4-5, patterns K): More dangerous; subnodal conduction abnormality (*QRS duration* with fixed PR interval and dropped beat in 2:1, 3:1, 4:1 pattern). Better with CSM, worse with atropine. Caused by anterior wall myocardial infarction (AWMI) (LAD distribution [see Figure 4-18 and Figure 4-10 A]), aortic valve surgery (repair or replacement), infiltrative cardiomyopathy, myocarditis degenerative conduction system disease. May progress to complete heart block without warning. Keep transcutaneous pacemaker backup leads on the patient.
    - **Temporary pacemaker** may be needed.
  - **Third-degree: complete heart block** (see Figure 4-5, pattern L) is a form of AV dissociation. Atrial activity is not transmitted to the ventricle because of AMI IWMI or AWMI infiltrative cardiomyopathy, degenerative conduction system disease. Neuromuscular diseases with AVB: myotonic muscular dystrophy, Kearns-Sayre syndrome, Erb dystrophy (limb-girdle), and peroneal muscular atrophy often progress to complete heart block. Transient block caused by IWMI may need no treatment or transcutaneous or pacemaker backup. Otherwise **permanent pacemaker** is indicated.

Pacemakers

- Indications
  - In AVB
  - Symptomatic third-degree AVB including intermittent (ACC/AHA class IC)
  - AVB with 3 sec or longer asystole or rate less than 40 bpm (ACC/AHA class IB)
  - Post catheter ablation (ACC/AHA class IB)
  - Neuromuscular diseases with AVB (ACC/AHA class IB)
  - In SSS
    - Symptomatic bradycardia including intermittent (ACC/AHA class IC) or with 3 sec or longer asystole or rate less than 40 bpm (ACC/AHA class IC)
- Most commonly used pacemaker is the dual-mode, dual-pacing, dual-sensing (DDD) pacemaker (the dual chamber paces both right atrium [RA] and RV, senses RA and RV spontaneous beats, and responds by inhibiting or triggering increasing rates). For patients who cannot increase their hearts rates with exercise, rate-adaptive pacemakers are available. The VVI (ventricular RV pacing, RV sensing inhibition by spontaneous beat) pacemaker is used in chronic atrial fibrillation with symptomatic bradycardia or asystole.
- A magnet can be used to shut the pacemaker off or convert to pacing (D or V) without sensing.
- **For complete ACC/AHA Guidelines** for Implantation of Cardiac Pacemakers and Antiarrhythmia Devices see http://circ.ahajournals.org/content/97/13/1325.full/ (accessed July 5, 2011).

Cardiomyopathy (CMP)

Dilated Cardiomyopathy (DCMP) (see Figures 4-23, 4-27A and B): LV (symmetrically) with poor LV function (LVEF decreased with normal or decreased intraventricular septum [IVS]/LV thickness).

- **Etiology**
  - **Idiopathic**
- Previous myocarditis most common; includes Takotsubo cardiomyopathy (a.k.a. transient apical ballooning syndrome, stress-induced cardiomyopathy, or "broken heart syndrome"): disproportional apical involvement (ballooning) (Figure 4-34) and see http://circ.ahajournals.org/cgi/content/full/108/16/2014 (accessed July 5, 2011).

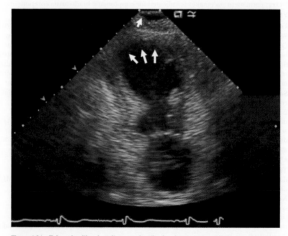

Figure 4-34   Takotsubo dilated cardiomyopathy ("broken heart syndrome"). Note disproportional apical involvement (ballooning [white arrows]). See color insert.

- **Ischemic:** severe CAD and infarctions
- **Infectious**
  - Mostly viral (coxsackievirus, echovirus, human immunodeficiency virus [HIV]); also tuberculosis, Lyme borreliosis, Chagas disease (suspect *Trypanosoma cruzi* in foreign-born patients with concomitant dysphasia and RBBB disproportional apical involvement); more than 30% of patients with sepsis of any origin may develop transient DCMP.
- **Toxic**
  - ETOH most common; cocaine, doxorubicin, and other anthracyclines, antiretroviral drug therapy, lead
- **Autoimmune**
  - May play part in infectious DCMP; connective tissue disorders (SLE, scleroderma, Wegener granulomatosis); postpartum and peripartum; eosinophilic
- **Malnutrition** and **endocrinopathies**
  - Hypothyroidism, acromegaly, pheochromocytoma, edematous beriberi (a.k.a. wet beriberi because of thiamine decrease in ETOH-abuser *(Do not confuse with toxic effect of ETOH.)*, carnitine decrease, hypophosphatemia, decreased selenium levels (ie, Keshan disease)
- **Sleep apnea** (central and obstructive sleep apnea)
- **End-stage** valvular, hypertensive, and infiltrative heart diseases
- **Neuromuscular diseases:** Duchenne muscular dystrophy, myotonic dystrophy
- **Tachycardia-induced**
- **Symptoms**
  - CHF, tachyarrhythmias, mural thrombus (see Figure 4-27B) leading to peripheral emboli
- **Physical examination**
  - JVD, rales, diffuse or dyskinetic LV apex, hepatomegaly, peripheral edema MVR and tricuspid regurgitation (TR) murmurs (see Tables 4-1, 4-2)
- **Laboratory test results**
  - Elevated BNP and pro-BNP suggest cardiac cause of dyspnea (CHF, acute pulmonary edema).
- **Special tests**
  - ECG: BBB common (see Figure 4-5, patterns P and R)
- **Chest x-ray**
  - Cardiomegaly (see Figure 4-2A and B), pulmonary vascular redistribution and pulmonary effusions (R > L)
- **Echo** is diagnostic (see Figure 4-27); RWMA (Figure 4-35)
  - May suggest CAD as an alternative diagnosis
- **ETT** may suggest CAD as an alternative diagnosis.

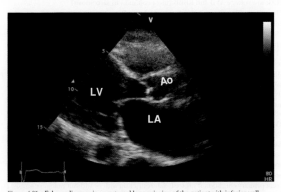

Figure 4-35   Echocardiogram in parasternal long axis view of the patient with inferior wall acute myocardial infarction and regional wall motion abnormalities. Ao, aorta; LA, left atrium; LV, left ventricle.

- **Cardiac MRI** to exclude myocarditis
- **Endomyocardial biopsy** gives low diagnostic yield.
- **Triage**
  - If arrhythmia, CHF, low blood pressure, or LVEF less than 30%, consider admission to ICU/CCU or monitored bed.
- **Therapy:** Standard treatment for acute and chronic heart failure.
  - **Chronic anticoagulation** for LVEF 25% or less
  - **Treat deficiency states:** thiamine, abstinence from ETOH, levocarnitine and phosphate supplement; treat Keshan disease with sodium selenite; consider checking selenium level in HIV DCMP
  - **Treat endocrine disorders**
  - **Immunosuppressive** therapy for autoimmune causes
  - **ICD:** if VT and failure of antiarrhythmic drugs (ACC/AHA class IB); if CHF alone (ACC/AHA class IIIC)
  - **Consider biventricular pacing**
    - RV, coronary sinus if symptomatic and QRS 130 msec or longer
  - **Cardiac transplantation** or **LVAD** in selected candidates

Restrictive Cardiomyopathy (RCMP)

- Decreased LV diastolic compliance indicates increased "stiffness," which indicates impaired LV relaxation with increased LV diastolic pressure (LVDP) and (usually decreased LV end diastolic [LVED] volume)
- **Etiology**
  - **Infiltrative diseases:** first-degree or second-degree amyloidosis most common, sarcoidosis
  - **Storage diseases:** Fabry disease, Gaucher disease, glycogen storage diseases, hemochromatosis (suspect in male patients of Scandinavian origin)
  - **Eosinophilic:** Loeffler endo- and myocarditis, endomyocardial fibrosis
  - **Carcinoid** and ergot alkaloids (because of serotonin toxicity)
  - **Idiopathic:** primary myocardial fibrosis, fibroelastosis
  - **Diabetes** mellitus: up to 5% of patients may have hemochromatosis
- **Symptoms**
  - Right-sided heart failure (ascites, peripheral edema) predominate, peripheral emboli, increased heart rate is poorly tolerated.
- **Physical examination**
  - JVD with or without Kussmaul sign (see Table 4-2), hepatomegaly, TR murmur (reflects RV failure)
  - **ECG:** low-voltage AVB and RBBB (most common in sarcoidosis)
  - **Chest x-ray:** RV increased (see Figure 4-2A and B)
  - **Echo**
    - Symmetrical wall thickening, small pericardial effusions common, speckled myocardial pattern in infiltrative diseases (particular amyloidosis), biatrial enlargement (see Figure 4-36); will differentiate from constrictive pericarditis
- **Cardiac CT and MRI**
  - May be useful for infiltrative diseases and to rule out constrictive pericarditis (which is surgically correctable)
- **Cardiac catheterization**
  - Increased right ventricular diastolic pressure (RVDP) with increased LVDP with "dip-plateau" pattern
  - **RV biopsy** may be of use in infiltrative diseases. *Rectal or fat pad biopsy is preferred if amyloidosis is suspected.*
- **Triage**
  - Consider admission to monitored bed if patient is hypotensive or if arrhythmia is present or suspected.
- **Therapy**
  - Treat primary condition if present. Salt restriction with or without *cautious* diuresis. *Do not use digitalis in amyloidosis.* RCMP increases sensitivity. May use in other RCMP to control VR. Avoid elevated heart rate. Use anticoagulates, particularly for eosinophilic RCMP.

HCMP (a.k.a. HOCM and idiopathic hypertrophic subaortic stenosis [IHSS])

Because obstruction is not always present, HCMP is a more appropriate term. Although HOCM is most well-known as a leading cause of sudden cardiac death in young athletes, it should be distinguished from athletic heart syndrome ("athlete's heart"; symmetrical wall thickness ≤12 mm although 16 mm has been reported; LV diastolic dimension ≥50 mm, normal LV relaxation). Also differentiate from second-degree LVH caused by systemic hypertension or aortic stenosis (AS) hypotension; hypovolemia may precipitate outflow obstruction in second-degree LVH.

- **Etiology:** two major forms
  - **Autosomal dominant (HOCM/IHSS)**
    - Mutation in 1 of 9 sarcomeric genes, most common heavy chain β-myosin locus 14, q11, resulting in myocardial fiber disarray resulting in asymmetrical septal hypertrophy (may be symmetrical), usually with outflow obstruction.
  - **Apical**
  - Usually nonobstructive (in 25% of Japanese patients with HCMP; a.k.a. Yamaguchi syndrome or "ace of spades heart"); less common in non-Japanese populations; diastolic dysfunction and atrial fibrillation are most common presentation.
- **HOCM** presents with decreased LV diastolic compliance, which appears as increased "stiffness," created by impaired LV relaxation with increased LVDP and decreased LVED volume with LV outflow tract obstruction (OTO), second-degree asymmetrical septal hypertrophy and MVR. Second-degree systolic anterior motion of the elongated anterior leaflet of the mitral valve also contributes to OTO. The degree of MVR is directly related to OTO. Hypovolemia precipitates OTO and leads to preload dependency.
- **Symptoms:** Dyspnea, increased excretion, syncope, arrhythmias, angina, *sudden death* may occur.
- **Physical examination**
  - Brisk carotid upstroke, systolic crescendo and decrescendo murmur at left sternal border, increases with Valsalva test (see Table 4-1); late-peaking holosystolic (MVR) murmur at the apex (see Table 4-1)
- **ECG:** LVH with septal Q waves in leads I, aVL, and V_5-V_6; atrial fibrillation and VT on Holter or loop monitor are common.
- **Echo (TTE)**
  - IVS thickness usually more than 1.5 mm (can be up to 60 mm!); IVS and postwall thickness more than 1.3 mm predicts genetic defect in 79% of patients (Figure 4-38). Elongated anterior leaflet of mitral valve with systolic anterior motion, Doppler during systole in the left ventricular outflow tract (Figures 4-37 and 4-38) demonstrate late peaking pattern and "jagged knife"-like pattern (subaortic gradient).
  - Apical variant: IVS hypertrophy toward the apex gives "ace of spades" appearance.
- **MRI**
  - Evaluation of patients suspected of having HOCM to diagnose phenotypic expression and possibly identify the subset of patients at risk of sudden cardiac death.
- **Cardiac catheterization**
  - Subaortic pressure gradient defines severity of obstruction; Brockenbrough-Braunwald-Morrow sign (a.k.a. HOCM sign), decreased pulse pressure (systolic pressure, aortic pressure), and pressure gradient postextrasystole.
- **Triage:** admit patient to monitored bed because of sudden death risk
- **Therapy**
  - Avoid hypovolemia and tachycardia (give fluids, avoid hot environments and strenuous exercise). Echo follow up. Genetic counseling with echo and MRI screening for first-degree relatives). Drug therapy: beta-blocker, CCB (drug grades II, IV; see Table 4-10); if arrhythmias, prefer disopyramide and sotalol (drug grades IA, III; see Table 4-10). Negative inotrope and chromotrope effects increase LVD volume.
  - *No digitalis in HOCM*; give with caution in apical variant; *diuretics with extreme caution* in both (because of potential to increase pressure gradient).
  - If pressure gradient is greater than 50 mm Hg, consider septal ETOH ablation, then surgical myectomy. *(Neither reduce VT.)* If failure of both, then consider cardiac transplantation in suitable candidates.

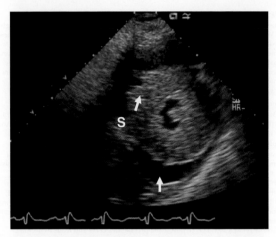

Figure 4-36   Echocardiogram in parasternal short axis view of a patient with restrictive cardiomyopathy (cardiac amyloidosis). Notice symmetrical nature of the left ventricle wall thickening, small pericardial effusion, and speckled (S) myocardial pattern. See color insert.

- **ICD** for recurrent VT (ACC/AHA class IC) and possibly sudden death prophylaxis in high-risk mutations (http://circ.ahajournals.org/content/97/13/1325.full [accessed July 5, 2011])
- **Other CMPs and special considerations**
  - **LV noncompaction:** (rare CMP) developmental arrest of LV compaction with resulting in communication of blood-filled sinusoidal recesses and endocardium (VT and CHF are common presentations); echo is usually diagnostic.

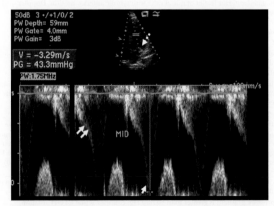

Figure 4-37   Pulsed-wave Doppler interrogation of left ventricle outflow tract of the patient with hypertrophic obstructive cardiomyopathy. Note late peaking (single white arrow) and a "jugged knife" appearance (double arrows).

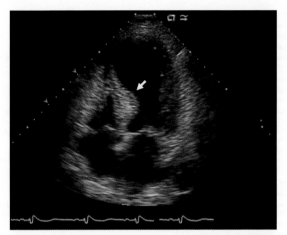

Figure 4-38 Echocardiogram (echo) in apical 4-chamber view of a patient with hypertrophic cardiomyopathy (HCMP). Note intraventricular septal thickness greatly exceeds free wall thickness. Two-dimensional echo differential diagnosis between acquired and congenital HCMP is difficult. See color insert.

- Arrhythmogenic right ventricular dysplasia (AVRD) is caused by autosomal dominant genetic defects of myocardial desmosomes. Most common in Italy. Of individuals with ARVD, 80% present with syncope or sudden cardiac death and 76% have LV involvement.
- **ECG:** epsilon wave
- **Treatment:** catheter ablation, ICD

Myocarditis

- **Etiology:** Most commonly viral, retroviral (HIV included), Lyme disease
  - May progress to DCMP (see above)
- **Symptoms:** fever, palpitations, CHF
- **Biomarkers** may be elevated.
- **Chest x-ray:** cardiomegaly
- **ECG:** ST-T changes
- **Echo:** decreased LVEF, sometimes pericardial effusion
- **RV biopsy** of questionable value; course unpredictable.
- **Triage**
  - Admit patient to monitored bed if arrhythmias or decreased LVEF. Consider ICU/ CCU if LVEF less than 30%, hemodynamically unstable, high-grade arrhythmias or if RV biopsy is considered.
- **Treatment**
  - Treat CHF, consider steroids plus azathioprine. If relentless rapid progression to extremely decreased LVEF consider cardiac transplantation in selected patients (but even then may reverse spontaneously).

Heart Failure

Definition: failure of the heart to meet body's metabolic demands (a.k.a. perfusion failure of cardiac origin)

Classification

- **Acute:** Pump failure leads to cardiogenic shock, acute pulmonary edema (Table 4-7)
- **Chronic:** CHF
- **Systolic:** decreased LV systolic performance (decreased LVEF)
- **Diastolic:** increased LVED volume, decreased LV diastolic compliance gives increased LV "stiffness"

Symptomatic (arbitrarily) May Distinguish

- **Right sided:** peripheral edema, ascites and hepatomegaly predominate
- **Left sided:** pulmonary edema predominates
  - *Caution:* Both ventricular systole and diastole are not a "squeeze/dilatation" but more of the spiral "wringing/unwringing of the wet towel" motion with difficult mathematical modeling. Present evaluation terminology (LVEF, LVED volume, etc.) are inadequate to describe physiologic events during systole and diastole.
  - **Newer echo** techniques, such as tissue Doppler and specular analysis are beyond spectrum of this book. For now, systolic and particular diastolic heart failure should be considered poorly understood.

Acute Pump Failure (patients are usually euvolemic)

- **Cardiogenic shock**
  - Severe LV failure with hypotension and oliguria less than 30 cc/h. MAP less than 60 mm Hg (MAP = [(2 × diastolic BP] + systolic BP] ÷ 3); usually from AMI, severe viral DCMP, end-stage valvular heart disease.
- **Precipitating events** ischemia, AMI.
- **Triage** to the ICU/CCU
- **Therapy**
  - **Monitoring:** Consider **cardiac output monitoring (normal limits:** 4.0–8.0 L/min). Pulmonary artery catheterization is invasive and does not improve survival (see the pulmonary artery catheter tutorial at http://emedicine.medscape.com/article/1824547-overview [accessed July 5, 2011]). NICOM, PiCCO and LiDCO cardiac sensor systems and TEE are minimally invasive; surface **echo**, TTE, and transesophageal Doppler are noninvasive. *At present, monitoring strategy largely depends on technology availability and institutional choice.*
    - **Arterial line (a.k.a. A-line)** placement for intraarterial blood pressure monitoring and central venous catheter (**a.k.a. CVP-line**) placement for central venous pressure (CVP) monitoring.
  - Systemic vascular resistance (SVR) calculations may help with management.
  - SVR = [(MAP − CVP) × 80] ÷ CO (normal limits: 800–1400 dyne × sec/cm^5, where CO is cardiac output.
  - Cardiac output and SVR may be indexed to body surface area.
    - **Increased SVR:** consider **vasodilators** (ie, nitroprusside)
    - **Decreased SVR:** consider **vasoconstrictors** (ie, norepinephrine, phenylephrine) (see Table 4-11)
  - Maintain cardiac output with inotropic drugs (see Table 4-11)
  - Oxygen by mask; if pulmonary edema coexists, use noninvasive positive pressure ventilation or intubation (positive pressure mechanical ventilation). *Note: Positive pressure mechanical ventilation may decrease MAP; keep airway pressure less than 25 mm Hg.*
  - If STEMI or ACS occurred less than 4 hours previously, perform rescue PCI
  - **Consider IABP** counterpulsation.
  - **Bridging LVAD:** if patient is a suitable candidate for cardiac transplantation.

Acute Pulmonary Edema (APE)

- **Etiology**
  - Usually AMI (*APE is AMI and acute ischemia until proven otherwise*), end-stage valvular heart disease, acute valvular disease (IWMI, SBE), myocarditis, hypertensive emergency end-stage CMP
- **Precipitating events**
  - Myocardial ischemia, AMI, renal failure (RF), therapy noncompliance, salt-restriction noncompliance (particularly in RF), arrhythmias, drugs (*nonsteroidal antiinflammatory*

TABLE 4-11. DRUGS COMMONLY USED IN ACUTE HEART (PUMP) FAILURE

Drug/Action	Dosage	Special Comments
Vasodilators[a]		
NTG	5–100 µg/min	May improve coronary flow (V > A)
Nitroprusside	0.5–10 µg/kg/min	*Thiocyanide toxicity* in decreased renal function; RF (V = A)
Nesiritide	2 µg/kg IVB, 0.01 µg/kg/min	Hypotension, renal disfunction (A > V)
Positive inotropic agents		
Dobutamine	2–10 µg/kg/min	CO increased, MAP may not increase
Dopamine	2–20 µg/kg/min and up	MAP increase dose-dependent action 2.5–10 positive inotrope, >10 vasoconstrictor
Milrinone	50 mg/kg IVB over 10 min, 0.375–0.75 µg/kg/min	PDEI Watch for VT
Amrinone	0.75 mg/kg IVB over 5 min, 5–15 µg/kg/min	Positive inotrope and vasodilator (PDEI) watch Plt count for decrease
Adrenergic (α, β) vasoconstrictors		
Norepinephrine	1–40 µg/min and up	$\alpha_1 > \beta_1$ Consider with caution for decreased SVR
Epinephrine	2–20 µg/min	$\alpha_{1,2} + \beta_{1,2}$
Phenylephrine	10–300 µg/min	α_1 consider with tachycardia
Vasopressin[b]	0.01–0.04 Units/min	Use IVB in ACLS only

A, arterial; ACLS, advanced cardiac life support; CO, cardiac output; IVB, intravenous bolus; MAP, mean arterial pressure; NTG, nitroglycerin; PDEI, phosphodiesterase inhibitor; Plt, platelet; RF, renal failure; SVR, systemic vascular resistance; V, venous.
[a]Consider if decreased SVR; use caution in hypotensive patients by combining with positive inotrope.
[b]Vasopressin may potentiate action of adrenergic vasoconstrictors.

drug [NSAID], CCB, beta-blocker), ETOH, sepsis and/or fever, anemia, thyrotoxicosis, PE, SBE, acute myocarditis.
- **Symptoms**: Dyspnea, tachycardia, tachypnea
- **Physical examination**
  - JVD, S_3 and S_4 (summation) gallop (S_4 absent in atrial fibrillation), with rales listen for new systolic murmurs (see Tables 4-1, 4-2)
  - **Chest x-ray:** pulmonary edema (rule out pulmonary causes of dyspnea)
  - **ECG** to rule out (in) ischemia or AMI
  - **Echo** to assess LV function and valvular apparatuses
- **Triage:** Admit patient to ICU/CCU
- **Therapy:** Head elevation, leg dangling if possible, loop diuretics (with caution in hypotensive patient, increase dose in RF, consider continuous renal replacement therapy [ultrafiltration] if creatinine clearance <15 cc/min)

- **NTG** (preload reduction), consider positive inotrope if decreased MAP (see Table 4-11).
- **Oxygen** by mask, **mechanical ventilation** (noninvasive positive pressure ventilation or intubation + positive pressure mechanical ventilation (action similar to NTG; mechanical preload reduction because of increased intrathoracic pressure)
- **Morphine** (reduces air hunger)

Chronic Heart Failure is CHF

- Most patients have hypervolemia (kidney salt retention in response to decreased cardiac output).
- Etiology
  - Cardiac causes: CAD, DCMP, valvular heart disease (not MVS), hypertension, congenital heart disease, RCMP, HOCM, pericardial disease, hypertensive heart disease, MVS-diastolic
- **Precipitating events** (see APE)
  - **Symptoms:** See APE; also fatigue, orthopnea, paroxysmal nocturnal dyspnea, peripheral edema.
- **Physical examination**
  - Dullness to chest percussion, edema, hepatomegaly, ascites
- **Chest x-ray**
  - Indicated for cardiomegaly, pulmonary vascular redistribution, pleural effusion (R > L more common), Kerley B lines (see Figure 4-2).
- **ECG:** LVH, arrhythmias, AVB, decreased voltage (DCMP), "sepal Qs"(HOCM)
- **Laboratory test results:** BNP more than 100 pg/mL in CHF (if persistent in spite of therapy, then increased poor prognosis). Poor prognosis with elevated blood urea nitrogen (BUN), creatinine, and liver function levels (end organ damage leading to RF, cardiac cirrhosis) and decreased serum glucose, thyroxine, thyroid-stimulating hormone, lipid profile, and serum sodium levels.

New York Heart Association (NYHA) Functional Classification

- **Symptoms: shortness of breath or angina, palpitation, fatigue**
  Class I: Above symptoms with above ordinary activity
  Class II: Above symptoms with ordinary activity, walking more than 100 m, climbing stairs and so forth
  Class III: Above symptoms with minimal activity, walking distances 20 to 100 m; comfortable only at rest
  Class IV: Above symptoms at rest (mostly bedbound)
- Echo
  - To assess LV function (LVEF), cardiac output, diastolic filling, valvular disease; RWMA indicates CAD, pericardial disease (ACC/AHA class IC)
- **CT, CTA, MRI:** may help to discover CMP
- **Cardiac catheterization** (ventriculography), coronary angiography for CAD (ACC/AHA class IIC)
- **ETT** with echo may rule out CAD.
  - Cardiopulmonary ETT helps to establish timing for cardiac transplantation in advanced CHF.
- **Triage**
  - Admit patient to monitored bed or ICU/CCU if mechanical ventilation is considered or hemodynamically unstable.
- **Therapy**
  - Nondrug
    - Restricted salt intake (<2 g/d) (ACC/AHA class IC), fluid restriction, *no NSAIDs,* prescribed exercise program (ACC/AHA class IB), influenza and pneumococcal vaccine, blood pressure control, therapy lipid disorders (ACC/AHA class IA), glucose control in patients with diabetes (ACC/AHA class IC)
  - **Drug Therapy (Table 4-12)**
  - **ACEI** in NYHA class II to IV and decreased LVEF (ACC/AHA class IA)
  - **ARB** in ACEI-intolerant patients and decreased LVEF (ACC/AHA class IA)
  - **Beta-blocker** in all stable patients and decreased LVEF unless contraindicated (ACC/AHA class IA)

- Addition of aldosterone antagonist (spironolactone [**Aldactone**] 25 mg PO/d) in selected patients with NYHA class II to III and decreased LVEF, who have preserved renal function and normal potassium concentration. Creatinine 2.5 mg/dL or less in men and 2.0 mg/dL or less in women, potassium less than 5.0 mEq/dL (ACC/AHA class IB).
- **Hydralazine plus nitrates** in ACEI- and ARB-intolerant patients with NYHA class III to IV function (may be more efficacious in African Americans [ACC/AHA class IIC])
- **Loop and thiazide diuretics** may offer symptomatic relief but no survival benefit.
- **Antiarrhythmic agents:** Only amiodarone and dofetilide have been shown *not to adversely affect survival*
- **Digoxin** guided by serum levels may reduce hospitalizations, but no survival benefit
- Consider **anticoagulation** if LV thrombus present, LV aneurysm (large akinetic aneurysms are located by echo), DCMP RCMP (particularly eosinophilic)
- For IV medications useful in CHF, see Tables 4-11 and 4-12; for beta-blocker use, see Tables 4-10 and 4-12

TABLE 4-12. DRUGS USEFUL IN THERAPY OF CHF ARTERIAL AND VENOUS VASODILATORS

Drug/Group	Dose (mg PO, unless specified)	Special Comments
ACEI, V = A, group side effects, angioedema, K⁺ increased, azotemia = decreased GFR, cough, A = V		
Captopril	6.25–50 TID	Leukopenia
Enalapril/Enalaprilet	2.5–10 BID	Decrease or discontinue diuretics
Lisinopril	5–40 TID	Longer half-life; decrease or discontinue diuretics
ARB, K⁺ increased, azotemia corresponds to decreased GFR, rhabdomyolysis, angioedema alternative to ACEI, A = V		
Losartan	25–100 Q day	Noninferior to ACEI; consider adding to ACEI in patients with diabetes
Valsartan	40–160 BID	
Beta-blocker (also see Table 4-10)		
Carvedilol	3.125 TID, double Q 2 weeks to 25 BID	Beta-blocker side effects
Nitrates: Drug tolerance develops (NTG see Table 4-10)		
Isosorbide dinitrate (V)	10–40 TID	Nitrates + hydralazine inferior to ACEI
Hydralazine (A)	50–200 TID	Drug-induced lupus, tachycardia, angina
Loop diuretics No survival benefit combine with thiazides and metolazone		
Furosemide	20–120 PO or IV	↓ K⁺, hypovolemia, hypotension
Bumetanide	0.25–1 PO or IV	Consider in P/Ts, decreased GFR

A; arterial; ACEI, angiotensin-converting enzyme inhibitor; ARB, angiotensin receptor blocker; BID, twice daily; CHF, congestive heart failure; GFR, glomerular filtration rate; NTG, nitroglycerin; PO, orally; Q, every; TID, 3 times daily; V; venous vasodilation.

- **Pacemaker therapy**
- ICD: Patients with NYHA class II to III function and LVEF less than 30%, undergoing optimal medical therapy and reasonable expectation of survival more than 1 year (ACC/AHA class IB).
- In ischemic CMP (ACC/AHA class IA)
- **Biventricular pacing** (resynchronization if LVEF ≤ 35%, sinus rhythm; NYHA class III or ambulatory class IV with optimal medical therapy and QRS duration >0.12 msec unless contraindicated [ACC/AHA class IA]).
- **Refractory end-stage CHF**
  - Therapy for acute pump failure. **Options for end-of-life care** and information about the option to inactivate defibrillation should be discussed with the patient and family when severe symptoms persist despite all recommended therapies (ACC/AHA class IC); positive inotropes may increase *mortality*, but in controlled environment can be used for palliation.
  - **LVAD: cardiac transplantation** in eligible patients
  - **Prognosis:** see Seattle Heart Failure Model at http://depts.washington.edu/shfm/app.php (accessed July 5, 2011)

Heart Failure with Preserved LVEF

- Diastolic dysfunction with decreased LV diastolic compliance corresponds to increased LV "stiffness."
- **Echo** is diagnostic; use coronary angiography if CAD is suspected.
- **Triage** as if CHF because of similar prognosis.
- **Therapy**
  - Because of absence of controlled clinical trials, management is based on control of factors known to impede ventricular relaxation. *No mortality improvement data.*
  - Control systolic and diastolic hypertension (ACC/AHA class IA)
  - Treat CAD (ACC/AHA class IA)
  - Prescribe diuretics to control pulmonary congestion and peripheral edema (ACC/AHA class IA). Use with caution so that LVED volume is not decreased.
  - ACEI, **ARB** (possible beneficial survival in 1 randomized study), beta-blocker, or CCB might be effective to minimize symptoms of heart failure (ACC/AHA class IIC).
- **Prognosis:** Mortality similar to those with decreased LVEF.

  For ACC/AHA practice guidelines for CHF evaluation and therapy, see http://circ.ahajournals.org/cgi/content/full/112/12/1825 (accessed July 5, 2011)

Valvular Heart Disease

For ACC/AHA guidelines for evaluation and therapy of patients with valvular heart disease, see http://www.scribd.com/doc/64904410/1/INTRODUCTION (accessed July 5, 2011)

Mitral Stenosis (Figure 4-39)

- **Etiology**
  - Most commonly **rheumatic fever** with history of rheumatic fever in foreign-born and *usually without in U.S.-born* patients.
  - **Functional** MVS because of LA myxoma, thrombus, or large SBE vegetation. Clot with prosthetic valve dysfunction after mitral valve replacement. Rarely caused by mitral annulus calcifications, Hunter and Hurler diseases, malignant carcinoid, ergot alkaloids therapy, or extrinsic LA compression by mediastinal tumor or abscess. *With pure MVS, SBE is uncommon.*
- **Symptoms**
  - Occurs in the fourth decade of life (second decade in foreign-born is not uncommon). Dyspnea on exertion, APE, atrial fibrillation embolic events (LA thrombus), frank hemoptysis is uncommon, but blood streaks in the sputum are caused by pulmonary hypertension (PH), pulmonary artery diastolic pressure has to be greater than left atrial pressure (see Table 4-1).
  - **Precipitating events:** Fever, anemia, tachycardia (commonly atrial fibrillation with increased VR), pregnancy for APE.

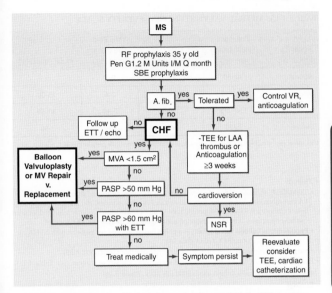

Figure 4-39 Approach to the patient with mitral valve stenosis. A. fib., atrial fibrillation; CHF, congestive heart failure; ETT, exercise tolerance test; I/M, intramuscular; LAA, left atrial abnormality; MS, mitral stenosis; MV, mitral valve; MVA, mitral valve area; NSR, normal sinus rhythm; PASP, positive airway systolic pressure; Pen G, penicillin G; Q, every; RF, renal failure; SBE, subacute bacterial endocarditis; TEE, transesophageal echocardiogram; VR, ventricular rate.

- **Physical examination** (see Tables 4-1, 4-2)
  - RV lift, loud sometimes palpable S_1, opening snap (see Figure 4-1). S_2-A_2 opening snap shortening (<80 msec) signifies worse MVS (increased LA/LV [transvalvular pressure gradient]) (see Figure 4-1, interrupted line and arrow). Low pitch middiastolic rumbling murmur at the apex increases prior to systole and corresponds to presystolic accentuation (absent in atrial fibrillation) duration correlates with increased LA/LV pressure gradient. (see Heart Sounds and Cardiac Arrhythmias at http://www.blaufuss.org [accessed July 5, 2011]).
  - **Chest x-ray:** Increased LA with straight left heart border. Later in disease with RAE corresponds to increased biatrial enlargement; increased RV, Kerley B lines (see Figure 4-2A and B)
  - **ECG:** LAE "p- mitrale" (see Figure 4-7) if in sinus, but atrial fibrillation is common (≈50% of patients)
  - **Echo**
    - **TEE** is often diagnostic; **TEE** is recommended for prosthetic valve and suboptimal TTE images and to assess for LA thrombus. LAE (possible spontaneous contrast ["smoke"] in LA). Mitral valve (MV) leaflets thickened more than 3 mm. Diastolic doming of the anterior leaflet "hokey stick" pattern is characteristic of RF-MVS. Doppler estimation of MV area by pressure half-time (most common) and transvalvular pressure gradient to assess MVS severity (Table 4-13). Tricuspid regurgitation (TR) correlates with RVSP and positive airway pressure is used to assess PH.
- **Triage:** Admit patient to monitored bed if in CHF or newly diagnosed and to ICU/CCU if APE present.

TABLE 4-13. MITRAL VALVE STENOSIS SEVERITY SCALE

Severity Criteria	Pressure Half-time (msec)	MVA (cm²)	TVG End Diastolic (mm Hg)	PASP (mm Hg)
Normal	30–60	4–6	0–2	<25
Mild	90–150	1.5–2.5	2–6	25–30
Moderate	150–219	1–1.5	7–10	30–50
Severe	≥220	<1	>10	>50

MVA, mitral valve area; PASP, positive airway systolic pressure; TVG, transvalvular pressure gradient.

- **Therapy**
  - **Treat CHF:** anticoagulation therapy in atrial fibrillation, history of thromboembolism, LA thrombus or LA diameter (by echo ≥5 cm; LA volume index ≥60 mL/m² may be a better indicator). RF and SBE prophylaxis. If atrial fibrillation is poorly tolerated, initiate cardioversion after 3 weeks or more of anticoagulation therapy; or TEE for clot.
  - **Percutaneous balloon valvuloplasty** is a preferred procedure for patients with NYHA class II to IV function (ACC/AHA class IA).
  - **Surgery:** MV repair; replacement if repair is not possible (see Figure 4-39).
- **Prognosis** depends on severity and candidacy for valvuloplasty or surgery (see Table 4-13).

Mitral valve regurgitation/insufficiency (MVR aka MR) (Figure 4-40)

- **Etiology**
  - **Chronic MVR**
    - Most common etiology: mitral valve prolapse (MVP) is myxomatous degeneration Because of pathological connective tissue weakening Second-degree myxomatous degeneration associated with systemic diseases is more extensive and involves other heart valves. RF (33%) usually with MVS, congenital; LV annular dilatation (ie, DCMP), HOCM caused by systolic anterior motion, mitral annulus calcification.
  - **Acute MVR**
    - Papillary muscle dysfunction, Iwma INFERIOR Wall Motion Abnormality (IWMA), chordae tendinea (chordal) rupture traumatic, first- or second-degree SBE.
- **Symptoms**
  - **Acute MVR** leads to APE, cardiogenic shock (Table 4-14)
  - **Chronic MVR** leads to progressive dyspnea on exertion, atrial fibrillation, PH.
- **Physical examination** (see Figure 4-1)
  - Hyperdynamic posterior myocardial infarct. Brisk carotid upstroke; decreased S_1, split S_2 and S_3.
  - High-pitched holosystolic murmur at apex moving to axilla, decreased with Valsalva test, increased with handgrip (see Table 4-4). Brief diastolic rumble (see Heart Sounds and Cardiac Arrhythmias at http://www.blaufuss.org).
  - *Acute MVR may have few or no physical findings, other than those of acute heart failure.*
  - **Chest x-ray:** Chronic shows increased LA and LV; pulmonary vascular redistribution (see Figure 4-3).
    - Acute: APE
  - **ECG:** LAE, LVH, atrial fibrillation is common. Figure 4-3, 4-5 Pattern F.
- **Echo**
  - Assess status of MV apparatus, LA, LV dimensions; *LVEF is falsely elevated* in MVR because of "pop-up" phenomenon (regurgitation into LA during systole [ie, LVEF <60% is a significant decrease in MVR]); Doppler regurgitant fraction, colored Doppler regurgitant jet area (RJA) and relationship to the LA (ie, LAW: Length, Area, Width). Effective regurgitant orifice; pulmonary vein (PV) systolic flow reversal.
  - TEE is superior to TTE for diagnosing papillary muscle dysfunction and chordal rupture.

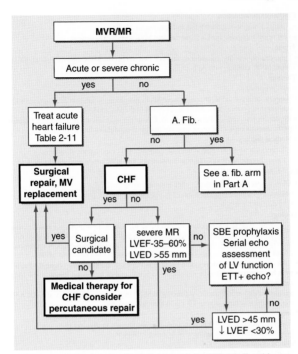

Figure 4-40   Approach to the patient with mitral valve regurgitation. A.Fib. and a.fib., atrial fibrillation; CHF, congestive heart failure; ETT, exercise tolerance test; LV, left ventricle; LVED, left ventricular end diastole; LVEF, left ventricular ejection fraction; MR, mitral valve regurgitation; MV, mitral valve; SBE, subacute bacterial endocarditis.

TABLE 4-14. MITRAL VALVE REGURGITATION SEVERITY SCALE

Severity Criteria	RJA (cm²)	RJA/LV (%)	ERO (mm²)	Reversal of PV Flow	LVEF (%) → LV Dysfunction[b]
Mild	<4	<20	<10	none	>60
Moderate	4–8	20–40	10–35[a]	?	30–60
Severe	>8	>40	>35	+	<30

ERO, effective regurgitant orifice; LV, left ventricular; LVEF, left ventricular ejection fraction; PV, pulmonary vein; RJA, regurgitant jet area.
[a]25–35 mm² is moderately severe ERO.
[b]LVED >45 mm is indicative of severe LV dysfunction.

- **Cardiac catheterization**
  - "Giant" V waves (suggestive but not specific for MVR)
  - Left ventriculogram for LV diameter and MVR severity assessment
- **Triage**
  - Depends on severity; consider monitored bed, if chronic MVR with CHF; ICU/CCU for acute MVR, chronic with APE
- **Therapy**
  - SBE prophylaxis
  - **Surgery** for acute MVR, chronic severe MVR, symptomatic patients or progressive LV dysfunction (*prior to development of significant CHF* [ACC/AHA class IB])
  - **Repair** is preferred to MV replacement. Consider minimally invasive surgery. Consider **percutaneous repair** for those who are marginal candidates for sternotomy.
  - **Medical therapy**
    - Surgery for acute MVR as acute heart failure (APE, cardiogenic shock)
    - Treat chronic MVR as CHF (see Table 4-12). For MVR treatment, see Figure 4-40.

Mitral Valve Prolapse (MVP)

- Barlow syndrome (a.k.a. systolic click-murmur syndrome)
- Definition: posterior displacement of any portion of the MV leaflet beyond mitral annular plane during LV systole.
- **Etiology**
  - "Classical" MVP (a.k.a. myxomatous MVP): redundant leaflets perhaps caused by excess of dermatan sulfate; chordal redundancy; and lengthening. Familial first-degree or associated with connective tissue diseases (Marfan, Ehlers-Danlos, Stickler syndromes; pseudoxanthoma elasticum; osteogenesis imperfecta). Often results in MVR.
  - "Nonclassical" MVP: (more common in women) likely *normal* variant (usually diagnosed by echo (superior leaflet displacement) with minimal or unrelated symptoms; seldom significant MVR.
  - Secondary or hemodynamic or functional MVP: in patients with CAD, CMP, RF, ASD, left-to-right shunting, severe TR (as in Ebstein anomaly).
- **Symptoms**
  - For classical MVP, see MVR, nonclassical asymptomatic or atypical chest pain palpitations. Secondary because of first-degree illness.
- **Physical examination**
  - May be associated with scoliosis, pectus excavatum carinatum; mid-late systolic click (sudden chordal tension) medium- to high-pitch late systolic murmur (MVR); earlier click with increased murmur on Valsalva test (see Table 4-2) (see Heart Sounds and Cardiac Arrhythmias at http://www.blaufuss.org [accessed July 5, 2011]).
  - **ECG:** T waves flat, inverted or biphasic in II, III and aVF.
  - **Echo**
    - TTE is diagnostic for MV leaflet prolapse (>2 mm beyond annular plane) in 2 or more standard views; scalloped appearance of MV, leaflet thickness more than 5 mm in PLAX view in diastole.
  - **Cardiac catheterization**
    - MVP with severe MVR requiring surgery, otherwise unnecessary
- **Triage**
  - Usually does not require admission; requires admission to the ICU /CCU if acute MVR develops
- **Therapy**
  - SBE prophylaxis is *not recommended*. Anticoagulation or ASA in concurring atrial fibrillation, if indicated see Figure 4-32; beta-blocker if palpitations with corresponding arrhythmia (on Holter monitor).

Aortic Stenosis (AS) (Figure 4-41; Table 4-15)

- **Etiology**
  - Calcific (a.k.a. degenerative) most common in patients older than 65 years of age. Congenital (ie, bicuspid AV) in patients younger than 65 years of age. RF in less than 10% of patients.

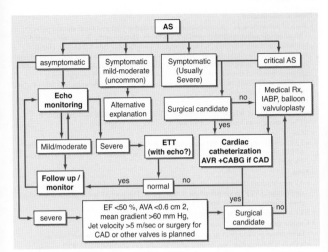

Figure 4-41   Approach to the patient with aortic stenosis (AS). AVA, aortic valve area; AVR, aortic valve replacement; CABG, coronary artery bypass graft; CAD, coronary artery disease; EF, ejection fraction; ETT, exercise tolerance test; IABP, intraaortic balloon pump; Rx, therapy.

- **Differential diagnosis:** subaortic obstruction fixed or dynamic (HOCM, subaortic membrane)
- **Symptoms**
  - CHF worse prognosis (50% of patients have 2-year mean survival without aortic valve repair); syncope (15% of patients have 3-year mean survival without aortic valve repair); angina (35% of patients have 5-year mean survival without aortic valve repair).
  - Acquired von Willebrand syndrome is seen in 21% of patients with severe AS (see http://www.nejm.org/doi/full/10.1056/NEJMoa022831 [accessed July 5, 2011]).
  - *Right heart failure is an ominous sign.*

TABLE 4-15. AORTIC STENOSIS SEVERITY SCALE

Severity Criteria	ASJV (msec)	AVMG (mm Hg)	AVA (cm²)	LVEF (%)
Normal	2–2.5	<10	>2	NL
Mild	<3	<30	1.6–2	NL
Mild-moderate			1.3–1.6	NL
Moderate	3–4	30–50	1–1.3	NL
Moderate-severe			0.7–1	NL
Severe	>4	>50	< 0.7	± mild ↓
Critical	May decrease 2 degrees with decreased LVEF	May decrease 2 degrees with decreased LVEF	<0.7	<50

ASJV, aortic stenosis jet peak velocity; AVA, aortic valve area; AVMG, aortic valve mean gradient; LVEF, left ventricular ejection fraction; NL, normal limits.

MEDICAL SPECIALTIES

- **Physical examination**
  - Narrow pulse pressure, carotid pulsus parvus et tardus (delayed small carotid pulse with anacrotic notch indicates severity), LV heave. Decreased S_2 (A_2) or unexpected splitting (indicates severity), S_4 (decreased LV compliance) (see Table 4-1). Harsh systolic crescendo- decrescendo murmur at right upper sternal border leading to sternal notch with or without carotids. Holosystolic (MVR) murmur in AS location (Gallavardin phenomenon); AS murmur decreased on Valsalva test, increased on leg raising (opposite to HOCM) (see Table 4-1). Concomitant aortic insufficiency (AI) murmur in 30% to 50% of patients.
- **Chest x-ray**
  - AV calcifications, left atrial abnormality, LVH, and poststenotic aortic dilatation ("swimming swan" pattern) corresponds to CHF (see Figure 4-2).
- **ECG**
  - LAE in 80% of patients; LVH with strain in 85% of patients; LAD, AVB, and/or BBB in 13% of patients; atrial fibrillation uncommon (see Figure 4-3, Figure 4-5 Patterns J,K,P,R).
- **Echo**
  - AV morphology (bicuspid), calcifications, cusp separation (PSAX), rule out HOCM membrane, LVEF (poor prognosis if decreased). Doppler AV mean gradient by AS jet peak velocity (ASJV), AV area (AVA).
- **ETT** to assess contractile reserve
- **Cardiac catheterization**
  - Determines peak-to-peak gradient (mean gradient – ∫AVA (by Gorlin formula).
  - AVA (cm^2) = (cardiac output mL/min ÷ systolic ejection gradient)/(43.3 × mean pressure gradient mm Hg)
  - Assess for concomitant CAD.
- **Therapy**
  - SBE prophylaxis.
  - **AV replacement**
    - AV replacement for symptomatic AS (ACC/AHA class IA); for asymptomatic critical or severe AS with ASJV greater than 5 msec; for AS that is moderate, moderate-severe, or moderate if CABG planned for concomitant CAD, other valvular or thoracic aortic surgery.
  - **Balloon valvuloplasty**
    - Bridging to AV replacement or destination (disappointing results) if poor surgical candidate.
  - **Percutaneous AV replacement**
  - **Ross procedure**
    - Patient's pulmonic valve is transplanted to the aortic position with PV replacement with human homograft in very selective patients (mostly children) and in selected centers.
  - **Drugs**
    - *Avoid drugs that increase transvalvular gradient* if possible (vasodilators), positive inotropes; and if LVEF is dramatically decreased, use beta-blocker and *cautious* diuretics for CHF. Forced "therapeutic minimalist" approach, IABP bridging to AV replacement (see Figure 4-41).

Aortic Insufficiency (AI) (Figure 4-42)

- AI is aortic regurgitation; three-quarters of patients are men
- **Etiology**
  - First-degree valve disease
  - RF usually with concomitant MV disease or AS, bicuspid AV, SBE, SLE, RA, percutaneous AS valvuloplasty, sinus of Valsalva aneurysm, perimembranous VSD, trauma, drugs (amphetamines and phentermine and fenfluramine [PHEN-FEN]).
  - Second-degree caused by aortic diseases, hypertension, aortic aneurysm, or type A dissection, Marfan syndrome, mucopolysaccharidoses, ankylosing spondylitis, syphilis, Takayasu disease, reactive arthritis, or giant cell arteritis.
- **Symptoms**
  - **Acute AI** (ie, trauma SBE, type A dissection, etc.) leads to acute pump failure, APE, cardiogenic shock (physical findings can be spare; high index of suspicion is key).
  - **Chronic AI** that is asymptomatic leads to CHF, palpitations, and angina (Table 4-16).

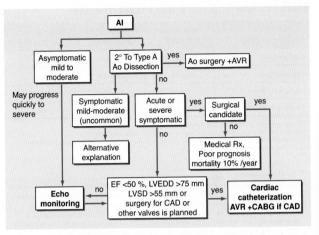

Figure 4-42   Approach to the patient with aortic insufficiency (AI). Ao, aorta; AVR, aortic valve replacement; CABG, coronary artery bypass graft; CAD, coronary artery disease; EF, ejection fraction; LVEDD, left ventricle end-diastolic diameter; LVSD, left ventricle systolic dimension; Rx, therapy.

TABLE 4-16. SUMMARY OF CLASSICAL SIGNS IN CHRONIC AORTIC INSUFFICIENCY

Signs	
Observational signs	
Muller	Uvula pulsation
Quincke	Blanching and flushing of the nail bed
De Musset	Head bobbing with heart beat
Landolfi	Systolic contraction and diastolic dilation of the pupil
Palpation signs	
Rosenbach	Liver pulsation
Gerhard	Spleen pulsation
Corrigan	Rapid rise and fall of carotid artery pulse. Watson water-hammer pulse same on the limb artery.
Auscultation signs	
Taube	Double sound when femoral artery compressed distally
Duroziez	Double bruit on femoral artery if compressed with stethoscope
Hill	Popliteal artery systolic BP; brachial systolic BP >60 mm Hg

BP, blood pressure.

TABLE 4-17. AORTIC INSUFFICIENCY SEVERITY SCALE

Severity Criteria	RJA (% of LVOT)	Pressure Half-Time (msec)	Regurgitant Fraction (%)
Mild grade 1+	<4	>500	<20
Moderate 2+[a]	4–24	350–500	20–40
Moderately severe 3+	25–59	200–350	40–55
Severe 4+[b]	>60	<200	>55

LVOT, left ventricular outflow tract; RJA, regurgitant jet area.
[a]Effective regurgitant orifice (ERO) >35 mm^2 indicates significant aortic insufficiency.
[b]LV end-diastolic dimension (LVEDD) >75 mm, LV systolic dimension (LVSD) >55 mm, decreased LVEF (<50%) indicate severe disease.

- **Physical examination**
  - Displaced hyperdynamic posterior myocardial infarct, wide pulse pressure (>50% systolic or diastolic <70 mm Hg may indicate significant disease), bounding peripheral pulse, bisferiens carotid pulse. Soft S_1 (premature MV closure). Systolic ejection click (dilated aortic or bicuspid AV), S_4 caused by LVH. High-pitched, blowing diastolic decrescendo murmur (best heard with diaphragm of the stethoscope) at left sternal border (right if aortic root is dilated) with patient leaning forward at the end-expiration (see Tables 4-1, 4-2).
  - Severe AI (Table 4-17) is indicated by low pitched mid to late diastolic rumble at the apex (Austin Flint murmur, MVS-like because of premature MV closure), "cooing dove" diastolic murmur (AV perforation with SBE) (see Figure 4-1 and Table 4-1).
  - **Chest x-ray:** Cardiomegaly (may be cor bovinum), ascending aortic dilatation, or widened mediastinum (may suggest Marfan or type A dissection). "Egg shell" aortic calcifications suggest syphilis.
  - **ECG:** LVH greater than 80%, LAD (ventricular ectopic arrhythmia, VT) AVB in acute AI.
  - **Echo:** TTE: Bicuspid valve, assess severity by RJA (as percentage of LV outflow tract), by color flow in PSAX and/or pressure half-time (color-weighted Doppler) and/or regurgitant fraction by pressure wave Doppler. TEE is better choice for aortic dissection.
  - **Cardiac CTA, MRI, and MRA:** Most effective in aortic disease. Test of *choice if dissection* is suspected.
  - **Cardiac catheterization**
    - Prior to surgery and to detect CAD. Diastolic pressure equalization with severe acute AI.
- **Triage**
  - *Patients with acute AI sent to ICU/CCU; immediate consultation regarding dissection cardiothoracic surgery.*
- **Therapy**
  - **Surgical**
    - **AV replacement** for acute decompensation, acute AI, symptomatic severe AI (ACC/AHA class IB), asymptomatic severe AI with LV end-diastolic dimension greater than 55 mm and/or LVEF less than 50% (Table 4-18)
  - **Medical**
    - Acute as APE, cardiogenic shock; *no vasoconstrictors or IABP*; chronic as CHF (see Figure 4-42).

Tricuspid Stenosis

- **Etiology**
  - RF (usually with MVS), congenital, carcinoid, right atrial myxoma or thrombus, Whipple disease, Fabry disease, ergot alkaloids therapy.
- **Symptoms:** CHF right-sided symptoms predominate.
- **Physical examination**
  - Jugular venous pressure slowly descending; diastolic rumbling murmur at left sternal border, increased with inspiration (see Table 4-1)
  - **Chest x-ray:** RAE with superior vena cava enlargement (see Figure 4-2)

- **ECG:** RAE, RAD (see Figures 4-3, 4-7)
- **Echo** is diagnostic.
- **Triage:** admit patient to monitored bed if CHF; admit patient to ICU/CCU if surgery is considered.
- **Therapy:** May need surgical repair or replacement.

Tricuspid Regurgitation (TR)

- **Etiology**
  - Almost invariably second-degree to PH (caused by increased RV compliance resulting in annular dilatation).
  - Other causes: Tricuspid valve prolapse usually with MVP and SBE (in IV drug users or patients with chronic indwelling venous catheters).
  - **Acute**
    - In massive PE, presentation of cardiogenic shock. TR severity by echo correlates with pulmonary artery systolic pressure and is used to judge PE and therapy for PE.
  - **Chronic**
    - In longstanding PH, first-degree primary PH or second-degree caused by repeated PEs, obstructive sleep apnea, pulmonary disease (chronic obstructive pulmonary disease, asthma, or congenital heart disease with right-to-left shunt, pulmonic valve or infundibular pulmonary artery stenosis [incomplete tetralogy]) systolic murmur at lower left sternal border is increased with inspiration. Right-sided **symptoms** of CHF predominate. **Echo** is diagnostic and used to grade PH
- **PH severity scale (judged by TR and pulmonary artery pressure in mm Hg)**
  - Normal 18–25
  - Mild 25–40
  - Moderate 40–70
  - Severe >70
  - Eisenmenger physiology >120 or > systolic systemic blood pressure
- **Triage:** Admit patient to ICU/CCU for acute TR and chronic TR if hemodynamically unstable
- **Therapy**
  - Treat primary disease, pulmonary embolectomy/endarterectomy (if because of repeated pulmonary emboli). May need PV homograft, or cardiopulmonary transplantation (primary PH). In rare cases without PH (tricuspid valve prolapse, SBE), repair or replace tricuspid valve. Excision is an option in SBE.

Prosthetic Heart Valves-A Comparative Assessment (see Table 4-18)

- **Bioprosthetic:** tissue valves
- **Heterograft:** (xenograft) mostly porcine placed on stents or stentless (used in older patients because of degeneration), occasional bovine pericardial (placed on stents or sewing ring)
- **Homograft:** (allograft) human cadaveric (least stenosis in AV position)
- **Auto-graft:** (self-self) via Ross procedure
- **Physical examination**
  - Soft ejection murmurs are normal, any regurgitant murmur is abnormal.

TABLE 4-18. A COMPARATIVE ASSESSMENT OF BIOPROSTHETIC HEART VALVES

Advantages	Disadvantages and Complications
May avoid anticoagulation (if no risk factors)	**Degeneration ≈ 30% fail in 10 years**
Failures occur slowly	SBE, dehiscence
Homograft in pulmonary position	Stenosis degenerative or thrombotic
May be hemodynamically superior (unstented)	Perivalvular leak may cause hemolysis
May be able to visualize by TTE	Thromboembolism

SBE, subacute bacterial endocarditis; TTE, transthoracic echocardiography.

MEDICAL SPECIALTIES

- **Chest x-ray** may be able to see stent (ring).
- **Echo:** Ring shadow may interfere with images.
- **Therapy**
  - If there are risk factors (atrial fibrillation, chamber dilatation), may require anticoagulation.
  - AV position INR 2 to 3 plus ASA 75 to 100 mg; MV position INR 2.5 to 3.5 plus ASA.
- **Mechanical valves:** More durable and therefore used in younger patients
  - **Ball in cage** (Star Edwards): very durable, see occasionally, single
  - **Tilting disk** (Medtronic Hall)
  - **Bileaflet tilting disk:** predominant type. (St. Jude)
- **Physical** examination: Crisp prosthetic click and some soft murmurs (including minimal central regurgitation) normal, ball in cage harsher murmurs normal
  - **Chest x-ray:** Valves may have diagnostic appearance.
  - **Fluoroscopy:** "Rocking" indicates dysfunction.
  - **Echo:** TEE preferred if abnormalities suspected.
- **Therapy**
  - SBE prophylaxis is all prosthetic valves.
  - Medical: **Require anticoagulation**
  - INR 2.5 to 3.5 plus ASA for 3 months then AV position INR 2 to 3 plus ASA indefinitely,
  - MV position or AV with risk factors (above) INR 2.5 to 3.5 plus ASA indefinitely.
    - Anticoagulation may be held (48 h prior, restart 24 h after) for surgery or procedures in AV position prosthesis without risk factors, otherwise "bridging" is required (UFH when INR ≤2 to APTT approximately 50–86 sec. Discontinue UFH 4–6 h prior surgery or invasive procedure, restart UFH and warfarin as soon as possible [feasible]).

Hypertension (systemic hypertension) (Figure 4-43)

See JNC7 (Table 4-19) guidelines at http://www.nhlbi.nih.gov/guidelines/hypertension/jnc7full.pdf. JNC8 new guidelines are under development.

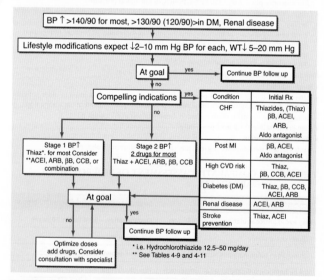

Figure 4-43   Approach to the patient with systemic hypertension. ACEI, angiotensin-converting enzyme inhibitor; ARB, angiotensin receptor blocker; βB, beta blocker; BP, blood pressure; CCB, calcium channel blocker; CHF, congestive heart failure; CVD, cardiovascular disease; DM, diabetes mellitus; MI, myocardial infarction; Rx, drug therapy; WT, weight.

TABLE 4-19. JNC7 CLASSIFICATION

Category	SBP (mm Hg)		DBP (mm Hg)
Normal	<120	and	<80
Prehypertension	120–139	or	80–90
Hypertension stage 1	140–159	or	90–99
Hypertension stage 2	≥160	or	≥100

DBP, diastolic blood pressure; SBP, systolic blood pressure.

- **Definition:** Chronic BP higher than 140/90 mm Hg; etiology is unknown in 90% or more cases (essential); approximately 5% of cases are second-degree (identifiable cause); consider in patients younger than 30 or older than 55 years of age at onset.
- **Prevalence:** approximately 60 million cases in the United States; higher incidence in African Americans than those of European origin.
- **Diagnostic** workup
  - Stage BP (see Table 4-28)
  - Assess risk factors and comorbidities:
    - Age (women >65 years; men >55 years), obesity (body mass index >30 kg/m², dyslipidemia, diabetes mellitus, smoking, family history of premature CAD (women <55 years; men <65 years)
  - Identify secondary causes of hypertension and reasons for persistent increased BP (see Table 4-20).
  - Identify presence of end-organ damage.
- **Symptoms**
  - Often none or nonspecific, sometimes related to 20 causes (clues) or end-organ damage.
- **Physical examination**
  - BP measurement techniques:
    - Measure BP with appropriate size cuff on both arms × 2 more than 5 min apart and legs; if coarctation is considered, ophthalmological examination for retinal changes, "clues" (Table 4-20). Consider patient BP self-check or BP monitoring if in doubt. S₂ (A₂), increased intensity, with S₄.
  - **Laboratory test results:** Electrolytes, BUN, creatinine (estimate GFR), glucose, urinalysis (including microalbumin), thyroid-stimulating hormone, lipid profile.
  - **ECG:** LVH
  - **Chest x-ray:** cardiomegaly but usually normal
- **Triage:** Patients seldom require admission
- **Treatment:** Goal BP less than 140/90; less than 130/80 in diabetes mellitus and renal disease. Most patients need more medications.
  - **Lifestyle modifications**
    - Decrease weight to achieve body mass index less than 25 kg/m²; decrease sodium chloride to less than 6 g daily; decrease ETOH consumption in men to 2 drinks per day or fewer, in women, 1 drink per day or fewer; initiate Dietary Approaches to Stop Hypertension (DASH) diet with increased fruits and vegetables and decreased fat intake; increase aerobic exercise to more than 30 min/d.
  - **Drug therapy** (see hypertensive urgency and Figure 4-43)
  - **Causes of resistant BP increase**
    - Improper BP measurement, increased salt intake, inadequate drug doses or drug (including herbal supplements) interactions, increased ETOH consumption, identifiable second-degree causes and consider printing out the JNC7 reference card at http://www.nhlbi.nih.gov/guidelines/hypertension/phycard.pdf).

TABLE 4-20.　IDENTIFIABLE CAUSES OF HYPERTENSION

Disease	Clue	Findings	Workup	Specific Therapy
Parenchymal renal disease	↑ or ↓ kidney DM, family history of renal failure	Polycystic kidney, glomerulonephritis, DM renal disease	Kidney ultrasound, CrCl, rheumatic markers	Treat primary disease, tight BP control (NaCl restriction, RRT if GFR <15 mL/min)
Renovascular disease and atherosclerosis in older men; fibromuscular dysplasia in young women	Recurrent APE, ↓ K⁺	Refractory ↑ BP, abdominal bruit, renal failure with ACEI	Doppler ultrasound, MRA, angiogram, aldosterone-to-renin ratio <10:1	Careful ACEI, ARB, CCB, renal artery angioplasty (±stenting), consider surgery
Coarctation in children and young adults	Delayed diminished femoral pulse	CXR indentation of aorta, BP: UE > LE	TTE, + in jugular-notch view, MRA	Surgery
Pheochromocytoma in young to middle aged adults	Peroxisomal, sweating, headache	Tachycardia, Wt ↓, orthostatic ↓ BP	↑ plasma metanephrine or 24 h catecholamine, CT, MRI	Surgery, phenoxybenzamine, labetalol (not pure beta-blocker)
Hyperaldosteronism	↓ K⁺	↓ K⁺ metabolic alkalosis	CT	Adenoma surgery
Cushing	Cushingoid appearance	↓ K⁺ metabolic alkalosis	CT, MRI	Disease specific
Sleep apnea	Snoring	Day somnolence, body habitus	Polysomno-graphy	C-PAP, BiPAP
Thyroid disease	Bradycardia	Myxedema	↓ T4, ↑ first-degree or ↓ second-degree TSH	Thyroid replacement
Parathyroid disease	Polyuria	Dehydration, altered MVS	↑ Ca, PTH	Therapy: ↑ Ca, surgery
Drugs: BCP, NSAIDs, licorice EPO, cyclosporine, steroid	History			Withdrawal if possible

ACEI, angiotensin-converting enzyme; APE, acute pulmonary edema; ARB, angiotensin receptor blocker; BCP, birth control pill; BiPAP, biphasic positive airway pressure; BP, blood pressure; Ca, calcium; CCB, calcium channel blocker; CPAP, continuous positive airway pressure; CrCl, creatinine clearance; CT, computed tomography; CXR, chest x-ray; DM, diabetes mellitus; EPO, evening primrose oil; GFR, glomerular filtration rate; LE, lower extremity; MRA, magnetic resonance angiography; MRI, ,magnetic resonance imaging; MVS, mitral valve stenosis; NaCl, sodium chloride; NSAID, nonsteroidal antiinflammatory drug; PTH, parathyroid hormone; RRT, relative retention time; T4, thyroxine; TSH, thyroid stimulating hormone; TTE, transthoracic echocardiography; UE, upper extremity; Wt, weight.

Hypertensive Emergency

- Increased BP with evidence of end-organ damage
- Central nervous system (CNS): encephalopathy, stroke, papilledema,
- Cardiovascular: aortic dissection, ACS, APE
- Renal: acute renal failure, scleroderma crisis, macroangiopathic hemolytic anemia, eclampsia
- **Symptoms** depend on end-organ damage
- **History and physical examination:** Question for cocaine and amphetamine abuse, clues for secondary hypertension (see Table 4-20), CHF, APE, ACS
- **Laboratory test results:** BUN, creatinine, CBC for schistocytes, cardiac biomarkers, urine drug screen
- **Chest x-ray:** Cardiomegaly, signs of end organ damage.
- **Echo:** LVH, RWMA, LVEF assessment
- **Triage:** Admit patient to the ICU
- **Treatment:** Decrease BP 25%, lower in cerebral hemorrhage and aortic dissection. See vasodilators in Tables 4-11 and 4-12; IV beta-blocker, CCB with labetalol 20 to 80 mg IVB every 10 min or 0.5 to 2 mg/min IV infusion. Hydralazine 10 to 20 mg IVB every 20 to 30 min (consider in eclampsia). Clevidipine is third-generation dihydropyridine CCB that has been developed for use in clinical settings in which tight BP control is crucial: IV 1 to 2 mg/h for initiation titrated by doubling the dose every 90 seconds; phentolamine 1- to 5-mg boluses, maximum 15-mg dose *(seldom used)*.
- **Special considerations in therapy**
  - Scleroderma crisis: ACEIs have increased antihypertensive efficacy and seem to be associated with improved survival.
  - Aortic dissection: labetalol, esmolol with nitroprusside
  - Preeclampsia and eclampsia: IV labetalol or nicardipine *(Hydralazine is associated with increased frequency of Cesarean section.)*
  - Cerebral hemorrhage: Nicardipine is an effective agent for the control of BP.
  - Postoperative hypertension, pain and anxiety control: labetalol, esmolol, nicardipine; consider clevidipine.
  - In pregnancy, use methyldopa 250 to 1000 mg PO BID/TID

Hypertensive Urgency

- No end-organ damage: BP higher than 180/120 mm Hg
- **Triage:** admit to the floor with frequent BP monitoring
- **Treatment:** Oral medications whenever possible; clonidine 0.2 mg PO, 0.1 mg every 1 h → transdermal patch every week.
- **Special considerations**
  - In pregnancy use methyldopa 250 to 1000 mg PO BID/TID; labetalol *(Hydralazine is associated with increased frequency of Cesarean section.)*

Pericardial Disease

- **Prevalence** more common in men than women.

Pericarditis and Pericardial Effusion

- **Etiology** (Table 4-21)
- **Symptoms**
  - Chest pain sharp, pleuritic, positional (decreased by leaning forward); fever and palpitations. *Pericardial effusion without pericarditis is largely asymptomatic until cardiac tamponade develops.*
- **Physical examination**
  - Pericarditis: Pericardial friction rub loudest leaning forward (classical tricomponent); premature contractions are common.
  - Pericardial effusion: distant (muffled) heart sounds, dullness to percussion left lower lung field (atelectasis , ie, Ewart sign)
- **Laboratory test results:** Cardiac biomarkers can be elevated (do not discriminate from AMI).
- **Chest x-ray:** With large (>250 mL) pericardial effusion, cardiac silhouette is increased with left heart border straight or convex "water bottle" configuration.
- **ECG:** See Figure 4-10B. Diffuse concave upward STE in all leads, but aVR and V_1, PR depression. STE persists for days. With large effusion "electrical alternans" and low QRS voltage.

MEDICAL SPECIALTIES

TABLE 4-21. COMMON ETIOLOGY OF PERICARDITIS AND
PERICARDIAL EFFUSION[a]

Type	Etiology	Comment
Idiopathic	Likely viral + autoimmune	Diagnosis of exclusion
Viral	Coxsackievirus B, echo adenoviruses, Enterovirus, HIV, EBV, HCV, VZV measles, influenza parainfluenza type 2, RSV, CMV, HSV	Most common Influenza, coxsackievirus B—seasonal epidemics
Granulomatous	<u>TB</u>, fungal (*Blastomyces dermatitidis*, Coccidioides, Aspergillus, Histoplasma, systemic Candida), RA, sarcoidosis	TB common outside the United States with high mortality[b] 11% of RA patients
Protozoa	Entamoeba, Toxoplasma, Trypanosoma	Amoeba common outside the United States[b]
Helminth	Echinococcus	Traditional sheepherders
<u>Bacterial</u>	*Streptococcus pneumoniae* and other streptococcus, staphylococcus, Salmonella, Shigella, *Neisseria meningitidis*, *Haemophilus influenzae*, anaerobes in children	Gram-positive more common but gram-negative increasing High percentage of patients develop constrictive pericarditis
Other infectious	*Borrelia burgdorferi* (Lyme disease), Nocardia, *Treponema pallidum* (syphilis), *Chlamydia psittaci*, actinomyces	Even less common: Listeria, Leptospira, rickettsial diseases
Neoplasia	Metastatic lung cancer, (adenocarcinoma squamous, small cell), breast cancer, leukemia, lymphoma (Hodgkin and non-Hodgkin), malignant melanoma	Most common presentation of CA in the heart, frequent cause of tamponade; mesothelioma in asbestos exposure.
Autoimmune/inflammatory	Scleroderma, SLE, RF, RA, Behçet syndrome, vasculitis, Wegener granulomatosis, reactive arthritis, inflammatory bowel disease	In scleroderma may coexist with RCMP
Metabolic/endocrine	**Uremic**, hypothyroidism, cholesterol pericarditis	
Cardiovascular	AMI, aortic dissection, **postcardiac injury syndrome** (especially after MVR)	AMI pericarditis is more common in STEMI
Drugs/iatrogenic	Hydralazine, ,procainamide, phenytoin, minoxidil, doxorubicin, and cyclophosphamide <u>Chest radiation</u>, pericardial placement of central line, invasive cardiac procedures	May occur >20 years after radiation. Various mechanisms for different drugs.

TABLE 4-21. COMMON ETIOLOGY OF PERICARDITIS AND PERICARDIAL EFFUSION[a] *(Continued)*

Type	Etiology	Comment
Miscellaneous + effusion without pericarditis	**Cardiac trauma**, cirrhosis, CHF, nephritic syndrome, amyloidosis, Takotsubo type CMP	

AMI, acute myocardial infarction; CA, cardiac arrest; CHF, congestive heart failure; CMP, cardiomyophaty; CMV, cytomegalovirus; EBV, Epstein-Barr virus; HCV, hepatitis C virus; HSV, herpes simplex virus; MVR, mitral valve repair or replacement; RA, rheumatoid arthritis; RCMP, restrictive cardiomyopathy; RF, rheumatic fever; RSV, respiratory syncytial virus; SLE, systemic lupus erythematosus; STEMI, ST-segment elevation myocardia infarction; TB, tuberculosis; VZV, varicella-zoster virus.

[a]Especially common causes in **bold**.

[b]Suspect in foreign-born or international traveler.

Bold: common causes of cardiac tamponade.

Underlined: common causes of constrictive pericarditis.

Underlined bold: cause cardiac tamponade and constrictive pericarditis.

- **Echo:** Most sensitive diagnostic of pericardial effusion and provides guidance for pericardiocentesis (Figure 4-44).
- **CT:** for effusion; helpful in late pericarditis.
- **Pericardiocentesis:** therapeutic if tamponade, diagnostic if malignant or infectious etiology is suspected.
- **Pericardial biopsy:** if strong suspicion of granulomatous pericarditis (see Table 4-30).
- **Triage**
  - Admit patient if low LVEF or significant pericardial effusion. Admit patient to ICU/CCU if suspicion of cardiac tamponade or significant arrhythmia is present.
- **Treatment**
  - Idiopathic and most viral pericardial diseases are self-limited. ASA, NSAIDs, colchicine 0.5 mg BID, prednisone 40 to 80 mg/d with taper in refractory cases. Pain may reoccur

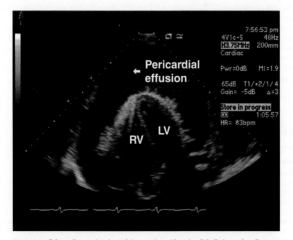

Figure 4-44 Echocardiogram in subcostal view a patient with pericardial effusion and cardiac (pericardial) tamponade. LV, left ventricle; RV, right ventricle. See color insert.

during taper. Surgical drainage if strong suspicion of nonviral infection. Pericardial window for recurrent effusion.

- **Cardiac tamponade** *does not correlate with volume of pericardial effusion due to low pericardial compliance* (compare Figure 4-44).
- **Etiology** same as pericardial effusion (see Table 4-21, especially common causes in **bold**).
- **Symptoms:** cardiogenic shock
- **Physical examination**
  - (see Figure 4-1) Tachycardia, tachypnea with clear lungs. Pulsus paradoxus (need manual BP cuff or arterial cannulation for diagnosis). Beck triad: hypotension (shock), muffled heart sounds, increased JVP (see Table 4-2).
- **Chest x-ray:** straight left heart border.
- **ECG:** may be pericarditis "electrical alternans" (see Figure 4-8)
- **Echo**
  - **Diagnostic:** (see Figure 4-44) (pericardial effusion as opposed to pleural is anterior to descending aorta and stops at coronary sinus) amount of fluid does not correlate with diastolic filling restriction (tamponade). Diastolic restriction corresponds to RA and later RV collapse during diastole, septal motion into LV with inspiration, decreased Doppler flow through MV and AV during inspiration (echo paradox). Dilated inferior vena cava more than 2 cm without inspiratory collapse, often pulsatile.
  - *BUT, pericardial effusion + shock = cardiac tamponade until proven otherwise.*
- **Pulmonary artery catheterization or cardiac catheterization**
  - Diastolic pressure is elevated more than 16 mm Hg (CVP, right atrial diastolic pressure, RVDP, pulmonary artery occluded pressure [a.k.a. wedge pressure; left atrial diastolic pressure/LVDP] all nearly (within 1–2 mm Hg) equal giving diastolic equalization (with intrapericardial pressure). Blunted Y-descent. All hemodynamic abnormalities (shock included) *should improve* with effusion drainage (does not have to be complete).

Treatment: Careful volume resuscitation and positive inotropes until pericardiocentesis is arranged (done).

Constrictive Pericarditis

- **Etiology:** See underlined causes in Table 4-21.
- **Symptoms:** fatigue and RV failure predominate
- **Physical examination:** Kussmaul sign (see Table 4-5), hepatomegaly ascites, pedal edema
- **Chest x-ray:** may see pericardial calcifications in 50% of patients.
- **ECG:** nonspecific low-limb-lead voltage.
- **Echo:** Biatrial enlargement, normal ventricular sizes and thickness (discriminate from RCMP and DCMP) (thickened pericardial and "septal bounce"—abrupt motion in early diastole, as if double systole). Low resting cardiac output.
- **CT and MRI** are often diagnostic and discriminate from RCMP.
- **Cardiac catheterization:** Atrial pressure, prominent X- and Y-descent. Rapid pressure decrease in early diastole, followed by rapid increase in the ventricles (dip-plateau, ie, "square root sign")

Treatment: careful diuresis, surgical pericardiectomy.

Diseases of Great and Large Vessels

Diseases of the Aorta

Aortic Aneurysm

- **Etiology**
  - Abnormal widening involving (opposed to false aneurysm) all layers of aortic wall. Most are abdominal aortic aneurysms (AAAs) located below the renal arteries and above aortic bifurcation, almost all are atherosclerotic. Thoracic aortic aneurysms (less common) can be second-degree to cystic median necrosis (Marfan, Loeys-Dietz, vascular Ehlers-Danlos, and Turner syndromes), aortic-syphilis (ascending aortic more common), and Behçet and Takayasu syndromes. Atherosclerotic (descending aortic more common) AAA risk of rupture is increased in smokers and if positive family history. Ascending thoracic aortic aneurysm (TAA) may be associated with bicuspid AV.

TABLE 4-22. SPORADIC AAA DIAMETER AND RISK OF RUPTURE

AAA Diameter (cm)	Risk of Rupture (%)
<4	0
4–5	0.5–5
5–6	3–15
6–7	10–20
7–8	20–40
>8	30–50

- **Symptoms** *May be none.*
  - TAA: pain, hoarseness, dysphasia, cough. AAA: abdominal pain and emboli to the legs.
- **Physical:** AAA, palpable mass; TAA, watch for other features of Marfan syndrome or other congenital conditions. Risk and features of syphilis.
- **Laboratory test results:** Serologic test for syphilis if suspected
- **Chest x-ray:** TAA, enlarged aorta (see Figure 4-2A and B). Thin-shell calcifications ascending aortic (syphilis).
- **Echo:** Often diagnostic; TEE more then TTE; watch for AI. For AAA, **aortic ultrasound** is nearly always diagnostic.
- **CTA and MRA** diagnostic for either TAA or AAA.
- **Contrast aortography** may be done for surgical evaluation.
- **Triage:** Admit patient to ICU if rupture suspected; admit patient to monitored bed if symptomatic; otherwise, or if found incidentally, patients seldom require admission.
- **Treatment**
  - **AAA screening** recommendations:
    - Routine screening is not recommended for women.
    - One time by ultrasound in all men 65 to 75 years of age who ever smoked (Agency for Healthcare Research and Quality [AHRQ] class IA) and maybe nonsmokers (AHRQ consensus); men older than 50 years of age with family history of AAA (AHRQ class IIA)
  - See AHRQ for details: http://www.guideline.gov/content.aspx?id=14577 (accessed July 5, 2011)
  - **Risk modification:** smoking cessation, treat hyperlipidemia
  - **Medications:** beta-blocker, ACEI
  - **Follow up:** expected diameter growth approximately 0.4 cm/y
  - **Surgery:** Emergency surgery for rupture; compare rupture risk with surgical risk; recommended for rapidly growing aneurysm or if AAA diameter is larger than 5.5 cm (see Table 4-22).
  - **Endovascular repair** in patients with high surgical risk.
  - Indications and risks summarized in http://www.geraldlawriemd.com/sections/aaa/JVS_AAA_Treatment_Guidelines.pdf (accessed July 5, 2011)
  - **TAA:** no screening guidelines; treatment as in AAA plus ARB in Marfan syndrome
    - **Surgery**
      - If TAA is growing more than 1 cm/y or of diameter larger than 5.5 cm in ascending aortic and larger than 6 cm in descending aortic). In Marfan and Loeys-Dietz syndromes, larger than 4.5 cm; vascular Ehlers-Danlos and Turner syndromes, larger than 5.0 cm (ACC/AHA class IC).
    - **Follow up:** expected diameter growth approximately 0.1 cm/y. See full guidelines at http://content.onlinejacc.org/cgi/content/full/55/14/e27#SEC117 (accessed July 5, 2011).
  - **Aortic Dissection**
    - Disruption of aortic intima, allowing dissection of blood into vessel wall forming "false lumen." *All aortic dissections are life-threatening.* See Figure 4-45 for classification.

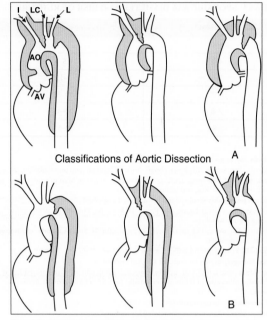

Figure 4-45   Classifications of aortic dissection. **A.** Stanford type A (involving ascending aorta) AV, aortic valve; Ao, aorta; I, innominate (brachiochephalic) artery; LC, left carotid artery; LS, left subclavian artery. **B.** Stanford type B (involving transverse and descending aorta).

- **Etiology**
  - Ascending aortic aneurysm: Hypertension, cystic median necrosis, Marfan syndrome, and so forth. (see TAA above), bicuspid AV, coarctation (Turner syndrome, neurofibromatosis [a.k.a. von Recklinghausen disease]) familiar aortic dissection, *third trimester of pregnancy in normal women.* Aortitis (syphilis + see TAA)
  - Descending aortic: atherosclerosis and hypertension.
  - Either descending, ascending, or both: Trauma, blunt chest or iatrogenic (cardiac catheterization, surgery, IABP, etc.), cocaine
- **Symptoms**
  - Sudden onset anterior or posterior chest pain (may be described as "ripping" or "tearing"); maximal point of pain may travel with the dissection; shock (pericardial tamponade , rupture); APE (caused by acute AI [see AI]); hypertension, CVA (carotid dissection or interruption of flow), syncope.
- **Physical examination**
- Asymmetry of carotid and brachial pulses, signs of tamponade, AI murmur, focal neurologic deficit.
- **Chest x-ray:** widened mediastinum is common
- **Echo:** TEE better then TTE; can be diagnostic and safely done in patient in shock; assess for presence of AI and tamponade
- **MRA** is superior to **CTA,** but both can be used
- **Aortography** if coronary dissection is suspected.

- **Triage:** admit patient to the ICU or cardiothoracic surgery or surgical ICU.
- **Treatment**
  - Reduce SBP approximately 110 mm Hg, and heart rate approximately 60 bpm. Use IV drugs: nitroprusside plus beta-blocker (see Table 4-10), labetalol 20 to 80 mg IVB every 10 min or 0.5 to 2 mg/min IV infusion.
  - Pain control with opiates if necessary. *Do not use hydralazine. Do not perform pericardiocentesis for pericardial effusion.*
  - Surgery: (see Figure 4-45) type A acute emergency aortic root replacement with or without aortic valve repair, type A chronic
  - Semielective if progression or AI
  - Type B if progression, TAA, branches involvement
  - Endovascular stenting usually with fenestration of false lumen
- **Prognosis:** Type A without surgery—mortality 1% an hour; type B, 10% an hour.

Other Diseases of the Aortic and Special Considerations

- **Takayasu arteritis**
  - Occurs predominantly in young women. Anorexia, fever, weight loss, branch involvement is common (claudication, cerebral ischemia). Loss of pulses ("pulseless disease"). Erythrocyte sedimentation rate is elevated. MRA is often diagnostic. Treat with glucocorticoids; immunosuppressive regimen, but mortality remains high.
- **Aortic atherosclerotic occlusive disease** (a.k.a. Leriche syndrome)
  - Risk factors: diabetes and smoking
  - Symptoms: buttocks and thigh claudication and impotence.
  - Physical examination: absent femoral pulses
  - Doppler, MRA diagnostic. Therapy aortic-femoral bypass.

Peripheral Vascular Disease

Arterial

- Occlusive disease of the arteries caused by atherosclerosis (most common in lower extremities) inflammation or vasospasm.
- **Arteriosclerosis**
  - **Etiology:** Atherosclerosis, arterial embolism
  - **Symptoms:** Intermittent claudication (muscular pain with exercise, relieved by rest) in the territory of the occluded artery. Later pain at rest, painful ulcers (*may be painless in patients with diabetes*) lead to gangrene of toes.
  - **Physical examination:** decreased peripheral pulses, ischemic ulcers or gangrene
  - **Vascular ultrasound** (arterial) with Doppler is diagnostic. May be done with exercise to induce claudication and flow gradient.
  - **CTA and MRA** are diagnostic.
  - **Arteriography** if angioplasty or surgery is planned
  - **Triage:** Admit patient to the floor if gangrene is suspected
  - **Treatment:** Mandatory smoking cessation. Foot care; prescribed exercise; treat hyperlipidemia. *Consider evaluation for CAD.*
  - **Surgery**
    - Ulcer debridement. **Bypass** (ie, aortic-femoral) or percutaneous angioplasty with or without stenting in patients with disabling claudication, rest pain, or gangrene.
  - **Arterial embolism** (from LA/LV thrombus, or paradoxical from RV venous system through right-to-left intracardiac shunt)
  - **Symptoms:** sudden onset of ischemic symptoms
  - **Physical examination:** pulseless, pale, cold extremity
  - **Triage:** admit patient to the ICU with vascular surgical consultation
  - **Treatment:** UFH via IV infusion. **Thrombolytic** therapy should be considered. For severe acute ischemia, surgical or endovascular **embolectomy** is often necessary.
- **Atheroembolism**
  - (see renal disease) after angiography or aortic surgery. Acute renal failure with possible gastrointestinal, CNS (confusion) or retinal ischemia, livedo reticularis (see Figure 4-22). Possible peripheral blood eosinophilia. *No anticoagulation.* Poor prognosis.

- **Thromboangiitis obliterans** (a.k.a. Buerger disease). Suspect in young men who are heavy smokers. Symptoms upper and lower extremity ischemia, ulcera, and gangrene. Lack of atherosclerotic lesions and smaller vessel involvement (including veins). **Mandatory smoking cessation.**

Venous (see pulmonary for venoembolic disease)

- **Superficial thrombophlebitis**
  - **Symptoms:** erythema and tenderness of the involve veins
  - **Triage:** admission is almost never necessary.
  - **Treatment:** Local heat, extremity elevation, ASA or NSAIDs
- **Deep venous thrombosis (DVT)**
  - Deep veins are defined as veins accompanying arteries, therefore the *superficial femoral vein is a deep vein.*
  - **Etiology** and risk factors: **Common DVT risk factors (risk factors in bold have strong association with DVT)**
  - Active cancer: **Pancreas**, lung, ovary, testes, **kidney**, breast stomach
  - Surgery: **Orthopedic**, thoracic, abdominal urological
  - Trauma to the extremity or spinal, **femoral, pelvic,** or tibia fractures
  - Immobilization: AMI, **CHF**, CVA
  - **Pregnancy** or estrogen use
  - Thrombophilia: decreased resistance to proteins C and S, **decreased antithrombin,** arterial and venous involvement (A + V), factor V Leiden
  - **Antiphospholipid antibody syndrome,** myeloproliferative disorders
  - Venulitis: homocystinuria, Behçet and Buerger diseases (A + V)
  - **Previous DVT**
  - **History and physical** are often unrevealing. *Probability analysis is essential.*
  - **Laboratory results:** D-dimer sensitive but not specific and should not be used to guide diagnosis.
  - **Vascular ultrasound** (venous) with Doppler is diagnostic; MRA may be useful in peripheral DVT, venography all but obsolete.
  - **Triage:** Admit patient to the floor; if proximal DVT or PE is suspected, admit patient to ICU
  - **Treatment:** Prevention is key. Systemic anticoagulation with unfractionated heparin UFH to activated partial thromboplastin time ×2 normal or low molecular weight heparin LMVH (American College of Chest Physicians [ACCP] class IA), followed by warfarin. DTIs for HIT. (Oral direct thrombin inhibitors are effective but not yet available.)
- **Phlegmasia alba dolens**
  - Near complete venous occlusion; **phlegmasia cerulea dolens.** complete venous occlusion causing ischemia; pregnancy (third trimester) and malignancy thought to be risk factors.
  - **Triage:** Admit patient to ICU with surgical consultation.
  - **Treatment:** anticoagulation and often **surgical thrombectomy**
  - For the latest ACCP guidelines see http://www.guideline.gov/content.aspx?id= 12957andsearch=anticoagulation (accessed July 5, 2011)
- **Suspected cardiac Syncope** (Figure 4-46)
  - Loss of consciousness because of reduction in cerebral blood flow
  - **Etiology:** Neurocardiogenic (a.k.a. vasovagal vasodepressor); orthostatic (a.k.a. postural) hypotension; cardiovascular neurologic (differentiate from seizures and loss of consciousness from other reasons hypoglycemia, hypoxemia, severe anemia psychiatric and factitious); past history of heart disease favors cardiac causes
  - **Symptoms:** Collapse with recovery without warning or with palpitations or chest pain favors cardiac prodrome sometimes described as faintness—favors vasovagal.
  - **Precipitation factors:** Exertion favors cardiac causes; position favors orthostatic hypotension. Cough, urination, defecation, emotional stress favors vasovagal.
  - **Duration** shorter than 5 seconds favors cardiac; longer than 5 seconds, neurocardiogenic.
  - **Medications:** CCB, ACEI,ARB, beta-blocker, hydralazine, diuretics, drugs causing QT prolongation, sedatives, hypnotics, virtually all antiarrhythmic drugs may cause syncope (see Tables 4-10).
  - **Physical examination:** Orthostatic BP measurements, orthostatic hypotension if SBP decreases more than 20 mm Hg in standing position. Good cardiac examination is

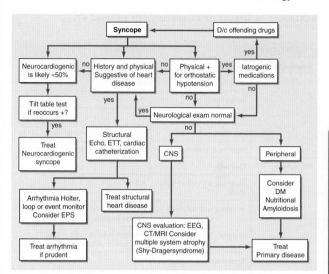

Figure 4-46 Approach to the patient with suspected cardiac syncope. CNS, central nervous system; CT, computed tomography; D/c, discontinue; DM, diabetes mellitus; EEG, electroencephalogram; EPS, electrophysiologic study; ETT, exercise tolerance test; MRI, magnetic resonance imaging.

MEDICAL SPECIALTIES

mandatory (ie, murmurs, heart failure, irregular pulse, pulse asymmetry), carotid bruits, focal neurologic deficit.

- **Chest x-ray:** aortic dilatation cardiac silhouette
- **ECG:** (see Figure 4-5) arrhythmia, AVB, BBB, bradycardia, pauses, QT prolongation, axis deviation, preexcitation pattern (see Figure 4-5, patterns N and O), Brugada syndrome (see Figure 4-11)
- **Monitoring:** Holter monitor (24–72 h), event recorder, loop recorder (external or implantable); pacemaker interrogation.
- **ETT:** If ischemia is suspected (may also help with preexcitation syndrome).
- **Echo:** evaluate for structural heart disease particularly for AS, RCMP, HOCM, PH.
- **EPS:** structural heart disease or arrhythmia.
- **Tilt table test** may help in neurocardiogenic causes.
- **CTA and MRA** may help in suspected aortic or pericardial diseases.
- **Triage:** Admit patient to monitored bed if cardiac cause is suspected.
- **Treatment:** Treat underlying disease causing syncope; discontinue all drugs with potential to cause syncope; vasovagal beta-blocker, fludrocortisone 0.05 to 0.2 mg/d PO; midodrine 5 to 10 mg BID or TID PO. Orthostatic hypotension lifestyle modifications, compressive stockings, volume repletion, fludrocortisone, midodrine (See Figure 4-46 for evaluation summary.)
- **Prognosis**

    One-quarter will reoccur at least once; vasovagal is a benign condition, cardiac syncope prognosis depends on the nature of primary disease, median survival approximately 6 years after diagnosis. Most individuals with multiple system atrophy causing orthostatic hypotension die within 7 to 10 years after the onset of symptoms (diagnosis is usually delayed).

    See a summary of evaluation and treatment of syncope at http://circ.ahajournals.org/cgi/reprint/106/13/1606 (accessed July 5, 2011).

TABLE 4-23. SUMMARY OF COMMON ADULT CONGENITAL HEART DISEASE

Classification		Conditions
Anatomical	**Level**	
	Atrial	ASD, PFO[a]
	Ventricular	VSD
	Aortic-pulmonary	PDA
	Left heart malformations	Bicuspid AV, great arteries transposition
	Right heart malformation	Tetralogy of Fallot[b], Ebstein anomaly[c]
Physiologic	**Cyanosis**	
	Acyanotic with left-to-right shunt	ASD,VSD, PDA
	Acyanotic without shunt	Bicuspid AV, great arteries transposition Ebstein anomaly
	Cyanotic	Tetralogy of Fallot, great arteries transposition, Eisenmenger tetralogy
Presentation	**Symptoms**	
	Asymptomatic murmur	ASD, PFO, small VSD, bicuspid AV
	Symptomatic	ASD (later), large VSD, tetralogy of Fallot great arteries transposition, Eisenmenger bicuspid AV(later) Ebstein anomaly

ASD, atrial septal defect; AV, atrioventricular; PDA, patent ductus arteriosus; PFO, patent foramen ovale; VSD, ventricular septal defect.
[a]For PFO, the most common is acyanotic.
[b]For Tetralogy of Fallot, the most common is cyanotic, which is a combination of infundibular pulmonary artery stenosis, overriding aorta, VSD, and right ventricular hypertrophy.
[c]Ebstein's anomaly tricuspid valve is displacement toward the apex of the right ventricle ("atriafication of the RV").

Common Cardiac Causes of Syncope

- **Bradyarrhythmias:** Sinus bradycardia, SSS, increase in degree of AVB, sinus arrest, pacemaker malfunction.
- **Tachyarrhythmias:** WPW, atrial fibrillation, atrial fibrillation SVT (if structural disease present),VT, VF
- **Fixed obstructions:** AS, subaortic membrane, MVS prosthetic valve thrombosis
- **Dynamic obstructions:** HOCM, atrial myxoma
- **LV failure:** AMI, DCMP, myocarditis
- **LV restriction or constriction:** RCMP, tamponade, constrictive pericarditis
- **RV failure: primary** RV MI; **secondary:** PE, severe PH, pulmonary stenosis including infundibular
- **Great vessels:** aortic dissection, subclavian steal (rare)

Common Adult Congenital Heart Diseases (Table 4-23)

Diagnosis

- **Echo:** TTE or TEE; **CT** may help.
- **Cardiac catheterization** often precedes surgery.
- **Treatment:** Usually **surgical,** for bicuspid AV ASD later in life.

See ACC/AHA guidelines for the Management of Adults with Congenital Heart Disease at http://circ.ahajournals.org/cgi/content/full/118/23/2395 (accessed July 5, 2011).

CHAPTER 5

Endocrinology

David J. Castaldo and Jody P. Boggs

GATHERING DATA

History (suggestive of endocrinopathies)

- General: fatigue, weight loss or gain
- Eyes, ears, nose, throat: visual disturbance (blurred vision, peripheral vision loss)
- Musculoskeletal: weakness
- Gastrointestinal (GI): abdominal pain, nausea and/or vomiting
- Genitourinary: polyuria, menstrual irregularities, infertility, impotence, changes in libido
- Psychiatry: depression, psychosis
- Skin: hyperpigmentation, striae, hirsutism, easy bruising

Physical Examination

- General: central obesity, moon facies, buffalo hump
- Eyes, ears, nose, throat: arcus senilis
- GI: tenderness
- Musculoskeletal: proximal weakness
- Skin: striae, hyperpigmentation in skin creases, excess hair, xanthomas, ecchymoses

Diagnostic Tests (laboratory test results)

- Hyper- or hypoglycemia, metabolic acidosis or alkalosis, hypo- or hyperkalemia, glucosuria, hormone-specific suppression or stimulation testing

Radiology

- Dual-energy x-ray absorptiometry (DEXA) scan (osteoporosis or osteopenia), magnetic resonance imaging (MRI) (pituitary or adrenal), computed tomography (CT) (adrenal)

GATHERING INFORMATION

Common Signs and Symptoms

- Diabetes mellitus (DM): polyuria, polydipsia, and blurred vision. Weight loss is seen in diabetes mellitus type 1 (DM-1).
- Diabetic ketoacidosis (DKA): nausea and vomiting, polyuria, polydipsia, abdominal pain, dyspnea.
- Hypoglycemia: palpitations, tremor, anxiety, sweating, hunger, and paresthesia; behavioral changes, confusion, fatigue, seizure, loss of consciousness and death.
- Hypothyroidism: fatigue, dry skin, cold intolerance, hair loss, difficulty concentrating and poor memory, constipation, weight gain (because of fluid retention), poor appetite, dyspnea, hoarse voice, menorrhagia, paresthesia, impaired hearing, depression.
- Hyperthyroidism: hyperactivity, irritability, worsening angina, dysphoria, heat intolerance and sweating, palpitations, fatigue and weakness, fine hair texture or alopecia, pruritus, urticaria, weight loss with increased appetite, increased stool frequency, diarrhea, polyuria, oligomenorrhea, and loss of libido. Fatigue, weight loss and depressive symptoms are seen in the older patients.
- Thyroid pain: acute or subacute thyroiditis, hemorrhage into a cyst, lymphoma, rarely amiodarone-induced thyroiditis or amyloidosis.
- Hypercalcemia: fatigue, depression, mental confusion, anorexia, nausea, constipation, polyuria.
- Hypocalcemia: muscle spasms, abdominal cramping, dyspnea.

History and Review of Systems

- DM: frequent infections, weight loss, family history, numbness and tingling, change in vision, polyuria, polydipsia, and any other personal or family history of autoimmune disease.
- DKA: recent illness, infection, ischemia, stress or change in insulin regimen
- Hypoglycemia: recent change in insulin regimen, weight changes, change in appetite
- Hyper- or hypothyroidism: weight changes, skin and hair changes, temperature intolerance, voice changes, constipation or frequent stools.
- Thyroiditis: recent iodine or amiodarone exposure, pregnancy, radiation, trauma or infection.
- Hypercalcemia: Establish chronicity. History of ingestion of vitamins or drugs, nephrolithiasis, peptic ulcer disease, osteoporosis. Check for symptoms of associated malignancy.
- Hypocalcemia: Establish chronicity. Investigate for malabsorption problems and nutritional history, family history, use of anticonvulsants, recent medications, recent surgery, alcohol history.

Physical Examination

- DM: acanthosis nigricans, signs of peripheral neuropathy, signs of retinopathy, superficial fungal infection.
- DKA and hyperglycemic hyperosmolar syndrome (HHONK) syndrome: hemodynamic stability, respiratory effort, abdominal tenderness, lethargy.
- Hypoglycemia: central nervous system changes, diaphoretic, tremor.
- Hypothyroidism: Check vital signs, appearance of skin, hair, and nails; temperature of extremities; edema; deep tendon reflexes; palpation of the thyroid.
- Hyperthyroidism: Check vital signs, signs of heart failure, palpate the thyroid, examine for audible thrill or bruit of the thyroid (increased vascularity), tremor, muscle strength and tone, deep tendon reflexes, examine the skin and nails.
- Thyroiditis: tenderness of the thyroid, palpation for presence of multinodular goiter, presence of fever.
- Hypercalcemia: Check vital signs, neurologic examination, bowel sounds, signs of underlying malignancy.
- Hypocalcemia: Check vital signs, electrocardiogram (ECG) (QT prolongation), arrhythmias, neuromuscular findings (muscle spasms, respiratory distress, Chvostek and Trousseau signs), mental status changes, abdominal cramping.

Diagnostic Tests

- Laboratory
  - DM: glycated hemoglobin (HbA_{1c}), basic metabolic panel, microalbumin-to-creatinine ratio; possibly islet cell antibodies (anti-glutamic acid decarboxylase, anti-insulin).
  - Hypoglycemia: insulin level, C-peptide, proinsulin, beta-hydroxybutyrate, sulfonylurea levels, cortisol, and ethanol.
  - DKA/HHONK: basic metabolic panel, urine ketones, plasma ketones (beta-hydroxybutyrate, acetoacetate), blood gas analysis, magnesium, phosphorus, fasting lipid panel, lipase, serum osmolality.
  - Thyroid: thyroid-stimulating hormone (TSH), free thyroxine (FT_4), free triiodothyronine (FT_3), antithyroid peroxidase (TPO), antithyroglobulin, fasting lipid panel, creatinine phosphokinase.
  - Thyroiditis: thyroid function test (TFTs), erythrocyte sedimentation rate (ESR), white blood cell count.
  - Hypercalcemia: Check calcium, phosphorus, vitamin D_2 (25-hydroxyergocalciferol [25OH-VitD]), vitamin D_3 (1,25-dihydroxycholecalciferol [1,25OH-VitD]), parathyroid hormone (PTH). Consider parathyroid hormone-related protein (PTHrP).
  - Hypocalcemia: PTH, 25OH-VitD, albumin.
- Radiology
  - Localizing insulinoma: MRI, transabdominal and endoscopic ultrasound
  - Hypothyroidism and hyperthyroidism: thyroid ultrasound
  - Thyroiditis: CT or ultrasound to evaluate for abscess
  - Hypercalcemia: depending on possible underlying malignancy

- Special Tests Specific to the Organ System
  - Hypoglycemia: food deprivation test
  - Localizing insulinoma: selective pancreatic arterial calcium injection
  - Thyroid: thyroidal radioactive iodine uptake scan, fine-needle aspiration (FNA) biopsy
  - Thyroiditis: possibly FNA

DIABETES MELLITUS

- Definitions
  - Normal glucose homeostasis
    - Fasting plasma glucose level less than 100 mg/dL
    - Plasma glucose level less than 140 mg/dL following an oral glucose challenge
    - HbA_{1c} level less than 5.6%
  - Impaired glucose homeostasis
    - Impaired fasting glucose (IFG): fasting glucose level 100 to 125 mg/dL
    - Impaired glucose tolerance (IGT): plasma glucose level 140 to 199 mg/dL following an oral glucose challenge
    - HbA_{1c} level: 5.7% to 6.4%
  - DM (Table 5-1)
- Pathophysiology
  - DM-1
    - Interactions of genetic, environmental, and immunologic factors.
    - Autoimmune destruction of beta cells occurring over months to years.
    - Most commonly develops before the age of 30 years, however, an autoimmune beta cell destructive process can develop at any age.
  - DM-2
    - Genetic and metabolic defects.
    - More typically develops with increasing age, however, it is being diagnosed more frequently in children and young adults.
    - Insulin resistance leads to compensatory hyperinsulinemia, which leads to IGT and a decline in insulin secretion and increased in hepatic glucose production leads to IFG.
- Etiologic Classifications
  - DM-1: typically autoimmune destruction of beta cells leading to complete or near-total insulin deficiency.
    - "Honeymoon" phase at initial presentation during which time glycemic control is achieved with modest doses of insulin.
  - DM-2: variable degrees of insulin resistance, impaired insulin secretion, and increased glucose production. Visceral or central obesity is very common.
  - Maturity-onset diabetes of youth
    - Autosomal dominant
    - Early onset of hyperglycemia, usually younger than 25 years of age
    - Impairment in insulin secretion

TABLE 5-1. CLASSIFICATION AND DIAGNOSIS OF DIABETES MELLITUS[1]

Symptoms of diabetes plus random blood glucose concentration >200 mg/dL
or
Fasting plasma glucose >126 mg/dL
or
HbA_{1c} >6.5%
or
Two-hour plasma glucose >200 mg/dL during an oral glucose tolerance test

Glycated hemoglobin, HbA_{1c}.

- Latent autoimmune diabetes of an adult: patients are usually lean, previously diagnosed with DM-2, have lower insulin secretory capacity and positive autoimmune markers (antiglutamic acid decarboxylase, anti-islet cell antibodies).[2,3]
- Flatbush diabetes (a.k.a. diabetes type 1b): patient with DM-2 who presents with DKA. Occurs in young African Americans. Antibodies are negative. Often does not require insulin following treatment of DKA.[4]
- Secondary causes of DM
  - Diseases of the exocrine pancreas: pancreatitis, pancreatectomy, cystic fibrosis, hemochromatosis ("bronze diabetes")
  - Endocrinopathies: acromegaly, Cushing syndrome, glucagonoma, pheochromocytoma, hyperthyroidism, somatostatinoma, aldosteronoma
  - Drugs or chemical-induced: glucocorticoids, nicotinic acid, diazoxide, beta-adrenergic agonists, thiazides, alpha-interferon, protease inhibitors, antipsychotics (atypical and others)
  - Infections: congenital rubella, cytomegalovirus, coxsackievirus
  - Other genetic syndromes associated: Down, Klinefelter, and Turner syndromes, Friedreich ataxia, Huntington chorea
- Clinical Manifestations
  - If symptomatic, complaints include polyuria, polydipsia, nocturia, blurred vision, weight loss, and frequent infections.
  - On physical examination:
    - Observe: acanthosis nigricans, central adiposity.
    - Signs of peripheral neuropathy: monofilament test, however, also test for vibration sensation, pressure sensation, and pain and temperature. Examine for ulcerations and signs of infection.
    - Signs of retinopathy: cotton wool spots, exudates, and neovascularization
- Screening Guidelines
  - Consider screening every 3 years beginning at age 45 years.
  - Consider screening earlier in patients with body mass index (BMI) more than 25 kg/m² with any of the following risk factors:
    - Physical inactivity
    - First-degree relatives with DM
    - High-risk ethnic group (Latino, Native American, African American, Asian American, Pacific Islander)
    - History of gestational diabetes
    - Hypertension (blood pressure ≥140/90 mm Hg)
    - Low high-density lipoprotein (HDL) cholesterol level (<35 mg/dL) and/or high triglyceride level (>250 mg/dL)
    - Polycystic ovarian syndrome
    - HbA$_{1c}$ level 5.7% or higher, IGT, or IFG on previous tests
    - Other clinical conditions associated with insulin resistance (eg, acanthosis nigricans, severe obesity)
    - History of cardiovascular disease
- Laboratory and Other Tests
  - Random glucose *or* fasting glucose *or* HbA$_{1c}$ *or* glucose tolerance test for diagnosis
  - For chronic complications: basic metabolic panel, urine microalbumin-to-creatinine ratio
  - Islet cell autoantibodies (anti-glutamic acid decarboxylase, anti-insulin) if autoimmunity is suspected
  - See section G for laboratory test results associated with acute complications.
- Triage Decisions
  - Identify acute complications of DM
    - DKA
    - HHONK
    - Hypoglycemia (secondary to antihyperglycemic regimen)
    - Infection: diabetic foot, osteomyelitis, urinary tract infection, mucormycosis, malignant external otitis, emphysematous cholecystitis, Fournier gangrene, and so forth
  - Differentiating DKA from HHONK (Table 5-2)

TABLE 5-2. DIABETIC KETOACIDOSIS AND HYPERGLYCEMIC HYPEROSMOLAR SYNDROME

	DKA	HHONK
Glucose	250–600 mg/dL	600–1200 mg/dL
Sodium	125–135 mEq/L	135–145 mEq/L
Potassium	Normal to elevated; however, total body stores are typically low	Normal
Creatinine	Slightly elevated	Moderately elevated
Osmolality	300–320 mmol/mL	330–380 mmol/mL
Plasma ketones	++++	±
Serum bicarbonate	<15 mEq/L	Normal to slightly low
Volume depletion	3–5 L	9–10 L
Arterial pH	6.8–7.3	>7.3
Arterial pCO$_2$, mmHg	20–30	Normal
Anion gap	Elevated	Normal to slightly elevated

DKA, diabetic ketoacidosis; HHONK, hyperglycemic hyperosmolar syndrome; pCO$_2$, partial pressure of carbon dioxide.

- Management of Acute Life-Threatening Complications
  - DKA: absolute and relative insulin deficiency with counterregulatory hormone excess (glucagon, catecholamines, cortisol, growth hormone) and volume depletion with acidosis and ketosis (from increase in free fatty acid release)
    - More common in DM-1
    - Precipitating events
      - Inadequate insulin administration
      - Infection
      - Infarction (cerebral, coronary, mesenteric)
      - Drugs (cocaine)
      - Pregnancy
    - Symptoms: nausea, vomiting, polyuria, polydipsia, abdominal pain, shortness of breath
    - Physical examination
      - Tachycardia
      - Hypotension and dehydration: secondary to osmotic diauresis
      - Tachypnea and Kussmaul respirations, fruity odor of the patient's breath and respiratory distress
      - Abdominal tenderness: may be severe
      - Lethargy, obtundation, cerebral edema, possibly coma
      - Signs of infection
    - Laboratory test results
      - Obtain basic metabolic panel, urine ketones, plasma ketones (beta-hydroxybutyrate, acetoacetate), blood gas analysis, magnesium, phosphorus, fasting lipid panel, lipase (if abdominal pain present).
    - Management[5–9]
      - Admission: Intensive care unit may be necessary for frequent monitoring, if pH less than 7, or patient is unconscious.
      - Initiate appropriate workup for precipitating event.
      - Replace fluids.

- Give 2 to 3 L 0.9% normal saline over the first 1 to 3 hours (at 15–20 mL/kg/h).
- Follow with 250 to 500 mL/h (4–14 mL/kg/h). If the corrected sodium is normal or elevated, give 0.45% normal saline. If the corrected sodium is reduced, give 0.9% normal saline. (See the Corrected Sodium calculator at http://www.medcalc.com/correctna.html.)
- Change to dextrose 5% injection, 0.45% normal saline at 150 to 250 mL/h when plasma glucose reaches 200 mL/dL.
  - Insulin reduces lipolysis, increases peripheral ketone body use, suppresses hepatic ketone body formation, and promotes bicarbonate regeneration.
    - Administer short-acting insulin: intravenously (IV) (0.1 unit/kg), then 0.1 unit/kg/h by continuous IV infusion.
    - Increase two- to threefold if no response in 2 to 4 h.
    - If the initial serum potassium is less than 3.3 mEq/L, do not administer insulin until the potassium is corrected.
    - If the initial serum potassium is more than 5.2 mEq/L, do not supplement potassium until it is corrected.
  - Electrolytes
    - Replace K^+ at 10 mEq/h when plasma K^+ is less than 5.0 to 5.2 mEq/L, ECG normal, urine flow and normal creatinine is documented.
    - Administer 40 to 80 mEq/h when plasma K^+ less than 3.5 mEq/L or if bicarbonate is given.
    - Administer sodium bicarbonate to patients with pH below 7.
      - If pH is between 6.90 and 7.00, give 50 mEq sodium bicarbonate plus 10 mEq of potassium chloride in 200 mL sterile water over 2 h.
      - If pH is below 6.90, give 100 mEq of sodium bicarbonate plus 20 mEq of potassium chloride in 400 mL sterile water over 2 h.
    - Initiate phosphate supplementation.
  - Monitoring
    - Assess capillary glucose every 1 to 2 h.
    - Measure electrolytes (K^+, bicarbonate, phosphate) and anion gap every 4 hours for the first 24 hours
    - Monitor blood pressure, pulse, respirations, mental status, fluid intake and output every 1 to 4 hours.
  - Follow-up
    - Continue the above until the patient is stable, glucose level 150 to 250 mg/dL, and acidosis is resolved.
    - At this point, insulin infusion may be decreased to 0.05 to 0.1 unit/kg/h.
    - Administer long-acting insulin as soon as the patient is eating. Overlap with insulin infusion.
- HHONK: DM-2 complication
  - Pathophysiology
    - Typically occurs in DM-2.
    - Usually precipitated by concurrent illness (myocardial infarction, stroke, serious infection), however, relative insulin deficiency and inadequate fluid intake are the underlying causes.
  - Clinical features
    - Several-week history of polyuria, weight loss, and decreased oral intake, culminating in mental confusion, lethargy, or coma.
  - Physical examination
    - Profound dehydration (osmotic diuresis), hypotension, tachycardia, and altered mental status.
    - Nausea and vomiting, and pain and Kussmaul respirations are *not* characteristic.
  - Management
    - Determine precipitating events.
    - Fluids
      - Give 1 to 3 L of 0.9% normal saline over the first 2 to 3 h.

- Because fluid deficits accumulate over days to weeks, too rapid a reversal may worsen neurologic function.
- If serum sodium level is higher than 150 mmol/L, 0.45% saline should be used.
- When hemodynamic stability is achieved, reverse free-water deficit with hypotonic fluids (0.45% saline initially, then 5% dextrose in water).
- Fluid deficit should be reversed over 1 to 2 days.
- Electrolytes
  - Potassium repletion
  - Phosphate repletion
- Insulin: for insulin deficiency, however, *not* needed for ketosis.
  - Insulin bolus 0.1 unit/kg followed by IV insulin at a rate of 0.1 unit/kg/h.
  - If the glucose does not decrease, increase the insulin infusion by twofold.
  - Glucose should be added to IV fluids when the plasma glucose falls to 250 to 300 mg/dL if patient is still not eating with the insulin infusion rate decreased to 0.05 to 0.1 unit/kg/h.
  - Continue insulin infusion until the patient has resumed eating, then transfer to subcutaneous delivery.
- Hypoglycemia (see next section)
- Management of Patients with DM during Hospitalization
  - Inpatient insulin therapy
    - Blood sugar goals: 140 to 180 mg/dL in critically ill patients. In noncritically ill patients, premeal target is less than 140 mg/dL and random glucose level less than 180 mg/dL.[10]
    - The "sliding scale" approach should no longer be used.
    - Basal-bolus approach:
      - If DM-1 and not eating:
        - Basal insulin (~0.2–0.3 unit/kg/day) with correctional insulin based on insulin sensitivity
      - If DM-1 and eating:
        - Basal insulin (~0.2–0.3 unit/kg/day) plus prandial insulin (~0.05–0.1 unit/kg/meal) with correctional insulin based on insulin sensitivity
      - If DM-2 and not eating:
        - Discontinue oral agents.
        - Begin correctional insulin based on insulin sensitivity.
      - If DM-2 and eating
        - Continue oral agents (if no contraindications) if well controlled.
        - If poorly controlled, discontinue oral agents and begin basal insulin (0.2–0.3 unit/kg/day) plus prandial insulin (0.05–0.1 unit/kg/meal) with correctional insulin based on insulin sensitivity.
      - If glucose still not well controlled:
        - Adjust basal insulin by approximately 10% to 20% every 1 to 2 days to achieve target, and adjust correctional insulin scale by 1 to 2 unit/dose every 1 to 2 days.
        - If response is still not sufficient, consider IV insulin.
    - Total daily dose (TDD) insulin:
      - DM-1: typically 0.4 to 1 unit/kg/day
      - DM-2: variable, can range from 0.2 to 1.5 unit/kg/day (for further discussion on management, see http://www.nejm.org/doi/full/10.1056/NEJMcp060094)
    - Calculating subcutaneous insulin dosing by IV insulin requirements:
      - Extrapolate TDD from the last 4 to 6 hours of insulin infusion. Average___ unit/h over the last 4 to 6 hours × 24 hours = ___unit as initial TDD.
      - 50% Basal = ___unit (given as glargine daily, detemir daily to twice daily, or NPH twice daily; maximum dose for the first 24 hours is 0.5 unit/kg)
      - 50% Prandial (*if eating*) = ___unit divided by 3 = ___unit/meal of rapid analogue (ie, lispro, aspart, glulisine; maximum dose for the first 24 hours is 0.1 unit/kg/meal)

TABLE 5-3. OUTPATIENT INSULIN THERAPY IN TYPE 2 DIABETES MELLITUS[13]

	Type of Insulin (Brand Name)	Onset (Hours)	Peak (Hours)	Duration (Hours)
Rapid-acting	Insulin lispro (Humalog)	0.25–0.5	1–2	3–4
	Insulin aspart (Novolog)	0.25–0.5	1–2	3–5
	Insulin glulisine (Apidra)	0.25–0.5	1–2	3–4
Short-acting	Regular (Humulin, Novolin R)	0.5–1	2–3	3–6
Intermediate-acting	NPH (Humulin, Novolin N)	2–4	4–6	8–12
Long-acting	Insulin detemir (Levemir)	0.8–2	–	6–24
	Insulin glargine (Lantus)	1.5–4	–	22–24

Source: Reference 7,26.

- Add correctional scale.
  - Correctional factor (the expected glucose-lowering response to 1 unit of insulin)
    - "Rule of 1700"
    - 1700/TDD = correction factor for lispro
  - Carbohydrate-counting factor (amount of carbohydrates 1 unit of insulin will cover[11]
    - "450 to 500 rule"
    - 450/TDD = for regular insulin
    - 500/TDD = for rapid-acting insulin
- For further discussion on inpatient and outpatient management guidelines, see http://endocrinology.yale.edu/patient/50135_Yale%20National%20F.pdf.
- On discharge and follow up (Table 5-3)
  - Tighter glucose control reduces microvascular complications (United Kingdom Prospective Diabetes Study and the U.S. National Institute of Diabetes and Digestive and Kidney Diseases Diabetes Control and Complications Trial).
  - It is controversial whether tighter glucose control prevents macrovascular complications.
  - American Diabetes Association (ADA) treatment goals
    - HbA$_{1c}$ level less than 7%: Consider following fructosamine in patients with anemia or hemoglobinopathies.
    - Preprandial plasma glucose level 70 to 130 mg/dL
    - Postprandial plasma glucose level less than 180 mg/dL
    - Blood pressure less than 130/80 mm Hg
    - Low-density lipoprotein (LDL) cholesterol level less than 100 mg/dL; less than 70 mg/dL in patients with overt cardiovascular disease
    - HDL level more than 40 mg/dL in men and more than 50 mg/dL in women
    - Triglyceride level less than 150 mg/dL (controversial)
  - Noninsulin antihyperglycemic medications used in DM-2 (Figure 5-1)
    - DM during pregnancy: metformin and sulfonylureas are safe and effective; however, insulin remains the mainstay of therapy.
- Chronic Complications of DM
  - Microvascular disease
    - Diabetic neuropathy: sensory, motor, and autonomic
    - Diabetic nephropathy: progresses slowly from microalbuminuria (30–300 mg/24 h) to macroalbuminuria (>300 mg/24 h) to nephrotic syndrome (>3.5 g/24 h). Manage

	Metformin (MET)	DPP4 Inhibitor	GLP-1 Agonist (Incretin Mimetic)	Sulfonylurea (SU)	Glinide**	Thiazolidinedione (TZD)	Colesevelam	Alpha-glucosidase inhibitor (AGI)	Insulin	Pramlintide
BENEFITS										
Postprandial glucose (PPG)-lowering	Mild	Moderate	Moderate to marked	Moderate	Moderate	Mild	Mild	Moderate	Moderate to marked	Moderate to marked
Fasting glucose (FPG)-lowering	Moderate	Mild	Mild	Moderate	Mild	Moderate	Mild	Neutral	Moderate to marked	Mild
Nonalcoholic fatty liver disease (NAFLD)	Mild	Neutral	Mild	Neutral	Neutral	Moderate	Neutral	Neutral	Neutral	Neutral
RISKS										
Hypoglycemia	Neutral	Neutral	Neutral	Moderate	Mild	Neutral	Neutral	Neutral	Moderate to severe	Neutral
Gastrointestinal symptoms	Moderate	Neutral	Moderate	Neutral	Neutral	Neutral	Moderate	Moderate	Neutral	Moderate
Risk of use with renal insufficiency	Severe	Reduce dosage	Moderate	Moderate	Neutral	Mild	Neutral	Neutral	Moderate	Unknown
Contraindicated in liver failure or predisposition to Lactic Acidosis	Severe	Neutral	Neutral	Moderate	Moderate	Moderate	Neutral	Neutral	Neutral	Neutral
Heart failure/Edema	Use with caution in CHF	Neutral	Neutral	Neutral	Neutral	Mild/Moderate — Contraindicated in class 3,4 CHF	Neutral	Neutral	Neutral unless with TZD	Neutral
Weight Gain	Benefit	Neutral	Benefit	Mild	Mild	Moderate	Neutral	Neutral	Mild to Moderate	Benefit
Fractures	Neutral	Neutral	Neutral	Neutral	Neutral	Moderate	Neutral	Neutral	Neutral	Neutral
Drug-Drug interactions	Neutral	Neutral	Neutral	Moderate	Moderate	Neutral	Neutral	Neutral	Neutral	Neutral

MEDICATIONS

** The term 'glinide' includes both repaglinide and nateglinide.

Figure 5-1   Glycemic control algorithm.[12]

with aggressive blood pressure control (angiotensin-converting enzyme inhibitor or angiotensin receptor blocker)
- Diabetic retinopathy: nonproliferative, proliferative, or macular edema
- Macrovascular disease
  - Coronary
  - Carotid and cerebral
  - Peripheral arteries
- For a comprehensive overview of the standards of medical care in diabetes by the American Diabetes Association (diabetes care 2012), see http://care.diabetesjournals.org/content/35/Supplement_1/S11.full.pdf+html?sid=96a0f77e-3b1d-4176-9b54-9da5eb047a7a.

METABOLIC SYNDROME

- Etiology, Definition, Pathophysiology
  - Insulin resistance with hypertension, dyslipidemia (decreased HDL level and elevated triglyceride level), central and visceral obesity, DM-2, or IGT/IFG
- Clinical Manifestations and Presentation
  - Abdominal obesity
  - Acanthosis nigricans
  - Also associated with hyperuricemia, polycystic ovarian syndrome, obstructive sleep apnea, and nonalcoholic steatohepatitis
- Laboratory and Tests
  - Diagnostic criteria (National Cholesterol Education Program guidelines establish diagnosis when at least three of the risk factors are present)
    - Abdominal obesity: waist circumference more than 40 inches in men and more than 35 inches in women
    - Triglyceride level 150 mg/dL or higher
    - HDL level less than 40 mg/dL in men and less than 50 mg/dL in women
    - Blood pressure 130/85 mm Hg or higher
    - Fasting glucose 100 mg/dL or higher
- Management
  - Lifestyle modification, diet and exercise 30 min/day five times per week per the Diabetes Prevention Program
  - Role of metformin
  - American Diabetes Association: "Metformin therapy for prevention of type 2 diabetes in those with impaired glucose tolerance (class A recommendation), impaired fasting glucose (class E recommendation), or an A1C of 5.7–6.4% (class E recommendation), especially for those with BMI >35 kg/m^2, age <60 years, and women with prior gestational diabetes mellitus (class A recommendation)."[14]

HYPOGLYCEMIA

- Definition
  - *Whipple's triad:* (1) symptoms consistent with hypoglycemia, (2) a low plasma glucose concentration, and (3) relief of symptoms after the plasma glucose level is raised.
- Etiology in an ill or medicated individual
  - Drugs
    - Insulin or insulin secretagogues
    - Alcohol
    - Others: angiotensin-converting enzyme inhibitors, angiotensin receptor antagonists, β-adrenergic receptor antagonists, quinolone antibiotics, indomethacin, quinine, sulfonamides, and so forth.
    - *Not* metformin, thiazolidinediones, α-glucosidase inhibitors, glucagonlike peptide-1 receptor agonists, and dipeptidyl peptidase-IV inhibitors unless combined with insulin secretagogues or insulin.

- Critical illness
  - Hepatic, renal or cardiac failure
  - Sepsis
  - Starvation
- Hormone deficiency
  - Cortisol
  - Glucagon and epinephrine (in insulin-deficient diabetes)
- Non-islet cell tumor
- Etiology in a seemingly well individual
  - Endogenous hyperinsulinism
    - Insulinoma
    - Functional beta-cell disorders (nesidioblastosis)
      - Noninsulinoma pancreatogenous hypoglycemia
      - Post-gastric bypass hypoglycemia
    - Insulin autoimmune hypoglycemia
      - Antibody to insulin
      - Antibody to insulin receptor
  - Insulin secretagogue
  - Accidental, surreptitious, or malicious hypoglycemia.
- Pathophysiology
  - Glucose normally kept 70 to 110 mg/dL
  - Glucose is maintained endogenously by hepatic glycogenolysis and hepatic and renal gluconeogenesis.
  - Hepatic glycogen stores maintain plasma glucose for approximately 8 h—shorter if demand is increased or stores are depleted by illness or starvation.
  - In hypoglycemia, the pituitary is stimulated to increase growth hormone and adrenocorticotropic hormone (ACTH), resulting in an elevation in cortisol.
  - Hypoglycemia also increases sympathoadrenal outflow, resulting in autonomic symptoms, as well as an increase in gluconeogenic precursors from muscle and fat (lactate, amino acids, fatty acids and glycerol).
- Risk Reduction
  - Normoglycemia in Intensive Care Evaluation Survival Using Glucose Algorithm Regulation (NICE-SUGAR) study showed increased mortality with attempts to control in-hospital plasma glucose values toward physiologic levels. Glucose goal in hospitalized patients are therefore 140 to 180 mg/dL.
  - Action in Diabetes and Vascular Disease (ADVANCE) and Action to Control Cardiovascular Risk in Diabetes (ACCORD) trials and Veterans' Administration Diabetes Trial (VADT) showed significant incidence of severe hypoglycemia in DM-2 with tighter glucose control attempts; little to no benefit in reducing macrovascular events as well.
- Clinical Manifestations and Presentation
  - Autonomic symptoms: release of catecholamines, glucagon, growth hormone, and cortisol. Palpitations, tremor, anxiety, sweating, hunger, and paresthesia.
  - Neuroglycopenic symptoms: lack of metabolic fuel for the brain. Behavioral changes, confusion, fatigue, seizure, loss of consciousness, and death.
  - Hypoglycemic unawareness: recurrent hypoglycemia shifts threshold for autonomic symptoms to lower levels. Therefore, the first manifestation is actually neuroglycopenia.
- Laboratory and Other Tests
  - Serum glucose should be drawn at the time of symptoms.
  - If the cause of hypoglycemia is unknown, obtain insulin level, C-peptide, proinsulin, beta-hydroxybutyrate, sulfonylurea levels, cortisol, and ethanol.
  - If hypoglycemia is not documented, overnight fasting or food deprivation during observation (inpatient 72-hour fast) may be required (standard test for insulinoma). Test is terminated if glucose level drops below 45 mg/dL with associated symptoms.

- Localizing an insulinoma may include MRI, transabdominal and endoscopic ultrasonography. May, if necessary, need selective pancreatic arterial calcium injection with measurements of hepatic venous insulin levels (distinguishes between insulinoma and islet cell hypertrophy and nesidioblastosis). *Class III recommendations.*[15]
- Management and Algorithmic Approach
  - Urgent treatment is necessary in patients with suspected hypoglycemia.
    - Administration of oral carbohydrates if feasible, or by parenteral glucagon or glucose if not feasible.
    - Hypoglycemia with sulfonylureas is often prolonged.
  - Approach to patient:
    - Diabetic patient: If patient has been treated with insulin, sulfonylurea, or other secretagogues, adjust the regimen and document improvement, and monitor.
    - Nondiabetic patient:
      - Look for clinical clues of a particular etiology: drugs, organ failure, sepsis, and so forth.
      - If no clues and apparently healthy, obtain fasting glucose level. Obtain 72-hour fast if initially more than 55 mg/dL and strong history.
        - If glucose level less than 55 mg/dL with elevated insulin, Whipple's triad, and elevated C-peptide, consider insulinoma, autoimmune, or sulfonylurea ingestion. Beta-hydroxybutyrate levels tend to be lower in insulinomas.
        - If glucose level less than 55 mg/dL with elevated insulin, Whipple's triad, and decreased C-peptide, consider exogenous insulin.
      - If glucose level during 72-hour fast is more than 55 mg/dL, apply mixed meal test. If Whipple's triad present, findings compatible with reactive hypoglycemia. If Whipple's triad is not present, hypoglycemia is excluded.

HYPOTHYROIDISM

- Definition: elevated TSH level, low FT_4 level
- Etiology: Iodine deficiency is the most common cause worldwide. In areas of iodine sufficiency, autoimmune disease (Hashimoto thyroiditis) and iatrogenic are the most common causes.
  - Primary hypothyroidism
    - Autoimmune: Hashimoto thyroiditis (marked lymphocytic infiltration) and atrophic thyroiditis (more extensive fibrosis, which is thought to be end-stage Hashimoto thyroiditis).
    - Human leukocyte antigen (HLA)-DR polymorphisms: genetic risk factors.
    - Anti-TPO, anti-thyroglobulin may be present. Approximately 20% have antibodies against thyrotropin receptor (TSH-R), preventing the binding of TSH.
    - Patients may present with a goiter (Hashimoto thyroiditis) or symptoms and signs of hypothyroidism (atrophic thyroiditis). Thyroid is nontender.
    - Iatrogenic: Iodine-131 (^{131}I) treatment, subtotal or total thyroidectomy, external irradiation of neck
    - Drugs: iodine excess (iodine-containing contrast media and amiodarone [Wolff-Chaikoff effect]), lithium, antithyroid drugs, p-aminosalicylic acid, interferon-α and other cytokines, aminoglutethimide, sunitinib, and so forth.
    - Congenital: absent or ectopic thyroid gland, dyshormonogenesis, TSH-R mutation
    - Iodine deficiency
    - Infiltrative disorders: amyloidosis, sarcoidosis, hemochromatosis, scleroderma, cystinosis, Riedel thyroiditis
    - Overexpression of type 3 deiodinase in infantile hemangioma
  - Transient hypothyroidism
    - Silent thyroiditis and postpartum thyroiditis
    - Subacute thyroiditis
    - Withdrawal of thyroxine treatment
    - After ^{131}I treatment or subtotal thyroidectomy for Graves disease

- Secondary hypothyroidism
  - Hypopituitarism: tumors, pituitary surgery and irradiation, infiltrative disorders, Sheehan syndrome, trauma, genetic forms of combined pituitary hormone deficiencies
  - Isolated TSH deficiency and inactivity
  - Hypothalamic disease: tumors, trauma, infiltrative disorders, idiopathic
- Wolff-Chaikoff effect: Excess iodine transiently inhibits thyroid iodine organification.
- Subclinical hypothyroidism: phase of compensation during reduction of thyroid function when normal thyroid hormone levels are maintained by a rise in TSH. Can be seen in autoimmune etiologies.
  - Patients may have mild symptoms, which become more apparent usually when TSH level is more than 10 mIU/L. Annual risk of developing clinical hypothyroidism is approximately 4% when associated with a positive TPO antibody.
- Clinical Manifestations and Presentation
  - Symptoms: Fatigue and generalized weakness, dry skin, cold intolerance, hair loss, difficulty concentrating and poor memory, constipation, weight gain (caused by fluid retention), poor appetite, dyspnea, hoarse voice, menorrhagia, paresthesia, impaired hearing, or depression.[16]
  - Signs: Dry, coarse skin; cool peripheral extremities; puffy hands, face, and feet with nonpitting pretibial edema (myxedema); diffuse alopecia; bradycardia; reduced myocardial stroke volume; hypertension; hyperlipidemia; peripheral edema; goiter; delayed tendon reflex relaxation; carpal tunnel syndrome; serous cavity effusions; dry, brittle hair; nail growth retardation; thinning of the outer third of the eyebrows; yellow appearance to skin.
    - If there is a sudden enlargement of the thyroid gland in a patient with chronic thyroiditis, there is a concern for lymphoma.
  - Signs and symptoms of other autoimmune diseases: Particularly vitiligo, pernicious anemia, Addison disease, alopecia areata, DM-1.
  - Polyglandular autoimmune syndrome type II: autoimmune thyroid disease with primary adrenal insufficiency and DM-1.
- Laboratory and other tests
  - Most valuable assay is TSH
  - Obtain a FT_4 if TSH is abnormal.
  - Obtain a FT_3 if TSH is elevated with normal FT_4.
  - Thyroid autoantibodies: anti-TPO, antithyroglobulin.
  - Thyroid scan, ultrasound, or both.
  - FNA biopsy can be used to confirm autoimmune thyroiditis.
  - Other abnormal laboratory findings:
    - Elevated creatinine phosphokinase, elevated cholesterol and triglyceride levels, and anemia.[16]
- Triage Decisions and Identifying Life-Threatening Complications
  - Myxedema coma: high mortality rate. Presents with reduced level of consciousness and/or seizures, hypothermia, hypotension, bradycardia, and hypoventilation. Almost always occurs in the older patients precipitated by factors that impair respiration.
  - Hashimoto encephalopathy: steroid-responsive syndrome associated with TPO antibodies, myoclonus, and slow-wave activity on electroencephalogram.
- Management
  - Immediate
    - Myxedema coma[17]
      - IV levothyroxine: single 500 μg IV loading dose, usually continued at 50 to 100 μg/day. May give the same initial dose by nasogastric tube.
      - Because of the concern for impaired thyroxine (T_4) to triiodothyronine (T_3) conversion during myxedema coma, T_3 IV or by nasogastric tube is used as an alternative (10–25 μg every 8–12 h) or in addition to T_4. Monitor for provoked arrhythmias.

- Another option: levothyroxine (200 μg) and liothyronine (25 μg) as a single IV bolus followed by daily levothyroxine (50–100 μg/d) and liothyronine (10 μg every 8 h). *Grade 2C recommendations.*
- Supportive therapy
  - Correct metabolic disturbances.
  - External warming is only indicated if temperature is less than 30°C (86°F), as it can result in cardiovascular collapse.
  - Parenteral hydrocortisone (50 mg every 6 h) should be administered, as there is impaired adrenal reserve in profound hypothyroidism.
  - Consider early broad-spectrum antibiotics.
  - Ventilatory support.
- Management issues during hospitalization:
  - Emergency surgery: generally safe in untreated hypothyroidism, however, routine surgery should be deferred until patient is euthyroid.
  - Euthyroid sick syndrome
    - An ill or starving body tends to decompensate by decreasing metabolic rates, resulting in a low FT_4 or triiodothyronine (T_3) estimate and a normal or low TSH level.
    - In addition, corticosteroids and dopamine may interfere with TFTs.
    - Treatment should be delayed until the underlying medical condition has resolved.
- On hospitalization and at follow-up
  - Levothyroxine replacement therapy
    - 1.6 μg/kg of body weight per day (if no thyroid function is present).
    - Dosing is traditionally started at lower initial doses depending on age, cardiac status, and the severity and duration of the hypothyroidism.
    - Treatment is indicated for clinical hypothyroidism, or possibly in patients with goiter and normal TSH.
  - Reassess and titrate after an interval of at least 6 weeks based on TSH. Adjust dosing in 12.5 to 25 μg increments.
  - Desiccated thyroid hormone, combinations (insufficient evidence present), or thyroid hormones, or T_3 should not be used as replacement therapy.
  - Thyroid absorption is affected by malabsorptive states and patient age.
  - Drug interactions: Certain drugs (cholestyramine, ferrous sulfate, sucralfate, calcium, and certain antacids) will affect absorption. Certain anticonvulsants will affect thyroid hormone binding. Rifampin and sertraline may accelerate levothyroxine metabolism, thus requiring a higher dose.
  - Treatment in subclinical hypothyroidism is controversial. Per 2002 American Association of Clinical Endocrinologists (AACE) guidelines, treatment is indicated in patients with TSH levels higher than 10 μIU/mL or in patients with TSH levels between 5 and 10 μIU/mL in conjunction with goiter or positive anti-TPO. Initial dosing is 25 to 50 μg/day.[16]

HYPERTHYROIDISM

- Definition
  - Thyrotoxicosis: state of thyroid hormone excess
  - Hyperthyroidism: excessive thyroid function
- Etiology
  - Primary hyperthyroidism
    - Graves disease: 60% to 80% of thyrotoxicosis
    - Toxic multinodular goiter
    - Toxic adenoma
    - Functioning thyroid carcinoma metastases
    - Activating mutation of the TSH receptor
    - Activating mutation of Gs_α (McCune-Albright syndrome)
    - Struma ovarii
    - Drugs: iodine excess (Jod-Basedow phenomenon)

- Thyrotoxicosis without hyperthyroidism
  - Subacute thyroiditis
  - Silent thyroiditis
  - Other thyroid destruction: amiodarone, radiation, infarction of adenoma
  - Ingestion of excess thyroid hormone (thyrotoxicosis factitia) or thyroid tissue
- Secondary hyperthyroidism
  - TSH-secreting pituitary adenoma: elevated TSH and FT_4 levels
  - Thyroid hormone resistance syndrome
  - Chorionic gonadotropin-secreting tumors (TSH level is low)
  - Gestational thyrotoxicosis (TSH level is low)
- Pathogenesis
  - Graves disease: thyroiditis caused by thyroid-stimulating immunoglobulin (TSI) produced in the thyroid, bone marrow, and lymph nodes.
    - TPO antibodies are present in up to 80% of patients.
    - Smoking, increase in iodine, postpartum state, immune reconstitution phase after receiving highly active antiretroviral therapy or alemtuzumab are all risk factors.
  - Thyroid-associated ophthalmopathy
    - Activated T cells infiltrate extraocular muscles and release interferon-γ, tumor necrosis factor, and interleukin-1 resulting in fibroblast activation and increased synthesis of glycosaminoglycans, which trap water and cause swelling.
    - Late in the disease, there is irreversible fibrosis of these muscles.
    - There is increased evidence that the TSH-R shares an autoantigen expressed in the orbit.
  - Other:
    - TBG is elevated in pregnant women or women taking estrogen-containing contraceptives, thus total T_4 and T_3 are elevated, however FT_4 and FT_3 are normal.
    - Mutations in TBG, transthyretin, and albumin may increase the binding affinity for T_3 and/or T_3, resulting in euthyroid hyperthyroxinemia or familial dysalbuminemic hyperthyroxinemia—increased total T_4 and/or T_3, but free FT_4 and FT_3 levels are normal.
- Clinical Manifestations and Presentation
  - Symptoms: hyperactivity, irritability, worsening angina, dysphoria, heat intolerance and sweating, palpitations, fatigue and weakness, fine hair texture or alopecia, pruritus, urticaria, weight loss with increased appetite, increased stool frequency, diarrhea, polyuria, oligomenorrhea, and loss of libido.
  - Apathetic thyrotoxicosis: seen in the older patients. Presents with fatigue, weight loss, and depressive symptoms.
  - Presentation
    - Cardiovascular: sinus tachycardia, atrial fibrillation (more common in the older patients), high cardiac output (bounding pulse, widened pulse pressure, aortic systolic murmur, heart failure)
    - Head, ears, eyes, nose, throat, and neck: goiter, signs of ophthalmopathy (see below). Diffusely enlarged firm thyroid in Graves disease—thrill or bruit may be heard because of increased vascularity of the gland and hyperdynamic circulation.
    - Neuro- and musculoskeletal: fine tremor, muscle weakness and wasting, proximal myopathy without fasciculations, hyperreflexia, osteopenia and bone fractures.
      - Thyrotoxicosis can sometimes be associated with a form of hypokalemic periodic paralysis.
    - Renal and electrolytes: mild hypercalcemia, hypercalciuria
    - Skin: warm, moist skin, gynecomastia, palmar erythema, onycholysis, acropachy (clubbing), thyroid dermopathy (a.k.a. pretibial myxedema—anterior and lateral aspects of the lower leg)
    - Thyroid-associated ophthalmopathy
      - Early signs: sensation of grittiness, eye discomfort, and excess tearing. Proptosis, diplopia, lid retraction, periorbital edema, conjunctival injection and optic neuropathy.

- • Can lead to corneal exposure and damage.
- • Must refer to ophthalmologist.
  - • "NO SPECS" scheme to assess extent and activity of orbital changes:
    - • 0 = No signs or symptoms
    - • 1 = Only signs (lid retraction or lag), no symptoms
    - • 2 = Soft-tissue involvement (periorbital edema)
    - • 3 = Proptosis (>22 mm)
    - • 4 = Extraocular-muscle involvement (diplopia)
    - • 5 = Corneal involvement
    - • 6 = Sight loss
- • Laboratory and Other Tests
  - • TSH, FT_4, FT_3.
  - • Diagnosis of Graves disease is confirmed in the setting of thyrotoxicosis, diffuse goiter on palpation, ophthalmopathy, and a personal or family history of autoimmune disorders.
  - • TSI antibody for thyrotoxicosis patients who lack the above features.
  - • Other laboratory test results: may see elevated bilirubin, liver enzymes, and ferritin along with microcytic anemia and thrombocytopenia.
  - • Radionuclide scan: when the clinical presentation of thyrotoxicosis is not diagnostic of Graves disease. *Class I recommendation.*[18]
    - • High (or normal) uptake
      - • Graves disease or Hashitoxicosis: diffuse homogeneous uptake
      - • Toxic adenoma: focal uptake
      - • Toxic multinodular goiter: diffuse heterogeneous uptake
    - • Low or no uptake: indicates destructive thyroiditis, iodine excess, and excess thyroid hormone and factitious thyrotoxicosis.
  - • Thyroid ultrasound (specify vascularity): will detect nodules or multinodular goiter. Low vascularity is commonly seen in thyroiditis.
  - • Subclinical hyperthyroidism: low TSH level with normal levels of FT_4 and FT_3. May resolve spontaneously. Deleterious effects on the cardiovascular and skeletal system.
- • Triage Decisions (Figure 5-2)
- • Management of acute life-threatening manifestations
  - • Thyrotoxic crisis and thyroid storm (Table 5-4): fever, delirium, seizures, coma, vomiting, diarrhea, and jaundice. May progress to cardiac failure, arrhythmia, or hyperthermia.
    - • Precipitated by acute illness (eg, stroke, infection, trauma, DKA), surgery, radioiodine treatment in patients with untreated hyperthyroidism.
  - • Treat precipitating causes.
    - • Supportive care; treating symptoms:
      - • Propranolol: reduce adrenergic manifestations. At high doses, will decrease T_4 to T_3 conversion.[20]
      - • Aggressive cooling with acetaminophen and cooling blankets, volume resuscitation, respiratory support, and monitoring in the intensive care unit. *Class I recommendations.*[18]
    - • Reduce thyroid hormone synthesis:
      - • Propylthiouracil (PTU) 600 mg loading dose, then 200 to 300 mg every 6 hours inhibits T_4 to T_3 conversion.
      - • Stable iodide and saturated solution of potassium iodide blocks thyroid hormone synthesis through Wolff-Chaikoff effect; given 1 hour after the first PTU dose so the iodine will not be incorporated into new hormone.
      - • Glucocorticoids may block T_4 to T_3 conversion. Prophylaxis against relative adrenal insufficiency.
- • Management during hospitalization
  - • Goal of treatment
    - • Reducing thyroid hormone synthesis (see above).

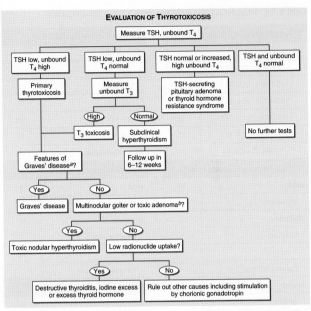

EVALUATION OF THYROTOXICOSIS

Measure TSH, unbound T₄

Figure 5-2 Evaluation of thyrotoxicosis. *Diffuse goiter, positive TPO antibodies, ophthalmopathy, dermopathy; *can be confirmed by radionuclide scan. T₃, liothyronine; T₄, thyroxine; TPO, thyroid peroxidase; TSH, thyroid-stimulating hormone. (From Jameson JL, Weetman AP. Disorders of the thyroid gland. In: Longo DL, et al., eds. *Harrison's Principles of Internal Medicine.* 18th ed. New York: McGraw-Hill; 2012:2911-2939.)

- Controlling symptoms: Beta-blockers should be given to patients with symptomatic thyrotoxicosis to help control adrenergic symptoms (class 1 recommendations of the AACE).
- Antithyroid drugs
  - Thioamides: PTU, carbimazole, methimazole.
    - Inhibits the function of TPO, reducing oxidation and organification of iodide. Reduces TSI levels. Inhibits deiodination of T₄ to T₃ conversion.
    - PTU: shorter half-life (90 min) than methimazole (6 h).
  - Preference
    - Methimazole should be used in patients who choose antithyroid drug therapy has treatment for Graves disease, *except:*
    - During the first trimester of pregnancy (aplasia cutis in infants, PTU is preferred).
    - In the treatment of thyroid storm (PTU is preferred).
    - In patients with minor reactions to methimazole who refuse radioactive iodine therapy. Class I recommendations of AACE.
  - Side effects: rash, urticarial, fever, arthralgias, hepatitis, systemic lupus erythematosus-like syndrome, agranulocytosis (<1%).
- Reducing the amount of thyroid tissue
  - Radioiodine (¹³¹I) treatment

TABLE 5-4. DIAGNOSTIC CRITERIA FOR THYROID STORM[19a]

Thermoregulatory Dysfunction		Cardiovascular Dysfunction	
Temperature (°F | °C)		**Tachycardia**	
99–99.9 | 37.2–37.7	5	99–109	5
100–100.9 | 37.8–38.2	10	110–119	10
101–101.9 | 38.3–38.8	15	120–129	15
102–102.9 | 38.9–39.4	20	130–139	20
103–103.9 | 39.4–39.9	25	≥140	25
≥104.0 | >40.0	30	**Atrial Fibrillation**	10
Central Nervous System Effects		**Heart Failure**	
Mild	10	**Mild**	5
Agitation		Pedal edema	
Moderate	20	**Moderate**	10
Delirium		Bibasilar rales	
Psychosis		**Severe**	15
Extreme lethargy		Pulmonary edema	
Severe	30	**Precipitant History**	
Seizure		Negative	0
Coma		Positive	10
Gastrointestinal-Hepatic Dysfunction			
Moderate	10		
Diarrhea			
Nausea/Vomiting			
Abdominal pain			
Severe	20		
Unexplained jaundice			

[a]A score of 45 or more is highly suggestive of thyroid storm; a score of 25 to 44 supports the diagnosis; and a score below 25 makes thyroid storm unlikely.
Adapted from: Burch HB, Wartofsky L, Endocrinol Metab Clin North Am 1993; 22;263.

- Small risk of thyrotoxic crisis, minimized by pretreating with antithyroid drugs for at least 1 month prior to treatment.
- Caution in patients with active ophthalmopathy, as this will be exacerbated. Recommend concurrent corticosteroids in patients with active ophthalmopathy undergoing treatment.
- Subtotal or near-total thyroidectomy
  - For patients who relapse after antithyroid drugs and prefer this treatment to radioiodine.

TABLE 5-5. SUBCLINICAL HYPOTHYROIDISM: WHEN TO TREAT[21]

Factor	TSH (<0.1 mU/L)	TSH (0.1–0.5 mU/L)
Age >65 years	Yes	Consider treating
Age <65 years with comorbidities		
Heart disease	Yes	Consider treating
Osteoporosis	Yes	No
Menopausal	Consider treating	Consider treating
Hyperthyroid symptoms	Yes	Consider treating
Age <65, asymptomatic	Consider treating	No

TSH, thyroid-stimulating hormone

- Possible preference in young patients or in those when the goiter is very large.
- Control of thyrotoxicosis with antithyroid drugs followed by potassium iodide is needed prior to surgery to reduce vascularity.
  - Risk: bleeding, damage to recurrent laryngeal nerves, hypoparathyroidism.
- On discharge and follow-up
  - Review TFTs and clinical manifestations 3 to 4 weeks after starting treatment. Dose is titrated based on unbound T_4 levels, *not* TSH levels (remain suppressed for several months).
- Subclinical hyperthyroidism: see Table 5-5 for when to treat.

THYROIDITIS

- Etiology and Pathogenesis
  - Acute: Mostly painful, acute onset
    - Bacterial (Staphylococcus, Streptococcus, Enterobacter)
    - Fungal (aspergillus, candida, coccidioides, histoplasma, pneumocystis)
    - Radiation thyroiditis following ^{131}I treatment
    - Drugs: (painless) amiodarone, interferon-α. More common in positive TPO.
    - Immunocompromised: fungal, mycobacterial, or *pneumocystis* thyroiditis
  - Subacute
    - Patchy inflammation infiltrate with disruption of thyroid follicles and multinucleated giant cells within some follicles, resulting in the release of preformed thyroid hormone (temporary). Progresses to granulomas accompanied by fibrosis. Thyroid returns to normal several months after onset.
    - Viral thyroiditis: (painful) mumps, coxsackie, influenza, adenovirus, echovirus.
    - Granulomatous thyroiditis (painful).
    - de Quervain thyroiditis (painful).
    - Silent thyroiditis (painless).
    - Postpartum thyroiditis (painless): 3 to 6 months after pregnancy. Brief thyrotoxicosis for 2 to 4 weeks, followed by hypothyroidism for 4 to 12 weeks, then resolution. Normal ESR, positive TPO. More common in DM-1.
    - Mycobacterial infection
  - Chronic
    - Autoimmunity
      - Focal thyroiditis: positive TPO
      - Hashimoto thyroiditis
      - Atrophic thyroiditis

- Riedel thyroiditis: insidious, painless hard goiter with compressive symptoms. Dense fibrosis disrupts the gland architecture.
  - Parasitic: echinococcus, strongyloidiasis, cysticercosis
  - Trauma: after palpation
- Clinical Manifestations and Presentation
  - Acute: fevers, dysphagia, tenderness and erythema over the thyroid, lymphadenopathy
  - Subacute: painful, radiating to the jaw or ear, enlarged thyroid, malaise, sometimes accompanied by fever.
    - May have symptoms of thyrotoxicosis or hypothyroidism depending on the phase of the illness. Upper respiratory infection may precede.
- Laboratory and Other Tests
  - TFTs are typically normal unless in the thyrotoxic phase or hypothyroid phase.
  - Thyroid antibodies are typically negative, except in silent thyroiditis.
  - ESR and white blood cell count are elevated in acute and subacute thyroiditis. ESR is normal in silent thyroiditis.
  - FNA reveals polymorphonuclear leukocytes in acute thyroiditis.
  - CT or ultrasound may be warranted to evaluate for abscess.
  - Radionuclide uptake: low in destructive subacute painless thyroiditis.
- Triage Decisions
  - Monitor for complications of acute thyroiditis: tracheal obstruction, septicemia, retropharyngeal abscess, mediastinitis, or jugular venous thrombosis.
- Management
  - During Hospitalization
    - Antibiotic treatment for bacterial acute thyroiditis.
    - Surgery may be required to drain an abscess.
    - For subacute thyroiditis: large doses of aspirin or nonsteroidal antiinflammatory drugs are used to control symptoms. If not improved, corticosteroids may be necessary, which are gradually tapered dose over 6 to 8 weeks.
    - For silent thyroiditis corticosteroids are not warranted. May use propranolol if symptomatic. Thyroid hormone may be required during hypothyroid phase.
    - Riedel thyroiditis: surgical relief and/or tamoxifen.
  - On discharge and follow-up
    - Thyroid function should be monitored every 2 to 4 weeks.

SPECIAL THYROID CONSIDERATIONS

- Sick Euthyroid Syndrome
  - Definition: abnormalities of circulating TSH or thyroid hormone levels in the setting of acute, severe illness and in the absence of underlying thyroid disease.
  - Etiology and Pathophysiology
    - From the release of cytokines such as IL-6.
    - Conversion of T_4 to T_3 through peripheral deiodination is impaired.
    - Decreased clearance of reverse triiodothyronine (rT_3), resulting in decreased T_3.
    - Rise in cortisol or administration of glucocorticoids may result in decreased TSH level.
  - Clinical manifestations and presentation: should be asymptomatic.
  - Laboratory and other tests: hormone pattern:
    - Most common is decreased total and FT_3 levels with normal FT_4 and TSH. Elevated rT_3.
    - Very ill patients: dramatic decrease in total T_4 and T_3 as well as TSH because of altered binding to TBG, which demonstrates a poor prognosis.
  - Triage decisions: Routine testing of thyroid function should be avoided in acutely ill patients.
  - Management
    - Immediate: do not treat with thyroid hormone unless there is historic or clinical evidence suggestive of hypothyroidism.

- During hospitalization observe for symptoms.
- On discharge and follow-up, recheck laboratory test results once acute illness has resolved.
- Amiodarone Effects on Thyroid Function
  - Etiology (three possible):
    - Acute, transient suppression of thyroid function
    - Hypothyroidism in patients susceptible to the inhibitory effects of a high iodine load (Wolff-Chaikoff effect)
    - Amiodarone-induced thyrotoxicosis (AIT) that may be caused by either a Jod-Basedow effect from the iodine load, in the setting of multinodular goiter, or incipient Graves disease, or a thyroiditis-like condition
  - Pathophysiology: Amiodarone contains a high (39%) iodine content by weight that persists for more than 6 months after discontinuation. It inhibits deiodinase activity, and its metabolites function as weak antagonists of thyroid hormone action.
    - Type 1 AIT: associated with an underlying thyroid abnormality (preclinical Graves disease and nodular goiter). Thyroid hormone synthesis becomes excessive from increased iodine exposure (Jod-Basedow phenomenon).
    - Type 2 AIT: no intrinsic thyroid abnormalities. Results from drug-induced lysosomal activation leading to destructive thyroiditis with histiocyte accumulation in the thyroid. Milder forms can resolve spontaneously or lead to hypothyroidism.
  - Clinical Manifestations and Presentation
    - Manifestations of hyperthyroidism, hypothyroidism, or asymptomatic
  - Laboratory and Other Tests
    - On initiation: transient decrease of T_4 levels (iodine load).
    - Soon thereafter: Thyroid hormone receptor action becomes predominant: increased T_4, decreased T_3, increased rT_3, and a transient TSH increase.
    - Within 1 to 3 months TSH levels normalize or are slightly suppressed.
    - Color-flow Doppler thyroid scanning
      - Type 1 AIT: increased vascularity
      - Type 2 AIT: decreased vascularity
  - Triage decisions
    - Whether to stop amiodarone
  - Management
    - Hypothyroidism: Unnecessary to discontinue amiodarone for the Wolff-Chaikoff effect. Levothyroxine can be used to normalize function.
    - AIT: Amiodarone should be stopped, if possible.
      - AIT type 1: High doses of antithyroid drugs can be used, but are often ineffective.
      - AIT type 2: Oral contrast agents (sodium ipodate or sodium tyropanoate) will rapidly reduce T_4 and T_3, decrease T_4 to T_3 conversion, and may block uptake of thyroid hormones. Glucocorticoids may have modest benefit. Lithium blocks thyroid hormone release.
  - On discharge and follow-up
    - Monitor TSH levels.

THYROID GOITER

- Definition, Etiology, and Pathophysiology
  - Goiter: enlarged thyroid from biosynthetic defects, iodine deficiency (most common cause worldwide), autoimmune disease (Graves and Hashimoto diseases), and nodular diseases.
    - Diffuse Nontoxic (Simple) Goiter
      - Absence of nodules and hyperthyroidism
      - More common in women
      - Prevalence of underlying autoimmune disease
    - Nontoxic Multinodular Goiter
      - More common in women.

- Increases in prevalence with age.
- Wide variation in nodule size: hypercellular to cystic areas as well as extensive fibrosis and areas of hemorrhage or lymphocytic infiltration.
- Develops over many years and is detected on routine physical examination or the individual notices a large neck.
- Risk of malignancy is similar to that of solitary nodules.
- Toxic Multinodular Goiter
  - Similar to nontoxic multinodular goiter except for the presence of functional autonomy
- Clinical Manifestations and Presentation
  - Simple Goiter and Multinodular goiter
    - Symptoms of thyrotoxicosis or hypothyroidism are possible.
    - If thyroid function is preserved, it is typically asymptomatic.
    - Localized pain and swelling if spontaneous hemorrhage into a cyst or nodule.
    - Sudden pain and/or hoarseness may also raise the possibility of invasive malignancy in multinodular goiter.
    - Monitor for tracheal or esophageal compression.
    - Substernal goiter may obstruct the thoracic inlet, presenting with *Pemberton sign*.
  - Toxic Multinodular Goiter
    - Features of goiter with subclinical hyperthyroidism or mild thyrotoxicosis.
    - Patient is usually older; may present with atrial fibrillation or palpitations, tachycardia nervousness, tremor, or weight loss.
    - May have had recent exposure to iodine.
- Laboratory and Tests
  - TFTs
  - TPO: Identify patients at risk for developing autoimmune thyroid disease.
  - Ultrasound is generally not indicated unless a nodule (or multinodular goiter) is palpable on physical examination.
  - Uptake scan is not generally necessary if thyroid function is preserved.
  - If toxic multinodular goiter present, thyroid scan typically shows heterogenous uptake with multiple regions of increased and decreased uptake; 24-hour uptake of radioiodine may not be increased.
  - CT and/or MRI, barium swallow and/or pulmonary function tests if compressive signs are present.
- Management
  - Large, dominant nodules or those with sonographic characteristics (microcalcifications, hypoechogenicity, increased vascularity), should be biopsied.
  - Iodine replacement or thyroid hormone if indicated (in simple goiters).
  - T_4 suppression is rarely effective for reducing multinodular goiter size and risks subclinical or overt thyrotoxicosis.
  - Contrast agents and other iodine-containing substances should be avoided in multinodular goiter because of risk of inducing the *Jod-Basedow effect*.
  - Surgery is rarely indicated unless tracheal compression or obstruction of the thoracic outlet. Glucocorticoids may be used in this setting as well.
  - Radioactive iodine reduces goiter size by approximately 50% in the majority of patients over 6 to 12 months.
  - Posttreatment autoimmune thyrotoxicosis is seen in up to 5% of patients.
  - In toxic multinodular goiters, antithyroid drugs can often stimulate growth of the goiter, and spontaneous remission does not occur. Radioiodine can be used to treat areas of autonomy. Radioiodine can be used to treat areas of autonomy and decrease the goiter mass, however some autonomy remains.

THYROID NODULES AND MASSES

- Definition
  - Toxic adenoma: solitary autonomously functioning thyroid nodule

- Pathogenesis
  - Toxic adenoma: acquired somatic, activating mutations in the TSH-R or the Gsα subunit gene, leading to enhanced thyroid follicular cell proliferation and function.
- Etiology: Thyroid Nodules
  - Benign nodular goiter, chronic lymphocytic thyroiditis, simple or hemorrhagic cysts, follicular adenomas, subacute thyroiditis, papillary carcinoma, follicular carcinoma, Hürthle cell carcinoma, poorly differentiated carcinoma, medullary carcinoma, anaplastic carcinoma, primary thyroid lymphoma, sarcoma, teratoma, and miscellaneous tumors, metastatic tumors
- Clinical Manifestations and Presentation
  - Toxic adenoma: usually mild thyrotoxicosis. Clinical features of Graves disease are absent.
  - Thyroid Nodule (AACE)
    - Record the following information (grade B):
      - Age, family history of thyroid disease or cancer, previous head or neck irradiation, rate of growth of the neck mass, dysphonia, dysphagia, or dyspnea, symptoms of hyperthyroidism or hypothyroidism, or use of iodine-containing drugs and/or supplements.
      - Most are asymptomatic.
      - Physical examination: examination is mandatory for the thyroid gland and cervical lymph nodes (grade C).
- Laboratory and Tests
  - Thyroid scan: definitive diagnostic test; demonstrates focal uptake in the hyperfunctioning nodule with diminished uptake in the remainder of the gland.
  - Thyroid nodule (AACE)
    - Always measure serum TSH (grade A).
    - Testing for antithyroglobulin antibodies should be restricted to ultrasound and clinical findings suggestive of chronic lymphocytic thyroiditis (grade C).
    - Measurement of calcitonin is mandatory in patients with a family history or clinical suspicion of medullary thyroid carcinoma or multiple endocrine neoplasia type 2 (MEN-2) (grade A).
    - Ultrasound should be performed in all patients with palpable thyroid nodules or multinodular goiters, patients at risk for thyroid malignancy, or patients with lymphadenopathy suggesting a malignant lesion (grade B).
    - Nodules that are hot on scintigraphy should be excluded from FNA biopsy (grade B).
    - MRI and CT are not indicated for routine thyroid nodule evaluation (grade D).
- Triage Decisions (Figure 5-3)
- Management
  - Toxic adenoma
    - Radioiodine ablation is usually the treatment of choice. ^{131}I concentrates in the nodule with minimal uptake in the normal thyroid tissue.
    - Limit surgical resection to enucleation of the adenoma or lobectomy, thereby preserving thyroid function.
    - Antithyroid drugs plus beta-blockers are not an optimal long-term treatment.
    - Ultrasound-guided ethanol injections or percutaneous radiofrequency thermal ablation.
  - Thyroid Nodules (AACE)
    - Clinical and ultrasound examination and TSH measured 6 to 18 months following initial benign FNA. (For further guidelines, please visit https://www.aace.com/files/thyroid-guidelines.pdf.)

HYPERCALCEMIA

- Etiology and Pathophysiology: Hyperparathyroidism and malignancy account for 90% of all cases.
  - Parathyroid

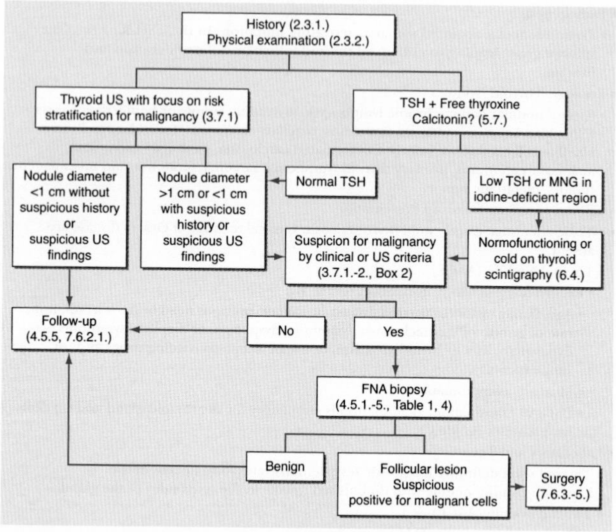

Figure 5-3 American Association of Clinical Endocrinologists, the Associazione Medici Endocrinologi (AME) and European Thyroid Association (ETA) thyroid nodule guidelines.[22] FNA, fine-needle aspiration; MNG, multinodular goiter; TSH, thyroid-stimulating hormone; US, ultrasound.

- Primary hyperparathyroidism: elevated secretion of PTH resulting in increased bone resorption enhancing calcium reabsorption, synthesis of 1,25OH-VitD, and GI calcium absorption. Typically asymptomatic. Peak incidence occurs between third and fifth decades of life and results from:
  - Adenoma: approximately 80% of patients. Typically inferior.
  - Hyperplasia: predominant chief cells.
  - Familial:
    - *MEN:* MEN 1 (Wermer syndrome—menin mutation) and MEN 2A (RET mutation) autosomal dominant
    - *Hyperparathyroidism jaw tumor syndrome:* parathyroid tumors in association with benign jaw tumors
    - *Nonsyndromic familial isolated hyperparathyroidism:* hereditary hyperparathyroidism without other endocrinopathies
  - Carcinoma: rare, and not often aggressive
- Lithium therapy: long-standing stimulation of parathyroid cell replication by lithium leads to development of adenomas. Lithium shifts the PTH secretion curve to the right in response to Ca^{++} (higher calcium levels are required to lower PTH secretion).
- Familial hypocalciuric hypercalcemia
  - Autosomal dominant.
  - An inactivating mutation in the calcium sensing receptor in the parathyroid and renal tubule, thus lowering the capacity of the sensor to bind calcium, resulting in inappropriately normal and/or elevated PTH secretion and excessive renal reabsorption of Ca^{++}.
  - Normal parathyroid size.

- Jansen disease
  - Autosomal-dominant activating mutations in the PTH/PTHrP receptor.
  - Short-limbed dwarfism because of abnormal regulation of chondrocyte maturation in the growth plates.
  - Multiple cystic resorptive areas.
- Malignancy
  - Squamous cell tumors are most frequently associated.
  - Solid tumor with metastasis (breast): local invasion and bone destruction
    - Humoral hypercalcemia of malignancy: solid tumor with humoral mediation of hypercalcemia (squamous cell lung, renal tumors).
      - Overproduction of PTHrP by cancer cells, which act like PTH.
    - Hematologic malignancies (multiple myeloma lymphoma, leukemia)
      - Direct bone marrow invasion
      - Activation of osteoclast activation factor as well as increased 1,25OH-VitD produced by certain lymphomas.
- Vitamin D
  - Vitamin D intoxication
  - Elevated 1,25OH-VitD; sarcoidosis, granulomatous disease (tuberculosis and fungal infections)
    - Excess of 25OH-VitD conversion to 1,25OH-VitD by macrophages and granulomas
  - Idiopathic hypercalcemia of infancy
    - *Williams syndrome*
    - Autosomal dominant (chromosome 7)
    - Supravalvular aortic stenosis, mental retardation, elfin facies
    - Abnormal sensitivity to vitamin D.
- High bone turnover
  - Hyperthyroidism caused by increased bone turnover with bone resorption exceeding bone formation.
  - Immobilization, particularly after spinal cord injury. Disproportion between bone formation and bone resorption.
    - Thiazides: secondary to hypocalciuric effect. Enhancement of proximal tubular resorption of sodium and calcium in response to sodium depletion.
    - Vitamin A intoxication.
- Renal Failure
  - Severe secondary hyperparathyroidism:
    - Resistance to normal PTH contributing to hypocalcemia, which stimulates parathyroid gland enlargement.
    - Increase in fibroblast growth factor-23 production by osteocytes, which inhibits renal α_1-hydroxylase.
  - Tertiary hyperparathyroidism:
    - PTH hypersecretion no longer responsive to medical therapy
    - Often requires surgery
  - Aluminum intoxication: patients on long-term dialysis who received aluminum-containing phosphate binders. Not typically used.
  - Milk-alkali syndrome:
    - Excessive ingestion of calcium and absorbable antacids such as milk or calcium carbonate.
- Clinical Manifestations and Presentation
  - History
    - Obtain dietary history and history of ingestion of vitamins or drugs.
    - History of nephrolithiasis: calcium oxalate or calcium phosphate.
    - History of peptic ulcer disease (MEN-1)
    - History of osteoporosis: hyperparathyroidism
    - Establish chronicity
      - Chronic hypercalcemia is most likely secondary to hyperparathyroidism.

- Consider occult malignancy if acute onset or no data as to the duration (hypercalcemia is a poor prognostic indicator).
- Review of Systems
  - Asymptomatic if hyperparathyroidism or familial hypocalciuric hypercalcemia.
  - Symptoms of associated malignancy.
  - Fatigue, depression, mental confusion, anorexia, nausea, vomiting, constipation, increase urination
  - Bone pain, ectopic calcification, and pruritus in secondary hyperparathyroidism.
  - Acute dementia, unresponsiveness and severe osteomalacia with bone pain, multiple nonhealing fractures and a proximal myopathy in aluminum toxicity.
  - Symptoms are more common at levels higher than 11.5 to 12 mg/dL
- Clinical Presentation
  - Reversible renal tubular defects because of calcium deposition and blocking antidiuretic hormone (ADH) activity.
  - *Osteitis fibrosa cystica*: increase in giant multinucleated osteoclasts in the scalloped areas on the surface of the bone and replacement by fibrous tissue; "salt and pepper" on x-ray.
  - Hypercalcemia plus alkalosis with renal failure is seen in milk alkali syndrome.
  - Short QT interval on ECG and sometimes cardiac arrhythmias.
  - At calcium levels higher than 13 mg/dL, metastatic calcification may occur.
  - Calcium levels 15 to 18 mg/dL can be a medical emergency as coma and cardiac arrest can occur.
- Laboratory and Tests
  - Verify true hypercalcemia versus hemoconcentration or elevated serum proteins (Table 5-6).
  - Obtain phosphorus, PTH, 25OH-VitD, and 1,25OH-VitD.
  - Consider PTHrP and/or bone scan if high suspicion for malignancy.
- Triage Decisions
  - *Hypercalcemic parathyroid crisis*: Rarely, hyperparathyroidism acutely worsens resulting in marked dehydration and coma. Most hyperparathyroidism is asymptomatic.

TABLE 5-6. LABORATORY EVALUATION OF HYPERCALCEMIA

	PTH	Phosphorus	Other Laboratory Test Results
Primary hyperparathyroidism	Elevated	Low (may be normal in setting of renal failure)	Elevated urine calcium and 1, 25OH-VitD
Familial hypocalciuric hypercalcemia	Elevated or low	Low	Low urine calcium
Humoral hypercalcemia of malignancy	Low/undetectable	Low/normal	Low/normal 1,25OH-VitD
Vitamin D intoxication	Low/normal	Elevated	–
Granulomatous disease	Low	Elevated/normal	Elevated 1,25OH-VitD
Hyperthyroidism	Low	Elevated	Elevated urine calcium

1,25OH-VitD, vitamin D₃ (1,25-dihydroxycholecalciferol).

- Guidelines for the management of asymptomatic primary hyperparathyroidism[23]
  - Guidelines for surgery
    - Serum calcium level more than 1 mg/dL above normal
    - Creatinine clearance less than 60 mL/min
    - Bone-density T score less than −2.5 at any of 3 sites
    - Age younger than 50 years
  - Follow-up for those who do not undergo parathyroid surgery
    - Serum calcium level test annually
    - Serum creatinine level test annually
    - Bone density scan every 1 to 2 years (3 sites)
  - For further management guidelines, see _____
    _____

- Management (Table 5-7)
  - Immediate (For more clinical opinions, see _____
    _____)
    - Mild hypercalcemia: Ca level less than 12 mg/dL
      - IV hydration.
      - Treat symptoms.
      - Correct hypophosphatemia if present.
    - Severe hypercalcemia: Ca level higher than 14 mg/dL
      - IV hydration and/or loop diuretics.

TABLE 5-7. TREATMENT OF HYPERCALCEMIA

Treatment	Onset	Details	Duration
Hydration (NS)	Hours	May require 3–6 L within the first 24 h	
Loop diuretics	Hours	Only after fluid volume is restored. Inhibits calcium reabsorption in the ascending limb of the loop of Henle.	
Bisphosphonates		Inhibits osteoclast-mediated bone resorption. Used extensively in cancer patients.	
Pamidronate	1–2 days	Monitor for hypocalcemia, hypophosphatemia, hypomagnesemia, or jaw necrosis	10–14 days to weeks
Zoledronate	1–2 days	As above	>3 weeks
Calcitonin	Hours	Blocks osteoclast-mediated bone resorption. Rapid onset—use in severe hypercalcemia. Monitor for rapid tachyphylaxis.	1–2 days
Glucocorticoids	Days	Increases urinary calcium excretion and decreases intestinal calcium absorption. Use in certain malignancies (multiple myeloma, leukemia, Hodgkin disease, other lymphomas, and carcinoma of the breast), vitamin D excess, and sarcoidosis.	Days, weeks
Hemodialysis	Hours	In renal failure	24–48 h after use

NS, normal saline.

- Bisphosphonates.
- Use calcitonin simultaneously for bone resorption inhibition while waiting for more sustained effects of bisphosphonates.
  - Hyperparathyroidism
    - Bisphosphonates: increase bone mineral density significantly without changing serum calcium.
    - Calcimimetics: lower PTH secretion, thus lowering calcium, but does not affect bone mineral density.
- During hospitalization and follow-up
  - Hyperparathyroidism
    - Concern remains for skeletal, cardiovascular, and neuropsychiatric disease.
    - Parathyroidectomy (see indications above):
      - Preoperative technetium 99m (^{99m}Tc) sestamibi scans with single-photon emission computed tomography.
      - Intraoperative sampling of PTH before and at 5-minute intervals after removal of a suspected adenoma to confirm a rapid fall (>50%) to normal levels of PTH.
      - For hyperplasia, remove 3 glands with partial excision of the fourth gland OR total parathyroidectomy with transplantation of a portion of the parathyroid gland into the muscles of the forearm.
      - Monitor for acute postoperative hypocalcemia.
    - Medical surveillance (see above)
  - Hypercalcemia of malignancy
    - Acute management of hypercalcemia as seen above
    - Reduction of underlying tumor mass
    - Glucocorticoids if underlying lymphoma
  - Vitamin D intoxication
    - Discontinue vitamin D.
    - Responsive to glucocorticoids, as levels persist for weeks after ingestion.
    - Severe intoxication may require intensive therapy.
  - Sarcoidosis and granulomatous disease
    - Limit vitamin D and calcium intake
    - Glucocorticoids: blocking excessive production of 1,25OH-VitD.
  - Severe secondary hyperparathyroidism
    - Restrict dietary phosphate.
    - Nonabsorbable antacids:
      - Calcium carbonate.
      - Aluminum-containing antacids are not frequently used.
    - Synthetic gels, which bind phosphagen:
      - Sevelamer
    - Calcitriol
  - Tertiary hyperparathyroidism
    - Parathyroid surgery
- On discharge and follow-up
  - Secondary hyperparathyroidism: Be wary of *aplastic* or *adynamic* bone disease during treatment, a low-bone-turnover state caused by excessive PTH suppression.

HYPOCALCEMIA

- Etiology and Pathophysiology
  - PTH Absent
    - Hereditary hypoparathyroidism
      - Developmental defects
      - Basal ganglia calcification and extrapyramidal syndromes
      - Papilledema and raised intracranial pressure
      - *DiGeorge syndrome*
        - Autosomal dominant microdeletions of chromosome 22q11.2
        - Infections, seizures, cardiovascular complications

- Mitochondrial dysfunction and myopathy
  - *MELAS (myopathy, encephalopathy, lactic acidosis, stroke-like episodes) syndrome*
  - *Kearns-Sayre syndrome*
- *Autosomal dominant hypocalcemic hypercalciuria*
  - Abnormalities in the calcium-sensing receptor
- *Bartter syndrome*
  - Inherited defect in the thick ascending limb of the loop of Henle.
  - Hypokalemia, alkalosis , and normal to low blood pressure, hypercalciuria
- *Autoimmune polyendocrine syndrome type 1 (Whitaker syndrome)*: candidiasis plus hereditary hypoparathyroidism with Addison disease
- Acquired hypoparathyroidism
  - Secondary to surgery
- Hypomagnesemia
  - Both deficient PTH release and impaired responsiveness to PTH
- PTH ineffective
  - Chronic renal failure
    - Impaired production of 1,25OH-VitD results in elevated fibroblast growth factor-23 production in bone leading to hypocalcemia, secondary hyperparathyroidism, and bone disease.
    - Calcium-elevating action of PTH is impaired.
  - Active vitamin D lacking
    - Decreased dietary intake or sunlight
      - PTH increased because of hypocalcemia, thereby promoting phosphaturia
    - Defective metabolism
      - Anticonvulsant therapy: increasing the conversion of vitamin D to inactive compounds
      - Vitamin D-dependent rickets type I: resistance to the action of vitamin D
      - Increased alkaline phosphatase
  - Active vitamin D ineffective
    - Intestinal malabsorption
    - Vitamin D-dependent rickets type II –
      - End-organ resistance to 1,25OH-VitD
      - Hypocalcemia, hypophosphatemia, secondary hyperparathyroidism
  - Pseudohypoparathyroidism
    - Defective PTH-dependent activation of proteins resulting in failure of PTH to increase intracellular cyclic adenosine monophosphate
    - Resembles hypoparathyroidism (PTH resistant)
    - Hypocalcemia and hyperphosphatemia, yet elevated PTH
    - Short stature, round facies, brachydactyly (short fourth and fifth metacarpals and metatarsals) and/or heterotopic calcification
    - Extrapyramidal manifestations: choreoathetotic movements and dystonia
- PTH overwhelmed by the loss of calcium
  - Severe, acute hyperphosphatemia: extensive tissue damage or cell destruction. Hypothermia, massive hepatic failure.
  - Acute pancreatitis.
  - Tumor lysis.
  - Acute renal failure.
  - Rhabdomyolysis.
  - After parathyroidectomy in osteitis fibrosa cystica
    - *Hungry bone syndrome*[24]
      - Temporary functional or relative hypoparathyroidism following parathyroidectomy or thyroidectomy.
      - Typically occurs in hyperparathyroidism patients who have bone disease preoperatively because of chronic increase in bone resorption.
- Medications
  - Protamine, heparin, glucagon

TABLE 5-8. LABORATORY AND TESTS OF HYPOCALCEMIA

	Phosphorus	25OH-VitD	PTH
Vitamin D deficiency	Low	Low/Low-normal	Elevated
Hypoparathyroidism	Elevated	–	Low
Pseudohypoparathyroidism	Elevated	–	Elevated
Vitamin D-dependent rickets	Low	I (low calcitriol) II (elevated calcitriol)	Elevated
Hypomagnesemia	Low	–	Low/Normal
Early secondary hyperparathyroidism	Normal/Elevated	1,25OH-VitD—Low	Elevated

25OH-VitD, vitamin D₂ (25-hydroxyergocalciferol)

- Clinical Manifestations and Presentation
  - Review of systems
    - Determine chronicity of hypocalcemia
    - Signs or symptoms of associated disorders
    - Nutritional history
    - Excessive alcohol intake: suggests magnesium deficiency
    - Recent surgery
    - Intestinal disorders
    - Developmental delays
  - Symptoms that typically occur in chronic hypocalcemia (Table 5-8)
    - Neuromuscular manifestations
      - Muscle spasms, carpopedal spasm, facial grimacing, laryngeal spasm, convulsions, respiratory arrest. Increased intracranial pressure may occur, and is often associated with papilledema.
      - Tetany: *Chvostek* and *Trousseau signs*
    - Mental status changes
      - Irritability, depression, psychosis
    - Cardiovascular manifestations
      - QT prolongation.
      - Arrhythmias.
      - Digitalis effectiveness may be reduced.
    - Gastrointestinal manifestations
      - Intestinal cramps, chronic malabsorption
      - Serum albumin: determine corrected calcium (see calculator at http://mdcalc.com/calcium-correction-for-hypoalbuminemia/)
- Triage Decisions
  - If hypocalcemia is chronic, suspect chronic renal failure, hereditary and acquired hypoparathyroidism, vitamin D deficiency, pseudohypoparathyroidism, and hypomagnesemia.
  - Acute transient hypocalcemia is seen in patients with severe sepsis, burns, acute renal failure, certain medications, and extensive transfusions with citrated blood.
- Management
  - Immediate
    - Parenteral calcium replacement initiated when hypocalcemia is symptomatic.
    - In severe, acute hyperphosphatemia:
      - Phosphate-binding antacids or dialysis.
      - Calcium administration tends to increase extraosseous calcium deposition and aggravate tissue damage.

- *Hungry bone syndrome*
  - Parenteral calcium.
  - Addition of calcitriol and oral calcium supplementation is sometimes needed for weeks to months.
- During hospitalization and follow-up
  - Oral calcium (2–4 g/d) plus vitamin D (calcitriol)
  - May need thiazide diuretic to avoid excessive urinary calcium excretion
  - Correct hypomagnesemia
  - Chronic renal failure
    - Replete vitamin D and calcitriol (more rapid onset)
    - Phosphate binders if hyperphosphatemia is present
    - Maintain PTH between 100 and 300 pg/mL, to prevent osteomalacia, severe secondary or tertiary hyperparathyroidism, or adynamic bone disease.
  - Vitamin D-dependent rickets type I
    - Calcitriol

CUSHING SYNDROME

Cushing syndrome is a state of cortisol excess, whereas Cushing disease is the syndrome caused by ACTH hypersecretion from the pituitary.

Epidemiology

1 to 2 per 100,000 people per year, women more than men (in pituitary adenoma)

Etiology

- ACTH-dependent: pituitary adenoma, ectopic secretion of ACTH by nonpituitary tumor (small cell lung cancer, carcinoid, pheochromocytoma, medullary thyroid cancer, islet cell tumor)
- ACTH-independent: adrenocortical adenoma, adrenocortical carcinoma, nodular adrenal hyperplasia
- Iatrogenic: exogenous glucocorticoids

Evaluation

- Twenty-four-hour urine output for free cortisol, overnight 1 mg dexamethasone suppression test, 11 PM salivary cortisol.
- Exclude exogenous steroid use; inhaled or injected steroid clearance can be delayed by ritonavir, megestrol acetate, herbal supplements (Figure 5-4).

Treatment

- Adenoma, tumor, ectopic-secreting tumor: surgical resection and/or pituitary irradiation.
- Nonresectable tumors: ketoconazole, metyrapone or etomidate (adrenal enzyme inhibition).
- Glucocorticoid replacement therapy.
- Exogenous: Stop steroids.

ADRENAL INSUFFICIENCY

- Adrenal crisis may be precipitated by:
- Sudden changes in supplemental synthetic steroid doses
  - Sudden loss of function (pituitary apoplexy, adrenal infarction, or hemorrhage)
- Symptoms of acute adrenal insufficiency
- Primary presentation is shock.
  - Other symptoms: nausea, vomiting, fatigue, lethargy, abdominal pain, fever, coma.
  - Hypoglycemia is rare in patients with primary-degree disease, but more common with secondary-degree disease, specifically with ACTH loss.

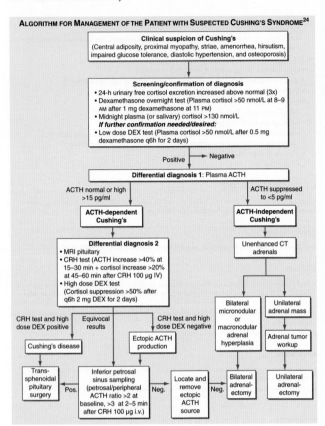

ALGORITHM FOR MANAGEMENT OF THE PATIENT WITH SUSPECTED CUSHING'S SYNDROME[24]

Figure 5-4 ACTH, adrenocorticotropic hormone; CRH, corticotropin-releasing hormone; CT, computed tomography; DEX, dexamethasone; MRI, magnetic resonance imaging.

- Chronic adrenal insufficiency may also cause hyperpigmentation, weight loss, hyperkalemia, hyponatremia, metabolic acidosis, azotemia, anemia, or eosinophilia.
- Primary clinical deficiency is the lack of mineralocorticoid hormones, which leads to hypotension.
- Patients with second-degree disease rarely have hypotension as aldosterone secretion is primarily dependent on angiotensin II

Etiology

Primary

- Autoimmune polyglandular syndrome or adrenalitis
  - Infection: tuberculosis, fungal, human immunodeficiency virus, Meningococcemia
  - Vascular: sepsis, trauma, hemorrhage, adrenal infarction and thrombosis

- Metastatic disease: lung, breast, melanoma
- Deposition: hemochromatosis, amyloidosis, sarcoidosis
- Drugs: ketoconazole, etomidate, rifampin, anticonvulsants

Secondary

- Loss of pituitary secretion of ACTH
  - Megestrol
  - Any cause of hypopituitarism

Diagnosis

- Cortisol level: 6 AM cortisol less than 3 mcg/dL; diagnostic (usually 10–20 mcg/dL at this time) more than 18 mcg/dL makes diagnosis unlikely.
  - Unreliable with altered albumin or cortisol binding globulin (estrogen use, nephrotic syndrome, or cirrhosis).
  - Septic shock makes diagnosis difficult as testing becomes unreliable and the patient may have "relative adrenal insufficiency."
  - Important to look for precipitating cause.
  - Standard testing is cosyntropin stimulation test: cortisol level 60 minutes after 250 mcg of cosyntropin (ACTH) given (normal ≥18 μg/dL).
  - Acute secondary adrenal insufficiency may yield normal results. Use early am cortisol level instead (Figure 5-5).

Alternative Testing

- Insulin-induced hypoglycemia
  - Metyrapone

Imaging

- Pituitary MRI
  - Adrenal CT: small adrenal glands in autoimmune disease; normal or large with other causes

Treatment

- Reasonable evidence (grade 2B) exists for adding corticosteroids therapy for all patients in severe septic shock.
- Dexamethasone 2 to 4 mg IV every 6 hours with fludrocortisone 50 mcg daily.
- When ACTH stimulation test performed, change to hydrocortisone 50 to 100 mg every 6 to 8 hours.
- Treatment of "relative" adrenal insufficiency is controversial.

Acute Insufficiency

- Normal saline plus IV hydrocortisone as above

Chronic Insufficiency

- Hydrocortisone 20 to 30 mg orally daily with two-thirds in the morning. Or prednisone 5 mg daily in morning.
  - Fludrocortisone (for primary insufficiency only) 0.05 mg to 0.10 mg orally every morning.
  - Consider dexamethasone 4 mg intramuscular syringe for emergency situations.

ADRENAL INCIDENTALOMAS

Epidemiology

- Abdominal CT scans: 4.4% find incidental adrenal mass. Increasing incidence with age.

Etiology

- Nonfunctioning
  - Functioning: pheo, adenoma (cortisol, aldosterone, sex hormones)
  - Malignancy (suspect if >4 cm)

ALGORITHM FOR THE MANAGEMENT OF THE PATIENT WITH SUSPECTED ADRENAL INSUFFICIENCY[24]

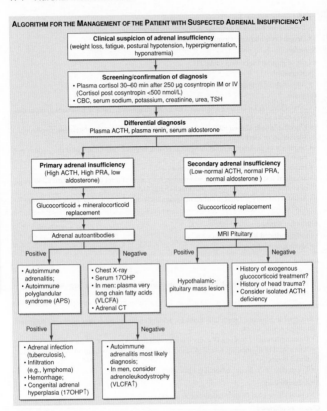

Figure 5-5 ACTH, adrenocorticotropic hormone; CBC, complete blood count; CT, computed tomography; IM, intramuscular; IV, intravenous; PRA, plasma renin activity; TSH, thyroid-stimulating hormone.

Laboratory: Rule out

- Subclinical Cushing syndrome (1 mg overnight dexamethasone suppression test). Requires confirmatory testing (ACTH, dehydroepiandrosterone-s and high-dose dexamethasone suppression).
- Pheochromocytoma (24-hour urine collection for fractionated metanephrines and catecholamines or plasma-free metanephrines).
- Hyperaldosteronism (if hypertensive, check plasma aldosterone and renin).

HYPOPITUITARISM

- Masses may cause headaches and/or visual disturbances.
  - Partial deficiency may manifest under stress.
  - Symptoms vary from hypotension to abdominal pain or fatigue.

Etiology

- Tumor: adenoma, craniopharyngioma, lymphoma, metastasis (breast, lung, colon), meningioma
- Infection: fungal, tuberculosis, parasitic, tertiary syphilis
- Vascular: Sheehan syndrome (infarction in postpartum hemorrhage), apoplexy (sudden hemorrhage), sickle cell disease
- Infiltrative: hemochromatosis, granulomatous disease (Sarcoidosis) or Wegener vasculitis, lymphocytic hypophysitis
- Genetic and developmental: Kallmann syndrome, Prader-Willi syndrome, aplasia, empty sella
  - Trauma: surgical, radiation, injury
- Most common causes: pituitary tumor 76%, extrapituitary tumor 13%, unknown 8%

Clinical Manifestations and Presentation

- Symptoms are related to specific hormone deficiencies or mass effect.
  - Partial hypopituitarism is more common than panhypopituitarism.
  - Acute: hypotension, fatigue, diabetes insipidus (polyuria and polydipsia), sudden headache (apoplexy), hypoglycemia.
  - Chronic: sexual dysfunction, weight loss, amenorrhea, headache or vision loss.

Laboratory and Other Tests

- Specific hormone deficiencies: Some or all may be present.
  - ACTH: similar to primary disorder, but without salt cravings, hypokalemia or hyperpigmentation
  - Prolactin: inability to lactate after delivery
  - TSH: inappropriately low/normal in setting of low FT_4
  - Follicle-stimulating hormone and luteinizing hormone: decreased libido, oligomenorrhea, infertility, impotence
  - Growth hormone: diagnose with insulin tolerance test, glucagon stimulation test
  - Vasopressin (ADH): polyuria, hypernatremia
- MRI of the pituitary

Treatment

- Treat specific hormone deficiency.
  - TSH: Treat with weight-based thyroxine (T_4) at 1.6 mcg/kg but only after correcting hypocortisolism to avoid precipitation of an adrenal crisis.
  - ACTH: Dexamethasone with a mineralocorticoid if needed until diagnosis is established to avoid interfering with serum cortisol measurements. Then hydrocortisone or prednisone is usually used at stress or physiologic levels.
  - Gonadotropins: can replace with gonadotropins or gonadotropin-releasing hormones if fertility desired. Testosterone supplement in men. Estradiol and progesterone in premenopausal women.
  - Vasopressin (ADH): Desmopressin acetate (5 mcg nasal spray to start) is the preferred treatment with IV fluid correction of volume.

HYPERLIPIDEMIA

Primary Etiology

- Genetic disorders

Secondary Etiologies

- Need to be excluded or evaluated (Table 5-9)

Evaluation and Treatment (Table 5-10)

- Fasting lipid panel after a 12-hour fast.
  - Calculate LDL, (Total Cholesterol—HDL—Triglyceride Level)/5

TABLE 5-9.   LIPID PROFILES OF SECONDARY ETIOLOGIES OF
             HYPERLIPIDEMIA

Cause	LDL	HDL	Triglycerides	Total Cholesterol
Obesity	H	L	–	–
DM-2	L	–	H	–
Thyroid disease	H	–	±	–
Nephrotic syndrome	H	–	–	H
ESRD	–	–	±	–
Alcohol	–	H	H	–
Cirrhosis	L	–	L	L
Hepatitis	–	–	H	H
Estrogen	–	H	H	–
Thiazides	H	–	–	–

DM-2, diabetes mellitus type 2; ESRD, end-state renal disease; H, high; HDL, high-density lipoprotein; L, low; LDL, low-density lipoprotein.

- If triglyceride level is more than 400 mg/dL, order direct measurement.
- Acute illness may alter lipid levels.
- See National Cholesterol Education Program Adult Treatment Panel III guidelines at http://www.nhlbi.nih.gov/guidelines/cholesterol/atglance.pdf.
- Lifestyle modification: diet and exercise

TABLE 5-10.   EFFECTS OF THERAPEUTIC AGENTS FOR
              HYPERLIPIDEMIA

Drug	Decrease LDL (%)	Increase HDL (%)	Decrease Triglycerides (%)	Side Effects
Statin	18–55	5–15%	7–30	Transaminitis, myalgias, rhabdomyolysis
Fibrate	5–20	10–20%	20–50	Myopathy with statin use, gallstones
Niacin	5–25	15–35%	20–50	Flushing (treat with ASA), pruritus, hyperglycemia, gout
Resins (Cholestyramine)	15–30	3–5	+/–	Bloating, binds other meds
Omega-3 fatty acids	5 increase	3	25–30	Dyspepsia

ASA, aspirin; HDL, high-density lipoprotein; LDL, low-density lipoprotein.

REFERENCES

1. American Diabetes Association. Position statement. *Diabetes Care*. 2011;34(suppl 1):S13.

2. Landin-Olsson M, Nilsson KO, Lernmark A, Sundkvist G. Islet cell antibodies and fasting C-peptid predict insulin requirement at diagnosis of diabetes mellitus. *Diabetologia*. 1990;33(9):561.

3. Niskanen LK, Tuomi T, Karjalainen J, Groop LC, Uusitupa MI. GAD antibodies in NIDDM. Ten-year follow-up from the diagnosis. *Diabetes Care*. 1995;18(12):1557.

4. Umpierrez G, Smiley D, Kitabchi AE. Narrative review: ketosis-prone type 2 diabetes mellitus. *Ann Intern Med*. 2006;144(5):350.

5. Sperling M. *Therapy for Diabetes Mellitus and Related Disorders*. Alexandria, VA: American Diabetes Association; 1998.

6. Kitabchi AE, Umpierrez GE, Miles JM, Fisher JN. Hyperglycemic crises in adult patients with diabetes. *Diabetes Care*. 2009;32(7):1335.

7. Rose BC, Post,TW. *Clinical Physiology of Acid-Base and Electrolyte Disorders*. 5th ed. New York: McGraw-Hill; 2001:809-815.

8. Barrett EJ, DeFronzo RA. Diabetic ketoacidosis: diagnosis and treatment. *Hosp Pract (Off Ed)*. 1984;19(4):89.

9. Kitabchi AE, Umpierrez GE, Murphy MB, et al. *Diabetes Care*. 2001;24(1):131.

10. Moghissi ES, Korytkowski MT, DiNardo M, et al. American Association of Clinical Endocrinologists and American Diabetes Association consensus statement on inpatient glycemic control. *Diabetes Care*. 2009;32(6):1119-1131.

11. Pastors JG, Waslaski J, Gunderson H. Diabetes meal-planning strategies. In: Ross TA, Boucher JL, O'Connell BS, eds. *Diabetes Medical Nutrition Therapy and Education*. Chicago: American Dietetic Association; 2005.

12. Rodbard HW, Jellinger PS, Davidson JA, et al. Statement by an American Asssociation of Clinical Endocrinologists/American College of Endocrinology consensus panel on type 2 diabetes mellitus: an algorithm for glycemic control. *Endocr Pract*. 2009;15(6) 540-559.

13. Whalen K, Mansour H. Pharmacotherapy of diabetes in the elderly. *U S Pharm*. 2009;43 (7):44-48.

14. American Diabetes Association. *Standards of medical care in diabetes*. Alexandria, VA: American Diabetes Association; 2012.

15. Cryer PE, Axelrod L, Grossman AB, et al. Evaluation and management of adult hypoglycemic disorders: an Endocrine Society Clinical Practice Guideline. *J Clin Endocrinol Metab*. 2009;94:709-728.

16. American Association of Clinical Endocrinologists. Medical guidelines for clinical practice: thyroid guidelines. *Endod Pract*. 2002;8(6):463.

17. Kim MI. Hypothyroidism in the elderly. In: Longo DL, et al. *Harrison's Textbook of Medicine*. 18th ed. New York: McGraw-Hill;2011.

18. Bahn RS, Burch HB, Cooper DS, et al. Hyperthyroidism and other causes of thyrotoxicosis: management guidelines of the American Thyroid Association and American Association of Clinical Endocrinologists. *Endocrine Practice*. 2011;17(3): e1-60.

19. Burch HB, Wartofsky L. *Endocrinol Metab Clin North Am*. 1993;22:263.

20. Perrild H, Hansen JM, Skovsted L, Christensen LK. Different effects of propranolol, alprenolol, sotalol, atenolol and metoprolol on serum T_3 and serum rT_3 in hyperthyroidism. *Clin Endocrinol (Oxf)*. 1983;18(2):139.

21. *Endod Pract*. 2010;16(suppl 1):7.

22. Bilezikian JP, Khan AA, Potts JT et al. Guidelines for the management of asymptomatic primary hyperparathyroidism: summary statement from the third international workshop. *J Clin Endocrinol Metab*. 2009;94(2):335.

23. Brasier AR, Nussbaum SR. Hungry bone syndrome: clinical and biochemical predictors of its occurrence after parathyroid surgery. *Am J Med*. 1988;84(4):654.

24. Arlt W. Disorders of the adrenal cortex. In: Longo DL, et al., eds. *Harrison's Principles of Internal Medicine*. 18th ed. New York: McGraw-Hill; 2012:2940-2691.

CHAPTER 6

Gastroenterology

Paul Marik

GATHERING DATA

Common Gastrointestinal (GI) Signs and Symptoms

Pain

(http://www.doctorslounge.com/gastroenterology/diagnosis/pain/abdominal.htm (accessed February 8, 2011).

- Abdominal pain is the most common and important abdominal symptom.
  - Visceral pain is usually dull and aching in character, although it can be colicky; it is often poorly localized. It arises from distention or spasm of a hollow organ such as the discomfort experienced early in intestinal obstruction or cholecystitis.
  - Parietal pain is sharp and very well localized. It arises from peritoneal irritation such as the pain of acute appendicitis with spread of inflammation to the parietal peritoneum.
  - With gastroesophageal reflux and peptic ulcer, the pain is burning or gnawing.
  - With gastroenteritis or intestinal obstruction, pain is colicky.
- Severity of pain
  - The pain of biliary or renal colic or mesenteric infarction is of high intensity, whereas the pain of gastroenteritis is less marked.
  - A patient taking corticosteroids may have significant masking of pain, and older patients often present with less intense pain.
  - It is helpful to ask a patient to compare this pain with previous painful experiences, grading on a 1 to 10 scale.
- Location of pain
  - Acute cholecystitis or hepatitis tends to occur in the right upper quadrant.
  - Appendicitis often produces pain in the periumbilical area and right lower quadrant.
  - Diverticulitis usually gives rise to lower abdominal pain in the midline or left lower quadrant.
  - Esophagitis and peptic ulcer disease usually cause discomfort substernally in the upper abdomen area.
  - Upper abdominal pain should always be considered a possible extension of cardiac pain, because myocardial infarction can present with referred pain.
- Radiation
  - Pancreatitis classically bores to the back.
  - Renal colic radiates to the groin.
- The onset, frequency, and duration of the pain are helpful features.
  - The pain of pancreatitis is typically gradual and steady.
  - The pain from rupture of a viscus with resultant peritonitis begins suddenly and is maximal from the onset.
  - Acute versus chronic pain: An arbitrary interval, such as 12 weeks, can be used to separate acute from chronic abdominal pain.
- Aggravating and relieving factors.
  - The pain of mesenteric ischemia usually starts within 1 hour of eating,
  - The pain of peptic ulcer disease is relieved by eating and recurs several hours after a meal when the stomach is empty.
  - The pain of pancreatitis is classically relieved by sitting up and leaning forward.
  - Peritonitis often causes patients to lie motionless on their backs because any motion causes pain.

- Associated symptoms include fevers, chills, weight loss or gain, nausea, vomiting, diarrhea, constipation, hematochezia, melena, jaundice, change in the color of urine or stool, change in the diameter of stool.
  - Weight loss may occur in association with malignancy.
  - Nausea and vomiting with bowel obstruction.
  - Change in bowel habits with a colonic lesion.
- Past medical and surgical history, including risk factors for cardiovascular disease and details of previous abdominal surgeries.
- Family history of bowel disorders.
- Alcohol intake.
- Intake of medications including over the counter medications such as acetaminophen, aspirin, and nonsteroidal anti-inflammatory drugs (NSAIDs).
- Women should be asked about their menstrual, obstetrical and gynecologic history, whether they engage in sexual activity, the number of sexual partners, whether any sexual partners are new, and whether any sexual partners are experiencing symptoms suggestive of a sexually transmitted infection.

Important Causes of Abdominal Pain

Pain originating in the abdomen

- Parietal peritoneal inflammation
  - Bacterial contamination
    - Perforated appendix or other perforated viscus
    - Pelvic inflammatory disease
  - Chemical irritation
    - Perforated ulcer
    - Pancreatitis
    - Mittelschmerz
- Mechanical obstruction of hollow viscera
  - Obstruction of the small or large intestine
  - Obstruction of the biliary tree
  - Obstruction of the ureter
- Vascular disturbances
  - Embolism or thrombosis (mesenteric ischemia)
  - Vascular rupture (abdominal aortic aneurysm or splenic artery)
  - Pressure or torsional occlusion
  - Sickle cell anemia
- Abdominal wall
  - Trauma
  - Infection of muscles (necrotizing fasciitis)
- Distension of visceral surfaces (eg, by hemorrhage)
  - Hepatic or renal capsules
- Inflammation of a viscus
  - Appendicitis
  - Typhlitis
  - Diverticulitis

Pain referred from extraabdominal source

- Cardiothoracic
  - Acute myocardial infarction
  - Myocarditis, endocarditis, pericarditis
  - Congestive heart failure
  - Pneumonia
  - Pulmonary embolus
  - Pleurodynia
  - Empyema
  - Esophageal disease, spasm, rupture, inflammation

- Genitalia
  - Torsion of testis

Metabolic causes

- Diabetes
- Uremia
- Hyperlipidemia
- Hyperparathyroidism
- Acute adrenal insufficiency
- Familial Mediterranean fever
- Porphyria
- C1 esterase inhibitor deficiency (angioneurotic edema)

Neurologic and Psychiatric causes

- Herpes zoster
- Causalgia
- Radiculitis from infection or arthritis
- Spinal cord or nerve root compression
- Functional disorders
- Psychiatric disorders

Toxic Causes

- Lead poisoning
- Insect or animal envenomations
  - Black widow spiders
  - Snake bites

Uncertain mechanisms

- Narcotic withdrawal
- Heat stroke

Differential Diagnosis of Abdominal Pain by Location

- Right upper quadrant
  - Cholecystitis
  - Cholangitis
  - Pancreatitis
  - Pneumonia, empyema
  - Pleurisy, pleurodynia
  - Subdiaphragmatic abscess
  - Hepatitis
  - Budd-Chiari syndrome
- Right lower quadrant
  - Appendicitis
  - Salpingitis
  - Inguinal hernia
  - Ectopic pregnancy
  - Nephrolithiasis
  - Inflammatory bowel disease
  - Mesenteric lymphadenitis
  - Typhlitis
- Diffuse nonlocalized pain
  - Gastroenteritis
  - Mesenteric ischemia
  - Bowel obstruction
  - Irritable bowel syndrome
  - Peritonitis
  - Diabetes
  - Malaria
  - Familial Mediterranean fever

- Epigastric
  - Peptic ulcer disease
  - Gastritis
  - Gastroesophageal reflux disease
  - Pancreatitis
  - Myocardial infarction
  - Pericarditis
  - Ruptured aortic aneurysm
  - Esophagitis
- Periumbilical
  - Early appendicitis
  - Gastroenteritis
  - Bowel obstruction
  - Ruptured aortic aneurysm
- Left upper quadrant
  - Splenic infarct
  - Splenic rupture
  - Splenic abscess
  - Gastritis
  - Gastric ulcer
  - Pancreatitis
  - Subdiaphragmatic abscess
- Left lower quadrant
  - Diverticulitis
  - Salpingitis
  - Inguinal hernia
  - Ectopic pregnancy
  - Nephrolithiasis
  - Irritable bowel syndrome
  - Inflammatory bowel disease

GI Bleeding

The history provides important clues as to the location (upper or lower GI tract) and cause of bleeding (Figure 6-1).

- Type of bleeding
  - Vomiting bright blood is characteristic of upper GI bleeding (UGIB)
  - Coffee-ground emesis is characteristic of UGIB
  - Melena stool is characteristic of UGIB (proximal to ligament of Treitz)
  - Maroon stool is usually caused by lower GI bleeding
  - Fresh blood per rectum suggests lower GI bleeding
- Previous GI bleeding; angiodysplasia, peptic ulcers, and so forth.
- The use of aspirin and other NSAIDs suggests peptic ulcer disease.
- Alcohol use is associated with cirrhosis and alcoholic gastritis.
- Occult GI blood loss is suggestive of a GI malignancy.
- History of chronic liver disease suggests esophageal varices.
- A history of diverticula suggests diverticular bleed.
- A history of an abdominal aortic aneurysm or graft increases concern regarding an aortoenteric fistula.

Nausea and Vomiting

- Abdominal pain with vomiting usually indicates an organic etiology (eg, cholelithiasis).
- Abdominal distension suggests bowel obstruction.
- Vomiting of food eaten several hours earlier suggests gastric obstruction or gastroparesis.
- Heartburn with nausea often indicates gastroesophageal reflux disease (gastroesophageal reflux disease)
- Early morning vomiting is characteristic of pregnancy.

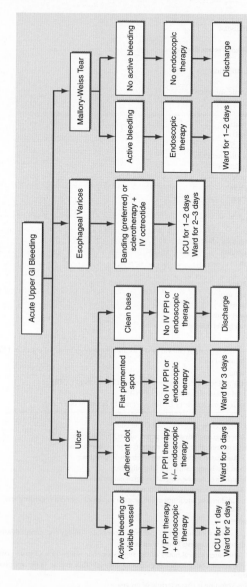

Figure 6-1 Suggested algorithm for patients with upper gastrointestinal bleed. PPI, proton pump inhibitor; ICU, intensive care unit; IV, intravenous.

- Feculent vomiting suggests intestinal obstruction or a gastrocolic fistula.
- Vertigo and nystagmus are typical of vestibular neuritis.
- Neurogenic vomiting may be positional, projectile, and is usually associated with other neurologic signs and symptoms. Sudden onset of severe headache is common.

Diarrhea

The history is essential to determine the nature of the diarrhea.

- Profuse watery diarrhea with signs of hypovolemia
- Stools containing blood and mucus
- Bloody diarrhea
- Number of stools per 24 hours

Important associated features include:

- Temperature
- Severe abdominal pain
- Recent hospitalization or use of antibiotics
- Systemic illness with diarrhea
- History of travel, contacts with diarrhoea

A food history may also provide clues to a diagnosis:

- Consumption of unpasteurized dairy products, raw or undercooked meat or fish, or organic vitamin preparations. Women who are pregnant have a 20-fold increased risk of developing listeriosis from meat products or unpasteurized dairy products.
- Symptoms that begin within 6 hours suggest ingestion of a preformed toxin of *Staphylococcus aureus* or *Bacillus cereus*.
- Symptoms that begin at 8 to 16 hours suggest infection with *Clostridium perfringens*.
- Symptoms that begin at more than 16 hours can result from viral or bacterial infection (eg, contamination of food with enterotoxigenic or enterohemorrhagic *Escherichia coli*).
- Syndromes that may begin with diarrhea but progress to fever and more systemic complaints such as headache, muscle aches, and stiff neck may suggest infection with *Listeria monocytogenes*, particularly in pregnant woman.

GI History and Review of Systems

A GI history should include the above symptoms as well as a history of weight loss and gain, abdominal bloating, detailed history of bowel habits, dietary habits and indiscretions, GI medications (antacids, laxatives, etc.), family history of GI diseases, previous surgical history and use of alcohol.

Physical Examination of the GI System

- See http://www.med-ed.virginia.edu/courses/pom1/pexams/Abdomen/ (accessed February 8, 2011).
- Gentle palpation to identify acute peritonitis and rebound tenderness as well as to identify organomegaly and other masses. Muscular rigidity or "guarding" is an important and early sign of peritoneal inflammation; it can be unilateral in a patient with a focal inflammatory mass such as a diverticular abscess or diffuse as in peritonitis.
- Auscultation of the abdomen may be helpful in the evaluation of abdominal pain. A complete lack of bowel sounds is found in advanced peritonitis or adynamic ileus. Abnormally active, high-pitched bowel sounds are a feature of early bowel obstruction.
- Percussion is also used to identify ascites, liver span, and bladder and splenic enlargement. Tympany signifies a distended bowel, while dullness may signify a mass. Shifting dullness is a reliable and fairly accurate sign for the detection of ascites.
- Rectal and pelvic examination: A rectal examination is generally required in all patients with acute abdominal pain, and a pelvic examination is generally required in all women with acute lower abdominal pain. Fecal impaction might be the explanation for signs and symptoms of obstruction in the older patient, while tenderness on rectal examination may be the only abnormal finding in a patient with retrocecal appendicitis. Stool for occult blood should also be obtained. The pelvic examination is critical for determining whether abdominal pain is caused by pelvic inflammatory disease, an adnexal mass or cyst, uterine pathology, or an ectopic pregnancy.

Diagnostic Tests

Laboratory

Patients with acute abdominal complaints should have the following laboratory tests performed:

- Complete blood count with differential.
- Electrolytes, blood urea nitrogen (BUN), creatinine, and glucose.
- Aminotransferases, alkaline phosphatase, and bilirubin.
- Lipase and amylase.
- Urinalysis.
- Pregnancy test in women of childbearing potential.
- In the presence of fever or unstable vital signs, blood and urine cultures should be performed.
- Coagulation profile in patients with GI bleed.
- Cardiac enzymes (troponins) and electrocardiogram (ECG) in patients older than 40 years of age.

Radiography (Plain Film, Barium Studies, Computed Tomography [CT], Ultrasound)

The appropriate radiographic tests will depend on the urgency of the case and the presenting signs and symptoms. Patients in need of urgent surgical intervention may proceed directly to the operating room for diagnosis and management, and some patients will need no further preoperative assessment because of a clear history consistent with a surgical disease such as appendicitis.

In patients with abdominal pain and or signs of obstruction, a supine and erect plain film of the abdomen is frequently obtained. While the diagnostic sensitivity of this test is low it may reveal free air under the diaphragm, dilated loops of bowel, free air in the bowel or kidney or evidence of fecal impaction. A CT scan of the abdomen usually with contrast is the diagnostic test of choice in patients with undiagnosed abdominal pain. CT angiography is indicated in patients with suspected vascular disease (mesenteric ischemia, aneurysms). Barium and Gastrografin studies are indicated in specific circumstances such as suspected esophageal rupture, fistula, and so forth. In patients with suspected cholecystitis and biliary tract disease, right upper quadrant ultrasonography is the initial diagnostic test of choice.

Special Tests (Endoscopy, Endoscopic Retrograde Cholangiopancreatography [ERCP], Hepatobiliary Iminodiacetic Acid [HIDA])

Patients with UGIB require upper endoscopy whereas those with lower GI bleeding require colonoscopy. Patients with biliary pancreatitis and biliary obstruction may require ERCP. Patients undergoing endoscopy require special preparation; the patients should be kept nothing by mouth (NPO) prior to the procedure (at least 8 hours), and a bowel prep is required for patients undergoing colonoscopy. HIDA scan may be required when the functional integrity of the biliary tract is under question.

Specific Diagnostic Scenarios

- Patients with UGIB require urgent endoscopy.
- Patients with suspected pancreatitis are best evaluated initially with an abdominal ultrasound.
- Patients with suspected mesenteric ischemia, diverticulitis are best evaluated with an abdominal CT.
- In the case of suspected partial or complete intestinal obstruction, a CT scan of the abdomen is more sensitive and more likely to yield a diagnosis than plain abdominal radiographs.
- Patients with ascites should undergo a diagnostic tap (Table 6-1). Paracentesis is preferably performed under ultrasound guidance to avoid "hitting" the bowel or superficial vessels.

Many patients will not have a firm diagnosis after initial assessment, and in these cases, careful observation of the patient's course will be the most important factor in their management, because severe pathology typically becomes more obvious with time, and benign conditions may spontaneously improve. In addition to watchful waiting

TABLE 6-1. CHARACTERISTICS OF ASCITIC FLUID IN VARIOUS DISEASE STATES

Condition	Gross Appearance	Protein (g/L)	Serum/Ascites Albumin Gradient	RBC (>10,000/μL)	WBC per μL	Other Tests
Cirrhosis	Straw-colored or bile stained	<25	>1.1	1%	<250 predominantly mesothelia	
Neoplasm	Straw-colored, hemorrhagic, mucinous, or chylous	>25	<1.1	20%	>1000 Variable cell types	Cytology, peritoneal biopsy
Tuberculous peritonitis	Clear, turbid, hemorrhagic, chylous	>25	<1.1	7%	>1000 usually >70 lymphocytes	Peritoneal biopsy, stain and culture for acid-fast bacilli
Pyogenic peritonitis	Turbid or purulent	If purulent, >25	<1.1	Unusual	Predominantly PMN	Gram stain and culture
Congestive heart failure	Straw-colored	Variable, 15–53	>1.1	10%	<1000 usually mesothelial, mononuclear	
Pancreatic ascites	Turbid, hemorrhagic, or chylous	Variable, often >25	<1.1	Variable, may be blood stained	Variable	Increased amylase in ascitic fluid

PMN, polymorphonuclear neutrophilic leukocyte; RBC, red blood cell; WBC, white blood cell.

(an important diagnostic test), the following additional investigations can also be considered:

- When clinical signs of peritonitis are present, but the etiology is not clear, an abdominal ultrasound is the test of choice, since it can effectively assess for appendicitis and abdominal abscess and obtains adequate views of intrapelvic pathology.
- Abdominal CT scan may be helpful as an alternative to ultrasound or in the clarification of equivocal ultrasound findings. In pregnant women with abdominal pain, ultrasound should be performed because it is not associated with radiation exposure or contrast, and pregnant patients may present with atypical history and physical findings of common pathologies.
- All barium studies should be avoided in patients with suspected obstruction because they may result in retention of barium and interference with subsequent diagnostic tests.
- In some patients, surgical intervention should be considered even before confirmatory testing. Patients with a painful pulsatile abdominal mass, with or without bruit, should be suspected to have a ruptured aortic aneurysm. In unstable patients with suspected aneurysm rupture, surgical referral should not be delayed. In stable patients, abdominal ultrasound is the preferred investigation, although CT scanning is also acceptable.

SPECIFIC GI CONDITIONS

UGIB (Table 6-2)

Approach to the Patient with UGIB

The urgency with which GI bleeding is managed is dictated by the rate of bleeding.

- The patient with trace heme-positive stools and without severe anemia can be managed as an outpatient.
- Visible blood requires hospitalization and inpatient evaluation.
- Persistent bleeding or re-bleed with hemodynamic instability necessitates intensive care unit (ICU) admission.
- Massive bleeding is defined as loss of 30% or more of estimated blood volume or bleeding requiring blood transfusion of 6 or more units over 24 hours.

Patient Assessment (Table 6-3)

- Blood pressure, pulse, postural changes, and assessment of peripheral perfusion.
- The presence of comorbid disease must be determined, especially coronary artery disease and cardiac failure.

TABLE 6-2. THE MAJOR CAUSES OF UPPER GASTROINTESTINAL BLEEDING

Source	Proportion of Patients (%)
Peptic ulcer disease Helicobacter pyloric and NSAIDs	31–59
Esophageal and gastric varices	7–20
Mallory-Weiss tear	4–8
Gastroduodenal erosions (gastritis)	2–7
Erosive esophagitis	1–13
Malignancy	2–7
Vascular ectasia	0–6
No source identified	8–14

NSAIDs, nonsteroidal anti-inflammatory drugs.

TABLE 6-3. CORRELATION BETWEEN PHYSICAL SIGNS AND SEVERITY
OF UPPER GASTROINTESTINAL BLEEDING

Physical Sign	Mild	Moderate	Severe
Blood Loss	<1 L	1–2 L	≥2 L
Blood pressure	Normal	Normal-borderline low	Hypotensive
Orthostasis	No	Possible	Likely
Tachycardia	None-mild	Moderate	Severe
Skin	Warm, perfused	Diaphoretic	Cool, clammy
Urine output	Normal	Diminished	Poor
Sensorium	Alert/anxious	Anxious	Confused/drowsy

- Estimating blood loss.
  - This can be estimated by measuring the return from a nasogastric (NG) tube.
  - An approximate estimate of blood loss can also be made by the hemodynamic response to a 2-L crystalloid fluid challenge:
    - If blood pressure (BP) returns to normal and stabilizes, blood loss of 15% to 30% has occurred.
    - If BP rises but falls again, blood volume loses of 30% to 40% has occurred.
    - If BP continues to fall, blood volume loss of more than 40% has probably occurred.

NG Tube Placement

- NG aspiration with saline lavage is beneficial to detect the presence of intragastric blood, to determine the type of gross bleeding, to clear the gastric field for endoscopic visualization, and to prevent aspiration of gastric contents.
- NG tube placement is essential to monitor ongoing bleeding and to decompress the stomach.
- Concerns that placement of a NG tube may induce bleeding in patients with coagulopathies are outweighed by the benefits of the information obtained.
- It should be noted that in approximately 15% of patients with UGIB, NG aspirate will fail to obtain blood or "coffee ground" material.

Initial Resuscitation

- Establish 2 large-bore intravenous (IV) lines or a large-bore central line.
- Insert NG tube and aspiration (by hand).
- Volume expansion with crystalloids.
- Monitor BP, pulse and urine output.
- Cross match blood. Blood products are the most efficient volume expanders and should be infused as soon as possible in patients with significant bleeds.
  - Transfusion requirements are determined by multiple factors, including patient age, presence of comorbidities, cardiovascular status, baseline hematocrit, and rate of the bleeding, along with the current hematocrit level.
  - Red blood cells (RBCs) are transfused in patients who have significant blood loss, continuing active bleeding, and those who manifest cardiac, renal, or cerebral ischemia (regardless of hematocrit).
  - The rate of blood transfusion is determined by the severity of the hypovolemia, by the rate of the bleeding, and by the presence of cardiac, renal, or cerebrovascular comorbidities.
  - Generally RBCs should be transfused to maintain a hemoglobin concentration between 8 and 10 g/dL.
  - It is important to note that it takes up to 72 hours for the hematocrit to reach its nadir after a single episode of bleeding (assuming no other intervention). Therefore a normal hemoglobin (on admission) does not exclude significant bleeding.

- Blood transfusion should not be withheld from actively bleeding patients, based on their hemoglobin and hematocrit. Conversely a falling hematocrit does not imply continued bleeding; but rather may represent equilibration of fluid between the intravascular and extracellular extravascular compartment.
  - Patients who have variceal bleeding should be transfused to a hematocrit of 25 to 27 (hemoglobin 8–9 g/dL) to avoid exacerbating the bleeding by increasing the portal pressure
- In patients with active bleeding, fresh frozen plasma FFP should be given if the international normalized ratio (INR) is more than 1.4. In addition, fresh frozen plasma should be given after 6 units of RBC's, and platelets after 10 units,
- Platelet transfusion is indicated if the platelet count is less than $50,000/mm^3$.
- Airway protection: The risk of aspiration is especially high in patients with massive bleeding or those who have an altered mental status. Endotracheal intubation is recommended in these patients. In addition, endotracheal intubation facilitates endoscopy. It may be advisable to place a NG tube prior to intubation in an attempt to empty the stomach and reduce the risk of aspiration during endotracheal intubation.
- In patients with severe UGIB and clinical evidence or a history of advanced liver disease or a history of previous variceal bleeding, an octreotide infusion should be commenced prior to endoscopy
- In patients with presumed UGIB, proton pump inhibitor (PPI) therapy is recommended before esophagogastroduodenoscopy (EGD). The rationale for PPI therapy is that the most common causes of UGIB, including ulcers, gastritis, duodenitis, and hemorrhagic reflux esophagitis, are medically treated with acid-suppressive therapy. PPI therapy is also useful, however, for hemostasis of lesions that are not caused by acid and are not in other circumstances treated by PPI therapy, probably because neutralization of intraluminal gastric acid promotes hemostasis by stabilizing blood clots.
- IV erythromycin (70–100 mg), through its effect as a motilin receptor agonist, has been shown to promote gastric motility and substantially improve visualization of the gastric mucosa on initial endoscopy.
- All patients who have acute GI bleeding require gastroenterology consultation.
- Surgical consultation is recommended for patients who have ongoing active bleeding, massive bleeding, recurrent bleeding, bleeding associated with significant abdominal pain, acute lower GI bleeding, and abdominal findings suggestive of an acute abdomen.

Triage of Patients. Who to Admit to the ICU?

At the time of triage the following criteria can stratify patients into a high-risk group (high risk of re-bleeding, requiring surgery, and dying).

- Systolic blood pressure of less than 100 mmHg on admission
- Severe comorbid disease
- Evidence of active, ongoing GI hemorrhage at the time of triage
- INR more than 1.4

The rate of rebleeding is approximately 3% in the low-risk group as compared to 25% in the high-risk group. Patients in the low-risk group do not usually require admission to an ICU and can be adequately managed on a general medical floor.

Endoscopy

Early upper GI endoscopy is the cornerstone of management of UGIB. Endoscopy within 12 to 24 hours of presentation is generally recommended. EGD is the prime diagnostic and therapeutic tool for UGIB. Early endoscopy serves 3 vital roles:

- Diagnosis
- Treatment
  - Nonvariceal bleeding: Endoscopic therapy has been shown to improve outcomes in patients with nonvariceal bleeding.
  - Variceal bleeding: Endoscopic sclerotherapy and/or band ligation is the method of choice in controlling active variceal hemorrhage.
- Risk stratification: Establishing an endoscopic diagnosis of the lesion and associated stigmata greatly enhances the ability to predict outcomes (ie, the risk of rebleeding).

TABLE 6-4. RECOMMENDED TREATMENT FOR *HELICOBACTER PYLORI*

Adjuvant	Antimicrobial 1	Antimicrobial 2	Duration of Therapy (days)
PPI twice daily	Clarithromycin twice daily	Amoxicillin twice daily or metronidazole twice daily	7–14
Ranitidine bismuth citrate twice daily	Clarithromycin twice daily	Amoxicillin twice daily or metronidazole twice daily	7–14
Bismuth four times daily	Tetracycline four times daily	Metronidazole three times daily	7–14

Further Management of Bleeding Peptic Ulcer Disease

- PPIs significantly decrease the risk of ulcer rebleeding, the need for urgent surgery, and the risk of death. An IV bolus followed by a continuous infusion of PPI for 72 hours after endoscopic hemostasis is recommended.
- Planned, second-look endoscopy that is performed within 24 hours after initial endoscopic therapy is not recommended.
- For most patients with evidence of persistent ulcer bleeding or rebleeding, a second attempt at endoscopic hemostasis is often effective, may result in fewer complications than surgery, and is the recommended management approach.
- Angiography with transcatheter embolization provides a nonoperative option for patients in whom a site of acute bleeding has not been identified or controlled by endoscopy.
- Patients should be tested and treatment of *Helicobacter pylori* infection (Table 6-4).
- Evaluation for any ongoing need for a nonsteroidal anti-inflammatory or antiplatelet agent and, if such treatment is indicated, appropriate coadministration of a gastroprotective agent are important.

Further Management of Esophageal Varices

- See http://www.aasld.org/practiceguidelines/Documents/Practice%20Guidelines/VaricesinGuidelinespg.pdf (accessed February 8, 2011).
- In patients with variceal hemorrhage, there remains a 40% chance of recurrent variceal bleeding within 72 hours and a 60% chance within 10 days if no additional treatment is used.
- Octreotide 50 µg bolus followed by an infusion of at a rate of 50 µg/h has been demonstrated to reduce the risk of early rebleeding.
- Endoscopic banding in combination with an octreotide infusion is more effective than endoscopic therapy alone for controlling bleeding and reducing the incidence of rebleeding.
- There is a close association between infection and variceal bleeding.
  - A complete microbiological workup, including blood cultures and diagnostic paracentesis when appropriate should be performed.
  - Antibiotic prophylaxis has been demonstrated to reduce the risk of infections in patients and to improve short-term survival.
  - Prophylaxis with a third-generation cephalosporin, quinolone, or amoxicillin-clavulanic acid is recommended.
- Paracentesis significantly decreases variceal pressure and tension. This suggests that ascites removal can be useful in the treatment of variceal bleeding in cirrhotic patients.
- There is a small chance that placement of a feeding tube or NG tube after variceal banding may dislodge the bands and/or cause bleeding. This should therefore be delayed for 48 to 72 hours.
- Balloon tamponade with a Minnesota or Sengstaken-Blakemore tube can be lifesaving in the presence of severe ongoing bleeding when carried out by experienced staff. However, placement by inexperienced staff is associated with an increased risk of death, largely because of esophageal perforation and pulmonary aspiration.

- Transjugular intrahepatic portosystemic shunt (TIPPS) is a radiological intervention that creates a portosystemic tract through the liver parenchyma, through which an 8 to 12 mm expandable metal stent is inserted.
  - TIPPS has become the treatment of choice as rescue therapy for the 10% to 20% of patients with variceal hemorrhage unresponsive to endoscopic management.
  - TIPPS has largely replaced emergency surgical shunting.
  - The main limitations of TIPPS are the development of encephalopathy in approximately 20% of patients and progressive development of shunt insufficiency (thrombosis).
- Gastric varices are the source of bleeding in 10% to 40% of patients with variceal hemorrhage. Unless the gastric varices are located on the proximal lesser curve, they are not amenable to endoscopic ligation, and for this reason early TIPPS is generally recommended.
- Nonselective beta-blockers (nadolol or propranolol) reduce the risk of rebleeding. A combination of endoscopic treatment together with beta-blockers reduces overall and variceal rebleeding more than either therapy alone.
- Recent data suggests that patients with acute variceal bleeding and at high risk for treatment failure, the early use of TIPPS was associated with a significant reduction in treatment failure and in mortality.

Management of Patients with Lower GI Bleeding (Table 6-5)

- Angiodysplasia and diverticular disease of the right colon account for the vast majority of episodes of acute lower GI bleeding. The spontaneous remission rate, even with massive bleeding is approximately 80%.
- In patients with ongoing lower GI bleeding, a radionuclide bleeding scan is indicated. There are two types of bleeding scan.
  - The first is a technetium-labeled sulfur colloid scan, which although very sensitive can only detect bleeding that occurs during the 1 to 2 hours following injection of the isotope.
  - Alternatively, a technetium labeled ("tagged") red blood cell bleeding scan can detect bleeding sites for up to 24 hours after the cessation of bleeding. If the result of either type of bleeding scan is positive angiography should then be performed.
- Selective mesenteric angiography detects arterial bleeding that occurs at a rate of 0.5 mL/min or faster. It can be both diagnostic and therapeutic. When active bleeding is seen selective arterial infusion of vasopressin arrests the hemorrhage in 90% of patients; adding sterile, absorbable gelatin powder further increases the efficacy of vasopressin. If bleeding continues and no source has been found, surgical intervention is warranted.
- Surgical intervention is also recommended in patients with recurrent diverticular bleeding.

TABLE 6-5. SOURCE OF LOWER GASTROINTESTINAL BLEEDING

Diagnosis	%
Diverticulosis	35
Colonic polyp or cancer	15
Benign anorectal conditions (including hemorrhoids)	10
Inflammatory bowel disease	15
Ischemic colitis	5
Angiodysplasia	10
Small bowel (including Meckel diverticulum)	1–2
Other (rectal ulcer radiation colitis, etc.)	10

Appendicitis

- Appendicitis occurs most frequently in the second and third decades of life. The incidence is highest in the 10- to 19-year-old age group.
- The diagnosis of appendicitis can be difficult, especially in patients younger than 3 years of age, pregnant, and older than 60 years of age.
- Appendiceal obstruction has been proposed as the primary cause of appendicitis. Appendiceal obstruction may be caused by fecaliths, calculi, lymphoid hyperplasia, infectious processes, and benign or malignant tumors.
- Bacterial overgrowth occurs within the diseased appendix. Aerobic organisms predominate early in the course, while mixed infection is more common in late appendicitis.
- The natural history of appendicitis is similar to that of other inflammatory processes involving hollow visceral organs. Initial inflammation of the appendiceal wall is followed by localized ischemia, perforation, and the development of a contained abscess or generalized peritonitis.

Diagnosis

- Abdominal pain is the most common clinical symptom of appendicitis and is found in nearly all confirmed cases. The classic signs of appendicitis include:
  - Periumbilical pain with subsequent migration to the right lower quadrant as the inflammation progresses
  - Anorexia
  - Nausea and vomiting
  - Fever and leukocytosis follow later in the course of illness
- Several findings on physical examination have been described to facilitate diagnosis:
  - McBurney point tenderness is described as maximal tenderness at 1.5 to 2 inches from the anterior superior iliac spine on a straight line from the anterior superior iliac spine to the umbilicus.
  - Rovsing sign refers to pain in the right lower quadrant with palpation of the left lower quadrant.
  - The psoas sign is indicative of a retrocecal appendix. This is manifested by right lower quadrant pain with right hip flexion.
  - The obturator sign is indicative of a pelvic appendix. This test is based on the principle that the inflamed appendix may lie again the right obturator internus muscle. When the clinician flexes the patient's right hip and knee followed by internal rotation of the right hip, this elicits right lower quadrant pain.
- Approximately 80% of patients with appendicitis have a preoperative leukocytosis (white cells >10,000 cells/μL) and a left shift in the differential.
- A pregnancy test should be performed for all women of childbearing age.
- Mild elevations in serum bilirubin (total bilirubin >1.0 mg/dL) have been noted to be a marker for appendiceal perforation.
- The diagnostic accuracy of clinical evaluation alone varies from 75% to 90% and is influenced by the experience of the examining clinician.
- The Alvarado score is the most widely used diagnostic aid for the diagnosis of appendicitis:
  - Migratory right iliac fossa pain (1 point)
  - Anorexia (1 point)
  - Nausea and vomiting (1 point)
  - Tenderness in the right iliac fossa (2 points)
  - Rebound tenderness in the right iliac fossa (1 point)
  - Fever higher than 37.5°C (99.5°F) (1 point)
  - Leukocytosis (2 points)
    - Score of 0 to 3. Low risk of appendicitis
    - Score of 4 to 6. Should be admitted for observation and reexamination. If the score remains the same after 12 hours, operative intervention is recommended.
    - Score 7 to 9.
  - A male patient should proceed to appendectomy.
  - A female patient who is not pregnant should undergo diagnostic laparoscopy, then appendectomy if indicated by the intraoperative findings.
    - Accuracy of the score appears to be lower in women.

- Over the last few decades, there has been increasing use of imaging modalities such as ultrasonography and CT in the diagnosis of acute appendicitis. Although the increased use of imaging has decreased the rate of negative appendectomies, many surgeons will proceed with surgical exploration, in the absence of imaging, if there is a strong clinical concern for appendicitis.

Management

- The great majority of patients with acute appendicitis are treated surgically, and surgery remains the gold standard.
- Supportive treatment includes:
  - Monitoring vital signs and urine output
  - Adequate hydration with IV fluids
  - Correction of electrolyte abnormalities
  - Antibiotics
    - Acute nonperforated appendicitis: A single preoperative antibiotic dose for surgical wound prophylaxis is adequate.
    - Perforated appendicitis: In patients with perforated appendicitis, the antibiotic regimen should consist of empiric broad-spectrum therapy with activity against gram-negative rods and anaerobic organisms pending culture.

Acute Cholecystitis

- Acute cholecystitis refers to a syndrome of right upper quadrant pain, fever, and leukocytosis associated with gallbladder inflammation, which is usually related to gallstone disease.
- Acalculous cholecystitis is clinically identical to acute cholecystitis but is not associated with gallstones, and usually occurs in critically ill patients. It accounts for approximately 10% of cases of acute cholecystitis and is associated with high morbidity and mortality.
- In 90% of cases, acute cholecystitis is caused by gallstones in the gallbladder. The pathogenesis of acute cholecystitis is not well understood, and only approximately 50% of patients have infected bile; the implicated pathogens include *E. coli*, Enterococcus, and Klebsiella. Acute cholecystitis causes bile to become trapped in the gallbladder.
- Patients with acute cholecystitis typically complain of abdominal pain, most commonly in the right upper quadrant or epigastrium. The pain may radiate to the right shoulder or back. Characteristically, acute cholecystitis pain is steady and severe. Associated complaints may include nausea, vomiting, and anorexia. There is often a history of fatty food ingestion approximately 1 hour or more before the initial onset of pain.
- Patients with acute cholecystitis are usually ill appearing, febrile, and tachycardic. Abdominal examination usually demonstrates voluntary and involuntary guarding. "Murphy sign" may be a useful diagnostic maneuver.
- The most common complication is the development of gallbladder gangrene (up to 20% of cases) with subsequent perforation. The risk of gangrenous cholecystitis is increased in the older patient and diabetic patients.
- The diagnosis must be based on a combination of clinical findings and imaging studies. Laboratory tests usually demonstrate a leukocytosis, with mild elevations in serum aminotransferases, amylase, and bilirubin.
- Ultrasonography is usually the first test obtained and can often establish the diagnosis. Nuclear cholescintigraphy (HIDA scan) may be useful in cases in which the diagnosis remains uncertain after ultrasonography.
- Supportive care
  - Initiate IV hydration and correction for electrolyte disorders.
  - Pain control: Opioid analgesia may be required, although effective analgesia can usually be accomplished with an intramuscular injection of ketorolac.
  - It is not clear that antibiotics are required for the treatment of uncomplicated cholecystitis. Although clear evidence of benefit is lacking, most patients who are hospitalized for an episode of acute cholecystitis are given antibiotics.
- Cholecystectomy
  - Patients who are at low-risk (American Society of Anesthesiologists classes I and II) benefit from an initial 24 to 48 hours of supportive therapy followed by cholecystectomy during the same hospital admission.

- Emergent surgery is usually required when gangrene or perforation are suspected, or if patients deteriorate while on supportive therapy.
- A nonsurgical supportive approach is generally preferred in high-risk patients. Patients who continue to have severe symptoms and show no improvement despite 1 to 2 days of medical management require gallbladder drainage by percutaneous cholecystostomy.

Diverticular Disease

- Colonic diverticular disease is common, and appears to be increasing in incidence. The prevalence is age dependent, increasing from less than 5% at age 40 years, to 30% by age 60 years, to 65% by age 85 years.
- Among all patients with diverticulosis, 70% remain asymptomatic, 15% to 25% develop diverticulitis, and 5% to 15% develop some form of diverticular bleeding.
- See http://www.fascrs.org/files/pp_sigmoid.pdf (accessed February 8, 2011).

Diverticulitis

- Diverticulitis represents micro- or macroscopic perforation of a diverticulum. A small perforation may be walled off by pericolic fat and mesentery. This may lead to a localized abscess or, if adjacent organs are involved, a fistula or obstruction. In comparison, poor containment results in free perforation and peritonitis.
- Clinical Presentation
  - The clinical presentation of diverticulitis depends on the severity of the underlying inflammatory process and whether or not complications are present.
  - Complicated diverticulitis refers to the presence of an abscess, fistula, obstruction, or perforation while simple diverticulitis refers to inflammation in the absence of these complications.
  - Left lower quadrant pain is the most common complaint in Western countries, occurring in 70% of patients.
  - Pain is often present for several days prior to admission, which aids in the differentiation of diverticulitis from other causes of acute abdominal symptoms. Up to one-half of patients have had 1 or more previous episodes of similar pain.
  - Physical examination usually reveals abdominal tenderness, characteristically in the left lower quadrant. A tender mass is palpable in approximately 20% of patients and abdominal distention is common. Generalized tenderness is indicative of free perforation and peritonitis.
  - Low-grade fever and mild leukocytosis are common.
- Diagnosis
  - The diagnosis of acute diverticulitis can often be made on the basis of the history and the physical examination. In the acute stage, it is helpful to perform further studies to confirm the diagnosis and to rule out other sources of acute abdominal signs.
  - CT scanning of the abdomen with IV and oral contrast is the diagnostic test of choice in patients suspected of having acute diverticulitis. CT can also identify the major complications of diverticulitis, including peritonitis, fistula formation and obstruction.
- Management
  - Approximately 25% of patients diagnosed with diverticulitis for the first time present with complicated diverticulitis. Nearly all of these patients require surgery.
  - The majority of patients with uncomplicated diverticulitis respond to medical therapy, although up to 30% require surgery.
  - Diverticulitis represents a localized infection that requires treatment with antibiotics. In the uncomplicated patient with acute diverticulitis, antibiotics should be continued for 7 to 10 days. The choice of antibiotics should be based on the usual bacteria, which are principally gram-negative rods and anaerobes (particularly *E. coli* and *Bacteroides fragilis*).
- See also www.fascrs.org, www.ssat.com, www.acg.gi.org, www.eaes-eur.org (all accessed February 8, 2011).

Diverticular Bleeding

- Diverticular bleeding is thought to result from progressive injury to the artery supplying that segment.
- The hallmark of diverticular bleeding is painless rectal bleeding, which is usually self-limited. Up to 50% of patients give a history of intermittent passage of maroon or bright red blood (hematochezia).

- Abdominal discomfort is usually not present, and it is rare for bleeding to coexist with acute diverticulitis.
- Approximately 5% of patients with diverticulosis present with massive hemorrhage, and hypovolemia.

Diverticular Colitis

- Diverticular colitis: A small subgroup of patients with diverticular disease develops a segmental colitis, most commonly in the sigmoid colon.

Mesenteric Ischemia

- Intestinal ischemia can be divided into acute and chronic, based on the rapidity and the degree to which blood flow is compromised.
- Acute mesenteric ischemia refers to the sudden onset of intestinal hypoperfusion, which can be caused by occlusive or nonocclusive obstruction of arterial or venous blood flow. It carries a high mortality (up to 60%).
  - Occlusive arterial obstruction is most commonly caused by emboli or thrombosis of mesenteric arteries, while occlusive venous obstruction is most commonly caused by thrombosis or segmental strangulation.
  - Risk factors include advanced age, atherosclerosis, low cardiac output states, cardiac arrhythmias, severe cardiac valvular disease, recent myocardial infarction, and intraabdominal malignancy.
- Chronic mesenteric ischemia (a.k.a. intestinal angina) refers to episodic or constant intestinal hypoperfusion, which usually develops in patients with mesenteric atherosclerotic disease.
- The major causes of acute mesenteric ischemia include:
  - Superior mesenteric artery embolism (50%)
    - Atrial fibrillation
  - Superior mesenteric artery thrombosis (15%–25%)
    - In patients with significant atherosclerotic vascular disease
  - Mesenteric venous thrombosis (5%)
    - Hypercoagulable states, usually an inherited thrombotic disorder
    - Portal hypertension
    - Abdominal infections
    - Blunt abdominal trauma
    - Pancreatitis
    - Splenectomy
    - Malignancy
  - Nonocclusive ischemia (20%–30%)
    - Patients with significant atherosclerotic vascular disease.
    - Inciting events include cardiac failure, sepsis, cardiac arrhythmias, and administration of medications such as digoxin and alpha-adrenergic agonists.
    - Several cases of nonocclusive mesenteric ischemia resulting from cocaine use have also been described.

Clinical Manifestations

- Classically, patients have rapid onset of severe periumbilical abdominal pain, which is often *out of proportion to findings on physical examination.*
- Nausea and vomiting are also common.
- The presentation may be more insidious with mesenteric vein thrombosis in which symptoms may have been present for weeks to months (typically 5–14 days) before diagnosis.
- Abdominal examination may be normal initially or reveal only abdominal distension or occult blood in the stool.
  - Signs of peritoneal inflammation, such as rebound tenderness and guarding, are absent.
  - As bowel ischemia progresses and transmural bowel infarction develops, the abdomen becomes grossly distended, bowel sounds become absent, and peritoneal signs develop.
  - A feculent odor to the breath may also be appreciated.
  - Mental status changes are reported to occur in approximately one-third of older patients with acute mesenteric ischemia.

Diagnosis

- The diagnosis of acute mesenteric ischemia depends on a high clinical suspicion, especially in patients with known risk factors (such as atrial fibrillation, congestive heart failure, peripheral vascular disease, or a history of hypercoagulability).
- Rapid diagnosis is essential to prevent the catastrophic events associated with intestinal infarction.
- Patients suspected of having acute mesenteric ischemia should be resuscitated after which a CT scan should be considered.
  - A CT scan of the abdomen may show focal or segmental bowel wall thickening or intestinal pneumatosis with portal vein gas.
  - Mesenteric arterial occlusions can be demonstrated as lack of enhancement of the arterial vasculature with timed IV contrast injections.
  - Emerging experience suggests that multidetector CT-angiography has a high degree of accuracy for diagnosing occlusive and nonocclusive acute mesenteric ischemia.
- If no alternative diagnosis is established and the clinical setting and radiographic findings do not warrant immediate laparotomy, patients should expeditiously undergo selective angiography of the superior mesenteric artery (SMA).
  - Mesenteric angiography remains the gold standard diagnostic study for acute arterial ischemia. Early and liberal implementation of angiography has been the major factor for the decline in the mortality of patients with acute mesenteric ischemia over the past 30 years.
  - Angiography is important even if surgery is planned because it cannot only identify the site of vascular compromise but also can be used to relieve mesenteric vasoconstriction with infusion of papaverine. Improvement in mesenteric vasoconstriction is essential for treatment of emboli, thromboses, and nonocclusive ischemia.
- A study suggested that elevation in the serum lactate was 100% sensitive but only 42% specific for intestinal ischemia and infarction. The specificity of an elevated serum lactate level does improve significantly when conditions such as shock, diabetic ketoacidosis, and renal and hepatic failure can be excluded.

Management

- Initial management should include aggressive fluid resuscitation, hemodynamic support, close hemodynamic monitoring, initiation of broad-spectrum antibiotics, and placement of a NG tube for gastric decompression.
- Vasoconstricting agents and digitalis should be avoided if possible because they can exacerbate mesenteric ischemia.
- Therapeutic options during angiography include the administration of intraarterial vasodilators or thrombolytic agents, angioplasty, placement of a vascular stent, and embolectomy depending on the cause of ischemia and the anatomy of the obstruction.
- Surgery should not be delayed in patients suspected of having intestinal infraction or perforation based on clinical, radiographic, or laboratory parameters.
  - Mesenteric arterial embolism: The traditional treatment of mesenteric arterial embolism has been early surgical laparotomy with embolectomy.
  - Mesenteric arterial thrombosis: Treatment of patients with acute mesenteric artery thrombosis is principally surgical. Thrombectomy alone is unlikely to offer a durable solution, because of the persistence of thrombogenic atherosclerotic plaques. As a result, various revascularization techniques, in conjunction with thrombectomy, and resection of nonviable segments have been advocated.
  - Mesenteric venous thrombosis: Standard initial treatment for acute mesenteric venous thrombosis includes heparin anticoagulation and resection of infarcted bowel.
  - Nonocclusive mesenteric ischemia: Primary therapy for patients with nonocclusive mesenteric ischemia involves papaverine infusion through the angiographic catheter and an attempt to reverse the underlying condition leading to splanchnic vasoconstriction.
- See also http://www.gastro.org/practice/medical-position-statements (accessed February 8, 2011).

Diarrhea

- Diarrhea is defined as passage of abnormally liquid or unformed stools at an increased frequency

- For adults on a typical Western diet, stool weight more than 200 g/day can generally be considered diarrheal.

- Diarrhea may be further defined as *acute* if less than 2 weeks, *persistent* if 2 to 4 weeks, and *chronic* if longer than 4 weeks in duration

- More than 90% of cases of acute diarrhea are caused by infectious agents; these cases are often accompanied by vomiting, fever, and abdominal pain. The remaining 10% or so are caused by medications, toxic ingestions, ischemia, and other conditions (Table 6-6).

Traveler's Diarrhea

- Traveler's diarrhea is gastroenteritis that is usually caused by bacteria endemic to local water.

  - Enterotoxigenic *E. coli* is most common.

- Symptoms include nausea, vomiting, borborygmi, abdominal cramps, and diarrhea begin 12 to 72 h after ingesting contaminated food or water.

- Diagnosis is mainly clinical.

- The mainstay of treatment is fluid replacement and an antimotility agent such as diphenoxylate or loperamide.

  - Antimotility agents are contraindicated in patients with fever or bloody stools and in children younger than 2 years of age.

  - Ciprofloxacin 500 mg orally twice daily for 3 days or levofloxacin 500 mg orally once daily is recommended in patients with severe disease and if fever and bloody stool are present.

- See also the health information for travelers' diarrhea at the Centers for Disease Control and Prevention website.

Clostridia Difficile Infection

- See http://www.cdc.gov/HAI/organisms/cdiff/Cdiff_infect.html (accessed February 8, 2011).

- *C. difficile* causes antibiotic-associated colitis; it colonizes the human intestinal tract after the normal gut flora have been altered by antibiotic therapy. It is one of the most common health care-associated infections and a significant cause of morbidity and mortality.

- Approximately 20% of hospitalized adults are *C. difficile* carriers who shed *C. difficile* in their stools but do not have diarrhea; in long-term care facilities, carriage rate may approach 50%. Although asymptomatic, these individuals serve as a reservoir for environmental contamination.

- The antibiotics most frequently implicated in predisposition to *C. difficile* infection are fluoroquinolones, clindamycin, cephalosporins, and penicillins, but virtually all antibiotics, including metronidazole and vancomycin, can predispose to *C. difficile*.

- Manifestations of *C. difficile*-associated diarrhea with colitis include:

  - Watery diarrhea up to 10 or 15 times daily
  - Lower abdominal pain
  - Cramping
  - Low-grade fever
  - Leukocytosis

- Physical examination generally demonstrates lower abdominal tenderness.

- Sigmoidoscopic or colonoscopic examination may demonstrate a spectrum of findings, from patchy mild erythema and friability to severe pseudomembranous colitis.

- Unexplained leukocytosis in hospitalized patients (even in the absence of diarrhea) may reflect underlying *C. difficile* infection.

- Pseudomembranous colitis: Patients with pseudomembranous colitis usually present with clinical manifestations of *C. difficile*-associated diarrhea with colitis. In addition, sigmoidoscopic examination in these patients demonstrates the presence of pseudomembranes, which is sufficient to make a presumptive diagnosis of *C. difficile* infection.

- Fulminant colitis: The manifestations of fulminant colitis typically include severe lower quadrant or diffuse abdominal pain, diarrhea, abdominal distention, fever, hypovolemia, lactic acidosis, and marked leukocytosis. Toxic megacolon is a clinical diagnosis based on the finding of colonic dilatation (>7 cm in its greatest diameter) accompanied by severe systemic toxicity.

TABLE 6-6. CAUSATIVE AGENTS AND CLINICAL FEATURES IN ACUTE INFECTIOUS DIARRHEA

Agent	Incubation Period	Vomiting	Abdominal Pain	Fever	Diarrhea
Toxin Producers (Preformed)					
Bacillus cereus, Staphylococcus aureus	1–8 h	3–4+	1–2+	0–1+	3–4+, watery
Clostridium perfringens	8–24				
Enterotoxin					
Vibrio cholera, enterotoxigenic Escherichia coli, Klebsiella pneumonia, Aeromonas species	8–72 h	2–4+	1–2+	0–1+	3–4+, watery
Enteroadherent					
E. coli, Giardia organisms, cryptosporidiosis, helminths	1–8 d	0–1+	1–3+	0–2+	1–2+, watery, mushy
Cytotoxin-Producers					
Clostridium difficile	1–3 d	0–1+	3–4+	1–2+	1–3+, usually watery, occasionally bloody
Hemorrhagic E. coli	12–72 h	0–1+	3–4+	1–2+	1–3+, initially watery, quickly bloody
Invasive (Minimal Inflammation)					
Rotavirus and Norwalk agent	1–3 d	1–3+	2–3+	3–4+	1–3+, watery
Variable Inflammation					
Salmonella, Campylobacter, Aeromonas species, Vibrio parahaemolyticus, Yersinia	12 h–11 d	0–3+	2–4+	3–4+	1–4+, watery or bloody
Severe Inflammation					
Shigella species, enteroinvasive E. coli, Entamoeba histolytica	12 h–8 d	0–1+	3–4+	3–4+	1–2+, bloody

MEDICAL SPECIALTIES

- Relapse or reinfection: Relapse or reinfection develops in 10% to 25% of treated *C. difficile* cases, and patients may experience several episodes of relapsing colitis. Relapse may present within days or weeks of completing treatment for *C. difficile*; the clinical presentation may be similar to or more severe than the initial presentation. Studies using molecular methods have shown that up to one-half of recurrent episodes are reinfections rather than relapses of infection with the original strain.
- Although *C. difficile* is the major infectious cause of antibiotic-associated diarrhea, it must be distinguished from other infectious and noninfectious causes of diarrhea. The diagnosis should be based on the presence of a positive stool toxin test or an endoscopic evaluation that demonstrates pseudomembranes in the colon.
- Toxin assays include cytotoxicity assay, enzyme immunoassay (EIA), and polymerase chain reaction (PCR). Most strains produce both toxins A and B, although some clinically relevant strains produce toxin A or B only.
  - Many laboratories use EIA testing for *C. difficile* toxins A and B, which is rapid but less sensitive than the cytotoxicity assay.
  - EIA for both toxins should be used because clinical cases may involve strains with a mutation in toxin A (rendering the EIA for toxin A ineffective) or strains that produce only toxin B. While the specificity of the EIA is good, the test has a relatively high false-negative rate because 100 to 1000 pg of toxin must be present for the test to be positive.
  - Up to 3 serial EIA tests may increase the diagnostic yield by as much as 10% if the initial test is negative.
- Patients with clinical manifestations of *C. difficile* and a positive diagnostic assay should receive antibiotics for treatment for *C. difficile*. Empiric therapy is appropriate pending results of diagnostic testing if the clinical suspicion is high. Treatment of *C. difficile* is not indicated in patients who have a positive toxin assay but are asymptomatic.
- Standard therapy consists of oral metronidazole or oral vancomycin for 10 to 14 days. Vancomycin is recommended for severe disease and for recurrent disease. The recommended regimen for metronidazole is 500 mg 3 times daily or 250 mg 4 times daily, whereas that of vancomycin is 125 mg 4 times daily.
- Repeat stool assays are not warranted following treatment. Up to 50% of patients have positive stool assays for as long as 6 weeks after the completion of therapy.

Chronic Diarrhea

- Diarrhea lasting longer than 4 weeks warrants evaluation to exclude serious underlying pathology.
- In contrast to acute diarrhea, most of the causes of chronic diarrhea are noninfectious.
- The classification of chronic diarrhea by pathophysiologic mechanism facilitates a rational approach to management (Figure 6-2).

Causes of Chronic Diarrhea According to Predominant Pathophysiologic Mechanism

- Secretory causes
  - Exogenous stimulant laxatives
  - Chronic ethanol ingestion
  - Other drugs and toxins
  - Endogenous laxatives (dihydroxy bile acids)
  - Idiopathic secretory diarrhea
  - Certain bacterial infections
  - Bowel resection, disease or fistula
  - Partial bowel obstruction or fecal impaction
  - Hormone-producing tumors
    - Carcinoid, VIPoma, medullary cancer of thyroid
    - Mastocytosis, gastrinoma, colorectal villous adenoma
  - Addison disease
  - Congenital electrolyte absorption defects
- Osmotic causes
  - Osmotic laxatives (Mg, PO_4, SO_4)
  - Lactase and other disaccharide deficiencies
  - Nonabsorbable carbohydrates
    - Sorbitol, lactulose, polyethylene glycol

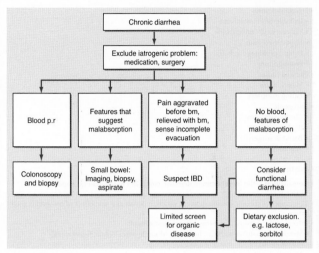

Figure 6-2 Approach to chronic diarrhea. bm, bowel movement; IBD, inflammatory bowel disease; p.r., per rectum.

- Steatorrheal causes
  - Intraluminal maldigestion
    - Pancreatic exocrine insufficiency
    - Bacterial overgrowth
    - Bariatric surgery
    - Liver disease
  - Mucosal malabsorption
    - Celiac sprue
    - Whipple disease
    - Infections
    - Abetalipoproteinemia
    - Ischemia
    - Postmucosal obstruction
      - Primary or secondary lymphatic obstruction
- Inflammatory causes
  - Idiopathic inflammatory bowel disease
    - Crohn disease
    - Ulcerative colitis
  - Lymphocytic and collagenous colitis
  - Immune related mucosal disease
    - Immunodeficiencies
    - Food allergy
    - Eosinophilic gastroenteritis
    - Graft-versus-host disease
  - Infections (invasive bacteria, viruses and parasites, Brainerd diarrhea)
  - Radiation injury
  - GI malignancies

- Dysmotile causes
  - Irritable bowel syndrome
  - Visceral neuromyopathies
  - Hyperthyroidism
  - Drugs (prokinetic agents)
  - Postvagotomy
- Factitial causes
  - Munchausen
  - Eating disorders
- Iatrogenic
  - Cholecystectomy
  - Ileal resection
  - Bariatric surgery
  - Vagotomy

Constipation

- Constipation is the most common digestive complaint in the general population (Table 6-7).
- The causes of chronic constipation are varied, it occurs as a side effect of commonly used drugs.
- Infrequently, constipation is the first manifestation of:
  - Metabolic (diabetes mellitus, hypothyroidism, hypercalcemia, heavy metal intoxication)
  - Neurologic disease
  - Obstructive intestinal disease
- Constipation is often treated on the basis of a patient's impression that there is a disturbance in bowel function. However, the term *constipation* has varied meanings for different people.

TABLE 6-7. CAUSES OF CONSTIPATION

Cause	Examples
Acute Constipation	
Acute bowel obstruction	Volvulus, hernia, adhesions, fecal impaction
Adynamic ileus	Peritonitis, head or spinal trauma, bed rest
Drugs	Anticholinergics (antipsychotics, antiparkinsonian), cations (iron, calcium, bismuth), opioids
Chronic Constipation	
Colonic tumor	
Metabolic disorders	Diabetes mellitus, hypothyroidism, uremia, hypercalcemia
CNS disorders	Parkinson disease, multiple sclerosis, stroke
Peripheral nervous system disorders	Autonomic neuropathy
Systemic disorders	Systemic sclerosis, amyloidosis, dermatomyositis
Functional	Colonic inertia, irritable bowel syndrome

CNS, central nervous system.

- Constipation has been defined as a stool frequency of less than 3 per week based on epidemiological studies in the United States and the United Kingdom.
- An international working committee recommended diagnostic criteria (Rome III) for functional constipation. The diagnosis should be based on the presence of at least 2 of the following for at least 3 months (with symptom onset at least 6 months prior to diagnosis).
  - Straining during at least 25% of defecations
  - Lumpy or hard stools in at least 25% of defecations
  - Sensation of incomplete evacuation for at least 25% of defecations
  - Sensation of anorectal obstruction or blockage for at least 25% of defecations
  - Manual maneuvers to facilitate at least 25% of defecations (eg, digital evacuation, support of the pelvic floor)

Causes

Treating Constipation (Table 6-8)

Irritable Bowel Syndrome (IBS)

Spastic Colon

- Irritable bowel syndrome consists of recurring upper and lower GI symptoms, including variable degrees of abdominal pain, constipation or diarrhea, and abdominal bloating.
- The cause is unknown, and the pathophysiology is incompletely understood.
- Some patients with IBS appear to have a learned aberrant illness behavior (ie, they express emotional conflict as a GI complaint, usually abdominal pain)
- Two major clinical types of IBS have been described.
  - In *constipation-predominant IBS*, most patients have pain over at least 1 area of the colon and periods of constipation alternating with a more normal stool frequency. Stool often contains clear or white mucus.
  - *Diarrhea-predominant IBS* is characterized by precipitous diarrhea that occurs immediately on rising or during or immediately after eating, especially rapid eating. Nocturnal diarrhea is unusual. Pain, bloating, and rectal urgency are common, and incontinence may occur.
- Diagnosis is clinical. The Rome criteria are standardized symptom-based criteria for diagnosing IBS; the criteria are met by the presence for at least 3 months of the following symptoms:
  - Abdominal pain or discomfort that is relieved by defecation or is associated with a change in frequency or consistency of stool, and
  - Disturbed defecation involving at least 2 of the following: altered stool frequency, altered stool form, altered stool passage, passage of mucus, and bloating or feeling of distention.
- Treatment is symptomatic, consisting of dietary management and drugs, including anticholinergics and agents active at serotonin receptors.

Inflammatory Bowel Disease (Table 6-9)

Diseases That Mimic IBD

Infectious

- Bacterial
  - *Salmonella*
  - *Shigella*
  - Toxigenic *E. coli*
  - *Campylobacter*
  - *Yersinia*
  - *C. difficile*
  - Gonorrhea
  - *Chlamydia trachomatis*
- Mycobacterial
  - Tuberculosis
  - *Mycobacterium avium*

TABLE 6-8. AGENTS USED TO TREAT CONSTIPATION

Type	Agent	Dosage	Side Effects
Fiber	Bran	Up to 1 cup/day	Bloating, flatulence, iron and Ca malabsorption
	Psyllium	Up to 30 g/day in divided doses of 2.5–7.5 g	Bloating, flatulence
	Methylcellulose	Up to 9 g/day in divided doses of 0.45–3 g	Less bloating than other fiber agents
	Ca polycarbophil	2–6 tablets/day	Bloating, flatulence
Emollients	Docusate Na	100 mg BID or TID	Ineffective for severe constipation
	Glycerin	2–3 g suppository once daily	Rectal irritation
	Mineral oil	15–45 mL PO once daily	Lipid pneumonia, malabsorption of fat soluble vitamins, dehydration
Osmotic Agents	Sorbitol	15–30 mL PO of 70% solution once daily or BID	Transient abdominal cramps, flatulence
	Lactulose	10–20 g once daily up to 4 times daily	Transient abdominal cramps, flatulence
	Polyethylene glycol	Up to 3.8 L during a 4-hour period	Fecal incontinence
Stimulants	Anthraquinone	Depends on brand used	Degeneration of Meissner and Auerbach plexus, malabsorption, abdominal cramps, dehydration
	Bisacodyl	5–15 mg/day PO; 10 mg suppositories up to 3 times weekly	Fecal incontinence, hypokalemia, abdominal cramps, rectal burning with suppository
Saline laxative	Mg	Mg sulphate 15–30 g/day or bid, milk of Mg 30–60 mL/day	Mg toxicity, dehydration, abdominal cramps
Enemas	Mineral- and olive-oil retention	100–150 mL/day rectally	Fecal incontinence, mechanical trauma
	Tap water	500 mL rectally	Mechanical trauma
	Phosphate	60 mL rectally	Damage to rectal mucosa, hyperphosphatemia, mechanical trauma

BID, twice daily; Ca, calcium; Mg, magnesium; Na, sodium; PO, by mouth; TID, three times daily.

**TABLE 6-9. DIFFERENT CLINICAL, ENDOSCOPIC, AND
RADIOGRAPHIC FEATURES**

	Ulcerative Colitis	Crohn Disease
Clinical		
Gross blood in stool	Yes	Occasionally
Mucus	Yes	Occasionally
Systemic symptoms	Occasionally	Frequently
Pain	Occasionally	Frequently
Abdominal mass	Rarely	Yes
Significant perineal disease	No	Frequently
Fistulas	No	Yes
Small-intestinal obstruction	No	Frequently
Colonic obstruction	Rarely	Frequently
Response to antibiotics	No	Yes
Recurrence after surgery	No	Yes
ANCA-positive	Frequently	Rarely
ASCA-positive	Rarely	Frequently
Endoscopic		
Rectal sparing	Rarely	Frequently
Continuous disease	Yes	Occasionally
Cobblestoning	No	Yes
Granuloma on biopsy	No	Occasionally
Radiographic		
Small bowel significantly abnormal	No	Yes
Abnormal terminal ileum	Occasionally	Yes
Segmental colitis	No	Yes
Asymmetric colitis	No	Yes
Stricture	Occasionally	Frequently

ANCA, antineutrophil cytoplasm antibody; ASCA, anti-*Saccharomyces cerevisiae* antibody.

- Parasitic
  - Amebiasis
  - *Isospora*
  - *Trichuris trichiura*
  - Hookworm
  - *Strongyloides*
- Viral
  - Cytomegalovirus (CMV)

- Herpes simplex
- Human immunodeficiency virus (HIV)
- Fungal
  - Histoplasmosis
  - Candida
  - Aspergillus

Noninfectious

- Inflammatory
  - Appendicitis
  - Diverticulitis
  - Diversion colitis
  - Collagenous/lymphocytic colitis
  - Ischemic colitis
  - Radiation colitis/enteritis
  - Solitary rectal ulcer syndrome
  - Eosinophilic gastroenteritis
  - Neutropenic colitis
  - Behçet syndrome
  - Graft-versus-host disease
- Neoplastic
  - Lymphoma
  - Metastatic carcinoma
  - Carcinoma of the ileum
  - Carcinoid
  - Familial polyposis
- Drugs and chemicals
  - NSAIDs
  - Phosphosoda
  - Cathartic colon
  - Gold
  - Oral contraception
  - Cocaine
  - Chemotherapy

Crohn Disease

- Crohn disease (CD) is a disorder of uncertain etiology that is characterized by transmural inflammation of the GI tract. CD may involve the entire GI tract from mouth to the perianal area.
  - Approximately 80% of patients have small bowel involvement, usually in the distal ileum, with one-third of patients having ileitis exclusively.
  - Approximately 50% of patients have ileocolitis, which refers to involvement of both the ileum and colon.
  - Approximately 20% have disease limited to the colon.
- The clinical manifestations of CD are much more variable than those of ulcerative colitis. Patients can have symptoms for many years prior to diagnosis.
  - Fatigue, prolonged diarrhea with abdominal pain, weight loss, and fever, with or without gross bleeding, are the hallmarks of CD.
  - Crampy abdominal pain is a common manifestation of CD, regardless of disease distribution.
  - The transmural nature of the inflammatory process results in fibrotic strictures. These strictures often lead to repeated episodes of small bowel, or less commonly colonic, obstruction.
  - Diarrhea is a common presentation, but often fluctuates over a long period of time.
  - Bleeding: Although stools frequently reveal the presence of microscopic levels of blood gross bleeding is less frequent than in ulcerative colitis. Transmural bowel inflammation is associated with the development of sinus tracts. Sinus tracts that penetrate the serosa can give rise to fistulas.

- Symptoms and signs related to perianal disease occur in up to one-third of patients with CD and may dominate the clinical picture. These include perianal pain and drainage from large skin tags, anal fissures, perirectal abscesses, and anorectal fistulas.
- Malabsorption: Bile acids are normally absorbed by specific receptors in the distal ileum. Bile salt malabsorption occurs when more than 50 to 60 cm of terminal ileum is diseased or resected.
- Severe oral involvement may present with aphthous ulcers or pain in the mouth and gums.
- Extra-intestinal manifestation
- Arthritis: Primarily involving large joints
- Eye manifestations include uveitis, iritis, and episcleritis
- Dermatologic manifestations include erythema nodosum and pyoderma gangrenosum
- Primary sclerosing cholangitis
- Renal stones: Calcium oxalate and uric acid kidney stones
- Bone loss and osteoporosis may result related to glucocorticoid use and impaired vitamin D and calcium absorption
- Vitamin B_{12} deficiency: A clinical picture of pernicious anemia can result from severe ileal disease because vitamin B_{12} is absorbed in the distal 50 to 60 cm of ileum.
- Secondary amyloidosis is a rare complication.
- The diagnosis of CD is usually established with endoscopic findings or imaging studies in a patient with a compatible clinical history.
- Colonoscopy with intubation of the terminal ileum is used to establish the diagnosis of ileocolonic CD. Endoscopic features include focal ulcerations adjacent to areas of normal appearing mucosa along with polypoid mucosal changes that give a cobblestone appearance.
- Imaging studies are most useful to evaluate the upper GI tract and allow documentation of the length and location of strictures in areas not accessible by colonoscopy. Imaging has traditionally involved barium studies, such as barium enema or upper GI series with small-bowel follow through.

Ulcerative Colitis (Table 6-10)

Liver Disease (Table 6-11 and Figure 6-3)

Causes of Liver Disease

- Inherited hyperbilirubinemia
  - Gilberts syndrome

TABLE 6-10. ULCERATIVE COLITIS—DISEASE PRESENTATION

	Mild	Moderate	Severe
Bowel movements	<4 day	4–6 day	>6 day
Blood in stool	Small	Moderate	Severe
Fever	None	<37.5°C (99.5°F) mean	>37.5°C (99.5°F) mean
Tachycardia	None	<90 bpm mean pulse	>90 bpm mean pulse
Anemia	Mild	<75%	>75%
Sedimentation rate	<30 mm		>30 mm
Endoscopic appearance	Erythema, decreased vascular pattern, fine granularity	Marked erythema, course granularity, absent vascular markings, contact bleeding, no ulcerations	Spontaneous bleeding, ulcerations

bpm, beats per minute.

TABLE 6-11. IMPORTANT DIAGNOSTIC TESTS IN COMMON LIVER DISEASES

Disease	Diagnostic Test
Hepatitis A	Anti-HAV IgM
Hepatitis B (acute)	HBsAg and anti-HBc IgM
Hepatitis B (chronic)	HBsAg, HBeAg, and/or HBV DNA
Hepatitis C	Anti-HCV and HCV RNA
Hepatitis D (delta)	HBsAg and anti-HDV
Hepatitis E	Anti-HEV
Autoimmune hepatitis	ANA or SMA, elevated IgG, and compatible histology
Primary biliary cirrhosis	Mitochondrial antibody, elevated IgM levels and compatible histology
Primary sclerosing cholangitis	p-ANCA, cholangiography
Nonalcoholic steatohepatitis	Ultrasound or CT evidence of fatty liver, high ferritin and compatible histology
α_1-antitrypsin disease	Reduced α_1-antitrypsin levels, phenotypes PiZZ or PiSZ
Wilson disease	Decreased serum ceruloplasmin and increased urinary copper; increased hepatic copper level
Hemochromatosis	Elevated iron saturation and serum ferritin; genetic testing for *HFE* gene mutations
Hepatocellular cancer	Elevated α-fetoprotein >500 ultrasound or CT image of mass

ANA, antinuclear antibody; CT, computed tomography; HAV, hepatitis A virus; HBc, antibody to hepatitis C; HBeAg, hepatitis B e antigen; HBsAg, hepatitis B surface antigen; HBV, hepatitis B virus; anti-HCV, antibody to hepatitis C virus; HDV, hepatitis D virus; anti-HEV, antibody to hepatitis E virus; IgG, immunoglobulin G; IgM, immunoglobulin M; p-ANCA, perinuclear antineutrophil cytoplasmic antibody; SMA, smooth muscle antibody.

- Crigler-Najjar syndrome, types I and II
- Dubin-Johnson syndrome
- Rotor syndrome
- Viral hepatitis
  - Hepatitis A
  - Hepatitis B
  - Hepatitis C
  - Hepatitis D
  - Hepatitis E
  - Others mononucleosis, herpes, adenovirus hepatitis
- Immune and autoimmune diseases
  - Primary biliary cirrhosis
  - Autoimmune hepatitis
  - Sclerosing cholangitis
  - Overlap syndromes
  - Graft-versus-host disease
  - Allograft rejection

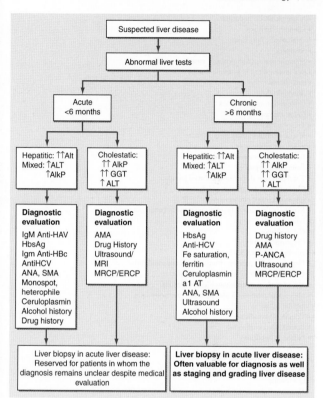

Figure 6-3   Approach to the evaluation of abnormal liver tests. AlkP, alkaline phosphatase; ALT, alanine aminotransferase; AMA, alkaline membrane assay; ERCP, endoscopic retrograde cholangiopancreatography; GGT, γ-glutamyltransferase; anti-HAV, antibody to hepatitis A virus; HBsAg, hepatitis B surface antigen; anti-HCV, antibody to hepatitis C virus; IgM, immunoglobulin M; MRCP, magnetic resonance cholangiopancreatography; MRI, magnetic resonance imaging; p-ANCA, perinuclear antineutrophil cytoplasmic antibody; SMA, smooth muscle antibody.

- Genetic liver diseases
  - α₁-Antitrypsin deficiency
  - Hemochromatosis
  - Wilson disease
  - Benign recurrent intrahepatic cholestasis
  - Progressive familial intrahepatic cholestasis
  - Others (galactosemia, tyrosinemia, cystic fibrosis, Newman-Pick, Gaucher disease)
- Alcoholic liver disease
  - Acute fatty liver

- Acute alcoholic hepatitis
- Laennec cirrhosis
- Nonalcoholic fatty liver
  - Steatosis
  - Steatohepatitis (nonalcoholic steatohepatitis)
- Liver involvement in systemic diseases
  - Sarcoidosis
  - Amyloidosis
  - Glycogen storage diseases
  - Celiac disease
  - Tuberculosis
  - Mycobacterium avium intracellulare
- Cholestatic syndromes
  - Benign postoperative cholestasis
  - Jaundice of sepsis
  - Total parenteral nutrition-induced jaundice
  - Cholestasis of pregnancy
  - Cholangitis and cholecystitis
  - Extrahepatic biliary obstruction (stone, stricture, cancer)
  - Biliary atresia
  - Caroli disease
  - Cryptosporidiosis
- Drug-induced liver disease
  - Hepatocellular pattern (isoniazid, acetaminophen)
  - Cholestatic pattern (methyltestosterone)
  - Mixed pattern (sulphonamides, phenytoin)
  - Micro- and macrovesicular steatosis (methotrexate)
- Vascular injury
  - Venoocclusive disease
  - Budd-Chiari syndrome
  - Ischemic hepatitis
  - Passive congestion
  - Portal vein thrombosis
  - Nodular regenerative hyperplasia
- Mass lesions
  - Hepatocellular carcinoma
  - Cholangiocarcinoma
  - Adenoma
  - Focal nodular hyperplasia
  - Metastatic tumors
  - Abscess
  - Cysts
  - Hemangioma

Chronic Liver Failure

- Cirrhosis is defined histologically as an advanced form of progressive hepatic fibrosis with distortion of the hepatic architecture and regenerative nodule formation.
- The major clinical consequences of cirrhosis are
  - Impaired hepatocyte function
  - An increased intrahepatic resistance (portal hypertension)
  - Development of hepatocellular carcinoma
- The clinical picture of chronic liver disease is frequently dominated by the complications of portal hypertension. In addition, infectious complications are common and associated with worsening of hepatocyte function and portal hypertension.

TABLE 6-12. CHILD-TURCOTTE-PUGH SCORING SYSTEM

Parameter	1	2	3
Ascites	Absent	Easily controlled	Poorly controlled
Bilirubin (mg/dL)	<2	2–3	>3
Albumin (g/dL)	>3.5	2.8–3.5	<2.8
INR	<1.7	1.7–2.3	>2.3
Encephalopathy	None	Grade 1–2	Grade 3–4

Cirrhosis represents a clinical spectrum, ranging from asymptomatic liver disease to hepatic decompensation. Manifestations of hepatic decompensation include:

- Variceal bleeding
- Ascites with spontaneous bacterial peritonitis
- Hepatic encephalopathy
- Hepatorenal syndrome
- Hepatopulmonary syndrome
- Portopulmonary hypertension
- Hepatocellular carcinoma
- Hepato-adrenal syndrome

The Child-Turcotte-Pugh (CTP) scoring system classifies chronic liver failure (CLF) into 3 categories based on severity (Table 6-12).

- A total CTP score of 5 to 6 is Child's class A, well-compensated disease;
- A CTP score of 7 to 9 is Child's class B, in which there is significant functional compromise.
- CTP score of 10 to 15 is Child's class C, advanced decompensated disease. The calculator for end-stage liver disease can be found at http://www.mdcalc.com/child-pugh-score-for-cirrhosis-mortality (accessed February 8, 2011).

The Model for End-Stage Liver Disease score provides another classification of the severity of CLF based on the readily obtainable laboratory values of serum creatinine, total bilirubin, and prothrombin time, expressed as the international normalized ratio. See the calculator at http://www.mdcalc.com/meld-score-model-for-end-stage-liver-disease-12-and-older (accessed February 8, 2011).

Causes of Cirrhosis

- Viral and infectious
  - Hepatitis B
  - Hepatitis C
  - Schistosomiasis
- Metabolic
  - Alcohol
  - Toxins
  - Medications
- Nonalcoholic steatohepatitis
- Genetic
  - Hereditary hemochromatosis
  - Wilsons disease
  - α_1-antitrypsin deficiency
  - Cystic fibrosis
- Autoimmune hepatitis
- Cholestatic
  - Primary biliary cirrhosis

- Primary sclerosing cholangitis
- Secondary biliary cirrhosis
- Vascular
  - Right heart failure
  - Budd-Chiari syndrome
- Sarcoid

Metabolic and Hematologic Derangements in Cirrhosis

- Hyperglycemia (portal-to-systemic shunting)
- Hypoglycemia (hepatocyte failure)
- Hypoalbuminemia
- Decreased synthesis of clotting factors, prolonged INR
- Decreased production of antithrombin, proteins S and C, thrombotic risk
- Increased ammonia
- Cholestasis
  - Impaired absorption of fat-soluble vitamins
- Anemia
  - Microcytic from iron deficiency
  - Macrocytic from folate and vitamin B_{12} deficiency
- Hyponatremia (Na <135 mmol/L)
- Thrombocytopenia
  - Hypersplenism
  - Alcohol
  - Marrow suppression
- "Low level" disseminated intravascular coagulation
- Renal dysfunction (hepatorenal)
- Impaired immunity

Spontaneous Bacterial Peritonitis

- Spontaneous bacterial peritonitis (SBP) is seen in up to 30% of patients with ascites. Patients who have SBP usually present with
  - Fever
  - Diffuse abdominal pain or tenderness
  - Altered mental status
  - Leukocytosis
  - Worsening renal function
- Approximately 15% of patients do not have any signs or symptoms of SBP.
- The diagnostic test of choice is abdominal paracentesis.
  - A neutrophil count higher than $250/mm^3$ is diagnostic of SBP.
  - Fluid cultures are positive in approximately half of the cases.
  - Almost all cases of SBP are secondary to a single microorganism, with *E. coli* and *Klebsiella pneumoniae* accounting for approximately half of the cases and gram-positive bacteria accounting for one-third.
- Treatment consists of a 5-day course of a third-generation cephalosporin, such as IV cefotaxime or ceftriaxone. For patients unable to take a cephalosporin, IV ciprofloxacin, followed by oral administration, is recommended.
- SBP is associated with the development of hepatorenal syndrome in approximately 30% of patients. The risk can be decreased by IV albumin infusion at a dose of 1.5 mg/kg at the time of SBP diagnosis and 1.0 mg/kg after 48 hours.
- Primary prophylaxis, defined as antibiotic treatment of patients without prior SBP, has been suggested in patients who have CLF and ascites who fulfill the following criteria:
  - Ascitic fluid protein concentration lower than 1 g/dL
  - Serum bilirubin level higher than 3.2 mg/dL, and
  - Platelet count higher than $98,000/mm^3$, as these patients have a threefold-increased risk of developing SBP within 1 year.

- A recent random clinical trial demonstrated that primary prophylaxis with norfloxacin significantly reduced the 1-year risk of developing SBP when compared with placebo (7% vs. 61%; $P < 0.001$)
- Following an initial episode of SBP, 1-year recurrence rate is 55%; 1-year survival is less than 50%, and antibiotic prophylaxis with fluoroquinolones is recommended. Amoxicillin-clavulanate and trimethoprim-sulfamethoxazole are acceptable alternatives in those unable to tolerate quinolones.

Hepatic Encephalopathy

- Hepatic encephalopathy has a wide range of clinical manifestations, from impaired memory and diminished attention to confusion and coma.
- Grading of mental status
  - Grade 0: No signs or symptoms
  - Grade 1: Trivial lack of awareness, euphoria or anxiety, shortened attention span impaired performance of addition
  - Grade 2: Lethargy or apathy, minimal disorientation for time or place, subtle personality change, inappropriate behavior, impaired performance of subtraction
  - Grade 3: Somnolence to semi-stupor, but responsive to verbal stimuli, confusion, gross disorientation
  - Grade 4: Coma (unresponsive to verbal or noxious stimuli)
- Acute worsening of hepatic encephalopathy should prompt an evaluation for reversible causes, such as GI bleeding, hypovolemia, hypoglycemia, hypokalemic metabolic alkalosis, infection, constipation, hypoxia, or excessive use of sedatives.
- The treatment of hepatic encephalopathy is with nonabsorbable disaccharides (eg, lactulose) to lower ammonia levels. The starting dose of lactulose is commonly 30 g give twice daily, titrated to two to three soft stools per day. The addition of nonabsorbable antibiotics such as rifaximin may further decrease intestinal ammonia production.
- Previously, aggressive protein restriction was recommended; however, this is now believed to worsen the nutritional status of patients and decreases overall survival. Guidelines published by the European Society for Clinical Nutrition and Metabolism (ESPEN) recommended that patients with cirrhosis should have an energy intake of 35 to 40 kcal/kg body weight per day and a protein intake of 1.2 to 1.5 g/kg body weight per day.
- Zinc deficiency impairs the activity of urea cycle enzymes and glutamine synthetase. Zinc deficiency has been implicated in the pathogenesis of hepatic encephalopathy as diminished serum zinc levels and their inverse correlation with blood ammonia levels have been reported.

Hepatorenal Syndrome

- Hepatorenal syndrome (HRS) is a functional form of renal failure that occurs in patients with end-stage liver disease. The pathophysiologic hallmark of HRS is vasoconstriction of renal circulation.
- In 1996 the International Club of Ascites established diagnostic criteria for the diagnosis of HRS. HRS was further classified as type 1 and type 2 according to the rate of decline of renal function.
  - Type 1 was arbitrarily defined as a 100% increase in serum creatinine reaching a value of more than 1.5 mg/dL in less than 2 weeks.
  - Patients who had a slower decline in renal function were deemed to have type 2 HRS.
  - Patients with type 1 HRS have a very poor prognosis compared to patients with type 2 HRS. The median survival time for type 1 HRS has been reported to be 14 days.
  - See http://www.icasites.org/about/guidelines/.
- Volume expansion with albumin and vasopressin analogues (ornipressin and terlipressin), norepinephrine and somatostatin have been used with variable success.
- Liver transplantation is considered the treatment of choice for patients with cirrhosis and type 1 HRS because it "allows for both the liver disease and associated renal failure to be cured."
- HRS is a frequent complication over overdiuresis (with furosemide [Lasix]), particularly in the setting of a contrast study or a therapeutic paracentesis. Patients who undergo a contrast study and or paracentesis require fluid loading (with albumin).

Hepato-Adrenal Syndrome

Adrenal dysfunction is common in critically ill patients with end-stage liver disease and treatment with corticosteroids may improve outcome.

Pulmonary Consequences of Portal Hypertension

Two distinct pulmonary vascular disorders can occur in cirrhosis:

- Hepatopulmonary syndrome (HPS) and portopulmonary hypertension. Both can coexist in the same patient.
- Portopulmonary hypertension is seen in 0.5% to 5% of patients with cirrhosis and/or portal hypertension and presents in similar ways to patients with pulmonary hypertension from other causes. Diagnosis is established by echocardiography and right-heart catheterization. Recent case reports and series have demonstrated improvement of pulmonary hypertension with oral sildenafil.
- HPS is defined as a defect in arterial oxygenation induced by intrapulmonary vascular dilatations. This entity is seen in 8% to 17% of patients with cirrhosis, and median survival is 11 months. Liver transplantation resolves HPS in the majority of patients.

Infection and Cirrhosis

Cirrhotic patients have several abnormalities that increase the susceptibility to bacterial infection. A National Hospital Discharge Survey demonstrated that hospitalized cirrhotics are more likely to develop sepsis (relative risk [RR] 2.6) and to die from sepsis (RR 2.0) than hospitalized noncirrhotic patients. Fifteen to thirty-five percent of cirrhotics develop nosocomial infection, with infection accounting for 30% to 50% of deaths in patients with cirrhosis.

- Usual infections
  - SBP
  - Pneumonia
  - Gram-negative bacteremia
  - Urinary tract infection
- Common pathogens
  - *E. coli*
  - *S. aureus*
  - *Enterococcus faecalis*
  - *Streptococcus pneumonia*
- Diagnosis of infection is difficult in patients with cirrhosis
  - Reduced white blood cell concentration because of hypersplenism.
  - Tachycardia and hyperdynamic circulation.
  - Hyperventilation caused by hepatic encephalopathy.
  - Blunted febrile response.
  - Cirrhosis itself results in low-grade fever.
- In patients with cirrhosis, infections further impair
  - Systemic and splanchnic hemodynamic derangements
  - Coagulation
  - Liver function
  - May trigger a variceal bleed

Supportive Care of the Hospitalized Cirrhotic

- Do not replace clotting factors or platelets unless bleeding.
- Feed with a 1 g/kg protein diet.
- Sequential compression devices for deep vein thrombosis prophylaxis.
- Exclude infection; culture blood, ascitic fluid.
- Prophylactic antibiotics in high-risk patients.
- *Do Not Diurese:* Give 25% albumin.
- Paracentesis in patients with tense ascites (replace albumin).
- Avoid nephrotoxic drugs.
- Lactulose for regular stool.
- Monitor venous ammonia.

- Adrenocorticotropic hormone stimulation test in all: Replace with hydrocortisone if adrenal insufficiency.
- Avoid sedatives (haloperidol okay).
- Ultrasound plus Doppler examination to exclude portal and splenic vein thrombosis and hepatocellular carcinoma.
- Test for α-fetoprotein level

Fulminant Liver Failure

See http://www.aasld.org/practiceguidelines/Documents/Bookmarked%20Practice%20 Guidelines/acute%20liver%20failure.pdf (accessed February 8, 2011).

Fulminant Hepatic Failure (FHF) (a.k.a. Acute Liver Failure)

- Defined as the development of impaired hepatic synthetic function with coagulopathy and the development of hepatic encephalopathy in the absence of underlying liver disease within a 2- to 3-month time period.
- This condition is uncommon but not rare; approximately 2000 cases annually in the United States with a mortality ranging 50% to 90% despite intensive care therapy.
- Although the clinical picture of chronic liver disease is frequently dominated by the complication of portal hypertension, the clinical picture of acute or fulminant hepatic failure is dominated by hepatocyte failure.
- Cerebral edema leading to intracranial hypertension complicates approximately 50% to 80% of patients with severe FHF (grade III or IV coma) in whom it is the leading cause of death.
- Recovery of functional liver mass in acute liver injury occurs more readily than in the chronic setting because of the lack of long-standing fibrosis and portal hypertension, and the host's overall better nutritional status. Therefore, if the individual can be supported throughout the acute event, and the inciting injury is removed or ameliorated, recovery will follow the rapid regeneration of liver cells. For those in whom spontaneous recovery is not possible, liver transplant may be lifesaving.
- Causes of fulminant hepatic failure
  - Viral hepatitis
    - Hepatitis B, C, and E, and rarely A and D infection
    - CMV infection
    - Viral hemorrhagic fevers
  - Drugs and toxins
    - Acetaminophen
    - Alcohol
    - Isoniazid
    - Valproic Acid
    - Phenytoin
    - Amanita phalloides
    - Carbon tetrachloride
    - Propylthiouracil
    - Methylenedioxymethamphetamine ("ecstasy")
  - Miscellaneous
    - Fatty liver of pregnancy
    - Reye syndrome
    - Wilson disease
    - Autoimmune chronic active hepatitis
    - Budd-Chiari syndrome (especially in patients with underlying hepatic disease)

Diagnostic Workup

- Blood and urine
  - Complete blood cell count with platelets
  - Electrolytes BUN and creatinine
  - INR
  - Liver panel

- Blood lactate
- Ammonia
- Blood gas with pH
- HIV testing (rapid)
- Hepatitis A, B, C, E (all markers)
- CMV PCR and antibody
- Herpes simplex virus PCR and antibody
- Epstein-Barr virus antibody
  - Autoimmune markers
  - Antinuclear antibody
  - Antismooth muscle antibody
  - Anti-liver kidney microsomal
- Metabolic markers
  - Uric acid
  - Serum copper and urine copper
- Hypercoagulable markers
  - Lupus anticoagulant, anticardiolipin
  - Factor V Leiden
- Toxicology screen and drug panel
  - Acetaminophen
  - Opiates
  - Barbiturates
  - Cocaine
  - Alcohol
- Pregnancy testing (women)
- Urine electrolytes and osmolarity
- Blood cultures
- Urine cultures
- Imaging and other testing
  - Chest radiograph
  - Abdominal ultrasound with Doppler study of the liver
  - ECG
  - Echocardiogram with estimation of pulmonary artery pressures

Indications for Liver Transplantation

The decision as to whether a patient will recover with conservative management or require transplantation has been the subject of many different reports and case series; however, the King's College Criteria remain the current standard for clinicians. These criteria are used to predict death in patients presenting with acute liver failure (ALF) in the setting of acetaminophen and other causes of ALF. Despite these criteria the decision as to when to "list" a patient with FHF is extremely difficult.

- King's College Criteria
  - Acetaminophen-induced ALF
    - Hepatic encephalopathy coma grades 3 to 4
    - Arterial pH less than 7.3
    - Prothrombin time (PT) more than 100 seconds
    - Serum creatinine more than 3.4 mg/dL
  - Non-acetaminophen-induced ALF
  - PT of more than 100 seconds or 3 of the following 5 criteria:
    - Age younger than 10 years or more than 40 years
    - ALF caused by non-A, non-B, or non-C hepatitis, halothane hepatitis, or idiosyncratic drug reactions
    - Jaundice present more than 1 week before onset of encephalopathy
    - PT more than 50 seconds
    - Serum bilirubin more than 17.5 mg/dL

Alcoholic Hepatitis

- See http://www.aasld.org/practiceguidelines/Documents/Bookmarked%20Practice%20 Guidelines/AlcoholicLiverDisease1–2010.pdf (accessed February 8, 2011).
- Alcoholic hepatitis is observed in approximately 20% of heavy drinkers and 50% of heavy drinkers who are admitted to an acute-care hospital.
- Alcoholic hepatitis is a serious disease, with a 28-day mortality of 35% in high-risk patients (Maddrey's discriminant function [mDF] ≥32).
- Alcoholic hepatitis is a clinical syndrome of jaundice and liver failure that generally occurs after decades of heavy alcohol use (mean intake, approximately 100 g per day). Not uncommonly, the patient will have ceased alcohol consumption several weeks before the onset of symptoms.
- The cardinal sign of alcoholic hepatitis is the rapid onset of jaundice. Other common signs and symptoms include
  - Fever
  - Ascites
  - Proximal muscle loss
  - Encephalopathy
  - Tender hepatomegaly
- Laboratory studies characteristically reveal:
  - Increased aspartate aminotransferase (AST) (but usually <300 IU)
  - AST-to-alanine aminotransferase (ALT) ratio more than 2
  - Increased white blood cell concentration with neutrophilia
  - Increased bilirubin (usually >5 mg/dL)
  - Increased INR
  - Increased creatinine
- A variety of scoring systems have been developed to assess the severity of alcoholic hepatitis and to guide treatment. The Glasgow alcoholic hepatitis score (Table 6-13) and the mDF help the clinician decide whether corticosteroids should be initiated. These scoring systems share common elements, such as the serum bilirubin level and prothrombin time (or INR).
- mDF is calculated as [4.6 × (patient's prothrombin time—control prothrombin time, in seconds)] + serum bilirubin level (mg/dL); see http://www.mdcalc.com/maddreys-discriminant-function-for-alcoholic-hepatitis (accessed February 8, 2011).

For more information, see the calculator at http://www.mdcalc.com/glasgow-alcoholic-hepatitis-score (accessed February 8, 2011).

Management

- Enteral feeding is recommended as the patients are frequently malnourished. A daily protein intake of 1.5 g per kilogram of body weight is recommended, even among patients with hepatic encephalopathy.
- Patients may develop alcohol withdrawal syndrome. While benzodiazepines are usually recommended, dexmedetomidine (in the ICU) or valproic acid (Depakote) may be

TABLE 6-13. GLASGOW ALCOHOL HEPATITIS SCORE

Score	1	2	3
Age	<50	>50	–
WCC	<15	≥25	–
BUN mg/dL	<14	≥14	–
INR	<1.5	1.5–2.0	>2.0
Bilirubin	<7.3	7.3–14.7	>14.7

BUN, blood urea nitrogen; WCC, white cell count.

particularly useful in this situation. NOTE: benzodiazepines may precipitate hepatic encephalopathy.

- Corticosteroid therapy abrogates the inflammatory process. However, the use of these agents has been controversial. An individual patient meta-analysis demonstrated that corticosteroids reduce mortality in patients with an mDF 32 or higher. Prednisolone at a dose of 40 mg/day for 28 days is usually recommended. A prompt decline in serum bilirubin indicates a favorable response to therapy. Patients who do not exhibit a reduction in serum bilirubin within 1 week are considered nonresponders and have a 6-month mortality rate of 50% or higher.

- One randomized, controlled trial showed that pentoxifylline (400 mg every 8 h), a phosphodiesterase inhibitor that modulates tumor necrosis factor (TNF)-α transcription, reduced short-term mortality among patients with alcoholic hepatitis. The survival benefit of pentoxifylline appears to be related to a significant reduction in the development of the hepatorenal syndrome.

- Direct TNF-α inhibitors have not been demonstrated to improve outcome.

Pancreatitis

- See http://www.acg.gi.org/physicians/guidelines/AcutePancreatitis.pdf (accessed February 8, 2011).

- Acute pancreatitis is a common disease that causes significant morbidity and mortality. More than 300,000 patients are admitted per year for pancreatitis and approximately 20,000 die from this disease per year in the United States.

- In developed countries, obstruction of the common bile duct by stones (38%) and alcohol abuse (36%) are the most frequent causes of acute pancreatitis. Gallstone-induced pancreatitis is caused by duct obstruction of gallstone migration. Obstruction is localized in the bile duct, the pancreatic duct, or both. Other well-established causes of acute pancreatitis include:
  - Hypertriglyceridemia
  - Post-ERCP
  - Drug induced
  - Autoimmune
  - Genetic
  - Abdominal trauma
  - Postoperative
  - Ischemia
  - Infections
  - Hypercalcemia and hyperparathyroidism
  - Posterior penetrating ulcer
  - Scorpion venom

- Abdominal pain is the cardinal symptom. It occurs in approximately 95% of cases. Typically it is generalized to the upper abdomen, but it may be more localized to the right upper quadrant, epigastric area, or, occasionally, left upper quadrant. The pain typically occurs acutely, without a prodrome, and rapidly reaches maximum intensity. It tends to be moderate to severe in intensity and tends to last for several days. The pain typically is boring and deep because of the retroperitoneal location of the pancreas.

- Approximately 90% of patients have nausea and vomiting, which can be severe and unremitting. The severity of the physical findings depends on the severity of the attack. Mild disease presents with only mild abdominal tenderness. Severe disease presents with severe abdominal tenderness and guarding, generally localized to the upper abdomen. Rebound tenderness is unusual.

Diagnosis

- Leukocytosis is common because of a systemic inflammatory response.

- Mild hyperglycemia is common because of decreased insulin secretion and increased glucagon levels.

- The serum lipase level is the primary diagnostic marker for acute pancreatitis because of its high sensitivity and specificity. Serum lipase is more than 90% sensitive for acute pancreatitis. The serum lipase level rises early in pancreatitis and remains elevated for several days.

- Serum amylase concentrations exceeding 3 times the normal upper limit support the diagnosis of acute pancreatitis. However, the serum amylase is within the normal range on admission in up to 20% of the patients.
- In a meta-analysis, a serum ALT level higher than 150 IU/L had a positive predictive value of 95% in diagnosing acute gallstone pancreatitis.
- Abdominal ultrasonography is the primary imaging study for abdominal pain associated with jaundice and for excluding gallstones as the cause of acute pancreatitis. It has the advantages of low cost, ready availability, and easy portability for bedside application in very sick patients When adequately visualized, an inflamed pancreas is recognized as hypoechoic and enlarged because of parenchymal edema. The pancreas is visualized inadequately in 30% of cases.
- Patients who present with severe pancreatitis or who present initially with mild to moderate pancreatitis that does not improve after several days of supportive therapy should undergo abdominal CT. CT scan with contrast is now standard for the diagnosis and workup of suspected severe pancreatitis. Patients should receive both IV and oral contrast. IV contrast is, however, contraindicated in the presence of renal insufficiency. Furthermore, patients must be "fully" volume resuscitated prior to receiving contrast.
  - Improvements in the contrast bolus techniques allow one to image the perfusion of the pancreatic parenchyma with accuracy. Areas of necrosis with diminished or no enhancement on contrast bolus are detected with an accuracy of 87% (see CT grading system below).
  - Except in cases of initial diagnostic uncertainty, it is advisable to wait 1 to 2 days to obtain the initial scan. Before this point, pancreatic necrosis may not be apparent, and in addition, the delay allows the patient to receive initial aggressive fluid resuscitation, thus reducing the risk of contrast-induced nephropathy.

Risk Stratification

- Most episodes of acute pancreatitis are mild and self-limiting, needing only brief hospitalization. However, 20% of patients develop severe disease with local and extrapancreatic complications characterized by early development and persistence of hypovolemia and multiple organ dysfunction.
- Risk stratification plays a key role in the management of patients with acute pancreatitis. Although amylase and lipase remain the standard for diagnosis, they are poor predictors of severity. A number of scoring systems have been developed to assess the severity of pancreatitis.
  - The Ranson Criteria was the first scoring system to be developed and remains commonly employed today.
  - More recently, the APACHE II Scoring System and the Imrie Score have been used to predict severity.
  - The Balthazar CT grading system is widely used in patients who have undergone CT scanning.
- Severe acute pancreatitis as defined by the Atlanta Symposium include a Ranson score of 3 or higher, APACHE-II score of 8 or higher, organ failure and/or local complications (necrosis, abscess or pseudocyst).

The calculator for Ranson's Criteria is available at http://www.mdcalc.com/ransons-criteria-for-pancreatitis-mortality (accessed February 8, 2011).

- At presentation
  - Age older than 55 years
  - Blood glucose level more than 200 mg/dL
  - White blood cell count more than 16,000/mm^3
  - Lactate dehydrogenase level more than 350 IU/L
  - Alanine aminotransferase level more than 250 U/L
- 48 hours after presentation
  - Hematocrit 10% decrease
  - Serum calcium less than 8 mg/dL
  - Base deficit more than 4 mEq/L
  - BUN increase more than 5 mg/dL
  - Fluid sequestration more than 6 L
  - Partial pressure of arterial oxygen (PaO$_2$) less than 60 mm Hg

Glasgow (Imrie) Severity Scoring System

- Age older than 55 years
- White cell count more than 15×10^9/L
- PaO_2 less than 60 mmHg
- Serum lactate dehydrogenase more than 600 units/L
- Serum aspartate aminotransferase more than 200 units/L
- Serum albumin less than 32 g/dL
- Serum calcium less than 2 mmol/L
- Serum glucose more than 10 mmol/L
- Serum urea more than 16 mmol/L

Balthazar CT Grading System

- A: Normal
- B: Gland enlargement, small intrapancreatic fluid collections
- C: Peripancreatic inflammation, more than 30% pancreatic necrosis
- D: Single extrahepatic fluid collection, 30% to 50% pancreatic necrosis
- E: Extensive extrapancreatic fluid collections, more than 50% pancreatic necrosis

Complications of Pancreatitis

- Renal dysfunction and failure
- Pulmonary complications
  - Acute respiratory distress syndrome
  - Pleural effusion
  - Atelectasis
  - Pneumonia
- Abdominal
  - Pancreatic necrosis is the most severe local complication because it is frequently associated with pancreatic infection.
  - Infection of pancreatic necrosis develops during the second or third week in 40% to 70% of patients.
  - Pancreatic abscess consists of a circumscribed collection of pus that arises around a restricted area of pancreatic necrosis.
  - Pseudocyst is a collection of pancreatic fluid enclosed by a wall of granulation tissue that results from pancreatic duct leakage.
  - Intraperitoneal hemorrhage
  - Splenic vein thrombosis (causing left-sided portal hypertension)
  - Obstructive jaundice
- Other
  - Disseminated intravascular coagulation/coagulopathy
  - UGIB
  - Hypocalcemia
  - Hyperglycemia
  - Hypertriglyceridemia

Management

- In mild forms of disease, besides the etiological treatment (mostly for gallstone-induced pancreatitis), therapy is supportive and includes fluid resuscitation, analgesia, oxygen administration, and antiemetics.
- Early fluid resuscitation to correct fluid losses in the third space and maintain an adequate intravascular volume is an important component of the management of patients with severe pancreatitis.
- Respiratory, cardiovascular, and renal function must be closely monitored.
- Morphine traditionally has been disfavored for acute pancreatitis because it increases the sphincter of Oddi pressure. Meperidine, 50 to 100 mg every 4 to 6 hours, has been the traditional opiate regimen of choice because it does not raise the sphincter pressure. Caution should be used with this agent as it active metabolite normeperidine accumulates with renal dysfunction and can cause seizures. Fentanyl is a useful alternative in this situation.

- NG tube aspiration traditionally was used to prevent pancreatic stimulation induced by gastric distention and acid secretion. Multiple clinical trials, however, have demonstrated no benefit from NG aspiration.
- Prophylactic antibiotics have previously been recommended to reduce the risk of pancreatic infection. However, recent meta-analyses have failed to demonstrate a benefit from prophylactic antibiotics. Recent guidelines issued by the American College of Gastroenterology do not recommend antibiotic prophylaxis to prevent pancreatic infection.
- Peritoneal lavage to remove toxic necrotic compounds is no longer recommended for severe pancreatitis. In a meta-analysis of eight random clinical trials involving a total of 333 patients, peritoneal lavage did not reduce morbidity or mortality.
- Adrenal insufficiency has been reported to occur in up to 35% of patients with severe pancreatitis. A cosyntropin stimulation test and treatment with hydrocortisones is recommended in those patients with adrenal insufficiency.
- To discriminate between sterile and infected pancreatic necrosis in patients who continue to deteriorate, ultrasound- or CT-guided fine-needle aspirations of pancreatic tissues should be performed. When infection is proven or in the presence of abscesses, targeted antibiotic therapy is warranted.
- Most patients with gallstone-induced pancreatitis present with mild disease and quickly recover after early resuscitation. ERCP is indicated for clearance of bile duct stones in patients with severe pancreatitis, in those with cholangitis, in those who are poor candidates for cholecystectomy, in those who are postcholecystectomy, and in those with strong evidence of persistent biliary obstruction.
- Probiotics should be avoided in patients with pancreatitis.
- Patients with acute pancreatitis have traditionally been treated with "bowel rest"; this included NG suction and NPO. Patients with mild pancreatitis were started on oral feeds once the pain subsided, whereas patients with severe pancreatitis were treated with parenteral nutrition until the disease process resolved. There is, however, *no scientific data to support this approach* to the management of patients with acute pancreatitis.
  - Both experimental and clinical data strongly support the concept that enteral nutrition started within 24 hours of admission to hospital reduces complications (primarily pancreatic infection), length of hospital stay and mortality in patients with acute pancreatitis.
  - Enteral nutrition should begin within 24 hours after admission and following the initial period of volume resuscitation and control of nausea and pain.
  - Patients with mild pancreatitis can take a low fatty diet by mouth while patients with severe pancreatitis should receive enteral tube feeds.
  - Clinical trials suggest that both gastric and jejunal tube feeding are well tolerated in patients with severe pancreatitis. However, postpyloric feeding is generally recommended.
  - Although there are limited data as to the optimal type of tube feed, a semi-elemental formula with omega-3 fatty acids and soluble fiber is recommended. Parenteral nutrition is associated with increased complications and mortality and *should be avoided* in patients with acute pancreatitis.

CHAPTER 7

Hematology

B. Mitchell Goodman, Jody P. Boggs, Sami G. Tahhan, and Armin Rashidi

ANEMIA

Gathering Data

History

- Seeks to define general etiology (ie, blood loss, decreased blood production, or destruction of red blood cells [RBCs]) (Table 7-1)
  - Common signs and symptoms
    - Fatigue, shortness of breath, palpitations, and tachycardia are common to most anemias.
    - Fever may help point to specific diagnosis (eg, thrombotic thrombocytopenic purpura [TTP], bone marrow infection, hemolytic anemias). Also, could suggest accompanying leukopenia and systemic infection
    - Dizziness, orthostasis: particularly if etiology is acute and/or accompanied by significant volume loss.
    - Abdominal pain may be present when splenomegaly is involved or in cases of hypercoagulability and associated vascular thrombosis (eg, paroxysmal nocturnal hemoglobinuria).
    - Bruising and bleeding suggests coincident platelet defect or deficiency or other coagulopathy. Site important, for example, hemarthrosis suggesting coagulopathy versus petechia or gingival bleeding suggesting platelet problem.
    - Melena or bright red blood per rectum: suggestive of lower or upper gastrointestinal blood loss.
    - Menorrhagia: may be hormonal or related to fibroid uterus.
  - Other important history
    - Family history of anemia: Various hemoglobinopathies, including thalassemias and sickle cell.
    - Nutritional: including alcohol use, as folate and cyanocobalamin deficiencies may be suggested.
    - Surgeries: including recent for acute blood loss, and remote, particularly those involving stomach and intestines, where important substrates for hematopoiesis are absorbed.
    - Exposures, for example, to children with parvovirus or to heavy metals.
    - Bone and joint pain may suggest increased erythropoiesis or etiologies such as sickle cell disease and myeloma.

Physical Examination

- Tachycardia and/or hypotension: particularly orthostatic, suggesting large volume or acute blood loss.
- Pale conjunctivae.
- Scleral icterus may suggest hemolysis and resultant indirect hyperbilirubinemia.
- Gingival petechia may be most notable under the tongue, where jaundice is also often evident.
- Lymphadenopathy may suggest infection or malignancy.
- Murmurs: usually systolic "flow" variety.
- Hepatosplenomegaly: More common in etiologies such as alcohol abuse and cirrhosis, and red cell or platelet disorders where spleen removes from circulating blood.
- Rectal examination for gross or occult blood: Ideally a voided stool sample is tested for blood so as not to confound results with trauma of digital rectal examination,

TABLE 7-1. CLASSIFICATION OF ANEMIAS BY PATHOPHYSIOLOGY

Decreased Production

Hemoglobin synthesis lesion: iron deficiency, thalassemia, anemia of chronic disease
DNA synthesis lesion: megaloblastic anemia
Stem cell lesion: aplastic anemia, myeloproliferative leukemia
Bone marrow infiltration: carcinoma, lymphoma
Pure red cell aplasia

Increased Destruction

Blood loss
Hemolysis (intrinsic)
Membrane lesion: hereditary spherocytosis, elliptocytosis
Hemoglobin lesion: sickle cell, unstable hemoglobin
Glycolysis: pyruvate kinase deficiency, etc.
Oxidation lesion: glucose-6-phosphate dehydrogenase deficiency
Hemolysis (extrinsic)
Immune: warm antibody, cold antibody
Microangiopathic: thrombotic thrombocytopenic purpura, hemolytic-uremic syndrome, mechanical cardiac valve, paravalvular leak
Infection: clostridial
Hypersplenism

From McPhee SJ, Papadakis MA, Rabow MW, eds. *Current Medical Diagnosis & Treatment 2012.* 51st ed. New York: McGraw-Hill; 2012:476.

- Bruising, petechiae, purpura.
- Confusion may be related to cerebral hypoperfusion or suggest an etiology such as TTP.

Diagnostic Tests

- Complete blood count (CBC) with differential: hemoglobin (Hb) less than 13.5 g/dL in men or 12 g/dL in women (hematocrit [Hct] <41% or 37% men and women, respectively) defines anemia. CBC may also identify comorbid leukopenia and thrombocytopenia. Mean corpuscular volume (MCV) and RBC distribution width can suggest iron deficiency, thalassemia, and so forth.
- Differential: Particularly helpful with certain oncologic disorders and leukemias.
- Peripheral smear can identify micro- and macrocytosis and hypochromia. Also important to detect deformities of red cells, such as sickled cells or spherocytes. Evidence of red cell destruction, including schistocytes also can be found. Rouleaux formation, although not very sensitive or specific, may suggest myeloma. Basophilic stippling may indicate lead toxicity (Figure 7-1).
- Electrophoresis: If hemoglobinopathy suspected.
- Chemistry panel identifies associated renal dysfunction, which may be a result of poor perfusion or may suggest etiologies such as TTP. Blood urea nitrogen elevation out of proportion to creatinine elevation suggests hypovolemia or upper gastrointestinal (GI) bleed and digestion of blood products.
- Liver function tests and enzymes: elevated indirect bilirubin, lactate dehydrogenase (LDH) and aspartate transaminase (AST) suggest hemolysis.
- Iron studies: Ferritin, serum iron, total iron binding capacity. Calculated iron saturation.
- Reticulocyte count is a marker of hematopoiesis. When elevated, it suggests hemolysis and resultant increased production of red cells. Must be corrected for degree of anemia (reticulocyte index). First calculate corrected reticulocyte percentage: Reticulocyte% × (Hct/Normal Hct). Then calculate reticulocyte index: Corrected Reticulocyte%/ Maturation Factor. Maturation factor is 1.5, 2.5, or 3 in mild, moderate, or severe anemia respectively (see http://www.accessmedicine.com/content.aspx?aID=6129411&searchStr= reticulocyte+count#6129411).
- Bone marrow biopsy

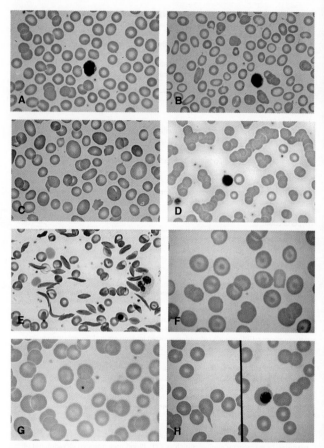

Figure 7-1   Peripheral blood smears. **A.** Normal peripheral blood smear. Small lymphocyte in center of field. Note that the diameter of the red blood cell is similar to the diameter of the small lymphocyte nucleus. **B.** Hypochromic microcytic anemia of iron deficiency. Small lymphocyte in field helps assess the red blood cell size. **C.** Macrocytosis. These cells are both larger than normal (mean corpuscular volume >100 femtoliters) and somewhat oval in shape. Some morphologists call these cells *macroovalocytes.* **D.** Rouleaux formation. Small lymphocyte in center of field. These red cells align themselves in stacks and are related to increased serum protein levels. **E.** Sickle cells. Homozygous sickle cell disease. A nucleated red cell and neutrophil are also in the field. **F.** Target cells. Target cells are recognized by the bull's-eye appearance of the cell. Small numbers of target cells are seen with liver disease and thalassemia. Larger numbers are typical of hemoglobin C disease. **G.** Howell-Jolly bodies. Howell-Jolly bodies are tiny nuclear remnants that normally are removed by the spleen. They appear in the blood after splenectomy (defect in removal) and with maturation and dysplastic disorders (excess production). **H.** Teardrop cells and nucleated red blood cells characteristic of myelofibrosis. A teardrop-shaped red blood cell (*left panel*) and a nucleated red blood cell (*right panel*) as typically seen with myelofibrosis and extramedullary hematopoiesis.

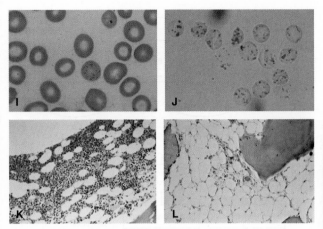

Figure 7-1 *(Continued)* **I.** Stippled red cell in lead poisoning. Mild hypochromia. Coarsely stippled red cell. **J.** Heinz bodies. Blood mixed with hypotonic solution of crystal violet. The stained material is precipitates of denatured hemoglobin within cells. **K.** Normal bone marrow. Low-power view of normal adult marrow (H and E stain), showing a mix of fat cells (clear areas) and hematopoietic cells. The percentage of the space that consists of hematopoietic cells is referred to as *marrow cellularity.* In adults, normal marrow cellularity is 35% to 40%. If demands for increased marrow production occur, cellularity may increase to meet the demand. As people age, the marrow cellularity decreases and the marrow fat increases. Patients older than 70 years of age may have a 20% to 30% marrow cellularity. **L.** Aplastic anemia bone marrow. Normal hematopoietic precursor cells are virtually absent, leaving behind fat cells, reticuloendothelial cells, and the underlying sinusoidal structure. (From Longo DL, et al., eds. *Harrison's Principles of Internal Medicine.* 18th ed. New York: McGraw-Hill; 2011.) See color insert.

SPECIFIC CONDITIONS

Anemias can be generally classified as microcytic, normocytic, or macrocytic. Hemolytic anemias are considered separately (Table 7-2 and Figure 7-2).

TABLE 7-2. CLASSIFICATION OF ANEMIAS BY MEAN CELL VOLUME

Microcytic
Iron deficiency
Thalassemia
Anemia of chronic disease

Macrocytic
Megaloblastic
Vitamin B_{12} deficiency
Folate deficiency

Nonmegaloblastic
Myelodysplasia, chemotherapy
Liver disease
Increased reticulocytosis
Myxedema

Normocytic
Many causes

From McPhee SJ, Papadakis MA, Rabow MW, eds. *Current Medical Diagnosis & Treatment 2012.* 51st ed. New York: McGraw-Hill; 2012:476.

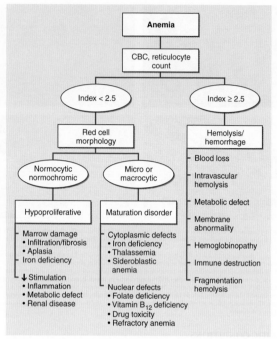

Figure 7-2 The physiologic classification of anemia. CBC, complete blood count. (From Longo DL, et al., eds. *Harrison's Principles of Internal Medicine.* 18th ed. New York: McGraw-Hill; 2011.)

Microcytic Anemias

Iron Deficiency Anemia [1]

- Epidemiology and etiology
  - Most common anemia: 30% of world population.
  - Women are more prone because of menstrual iron losses.
  - Causes range from dietary to malabsorptive to blood loss (Table 7-3).
    - Acute or chronic hemorrhage, particularly GI bleed or menses
    - Malabsorption caused by gastrectomy or gastric bypass
    - Poor dietary intake
    - Celiac disease
    - Inflammatory bowel disease
    - Elevated gastric pH
    - Pregnancy

TABLE 7-3. CAUSES OF IRON DEFICIENCY

Increased Demand for Iron
Rapid growth in infancy or adolescence
Pregnancy
Erythropoietin therapy

Increased Iron Loss
Chronic blood loss
Menses
Acute blood loss
Blood donation
Phlebotomy as treatment for polycythemia vera

Decreased Iron Intake or Absorption
Inadequate diet
Malabsorption from disease (sprue, Crohn disease)
Malabsorption from surgery (postgastrectomy)
Acute or chronic inflammation

From Longo DL, et al., eds. *Harrison's Principles of Internal Medicine*. 18th ed. New York: McGraw-Hill; 2012:846.

- Pathophysiology
  - Total body iron approximately 45 mg.
  - Two-thirds involved with cellular Hb.
  - One-third in storage form (ferritin).
  - Approximately half recycled from older red cells and returned by transferrin to bone marrow for new hematopoiesis.
  - Dietary requirement is approximately 1 to 2 mg to replace that excreted. Normal Western diet supplies approximately 15 mg, with 3 mg absorbed in the duodenum, but only 1 mg ultimately entering circulation.
  - Iron deficiency and decreased marrow iron precede overt anemia and microcytosis.
- Presentation
  - Slow, chronic blood loss and other causes of gradual iron loss generally present as fatigue, dyspnea, and pallor.
  - Rapid blood loss may present with dizziness and orthostasis.
  - Hair loss rarely.
  - Pica, particularly ice or clay.
  - Plummer-Vinson syndrome: dysphagia, esophageal web, atrophic glossitis; rare in developed countries.
  - Koilonychia: spoon nails; also rare.
- Diagnosis
  - CBC showing anemia and low MCV
  - Peripheral smear with microcytosis and hypochromia
  - Serum ferritin
    - Usually the first test.
    - Level less than 15 to 30 mcg/L is diagnostic of iron deficiency.
    - Can be falsely normal or even elevated despite iron deficiency in inflammatory conditions, malignancy, or liver disease.
  - Transferrin saturation
    - Serum iron; total iron-binding capacity (TIBC)
    - Less than 15% consistent with iron deficiency.
    - Significant diurnal variation and susceptibility to alteration from other conditions limits utility.

- Bone marrow aspiration
  - Stain for iron.
  - Previously considered gold standard.
  - Invasiveness and operator dependence limit utility.
- Soluble transferrin receptor
  - Increasingly available.
  - Particularly useful to diagnose iron deficiency in setting of chronic disease or inflammation.
  - Level is proportional to degree of iron deficiency (high levels suggest iron deficiency).
- Other tests
  - Inappropriately low reticulocyte count
  - Thrombocytosis
- Management
  - Identify underlying cause.
  - Rule out GI malignancy, particularly in men and nonmenstruating women and patients older than 50 years of age.
  - Oral iron supplementation:
    - Preparations include ferrous sulfate, ferrous gluconate, ferrous fumarate.
    - Generally ferrous sulfate preferred as it contains twice the elemental iron per tablet of the others.
    - Reticulocytosis may be induced within a week.
    - For Hb more than 11 g/dL, generally 4 weeks of ferrous sulfate 324 mg (containing 65 mg elemental iron per tablet, anticipating 10% absorption) thrice daily is sufficient to normalize Hb. More severe anemia requires longer courses or higher doses.
    - Several months of therapy may be required to replenish bone marrow stores
    - Antacids, carbonated beverages with phosphorous, multivitamins with calcium, magnesium, or phosphorous can impair absorption.
    - Dosing between meals and with vitamin C can improve absorption.
    - Tests to measure iron absorption are available. If malabsorption suspected, evaluate for *Helicobacter pylori*, celiac disease, autoimmune gastritis.
    - Side effects may limit dosing and include nausea, vomiting, and diarrhea.
  - Parenteral replacement
    - Used in failure or intolerability of oral iron
    - Three preparations
      - Iron dextran requires test dose because of significant risk of anaphylaxis.
      - Sodium ferric gluconate—no test dose.
      - Iron sucrose—no test dose required.
- Follow-up
  - Dependent on etiology.
  - Reassessment of iron stores at approximately 4 weeks is reasonable in patients receiving conventional thrice daily oral therapy. Later reassessment indicated if dose is decreased and administration prolonged.

Anemia of Acute or Chronic Inflammation [2]

- Common etiologies include infection, cancer, and rheumatoid arthritis.
- May be microcytic or normocytic.
- May coexist with iron deficiency and important to distinguish (Table 7-4). Ferritin levels can increase 2 to 3 times baseline.
- Involves impaired iron recycling at the macrophage or transferrin level. This is believed to withhold iron from pathogenic organisms, impairing their vitality.
- Also, inflammatory cytokines may decrease erythropoietin (EPO) production or marrow response to EPO.
- Serum iron levels and TIBC may be low.
- Ferritin may be normal or high.
- Serum transferrin receptor levels are normal.

TABLE 7-4. DIAGNOSIS OF HYPOPROLIFERATIVE ANEMIAS

Tests	Iron Deficiency	Inflammation	Renal Disease	Hypometabolic States
Anemia	Mild to severe	Mild	Mild to severe	Mild
MCV (fL)	60–90	80–90	90	90
Morphology	Normo-microcytic	Normocytic	Normocytic	Normocytic
SI	<30	<50	Normal	Normal
TIBC	>360	<300	Normal	Normal
Saturation (%)	<10	10–20	Normal	Normal
Serum ferritin (μg/L)	<15	30–200	115–150	Normal
Iron stores	0	2–4+	1–4+	Normal

MCV, mean corpuscular volume; SI, serum iron; TIBC, total iron-binding capacity.
From Longo DL, et al., eds. *Harrison's Principles of Internal Medicine.* 18th ed. New York: McGraw-Hill; 2012:850.

- Anemia, and therefore symptoms, are typically mild.
- Treatment is aimed at the causative pathology.

Anemia of Chronic Disease

- Essentially a subset of anemia of chronic inflammation.
- Usually normocytic.
- Chronic kidney disease is most common example, with decreased EPO production.
- Particularly in chronic kidney disease, EPO supplementation can be used, after confirmation of adequate iron stores.

Sideroblastic Anemia [3]

- Etiology (Table 7-5):
  - Most often acquired: Isoniazid, ethanol, zinc excess, copper deficiency
  - May be hereditary: Usually X-linked
  - May be a subtype of myelodysplasia
- Involves impaired incorporation of iron into heme.
- This ineffective erythropoiesis leads to anemia, increased iron absorption. Can be microcytic, normocytic, or macrocytic.
- Symptoms are dependent on the degree of anemia.
- Diagnosis:
  - Anemia is moderate with Hct in the 20% to 30% range.
  - Smear may show dimorphic red cell population, with hypochromic and normochromic cells.
  - Serum ferritin, iron and transferrin saturation are high.
  - TIBC is normal.
  - Bone marrow may show mitochondria with abnormal "ring" of iron at periphery (ie, a ringed sideroblast).
- Management:
  - Usually supportive; transfusion may be required if symptomatic.
  - Phlebotomy or iron chelation may have a role depending on degree of anemia and iron overload.
  - Pyridoxine may be of use at 50 to 200 mg per day orally.

TABLE 7-5. CLASSIFICATION OF SIDEROBLASTIC ANEMIAS

I. Acquired
    A. Primary sideroblastic anemia (myelodysplastic syndromes)
        1. Subunit 1 of the mitochondrial cytochrome oxidase
    B. Sideroblastic anemia secondary to
        1. Isoniazid
        2. Pyrazinamide
        3. Cycloserine
        4. Chloramphenicol
        5. Ethanol
        6. Lead
        7. Chronic neoplastic and inflammatory disease
        8. Zinc
II. Hereditary
    A. X chromosome linked
        1. *ALAS2* deficiency
        2. Hereditary sideroblastic anemia with ataxia: mitochondrial ATP binding cassette
           (*ABCB7*) mutations
    B. Autosomal
        1. Mitochondrial myopathy and sideroblastic anemia (*PSU1* mutations)
    C. Mitochondrial
        1. Pearson marrow-pancreas syndrome

From Lichtman MA, Kipps TJ, Uri Seligsohn U, et al. *Williams Hematology*. 8th ed. New York: McGraw-Hill; 2010.

Thalassemias (see Hemolytic Anemias)

Normocytic Anemias

• Anemia of chronic inflammation and chronic disease (see above)
• Sideroblastic anemia (see above)
• Pure red cell aplasia [4]
  • Epidemiology, etiology, and pathophysiology
    • Rare, autoimmune disorder in adults.
    • T-lymphocytes or immunoglobulin G (IgG) antibodies to erythroid
      precursors.
    • More rarely, anti-EPO antibodies may develop in patients receiving chronic
      EPO.
    • Disease associations include systemic lupus erythematosus, chronic lymphocytic
      leukemia, thymoma, lymphoma.
    • Medication causes include phenytoin and chloramphenicol.
    • Infections: parvovirus B-19.
  • Presentation: Anemia, and therefore symptoms, may be profound.
  • Diagnosis:
    • CBC and peripheral smear should demonstrate normocytic anemia with other cell
      lines intact.
    • Normal red cell morphology.
    • Bone marrow is normocellular except erythroid precursors are absent or severely
      diminished (contrast to myelodysplastic syndrome [MDS] below).
    • Consider imaging of chest for thymoma.
  • Management
    • Supportive transfusions
    • Parvovirus infection treated with intravenous immunoglobulin (IVIG)

- Other cases treated with immunosuppression, including combo therapy with cyclosporine and antithymocyte globulin

Macrocytic Anemias [5]

Megaloblastic

- Defective DNA synthesis results in large erythrogenic precursors.
- Most often caused by deficiency of folate, vitamin B_{12}, or both.
- CBC demonstrates elevated MCV, typically more than 100 to 110 femtoliters.
- LDH and indirect bilirubin may be modestly elevated because of intramedullary destruction of abnormal erythroid cells.
- Smear shows macroovalocytes and hypersegmented neutrophils.
- Bone marrow aspirate (rarely necessary) shows erythroid hyperplasia with retarded nuclear development while cytoplasm develops normally. Reversal of usual 2:1 myeloid-to-erythroid ratio. Also giant metamyelocytes.
- Causes are essentially vitamin B_{12} and folic acid deficiency
  - Vitamin B_{12} (cobalamin) deficiency
    - Etiology and pathophysiology (Table 7-6)
      - Vitamin B_{12} from diet (typically animal sources) absorbed in ileum with aid of intrinsic factor produced by parietal cells of gastric mucosa.
      - Deficiency caused by malnutrition (typically vegans or alcoholics) or abnormalities or disruption of absorption.
      - Antibodies to intrinsic factor or parietal cells (pernicious anemia) associated with autoimmune atrophic gastritis.
      - Zollinger-Ellison syndrome and *H. pylori* may damage parietal cells as well.
      - Gastrectomy.
      - Small bowel surgery.
      - Inflammatory bowel disease.
      - Fish tapeworm (*Diphyllobothrium latum*).
      - Human immunodeficiency virus (HIV) and drugs: Including metformin, colchicine, and antiepileptics; unlikely to be symptomatic deficiency.

TABLE 7-6. CAUSES OF VITAMIN B_{12} DEFICIENCY

Dietary deficiency (rare)

Decreased production of intrinsic factor
  Pernicious anemia
  Gastrectomy

Helicobacter pylori infection

Competition for vitamin B_{12} in gut
  Blind loop syndrome
  Fish tapeworm (rare)

Pancreatic insufficiency

Decreased ileal absorption of vitamin B_{12}
  Surgical resection
  Crohn disease

Transcobalamin II deficiency (rare)

From McPhee SJ, Papadakis MA, Rabow MW, eds. *Current Medical Diagnosis & Treatment 2012.* 51st ed. New York: McGraw-Hill; 2012:481.

- Deficiency takes years to manifest after absorption impaired because of large stores in liver.
- Presentation
  - Largely related to peripheral neuropathy, followed by posterior and pyramidal spinal cord damage and cerebral cortical disease
    - Paresthesias, peripheral neuropathy, loss of vibratory sense, decreased proprioception
    - Ataxia
    - Memory loss, dementia
  - Oral stomatitis
  - Glossitis
- Diagnosis
  - CBC showing anemia and/or macrocytosis.
  - May have thrombocytopenia and, less often, leukopenia.
  - Peripheral smear and bone marrow (seldom necessary) as above.
  - Serum vitamin B_{12} level:
    - Abnormally high in liver disease.
    - Severe deficiency with levels less than 74 pmol/L (100 ng/L).
    - 74 to 148 pmol/L or 100 to 200 ng/L represents borderline deficiency.
    - Follow up borderline levels with methylmalonic acid.
  - Methylmalonic acid (MMA):
    - Elevated in vitamin B_{12} deficiency
    - May also elevate in renal disease
  - Homocysteine:
    - May be elevated with vitamin B_{12} or folate deficiency.
    - Also elevated in a number of other disease states. Therefore, do not order.
  - Intrinsic factor and parietal cell antibodies to diagnose pernicious anemia.
  - Serum gastrin level high in pernicious anemia.
  - Schilling test: Measures absorption of oral vitamin B_{12}; no longer widely used.
  - Bone marrow biopsy may be indicated if vitamin B_{12}, RBC folate, and MMA levels normal.
- Management
  - Intramuscular vitamin B_{12} 100 mcg daily for 1 wk, weekly for 1 month, then monthly for life unless reversible cause identified.
  - Oral therapy likely adequate, even in pernicious anemia where only 1% absorbed; dose is 100 mcg/day for life.
- Folate deficiency
  - Etiology and pathophysiology (Table 7-7)
    - Absorbed from dietary intake throughout most of GI tract: mostly green leafy vegetables and citrus fruits.
    - Deficiency takes only a few months to manifest.
    - Major cause is inadequate dietary intake (eg, alcoholics, overcooking vegetables).
    - Other causes of malabsorption include sprue, Crohn disease, and medications such as phenytoin, metformin, cholestyramine, and trimethoprim-sulfamethoxazole.
    - Methotrexate causes deficiency through interfering with conversion to active form through dihydrofolate reductase.
    - Increased folic acid requirements in pregnancy and hemolytic anemia may outstrip normal dietary supply.
  - Presentation
    - Mucosal disease similar to that in vitamin B_{12} deficiency
    - No neurologic sequelae
  - Diagnosis
    - Again, CBC with anemia and macrocytosis.

TABLE 7-7. CAUSES OF FOLATE DEFICIENCY

Dietary deficiency

Decreased absorption
  Tropical sprue
  Drugs: phenytoin, sulfasalazine, trimethoprim-sulfamethoxazole

Increased requirement
  Chronic hemolytic anemia
  Pregnancy
  Exfoliative skin disease

Loss: dialysis
Inhibition of reduction to active form   Methotrexate

From McPhee SJ, Papadakis MA, Rabow MW, eds. *Current Medical Diagnosis & Treatment 2012*. 51st ed. New York: McGraw-Hill; 2012:482.

- • RBC folate, not serum folate preferred.
  - • Serum folate varies significantly with dietary intake and therefore not useful for assessment of deficiency.
  - • RBC folate less than 150 ng/mL diagnostic of deficiency.
  - • As above, if megaloblastic anemia and normal RBC folate, vitamin B_{12}, and MMA, bone marrow examination may be indicated.
- • Management
  - • Oral replacement of 5 mg/day for 4 months is generally sufficient.
  - • All patients should be evaluated for vitamin B_{12} deficiency, as folic acid replacement can reverse the RBC morphologic changes of vitamin B_{12} deficiency, thereby masking it and placing patients at risk for severe neurologic sequelae.
  - • Certain populations may benefit from folic acid prophylaxis:
    - • Pregnant women to decrease risk of neural tube defects in fetus
    - • Sickle cell disease
    - • Other hemolytic anemias

Nonmegaloblastic

- • Typically less dramatic elevation of MCV
  - • Alcohol abuse: even without cirrhosis or vitamin deficiency.
  - • Medications: reverse transcriptase inhibitors (zidovudine).
  - • Myelodysplasia more common in older patients (see above).
  - • Liver disease.
  - • Hypothyroidism.
  - • Chronic hemolysis or hemorrhage with associated reticulocytosis.
  - • Chronic obstructive pulmonary disease.
  - • Splenectomy.

Pancytopenia

Includes disorders of hypocellular and normocellular bone marrow, infiltrative bone marrow diseases, and systemic diseases such as alcoholism, hypersplenism, and sepsis

Aplastic Anemia [6]

- • Epidemiology, etiology, and pathophysiology
  - • A bone marrow failure syndrome.
  - • Incidence 2 to 7 per million per year; same in men and women; biphasic peaks (second and third decades of life, then again in older adults).

- May be hereditary, including Fanconi anemia.
- Other causes include radiation or chemotherapy, drugs (chloramphenicol, phenytoin, carbamazepine), viruses (Epstein-Barr virus, cytomegalovirus, hepatitis), defects in telomere length (including congenital dyskeratosis) and autoimmune (systemic lupus erythematosus).
- Two-thirds are idiopathic.
- Presentation
  - Fatigue related to anemia
  - Bleeding related to thrombocytopenia
  - Infection related to leukopenia
- Diagnosis
  - One of exclusion
  - Pancytopenia on CBC: early on, 1 or 2 cell lines may be involved, ultimately progressing to all 3.
  - Severe aplastic anemia defined as white blood cell (WBC) count less than 500; platelet count less than 20,000; $10^3/\mu L$ and per microliter respectively less than 1%; bone marrow cellularity less than 20% (3 out of 4 of these features).
  - Morphologically normal cells on smear.
  - Bone marrow shows replacement of normal hematopoietic cells with fat. Any cells present are normal in appearance.
  - Absence of hepatosplenomegaly, lymphadenopathy, or bone pain.
- Management
  - Initially supportive, with red cell and platelet transfusions and prophylactic antimicrobials.
  - Severe aplastic anemia, treated only supportively, has median survival of 3 months and 1-year survival of 20%.
  - Treatment of choice for patients younger than 40 to 50 years of age with severe aplastic anemia is sibling-donor bone marrow or stem cell transplant. Response rate up to 80%.
  - Unrelated donor transplants are typically reserved for younger patients not responding to other therapy. Response rate near 50%.
  - Older patients or those with severe disease or those without sibling-donors should receive antithymocyte globulin plus cyclosporine. Long-term response rate near 75%, although recovery of cell counts is incomplete.
  - May also use granulocyte colony-stimulating factor, although may increase risk of later MDS.
  - Other treatment options include cyclosporine and oxymetholone.
  - Paroxysmal nocturnal hemoglobinuria, acute myeloblastic leukemia (AML), MDS develops in 25% of untransplanted long-term survivors.
- Prognosis: Dependent on age at diagnosis and severity of cytopenias.

Myelodysplastic Syndromes

(see http://asheducationbook.hematologylibrary.org/content/2002/1/136.full.pdf+html and http://pdn.sciencedirect.com/science?_ob=MiamiImageURL&_cid=71074&_user= 960061&_pi=S0140673600020997&_check=y&_origin=article&_zone=toolbar&_coverDate =08-Apr-2000&view=c&originContentFamily=serial&wchp=dGLbVlV-zSkzV&md5= 83166e090ea588ad5fd8970bac00669b/1-s2.0-S0140673600020997-main.pdf and http:// annonc.oxfordjournals.org/content/21/suppl_5/v158.full [all accessed February 1, 2012].) [7]

- Epidemiology, etiology, pathophysiology
  - Mean age at onset older than 70 years of age.
  - Incidence is 40 to 50 per million in general population and 400 to 600 per million in adults older than 60 years of age.
  - Acquired clonal bone marrow disorder.
  - Ineffective hematopoiesis resulting in destruction of cells in the bone marrow and resultant peripheral cytopenias.

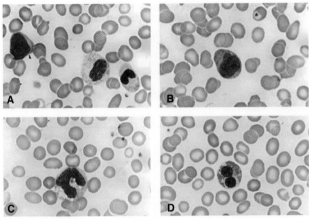

Figure 7-3   Myelodysplastic syndrome (oligoplastic myelogenous leukemia). **A**. Blood film. Blast, monocyte, and pseudo-Pelger-Huët cell. **B**. Blood film. Monocyte. **C**. Blood film. Monocyte. **D**. Blood film. Dysmorphic eosinophil with very small granules. (From Lichtman MA, et al. *Lichtman's Atlas of Hematology*. New York: McGraw-Hill; © 2007 by The McGraw-Hill Companies, Inc. All rights reserved.) See color insert.

- Causes include radiation and benzene exposure, alkylating chemotherapeutic agents, and DNA topoisomerase inhibitors.
- Disease may also arise de novo.
- Presentation
  - Many diagnosed by chance in an asymptomatic phase (2%).
  - Anemia more common in early course.
  - Fatigue, bleeding, infections caused by cytopenias.
- Diagnosis (Tables 7-8 and 7-9)
  - CBC with cytopenias (often pancytopenia).
  - Normo- or macrocytosis.
  - Peripheral smear with macro-ovalocytes and abnormal neutrophils showing Pelger-Huet abnormality (Figure 7-3). May see left shift and blasts as well.
  - Atypical cells on bone marrow examination:
    - Usually hypercellular
    - Erythroid hyperplasia
    - Megaloblastic features
  - Subtype determined by bone marrow examination, blast cell counts, ringed sideroblasts, and other features. World Health Organization classification has replaced older French-American-British classification (Table 7-10; see 7-8).
- Treatment
  - Largely dependent on prognostic score and requires experienced hematology input.
  - Supportive transfusions, EPO, colony-stimulating factors have some role.
  - Lenalidomide treatment of choice in patients with chromosome 5q-deletion syndrome.
  - Azacitidine treatment of choice for those with high-risk MDS.
  - Only stem cell transplant is curative, but available to a minority of patients.

TABLE 7-8. WORLD HEALTH ORGANIZATION (WHO) CLASSIFICATION OF MYELODYSPLASTIC SYNDROMES AND NEOPLASMS

Name	WHO Estimated Proportion of Patients with MDS (%)	Peripheral Blood: Key Features	Bone Marrow: Key Features
Refractory cytopenias with unilineage dysplasia (RCUD):			
Refractory anemia (RA)	10–20	Anemia <1% of blasts	Unilineage erythroid dysplasia (in ≥10% of cells) <5% blasts
Refractory neutropenia (RN)	<1	Neutropenia <1% blasts	Unilineage granulocytic dysplasia <5% blasts
Refractory thrombocytopenia (RT)	<1	Thrombocytopenia <1% blasts	Unilineage megakaryocytic dysplasia <5% blasts
Refractory anemia with ring sideroblasts (RARS)	3–11	Anemia	Unilineage erythroid dysplasia ≥15% of erythroid precursors are ring sideroblasts <5% blasts
		No blasts	
Refractory cytopenias with multilineage dysplasia (RCMD)	30	Cytopenia(s) <1% blasts	Multilineage dysplasia ± ring sideroblasts <5% blasts
		No Auer rods	No Auer rods
Refractory anemia with excess blasts, type 1 (RAEB-1)	40	Cytopenia(s) <5% blasts	Unilineage or multilineage dysplasia
		No Auer rods	
Refractory anemia with excess blasts, type 2 (RAEB-2)		Cytopenia(s) 5%–19% blasts	Unilineage or multilineage dysplasia 10%–19% blasts
		± Auer rods	± Auer rods
MDS associated with isolated Del(5q) (Del(5q))	Uncommon	Anemia	Isolated 5q31 chromosome deletion
		Normal or high platelet count	Anemia; hypolobated megakaryocytes
		<1% blasts	<5% blasts

TABLE 7-8. WORLD HEALTH ORGANIZATION (WHO)
CLASSIFICATION OF MYELODYSPLASTIC
SYNDROMES AND NEOPLASMS *(Continued)*

Name	WHO Estimated Proportion of Patients with MDS (%)	Peripheral Blood: Key Features	Bone Marrow: Key Features
Childhood MDS, including refractory cytopenia of childhood (*provisional*) (RCC)	<1	Pancytopenia	<5% marrow blasts for RCC
			Marrow usually hypocellular
MDS, unclassifiable (MDS-U)	?	Cytopenia	Does not fit other categories
		≤1% blasts	Dysplasia
			<5% blasts
			If no dysplasia, MDS-associated karyotype

Note: If peripheral blood blasts are 2%–4%, the diagnosis is RAEB-1 even if marrow blasts are less than 5%. If Auer rods are present, WHO considers the diagnosis RAEB-2 if the blast proportion is less than 20% (even if less than 10%), acute myeloblastic leukemia (AML) if at least 20% blasts. For all subtypes, peripheral blood monocytes are less than 1×10^9/L. Bicytopenia may be observed in RCUD subtypes, but pancytopenia with unilineage marrow dysplasia should be classified as MDS-U. Therapy-related MDS (t-MDS), whether caused by alkylating agents, topoisomerase II (t-MDS/t-AML) in the WHO classification of AML and precursor lesions. The listing in this table excludes MDS/myeloproliferative neoplasm overlap categories, such as chronic myelomonocytic leukemia, juvenile myelomonocytic leukemia, and the provisional entity RARS with thrombocytosis.
MDS, myelodysplastic syndrome.
From Longo DL, et al., eds. *Harrison's Principles of Internal Medicine*. 18th ed. New York: McGraw-Hill; 2012:895.

TABLE 7-9. INTERNATIONAL PROGNOSTIC SCORING SYSTEM (IPSS)

Prognostic Variable	Score Value				
	0	0.5	1	1.5	2
Bone marrow blasts (%)	<5%	5%–10%		11%–20%	21%–30%
Karyotype[a]	Good	Intermediate	Poor		
Cytopenia[b] (lineages affected)	0 or 1	2 or 3			

Risk Group Scores	Score
Low	0
Intermediate-1	0.5–1
Intermediate-2	1.5–2
High	≥2.5

[a]Good, normal, -Y, del(5q), del (20q); poor, complex (≥3 abnormalities) or chromosome 7 abnormalities; intermediate, all other abnormalities.
[b]Cytopenias defined as hemoglobin <100 g/L, platelet count <100,000/µL, absolute neutrophil count <1500/µL.
From Longo DL, et al., eds. *Harrison's Principles of Internal Medicine*. 18th ed. New York: McGraw-Hill; 2012:896.

TABLE 7-10. CLASSIFICATIONS OF MDS

FAB	WHO-2001	WHO-2008	WHO-2008 Diagnostic Criteria
RA	RA	RCUD	
(n/a)	RA	RA	Anemia (Hb <10 g/dL); ± neutropenia or thrombocytopenia; <1% circulating blasts; <5% medullary blasts; unequivocal dyserythropoiesis in ≥10% erythroid precursors; dysgranulopoiesis and dysmegakaryopoiesis, if present, in <10% nucleated cells; <15% RS; no Auer rods
(n/a)	(n/a)	RN	Neutropenia (absolute neutrophil count <1.8 × 10^9/L); ± anemia or thrombocytopenia; <1% circulating blasts; <5% medullary blasts; ≥10% dysplastic neutrophils; <10% dyserythropoiesis and dysmegakaryopoiesis; <15% RS; no Auer rods
(n/a)	(n/a)	RT	Thrombocytopenia (platelet count <100 × 10^9/L); ± anemia or neutropenia; <1% circulating blasts; <5% medullary blasts; R10% % dysplastic megakaryocytes of ≥30 megakaryocytes; <10% dyserythropoiesis and dysgranulopoiesis; <15% RS; no Auer rods
RARS	RARS	RARS	Anemia; no circulating blasts; <5% medullary blasts; dyserythropoiesis only, with RS among >15% of 100 erythroid precursors; no Auer rods
(n/a)	RCMD	RCMD	Cytopenia(s); <1 × 10^9/L circulating monocytes; <1% circulating blasts; <5% medullary blasts; dysplasia among >10% cells of ≥2 lineages; no Auer rods
	and RS	(n/a)	(n/a)
RAEB	RAEB-1	RAEB-1	Cytopenia(s); <1 × 10^9/L circulating monocytes; <5% circulating blasts; 5%–9% medullary blasts; dysplasia involving ≥1 lineage(s); no Auer rods
(n/a)	RAEB-2	RAEB-2	Cytopenia(s); <1 × 10^9/L circulating monocytes; 5%–19% circulating blasts; 10%–19% medullary blasts; dysplasia involving ≥1 lineage(s); ± Auer rods
(n/a)	(n/a)	RAEB-F	Similar to RAEB-1 or RAEB-2, with at least bilineage dysplasia and with diffuse coarse reticulin fibrosis, with or without collagenous fibrosis
RAEB-T	(AML)	(AML)	(n/a)

TABLE 7-10. CLASSIFICATIONS OF MDS *(Continued)*

FAB	WHO-2001	WHO-2008	WHO-2008 Diagnostic Criteria
(n/a)	MDS, U	MDS, U	Pancytopenia; <1 × 10⁹/L circulating monocytes; ≤1% circulating blasts; <5% circulating blasts; dysplasia in <10% cells of ≥1 lineage(s); demonstration of MDS-associated chromosomal abnormality(ies), exclusive of 18, del(20q), and -Y
	MDS, isolated del(5q)	MDS, isolated del(5q)	Anemia; platelet count may be normal or increased; <1% circulating blasts; <5% blasts; medullary blasts; megakaryocytes with characteristic nuclear hypolobulation; isolated del(5q) cytogenetic abnormality involving bands q31-q33
CMML	(MDS/MPN)	(MDS/MPN)	(n/a)
(n/a)	(n/a)	RCC	Thrombocytopenia, anemia, and/or neutropenia; <2% circulating blasts; <5% medullary blasts; unequivocal dysplasia in ≥2 lineages, or in >10% cells of one lineage; no RS

Abbreviations: CMML, chronic myelomonocytic leukemia; FAB, French-British-American; MDS, U, myelodysplastic syndrome, unclassifiable; MPN, myeloproliferative neoplasm; n/a, not applicable; RAEB-F, refractory anemia with excess blasts with fibrosis; RAEB-T, refractory anemia with excess blasts in transformation; RCC, refractory cytopenia of childhood; RN, refractory neutropenia; RS, ring sideroblasts; RT, refractory thrombocytopenia; WHO, World Health Organization. From Nguyen PL. The myelodysplastic syndromes. *Hematol Oncol Clin North Am.* 2009;23(4):675–91.

- Prognosis
  - Prognosis is determined by subtype (see Table 7-9).
  - Biggest risk is progression to acute leukemia.

Myelophthisis [8]

- Etiology, epidemiology, and pathophysiology (Table 7-11)
  - Can be a primary hematologic disease (see Primary Myelofibrosis) or secondary to marrow infiltration from extramedullary source. The term *myelophthisis* is usually reserved for secondary forms.
  - Table 7-11 lists most common causes.
  - Three distinct pathophysiologic features:
    - Myelofibrosis: fibroblast proliferation in marrow
    - Myeloid metaplasia: extramedullary hematopoiesis in spleen, liver, lymph nodes
    - Ineffective erythropoiesis
- Presentation
  - May be related to anemia with fatigue, and so forth
  - May be related to underlying cause, such as metastatic cancer or granulomatous disease
- Diagnosis
  - Anemia: normocytic, normochromic.
  - WBC and platelet counts are variable.
  - Leukoerythroblastic peripheral smear (Figures 7-4 and 7-5):
    - Nucleated red cells
    - Immature myeloid precursors
  - RBC morphologies include tear drops, nucleated RBCs, and distorted RBCs.
  - Platelets may be giant.

TABLE 7-11. CAUSES OF MARROW INFILTRATION

  I. Fibroblasts and Collagen
    A. Primary myelofibrosis
    B. Fibrosis of other myeloproliferative disorders
    C. Fibrosis of hairy cell leukemia
    D. Metastatic malignancies
    E. Sarcoidosis
    F. Secondary myelofibrosis with pulmonary hypertension
 II. Other Noncellular Material
    A. Oxalosis
III. Tumor Cells
    A. Carcinoma (lung, breast, prostate, kidney, thyroid, and neuroblastoma)
    B. Sarcoma
IV. Granulomas (inflammatory cells)
    A. Miliary tuberculosis
    B. Fungal infections
    C. Sarcoidosis
 V. Macrophages
    A. Gaucher disease
    B. Niemann-Pick disease
VI. Marrow Necrosis
    A. Sickle cell anemia
    B. Septicemia
    C. Tumors
    D. Arsenic therapy
VII. Failure of Osteoclast Development
    A. Osteopetrosis

From Lichtman MA, Kipps TJ, Uri Seligsohn U, et al. *Williams Hematology.* 8th ed. New York: McGraw-Hill; 2010.

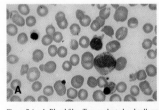 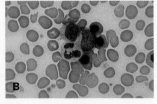

Figure 7-4   A. Blood film. Two nucleated red cells and a promyelocyte and a lymphocyte. The red cells show occasional but increased poikilocytosis. The patient had metastatic renal carcinoma to several sites including marrow. **B.** Blood film. White cell concentrate (buffy coat). Three nucleated red cells, 2 myelocytes, and a segmented neutrophil are evident. Another nucleated red cell can be partially visualized at right margin of field. In this case the blood film did not have evidence of a leukoerythroblastic reaction, but evidence was found in a film of the white cell concentrate. Because the white cell concentrate is the layer between the red cells and plasma in centrifuged blood, the red cells aspirated with the white cells are usually of lower density than average and reticulocyte rich, as evident here. Red cell morphology is not representative of the direct blood film. Patient had carcinoma of the lung metastatic to marrow. In leukoerythroblastic reactions, the red cell precursors that escape the marrow are usually orthochromatic erythroblasts, although occasionally earlier precursors may be seen. (From Lichtman MA, et al. *Lichtman's Atlas of Hematology.* New York: McGraw-Hill; © 2007 by The McGraw-Hill Companies, Inc. All rights reserved.) See color insert.

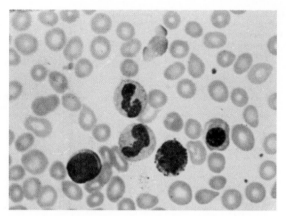

Figure 7-5 Teardrop-shaped red blood cells indicative of membrane damage from passage through the spleen, a nucleated red blood cell, and immature myeloid cells indicative of extramedullary hematopoiesis are noted. This peripheral blood smear is related to any cause of extramedullary hematopoiesis. (From Longo DL, et al., eds. *Harrison's Principles of Internal Medicine.* 18th ed. New York: McGraw-Hill; 2011.) See color insert.

- WBCs include myelocytes, promyelocytes, and myeloblasts.
- Bone marrow aspiration by yield nothing (a "dry tap")
- Magnetic resonance imaging may be used to estimate degree of marrow replacement and to identify suitable site for biopsy.
- Splenomegaly, often massive in primary myelofibrosis, usually absent.
- Treatment
- Aimed largely at underlying disease.
- Supportive RBC transfusion may be indicated.
- Prognosis dependent on underlying disease. If related to malignancy, myelophthisis portends extremely poor prognosis.

Other Anemias [9]

- Endocrine disorders
  - Hypothyroidism
  - Addison disease
  - Hyperparathyroidism
- Protein starvation
- Chronic liver disease (from multiple etiologies)
- Medication effects

Hemolytic Anemias

(Harrison's Online, Williams hematology, Current diagnosis & treatment)

- **Definition/pathophysiology/classification**
  - **Definition**
    - Hemolysis – Increased red cell turnover in which the rate of red cell destruction exceeds the bone marrow's normal capacity to produce more red cells.
    - Compensated hemolysis – Red cell destruction stimulates release of erythropoietin (EPO) by the kidney resulting in enough of an increased output of red cells from the bone marrow to balance the increased destruction. There is no anemia in compensated hemolysis.

- Decompensated hemolysis – Anemia onset is so sudden, it interferes with adequate EPO production.
- **Etiologies/pathophysiology**
- **Intracorpuscular defects**
  - **Hereditary**
    - Hemoglobinopathies
      - Sickle cell anemia
      - Thalassemia
    - Enzymopathies – Red cell enzymes normally provide energy in the form of ATP and prevent oxidative damage to hemoglobin and other proteins. When defective, the RBC is susceptible to oxidative stress.
      - Pyruvate kinase deficiency
      - G6PD deficiency
    - Membrane–cytoskeletal defects – Membrane consists of a lipid bilayer spanned by a number of proteins. Underneath the membrane is a network of other proteins that make up the cytoskeleton: the main being spectrin (consisting of α-spectrin and β-spectrin). The membrane is linked to the cytoskeleton by ankyrin, band 4.1 and band 4.2.
      - Hereditary spherocytosis
      - Hereditary elliptocytosis
      - Paroxysmal nocturnal hemoglobinuria
  - **Acquired**
    - Paroxysmal nocturnal hemoglobinuria (PNH)
- **Extracorpuscular factors**
  - **Hereditary**
    - Familial (atypical) hemolytic uremic syndrome –
      - Typically seen in children.
      - Inherited cause of HUS characterized by microangiopathic hemolytic anemia with fragmented erythrocytes, thrombocytopenia, and acute renal failure.
  - **Acquired**
    - Mechanical destruction
    - (microangiopathic/prostheses)
    - Toxins
    - Drugs
    - Infectious
      - Malaria – most frequent cause of hemolytic anemia in endemic areas
      - Shiga toxin-producing *Escherichia coli* O157:H7 – the main etiologic agent of the hemolytic-uremic syndrome
      - *Clostridium perfringens* sepsis
      - *Haemophilus influenza* type b
      - Babesiosis
    - Autoimmune
    - Entrapment

CAUSES OF HYPERSPLENISM

Congestive	Cirrhosis, portal or splenic vein obstruction
Neoplasm	Leukemia, metastatic carcinoma
Inflammatory	Sarcoidosis, SLE, Felty syndrome
Infections	Tuberculosis, brucellosis, malaria
Storage diseases	Gaucher disease, letterer-siwe disease, amyloidosis
Chronic hemolytic diseases	Spherocytosis, thalassemia, G6PD deficiency, elliptocytosis
Myeloproliferative	Myelofibrosis with myeloid metaplasia

- **Clinical manifestations/presentation**
  - **Gathering information**
    - Inquire as to onset of symptoms
      - Abrupt (as seen in autoimmune hemolytic anemia vs. gradual (as seen in hereditary spherocytosis or cold agglutinin disease)
    - Obtain family history
    - History of cholelithiasis
    - Recent history of stress, trauma, or infection
    - History of malignancy
    - Medication history
    - History of or family history of autoimmune disease
  - **Clinical manifestations**
    - Skin discoloration: pale vs. jaundiced
    - Fatigue
    - Tachycardia
    - Dyspnea
    - Angina
    - Discoloration of the urine
  - **Physical exam findings**
    - Splenomegaly
    - Hepatomegaly
    - Jaundice
    - Pallor
    - Skeletal changes – due to overactivity of the bone marrow as seen in thalassemia
- **Laboratory and tests**
  - Hemoglobin – normal to severely reduced
  - MCV/MCH – typically elevated due to an increased number of reticulocytes.
  - Reticulocyte count – increased – main sign of the erythropoietic response by the bone marrow.
    - Reticulocyte index (RI) = http://mdcalc.com/absolute- reticulocyte-count-index/
    - RI >2 represents an adequate red blood cell production from the bone marrow.
  - Lactate Dehydrogenase (LDH) – increased
  - Haptoglobin – reduced to absent
  - Indirect bili – increased
  - Urobilinogen – increased in both urine and stool
  - Hemoglobinuria – indicates an intravascular cause
  - Coombs' test – antisera against Ig or C3 applied to patient's RBCs.
    - Agglutinates in autoimmune hemolysis
  - Blood smear – may reveal macrocytes, polychromasia, occasional nucleated red cells. Examine for schistocytes.
  - Iron studies – deficient, normal or elevated
  - Folic acid – an erythropoietic factor – deficient due to increased requirement.
- **Complications**
  - Increased bilirubin production may produce gallstones
  - Persistent hemoglobinuria from chronic intravascular hemolysis may lead to considerable iron *loss*
  - Chronic extravascular hemolysis may lead to iron *overload*, especially if the patient needs frequent blood transfusions. This may lead to cirrhosis or cardiomyopathy.
- **Thalassemia**
  - **Pathogenesis**
    - Inherited disorders of α- or β-globin biosynthesis, thus diminishing production of hemoglobin tetramers.
    - Results in hypochromia and microcytosis
    - Highly unpaired α- or β-chains accumulate and form toxic inclusion bodies that kill developing erythroblasts in the marrow.

- Few proerythroblasts survive, and those that do have inclusion bodies that are detected in the spleen, thus shortening their life span.
- If profound anemia is present, it stimulates erythropoietin release and compensatory erythroid hyperplasia.
- However, marrow response is limited due to ineffective erythropoiesis, therefore anemia persists.
- Erythroid hyperplasia can become so significant that masses of extramedullary erythropoietic tissue are produced in the liver and spleen.
- Hemoglobin F persists to various decrees in β-thalassemia
- Epidemiology;
  - α-thalassemia = southeast Asia and China, less commonly in Blacks
  - β-thalassemia = Mediterranean origin, lesser extent in Asians and Blacks
- **Clinical manifestations/presentation**
  - α-Thalassemia – deletion(s) in α-globin gene(s).
    - If 3 or 4 α-globin genes are normal = α-thalassemia-2 trait
      - Asymptomatic, silent carrier
      - Only manifestation is hypochromia and microcytosis
    - If 2 of 4 α-globin genes are normal = α-thalassemia-1 trait or α-thalassemia minor
      - Mild microcytic Anemia
      - Hematocrit typically 28–40%
    - If 1 of 4 α-globin genes are normal = HbH (β4) disease
      - Moderate hemolytic anemia, but milder ineffective erythropoiesis.
      - Hematocrit typically 22–32%
      - Survival commonly occurs into mid-adulthood without transfusions.
      - Splenomegaly
    - If 0 of 4 α-globin genes are normal = Hb Barts (γ4)
      - Fetal hypoxia
      - Congestive heart failure
      - Edema (hydrops fetalis)
      - Death in utero
  - **β-Thalassemia** – point mutations in the β-globin gene (on chromosome 11) resulting in absent (β°) or decreased gene product (β+) http://www.accessmedicine.com/popup.aspx?aID=5535
    - Homozygous β
    - normal
    - Heterozygous β° or β+ = trait/thalassemia minor
      - 1 mutated β-globulin gene
      - Asymptomatic
      - Only abnormality is hypochromia and microcytosis with target cells on blood smear. Anemia is minimal
      - Hematocrit is rarely <30–33%
    - Homozygous β+ (mild) = thalassemia intermedia
      - 2 mutated β-globulin genes – mild mutation resulting in a milder course than Thalassemia major
      - Chronic hemolytic anemia
      - Iron overload may be present
      - Factors can aggravate the anemia – infection, puberty onset, stress
      - May have hepatosplenomegaly and bony deformities.
    - Homozygous β° or β+ (severe) = Thalassemia major/Cooley's anemia
      - Significant amount of unpaired α-chains resulting in severe and profound anemia.
      - Massive ineffective erythropoiesis: hepatosplenomegaly, profound microcytosis
      - Elevated levels of HbF, HbA2, or both.
      - Children may be normal at birth, but after 6 months (when HbF switches to HbA):
        - Severe anemia
        - "Chipmunk" facies

- Thinning and pathologic fractures of the long bones and vertebrae, resulting in profound growth retardation in severe cases.
- Physical examination may reveal hepatosplenomegaly, leg ulcers, and high-output congestive heart failure.
- All calorie intake goes to support erythropoiesis, leading to severe malnutrition with susceptibility of infection, endocrine dysfunction, and possibly death within the first few decades of life.
- Laboratory/studies

	HCT	MCV	Reticulocyte	Hb electrophoresis
α-thalassemia trait	28–40%	60–75	Normal	Normal
HbH disease	22–32%	60–70	Elevated	Fast migrating hemoglobin (hemoglobin H)
β-thalassemia minor	28–40%	55–75	Normal or slightly elevated	Elevated hemoglobin A2 to 4–8% and occasional elevations of hemoglobin F to 1–5%
β-thalassemia major	Severe, may fall to <10%	55–75	Elevated	Little to no hemoglobin A. Variable amounts of hemoglobin A2. The major hemoglobin present is hemoglobin F.

MEDICAL SPECIALTIES

- Mentzer's index =
  - MCV/RBC ratio < 13 = thalassemia
  - MCV/RBC ratio >13 = iron-deficiency anemia
  - *Mentzer WC. differentiation of iron deficiency from thalassemia trait. Lancet. 19731882*
- Iron
  - Normal or elevated (in chronic transfusions)
- Peripheral blood smear
  - α-thalassemia trait = microcytes, hypochromia, occasional target cells, acanthocytes http://www.accessmedicine.com/popup.aspx?aID = 23331
  - HbH disease = hypochromia, microcytosis, target cells and poikilocytosis http://www. accessmedicine.com/popup.aspx?aID = 23332
  - β-thalassemia minor = hypochromia, microcytosis, target cells, possible basophilic stippling http://www.accessmedicine.com/popup.aspx?aID = 23333
  - β-thalassemia major = severe poikilocytosis, hypochromia, microcytosis, target cells, basophilic stippling, and nucleated red blood cells. http://www.accessmedicine.com/popup.aspx?aID = 233334
- Management
  - β-thalassemia major
    - Chronic transfusions to maintain hematocrit at least 27–30%, so erythropoiesis is suppressed
    - Splenectomy may be required if the annual transfusion requirement increases by >50%. Pneumovax prior to splenectomy
    - Folic acid supplementation
    - Monitor for iron overload – may need a chelator
    - Allogeneic HSCT
  - β-thalassemia intermedia
    - Can survive without transfusion
    - May benefit from splenectomy
    - Monitor for iron overload and hemosiderosis
  - β-thalassemia minor or α-thalassemia trait
    - Requires no treatment
    - Identify as to avoid inappropriate iron replacement.

- HbH disease
  - Folic acid
  - Possibly splenectomy
  - Avoid oxidative drugs (i.e., sulfonamides)

Sickle Cell Disease (SCD) [10]

- Genetics and epidemiology
  - Autosomal recessive.
  - Results from single substitution of valine for glutamine on the β-globin chain.
  - Gene is carried by 8% of African Americans; 1 in 400 African American children are born homozygous for the gene and have sickle cell anemia.
  - Variants exist, including sickle cell hemoglobin C (HbSC) disease, the sickle thalassemias (α and β$^+$ or β^0), and sickle cell trait:
    - HbSC very similar to SCD, but milder except for higher incidence of retinopathy. Typical Hct nearer 30% or more.
    - Sickle α-thalassemia has similar morbidity to sickle cell anemia with milder anemia.
    - Sickle β-thalassemia phenotype depends on proportion of HbA, typically higher with sickle β$^+$, and therefore a milder disease.
    - Sickle trait (heterozygous for HbS and HbA) is generally asymptomatic. May have painless hematuria. High altitudes and extreme exertion may precipitate symptomatic vasoocclusion.
    - Hereditary persistence of HbF may yield a milder variant of SCD.
- Pathophysiology
  - Resultant Hb loses affinity for oxygen, becoming deformed and "sticky." Typical stimuli for release of oxygen by Hb (elevated temperature, increased CO_2 production, etc.) will potentiate this process.
  - As distinct Hb molecules contact one another within the RBC, they polymerize and deform the cell. Cell membrane function is also disrupted.
  - Cellular dehydration is promoted in part by hyperactivity of the calcium-activated potassium channel (Gardos channel) which facilitates extracellular movement of potassium chloride (KCl) and water (see http://sickle.bwh.harvard.edu/clt.html).
  - The resultant sickled RBCs are more adherent to each other and vascular endothelium. They are rigid, and flow is disrupted, particularly in smaller caliber vessels.
  - Deformed cells are lysed, causing hemolytic anemia and releasing cellular free Hb, which scavenges nitric oxide, thereby impairing vasodilation.
  - The entire process creates a proinflammatory state that increases WBC and platelet counts and promotes hypercoagulability.
- Clinical manifestations
  - Hemolytic anemia with Hct ranging from 15 to 30%.
  - Baseline leukocytosis and reticulocytosis.
  - Other manifestations protean and related to vasoocclusion and resultant hypoperfusion and hypoxia in various vascular territories.
  - Symptom onset in first year of life as fetal Hb replaced by sickle Hb.
  - Autosplenectomy (from repeated microinfarction of the vascular bed causing organ damage) occurs in first few years of life typically, rendering susceptibility to infection with encapsulated organisms (*Haemophilus influenza*, pneumococcus, etc.).
  - Most common manifestation is **acute painful episode** or **"crisis"** caused by microinfarction in bones and connective tissues. Accounts for 90% of hospitalizations. Patients with more than 2 to 3 acute painful episodes (requiring acute medical evaluation) have increased mortality.
    - Fever (even in absence of infection).
    - Tachycardia.
    - Severe acute pain.
    - Leukocytosis.
    - Worsening of baseline anemia and reticulocytosis

- Other markers of hemolysis as well, including elevated levels of LDH and AST, and decreased haptoglobin level.
- May last hours to approximately 2 weeks.
- Precipitators may include infection, exertion, fever, anxiety, temperature changes, hypoxia, and hypertonic x-ray dyes.
- Absence of objective evidence of painful crisis does not preclude its existence in patients with SCD complaining of acute painful episodes.
- **Acute chest syndrome:** responsible for about 25% of sickle cell deaths [11] and is the leading cause of death in SCD. It is the second most common reason for hospitalization. Also a major complication of surgery in general.
  - Fever.
  - Chest pain.
  - Tachypnea, cough, and shortness of breath.
  - Hypoxia.
  - Likely bronchial hyperactivity and spasm.
  - May be indistinguishable from pneumonia.
  - Multilobar or worsening infiltrates and/or hypoxia are ominous signs and may warrant specialized therapy (see below).
  - Regional hypoxia within the lung potentiates sickling, microinfarction, and pain, and leads to splinting and atelectasis. This potentiates further hypoxia and tissue damage within the lung and elsewhere.
- Other clinical manifestations
  - Bone infarction
    - May increase susceptibility to infection and osteomyelitis (*Staphylococcus aureus* most common, but salmonella not uncommon)
    - May lead to avascular necrosis of large joints (shoulders, hips) ultimately requiring joint replacement
  - Stroke [12]
    - Ischemic stroke most common
      - 11% of patients have stroke by age 20 years; 20% by age 45 years.
      - Children with stroke history are maintained on exchange transfusion protocol with target HbS less than 30%. Data on adults lacking and applicability a challenge given loss of vascular access, transfusional iron overload, and development of antibodies to RBC antigens.
    - Hemorrhagic stroke risk may exceed ischemic risk in third decade of life.
  - Priapism
    - Repeated or prolonged may result in permanent loss of function.
  - Aplastic crisis
    - Most often associated with parvovirus B-19.
    - Reticulocyte count will be inappropriately low.
  - Chronic nondecubitus skin ulcers
    - Usually distal lower extremities.
    - May be associated with infection.
    - Some note a role of hydroxyurea in susceptibility to ulcers. This is unclear.
  - Hepatic manifestations
    - Acute hepatic crisis
      - Right upper quadrant pain and marked elevation in transaminases and bilirubin
      - Low-grade fever
    - Hepatic sequestration
      - Large volumes of RBCs sequestered in liver
      - Acute and large drop in Hb
      - Right upper quadrant abdominal pain as well
    - Cholelithiasis
      - Pigmentary gall stones
      - May lead to acute cholecystitis and require cholecystectomy

- Renal manifestations
  - Papillary infarct and necrosis and renal infarction
    - Symptoms range from microscopic hematuria to painless gross hematuria to flank pain, fever, vomiting, and loss of renal function.
  - Isosthenuria.
    - Impaired concentrating ability
    - Leads to dehydration and further tissue damage
  - Proteinuria.
  - Renal tubular acidosis, typically distal type causing hyperkalemia.
  - Ultimately, the parenchymal damage may lead to progressive loss of renal function and renal failure.
- Cardiac complications
  - Chronic high output related to anemia and relative hypoxia may cause cardiomyopathy and chamber enlargement.
  - Myocardial infarction may occur in absence of major epicardial coronary artery disease.
- Pulmonary complications [13]
  - Pulmonary hypertension
    - May be asymptomatic.
    - May result from repeated bouts of acute chest syndrome or arise spontaneously.
    - Pulmonary pressure varies tremendously in and out of acute vasoocclusive episodes.
    - Tricuspid regurgitant jet more than 2.5 m/s associated with 10-fold increase in mortality.
  - Restrictive, and less commonly, obstructive lung diseases [14]
- Retinopathy, hemorrhage, retinal artery occlusion, retinal detachment
- Transfusional iron overload: Elevated ferritin and iron saturation. Ferritin may rise and fall with pain crisis and should be assessed in steady state when possible.
  - Long-term sequelae not well studied.
  - Iron chelation therapy (deferoxamine subcutaneously or intravenously and deferasirox orally) is available.
- Chronic pain
  - Complex entity that has physiologic and biopsychosocial components.
  - Chronic skin ulcers, avascular necrosis of bone are common causes.
- Laboratory and other tests: As the overwhelming majority of patients present with acute pain of some variety, we will focus on evaluation of such here. The primary goal of laboratory assessment is to evaluate for acutely reversible causes of the presentation, such as profound anemia warranting transfusion or infection requiring antibiotics. (Between such episodes, periodic monitoring of blood counts and renal and hepatic function is advised. Also, some advocate annual echocardiography to screen for pulmonary hypertension, though evidence of benefit is lacking.)
  - CBC with differential: Evaluate for leukocytosis beyond baseline and worsening of chronic anemia. Marked leukocytosis may suggest acute infection. Marked drop in Hb level can be seen with vasoocclusion and increased hemolysis and may point to specific entities such as hepatic sequestration.
  - Peripheral blood smear can give idea of degree of RBC sickling.
  - Serum chemistry: May exhibit hyperkalemia associated with distal type renal tubular acidosis. Also a general screen for renal failure as a comorbidity.
  - Liver function tests and transaminases: particularly in patients with abdominal pain and marked drop in Hb level:
    - Elevations in bilirubin, LDH, transaminases, alkaline phosphatase levels may portend hepatic crisis or sequestration or cholecystitis.
    - AST, LDH, indirect bilirubin levels may be elevated in hemolysis independent of hepatic function.
  - Urinalysis: particularly if febrile or symptomatic and concern for infection:
    - Typically will be isosthenuric because of repeated papillary infarction over time.

- Blood cultures: if infection suspected or the patient has indwelling vascular access device.
- Hb electrophoresis may be useful for diagnosis of SCD if history uncertain or to monitor effect of therapy (see below).
- Most patients should have chest x-ray to evaluate for infiltrates suggestive of infection or acute chest syndrome.
- If suspicion of venous thromboembolism, evaluation as with nonsickle cell patients is appropriate. However, patients will have abnormalities in ventilation and perfusion at baseline. Also, hypertonic contrast dye may precipitate cellular sickling and should be used with caution.
- Other laboratory and imaging modalities are used given particular presenting concerns as in patients without SCD.
- Management of most common presentations (see http://scinfo.org/problem-oriented-clinical-guidelines/ and http://www.nhlbi.nih.gov/health/prof/blood/sickle/sc_mngt.pdf and http://sickle.bwh.harvard.edu/)
  - Acute painful crisis [15]
    - Focused screen for reversible cause, such as infection, dehydration, worsening of baseline anemia.
    - Initiate supplemental oxygen to maintain normal oxygen saturation.
    - Intravenous fluid hydration: If hypovolemic, start with normal saline (NS). Transition to hypotonic (50% NS or 25% NS) as early as feasible given at least theoretic benefit to cellular rehydration.
      - Use with caution in patients with comorbid cardiopulmonary compromise.
      - Use with caution in patients with renal impairment.
      - Monitor for electrolyte abnormalities.
    - Limited randomized, controlled data to favor one analgesic or route over another. Reasonable approach is parenteral narcotics through scheduled bolus or patient-controlled analgesia system.
    - Nonsteroidal antiinflammatory drugs, particularly ketorolac, acutely may be of added benefit. Use with caution in patients with renal disease.
    - Patients receiving regular narcotics and those with chest pain should have incentive spirometry to decrease pulmonary complications.
    - Exchange transfusion may be of benefit in severe refractory acute pain crisis, although again, evidence is limited.
  - Acute chest syndrome [16]
    - Difficult to distinguish from pneumonia.
    - Defined as chest pain, fever, pulmonary infiltrate, and tachypnea.
    - Treat as community-acquired pneumonia with coverage for atypical pathogens, as these are suspected to have a role in etiology, particularly chlamydia pneumonia.
    - Bronchodilators may help as bronchial hyperactivity has been shown.
    - Exchange transfusion is indicated for worsening hypoxia or infiltrates. Simple transfusion is reasonable alternative if timely exchange cannot be achieved. These patients should be managed in an intensive care unit.
    - Analgesia important to promote adequate tidal volume of respirations
  - Stroke [17]
    - Most robust data is in children.
    - Children at risk for or with history of ischemic stroke are maintained on exchange transfusion protocols to maintain HbS percentage less than 30.
    - Adults are treated similarly when possible and not limited by venous access, iron overload, or antibodies to transfused blood.
  - Disease modifying therapies
    - Hydroxyurea [18]
      - Only drug that modifies disease process.
      - Increases Hb, fetal Hb, MCV.
      - A major mechanism of action is increased production of fetal Hb, which has higher affinity for oxygen and does not participate in sickling process.
      - Also decreases WBC count, thereby tempering inflammatory cascade.

- Decreases reticulocytosis.
- Decreases pain crisis, hospitalization, transfusion, acute chest syndrome, mortality.
- Strongest indication is patients with more than three painful crises per year (level 1 evidence [19]). National Institutes of Health Consensus Conference 2008 http://www.guideline.gov/content.aspx?id=12656 concluded it is grossly underused.
- Dose usually begun at 500 mg and titrated to 30 to 35 mg/kg. Monitor CBC and reticulocyte count every 2 to 6 weeks myelosuppression. [20]
- Blood transfusion: [21] Typically aim not to exceed Hb of 10 mg/dL to avoid hyperviscosity. Ideally use sickle negative, leukoreduced, phenotype-specific blood.
  - Exchange transfusion
    - Strongest evidence for exchange transfusion in primary and secondary stroke prevention in children with target HbS less than 30%. Adults with history of stroke typically maintained on this regimen as no safe stop time identified. [22]
    - Exchange also used in cases of acute chest syndrome and worsening infiltrates or hypoxia.
    - Acute multiorgan failure.
    - Exchange may decrease iron burden compared to simple transfusion.
  - Simple transfusion
    - Acute treatment of a variety of conditions
      - Symptomatic anemia
      - Preparation for major surgery (that requiring general anesthesia)
      - Acute splenic or hepatic sequestration
      - Acute chest syndrome or stroke if exchange unavailable or delayed
    - Chronic scheduled transfusions
      - Chronic heart failure
      - Chronic pulmonary hypertension or hypoxia
      - Anemia of chronic kidney disease not responding to EPO
- Stem cell transplant (see http://asheducationbook.hematologylibrary.org/content/2011/1/273.full.pdf+html)
  - Only curative therapy available.
  - Most data on children younger than 16 years of age.
  - Complications increase with comorbidities.
  - Not widely available.
- General management and health maintenance
  - Penicillin for prophylaxis of pneumococcal infections, beneficial in young children, but has not been shown to be necessary in adults.
  - Subacute bacterial endocarditis prophylaxis prior to dental procedures is still generally employed.
  - Important immunizations (in addition to usual adult immunization schedule; see http://www.annals.org/content/154/3/168.full.pdf+html)
    - Pneumococcal (efficacy may be limited given asplenia)
    - Meningococcal
    - Varicella
    - Zoster
    - Some advocate hepatitis A and B vaccines based on possibility of chronic liver disease
    - *Haemophilus influenza*
  - Folic acid supplementation
  - Vitamin D supplementation
    - Up to 98% of patients found to be deficient
    - Important for bone health and myriad other putative benefits
- Prognosis: life expectancy generally into fifth or sixth decades of life
- **Pyruvate kinase deficiency**
  - **Epidemiology**

- Prevalence ~1:10,000
- Autosomal recessive
- **Clinical manifestations/presentation**
  - Often presents in the newborn with neonatal jaundice, which persists with a very high reticulocytosis
  - Variable anemia – If mild, it is typically compensated and generally well tolerated. Symptoms may be severe enough to warrant regular blood transfusions.
- **Lab/studies**
  - Chronic normo-macrocytic anemia
  - Coombs-negative
- **Management**
  - Supportive
  - Folic acid supplementation
  - Transfusion if necessary +/− iron chelation
  - Splenectomy may be beneficial in severe disease
  - Consider bone marrow transplantation from HLA-identical Pyruvate Kinase-normal sibling in severe cases.
- **G6PD deficiency**
  - **Pathogenesis/etiology/definition**
    - Glucose 6-phosphate dehydrogenase (G6PD) is a housekeeping enzyme critical in the redox metabolism of all aerobic cells. It is the only source of NADPH in RBCs that directly and via glutathione defends them against oxidative stress.
    - G6PD deficiency causes an increase in oxidative damage vulnerability and accelerated red cell aging.
    - X-linked, therefore most common in males
      - Some heterozygous females can be just as affected as hemizygous males.
    - Seen in tropical and subtropical areas (Africa, Southern Europe, the Middle East, and Southeast Asia)
    - Provides a relative resistance against *Plasmodium falciparum*
    - Precipitated by oxidative agents:
      - Fava beans
      - Infections
      - Drugs – Primaquine, Dapsone, Sulfamethoxazole, Nitrofurantoin, Phenazopyridine, Methylene blue
  - **Clinical manifestations/presentation**
    - Mostly asymptomatic
    - Develops acute intravascular hemolytic attack when challenged by oxidative agents:
      - Starts with malaise, weakness, and abdominal or lumbar pain
      - After an interval of several hours to 2–3 days, the patient develops jaundice and often dark urine due to hemoglobinuria.
    - Full recovery following acute hemolytic attack
    - May develop gallstones and/or splenomegaly
  - **Lab/studies**
    - Acute hemolytic attack:
      - Normocytic normochromic anemia is moderate to extremely severe.
      - Indirect hyperbilirubinemia
      - Reticulocytosis
      - Evidence of intravascular hemolysis: hemoglobinemia, hemoglobinuria, high LDH, low/absent haptoglobin
    - Peripheral blood smear
      - Anisocytosis, polychromasia, and spherocytes.
      - Bizarre poikilocytes
      - Heinzi bodies – denatured hemoglobin – signature of oxidative damage to red cells.
      - Bite cells

- May develop acute renal failure
- Decreased G6PD levels
- **Management**
  - Avoid exposure to triggering factors.
  - Prevent drug-induced hemolysis by testing for G6PD deficiencies before prescribing.
  - Most acute hemolytic attacks are treated supportively; however, severe anemias may require blood transfusion.
  - Folate supplementation is used in chronic nonspherocytic hemolytic anemia (a subset of G6PD deficiencies)
  - Splenectomy may be beneficial in severe cases.
  - Hemodialysis may be necessary if acute renal failure is present.
- **Hereditary Spherocytosis**
  - **Pathogenesis/epidemiology**
    - Estimated frequency of 1/5000.
    - Typically seen in Northern Europeans
    - Will usually have positive family history
    - Autosomal dominant – some severe forms are autosomal recessive.
    - Mutations are seen in the membrane-cytoskeleton structure – α-Spectrin, β-Spectrin, Ankyrin, Band 3 (the anion channel), or Band 4.1/4.2
    - Majority of destruction occurs in the spleen. Transit through the splenic circulation makes the red cells more spherocytic, thereby accelerating their demise.
  - **Clinical manifestations/presentation**
    - Anemia – mild to severe. Usually normocytic
    - Jaundice
    - Splenomegaly
    - Pigmented gallstones
  - **Lab/studies**
    - Peripheral blood smear reveals spherocytes http://www.accessmedicine.com.evms.idm. oclc.org/popup.aspx?aID=9117922
    - Increased mean corpuscular hemoglobin concentration (MCHC)
    - Increased reticulocytes
    - Abnormal Osmotic fragility test
  - **Management**
    - Avoid splenectomy in mild cases
    - Delay splenectomy until at least 4 years of age, after the risk of severe sepsis has peaked
    - Antipneumococcal vaccination before splenectomy; however, penicillin prophylaxis postsplenectomy is controversial.
    - May require cholecystectomy
    - For more guidelines on diagnosis and management of HS: http://www.bcshguidelines. com/documents/HS_BCSH_Sept_2011 final.pdf
- **Hereditary elliptocytosis**
  - **Pathogenesis/etiology/definition**
    - Mostly autosomal dominant
    - Mild or asymptomatic
    - Severe cases – bizarre poikilocytes predominant.
  - **Clinical manifestations/presentation**
    - Same as HS
  - **Lab/studies**
    - Elliptocytes on peripheral blood smear.
  - **Management**
    - Splenectomy may be beneficial in severe cases, otherwise simply observation.
- **Paroxysmal nocturnal hemoglobinuria**
  - **Pathogenesis**

- Acquired chronic hemolytic anemia characterized by persistent intravascular hemolysis.
- A mutation in the X-linked PIG-A gene, a gene which participates in the synthesis of glycosylphosphatidyl-inositol (GPI). GPI anchors surface proteins to RBCs. Surface proteins normally protect RBCs from activated complement.
- When PIG-A is mutated, RBCs have an increased susceptibility to complement due to the lack of surface proteins (particularly CD59 and CD55).
- Patients have recurrent exacerbations.
- Increased risk for venous thrombosis – unknown mechanism; however, there may be inappropriate platelet activation through CD59 deficiency.
- Without treatment, the median survival is ~8–10 years. The most common cause of death being venous thrombosis, followed by infection and hemorrhage.
- **Clinical manifestations/presentation**
  - Dark urine
  - Venous thrombosis
  - May present with recurrent attacks of severe abdominal pain (indicating intraabdominal thrombosis)
  - Acute hepatomegaly and ascites (due to hepatic vein thrombosis/Budd-Chiari syndrome) in the absence of liver disease.
  - May evolve into an aplastic anemia. Rarely it may terminate into acute myeloid leukemia.
  - Iron deficiency secondary to hemoglobinuria
- **Lab/studies**
  - Normo-macrocytic anemia – mild to moderate to severe. However, may be microcytic due to iron deficiency from chronic urinary blood loss.
  - Possibly pancytopenia
  - Unremarkable red cell morphology.
  - May have elevated MCV secondary to reticulocytosis
  - Elevated unconjugated bilirubin
  - LDH is markedly elevated
  - Haptoglobin is undetectable
  - Hemoglobinuria – can vary from day to day.
  - Bone marrow reveals a cellular pattern, with marked to massive erythroid hyperplasia, often with mild to moderate dyserythropoietic features. Bone marrow may become hypocellular or even aplastic.
  - Definitive diagnosis: Flow cytometry reveals a discrete population of cells deficient in CD55 and CD59.
  - Sucrose hemolysis test is unreliable. The acidified serum (Ham) test is seldom carried out.
- **Management**
  - Folic acid supplements are mandatory
  - Check serum iron periodically and supplement when appropriate
  - Transfusion when appropriate
  - Eculizumab – humanized monoclonal antibody against the complement component C5. Administered IV every 14 days.
  - Glucocorticoids do not have any effect, and actually tend to be contraindicated.
  - The only definitive cure is allogeneic bone marrow transplantation, and may be considered in young patients with severe PNH.
- **Mechanical destruction (microangiopathic/prosthesis)**
  - **Pathogenesis/etiology/definition**
    - RBCs succumb to shearing or wear and tear resulting in intravascular hemolysis
    - **Etiologies:**
      - Hemolytic-Uremic Syndrome (HUS) – see HUS section
      - Thrombotic thrombocytopenic purpura (TTP) – see TTP section
      - Disseminated intravascular coagulation (DIC)

- Pathophysiology: Widespread intravascular fibrin formation in response to excessive blood protease activity that overcomes the natural anticoagulant mechanism.
  - Exposure of blood to phospholipids from damaged tissue, hemolysis, and endothelial damage.
  - Consumption of platelets and coagulation factors
  - Release of several proinflammatory cytokines (interleukin-6 and tumor necrosis factor) http://www.accessmedicine.com.evms. idm.oclc.org/popup.aspx?alD= 9100911
- Etiology:
  - The most common causes are bacterial sepsis, malignant disorders, and obstetric causes.

CAUSES

Sepsis	Bacterial – Staphylococci, Streptococci, Pneumococci, Meningococci,
	Gram-negative bacilli
	Viral
	Mycotic
	Parasitic
	Rickettsial
Immunologic	Acute hemolytic transfusion reaction
	Organ/tissue transplant rejection
	Graft-versus-host disease
Trauma/Tissue injury	Brain injury
	Extensive burns,
	Fat embolism
	Rhabdomyolysis
Drugs	Fibrinolytic agents
	Warfarin (especially in protein C deficiency)
	Aprotinin
	Prothrombin complex concentrates
	Recreational drugs (amphetamines)
Vascular	Giant hemangiomas
	Large vessel aneurysms
Envenomation	Snake
	Insects
Obstetrical	Abruptio placentae
	Amniotic-fluid embolism
	Dead fetus syndrome – can produce a chronic DIC
	Septic abortion
Liver disease	Fulminant hepatic failure
	Cirrhosis
	Fatty liver of pregnancy
Malignancy	Acute promyelocytic leukemia
	Metastatic carcinoma & hemangioma – chronic DIC

- Clinical manifestations:
  - Fibrin deposition in small and midsize vessels results in multisystem organ failure (the lung, kidney, liver, and brain)
  - Systemic bleeding – oozing, petechiae, and ecchymoses to severe hemorrhage.
  - Thrombosis of large vessels and cerebral embolism.
  - Hemodynamic complications and shock
  - Purpura fulminans results from thrombosis of extensive areas of the skin.
  - Mortality 30–80%
- Labs/studies
  - Prolonged coagulation tests (PT and/or PTT, thrombin time)
  - Elevated fibrin degradation products/D-dimer
  - Diminished fibrinogen only in severe cases of DIC
  - Schistocytes on peripheral blood smear.
  - Thrombocytopenia (typically <100,000) – repeat platelet count every 6–8 hours
  - RBC count

DIAGNOSTIC ALGORITHM

- Taylor, Fletcher B, Cheng-Hock Toh, Hoots, W. Keith, Wada, Hideo. *Towards a Definition, Clinical and Laboratory Criteria, and a Scoring System for DIC.* International Society on Thrombosis and Haemostasis. Thromb Haemost 2007, 5(3): 604–606
- Risk assessment: Does the patient have an underlying disorder known to be associated with overt DIC? *If yes, proceed. If no, do not use this algorithm*
- Order global coagulation tests (platelet count, prothrombin time (PT), fibrinogen, soluble fibrin monomers or fibrin degradation products.
- Score global coagulation test results:

	0	1	2	3
Platelet count	>100	<100	<50	–
Elevated fibrin-related marker	No increase	–	Moderate increase	Strong increase
Prolonged prothrombin time	<3 sec	>3 sec but <6 sec	>6 sec	–
Fibrinogen level	>1.0 gram/L	<1.0 gram/L	–	–

- If the score is >5, symptoms are compatible with overt DIC. Scoring should be repeated daily.
- If the score is <5, not affirmative for overt DIC. Repeat over the next 1–2 days. http://www.isth.org/default/assets/File/defdictable2.pdf
  - Management
    - Treat the underlying cause
    - Hemodynamic and respiratory support
    - Control of bleeding in DIC patients with marked thrombocytopenia (platelets <10,000–20,000/μL^3) and coagulopathy will require replacement
      - FFP
      - Cryoprecipitate if low levels of fibrinogen or brisk hyperfibrinolysis – replace 10 units of cryo for every 2–3 units of FFP
      - Adjust according to the patient's clinical and laboratory evolution.
      - Platelets at 1–2 units/10 kg body weight
    - Low doses of continuous IV heparin (5–10 units/kg per hour) may be effective in patients with low-grade DIC associated with solid tumor, acute promyelocytic leukemia, in the setting of recognized thrombosis, for the treatment of purpura fulminans, during surgical resection of giant hemangiomas and during the removal of a dead fetus. It is not appropriate for acute DIC.

- Antifibrinolytics (EACA or tranexamic acid) may reduce bleeding episodes in patients with DIC and confirmed hyperfibrinolysis. Can increase the risk of thrombosis.
- Protein C – may be considered to treat purpura fulminans associated with protein C deficiency or meningococcemia; however otherwise, data are lacking.
- For further guidelines on diagnosis and management: http://www.bcshguidelines.com/documents/intravascular_coagulation_bjh_26Oct09.pdf
- Malignant hypertension
- HELLP
- Prosthetic heart valves – especially when paraprosthetic regurgitation is present.
- March hemoglobinuria – acute and self-inflicted. Seen in marathon runners.
- **Clinical manifestations/presentation**
  - May be asymptomatic if hemolysis is mild and iron stores are normal.
  - Otherwise, as seen above based on particular etiology.
- **Lab/studies**
  - Schistocytes on peripheral blood smear
  - Hemoglobinuria
  - Platelets low or normal

	PT(INR)	PTT	Platelets	Creatinine	LFTs
HUS	–	–	Low	Elev	–
TTP	–	–	Low	Elev	–
DIC	Elev	Elev	Low	–	–
HELLP	–	–	Low	Nl/Elev	Elev

- **Management**
  - Treat underlying etiology and provide supportive care – see above
- **Toxic agents & drugs**
- **Pathogenesis/etiology**
  - Caused by chemicals with oxidative potential even in patients who are not G6PD-deficient OR by chemicals that are nonoxidative.
  - Mechanism of hemolysis:
    - Occurs by a direct chemical action on red cells.
    - A drug behaves as a hapten and induces antibody production – ex: penicillin. Upon subsequent exposure, the red cells are affected by the penicillin–antipenicillin reaction. Subsides as soon as drug administration is stopped.
    - The drug triggers, through mimicry, the production of an antibody against a red cell antigen – ex: methyldopa
  - Chemicals with oxidative potential:
    - Hyperbaric oxygen
    - Nitrates
    - Chlorates
    - Methylene blue
    - Dapsone
    - Cisplation
    - Aromatic (cyclic) compounds.
  - Nonoxidative chemicals:
    - Arsine
    - Copper
    - Lead – basophilic stippling.
  - Others:
    - Snake venom – cobras and vipers
    - Spider bites

- **Management**
  - Removal of causative agent.
- **Autoimmune**
  - **Pathogenesis/etiology/definition**
    - The most common form of acquired hemolytic anemia.
    - Autoantibody binds to red cells, resulting in red cell destruction by
      - Erythrophagocytosis by macrophages (and perhaps monocytes) – takes place in the spleen, liver, and bone marrow (i.e., extravascular hemolysis).
      - Antigen–antibody complex on the RBC activates complement, thus resulting in a large membrane attack complex to form and causing direct destruction (i. e., intravascular hemolysis).
    - Etiology:
      - **Warm AIHA** – IgG binds to the red blood cell membrane most avidly at body temperature.
        - Idiopathic
        - Autoimmune (SLE)
        - Lymphoproliferative – CLL or lymphomas
        - Drugs (Penicillin)
      - **Cold AIHA** – An acquired hemolytic anemia due to an IgM autoantibody usually directed against the I antigen on RBCs. Antibodies react with cells at lower <37°C temperatures.
        - Idiopathic
        - Waldenstrom macroglobulinemia – monoclonal IgM paraprotein is produced.
        - Postinfectious following mycoplasma pneumonia or infectious mononucleosis.
  - **Clinical manifestations/presentation**
    - Very abrupt onset and can be dramatic
    - Fatigue
    - Angina or congestive heart failure
    - Jaundice
    - Splenomegaly
    - Hemoglobinuria – if intravascular destruction
    - Mottled or numb fingers or toes, episodic low back pain and dark colored urine in cold AIHA
  - **Lab/studies**
    - Anemia may be severe (hematocrit <10%)
    - Reticulocytosis
    - Peripheral blood smear reveals spherocytes and possibly nucleated red blood cells
    - Increased indirect bilirubin
    - ~10% have immune thrombocytopenia = Evan's syndrome
    - Coomb's test –
      - Direct Coombs = patient's RBC with Coombs reagent – + agglutination indicates the presence of an antibody (IgG, complement, or both) on the red blood cell surface.
      - Indirect Coombs = patient's serum with type O RBCs. After incubation, Coombs reagent is added – + agglutination indicates the presence of free antibody in the patient's serum.
      - Autoimmune hemolytic anemia commonly has a positive direct Coombs and the indirect Coombs may or may not be positive. A positive indirect Coombs indicates the presence of a large amount of autoantibody that has saturated binding sites in the RBC and consequently appears in the serum.
      - Serum cold agglutinin titers
  - **Triage decisions**
    - Transfusion
      - If symptomatic from anemia
      - Proves to be difficult, as antibodies are often unspecific, resulting in incompatible cross-matched blood.
      - Transfuse incompatible blood if emergent

- **Management**
  - Corticosteroids – first-line treatment
    - Prednisone 1–2 mg/kg/day in divided doses may produce prompt remission; however, relapses are not uncommon.
  - If the patient has relapsed, or not responded to corticosteroids, second-line treatments include:
    - Rituximab – can produce remissions in up to 80% of patients.
    - Splenectomy – benefits by removing a major site of hemolysis.
  - Third-line agents:
    - Azathioprine
    - Cyclophosphamide
    - Cyclosporine
    - IVIg
  - In severe refractory cases, consider auto- or allohematopoietic stem cell transplantation.
  - Treat underlying diseases
  - Avoid cold temperatures in cold AIHA
  - For further guidance regarding treatment: http://bloodjournal.hematologylibrary. org/content/116/ll/1831.full.pdf

MYELOPROLIFERATIVES DISORDERS [23]

General Features

- Clonal stem cell disorders.
- May have typical chromosomal abnormalities evident on cytogenetics.
- May involve myeloid, erythroid, or platelet cell lineages.
- May involve extramedullary hematopoiesis.
- World Health Organization classification includes 8 disorders (Tables 7-12 and 7-13); this review focuses on 4 major disorders:
  - Polycythemia vera
  - Essential thrombocytosis
  - Primary myelofibrosis
  - Chronic myelogenous leukemia (CML)
- All have some potential to evolve into acute leukemia.

TABLE 7-12. WORLD HEALTH ORGANIZATION CLASSIFICATION OF CHRONIC MYELOPROLIFERATIVE DISORDERS

Chronic myelogenous leukemia, bcr-abl–positive
Chronic neutrophilic leukemia
Chronic eosinophilic leukemia, not otherwise specified
Polycythemia vera
Primary myelofibrosis
Essential thrombocytosis
Mastocytosis
Myeloproliferative neoplasms, unclassifiable

From Longo DL, et al., eds. *Harrison's Principles of Internal Medicine.* 18th ed. New York: McGraw-Hill; 2012:898.

TABLE 7-13. WHO DIAGNOSTIC CRITERIA FOR POLYCYTHEMIA VERA, ESSENTIAL THROMBOCYTHEMIA, AND PRIMARY MYELOFIBROSIS

		2008 WHO Diagnostic Criteria		
		Polycythemia vera[a]	Essential Thrombocythemia[a]	Primary Myelofibrosis[a]
Major criteria	1	Hb > 18.5 g/dL (men) > 16.5 g/dL (women) or[b]	Platelet count ≥ 450 × 10⁹/L	Megakaryocyte proliferation and atypical accompanied by either reticulin and/or collagen fibrosis, or[d]
	2	Presence of JAK2V617F or JAK2 exon 12 mutation	Megakaryocyte proliferation with large and mature morphology.	Not meeting WHO criteria for CML, PV, MDS, or other myeloid neoplasm
	3		Not meeting WHO criteria for CML, PV, PMF, MDS or other myeloid neoplasm	Demonstration of JAK2V617F or other clonal marker or no evidence of reactive marrow fibrosis
	4		Demonstration of JAK2V617F or other clonal marker or no evidence of reactive thrombocytosis	
Minor criteria	1	BM trilineage myeloproliferation		Leukoerythroblastosis
	2	Subnormal serum EPO level		Increased serum LDH level
	3	EEC growth		Anemia
				Palpable splenomegaly

BM, bone marrow; Hb, hemoglobin; Hct, hematocrit; EPO, erythropoietin; EEC, endogenous erythroid colony; WHO, World Health Organization; CML, chronic myelogenous leukemia; PV, polycythemia vera; PMF, primary myelofibrosis; MDS, myelodysplastic syndromes; LDH, lactate dehydrogenase.

[a] PV diagnosis requires meeting either both major criteria and 1 minor criterion or the first major criterion and 2 minor criteria. ET diagnosis requires meeting all 4 major criteria. PMF diagnosis requires meeting all 3 major criteria and 2 minor criteria.

[b] or Hb or Hct >99th percentile of reference range for age, sex, or altitude of residence or red cell mass >25% above normal mean predicted or Hb >17 g/dL (men)/ >15 g/dL (women) if associated with a sustained increase of ≥2 g/dL from baseline that cannot be attributed to correction of iron deficiency.

[c] Small to large megakaryocytes with aberrant nuclear/cytoplasmic ratio and hyperchromatic and irregularly folded nuclei and dense clustering.

[d] In the absence of reticulin fibrosis, the megakaryocyte changes must be accompanied by increased marrow cellularity, granulocytic proliferation and often decreased erythropoiesis (ie, prefibrotic PMF).

From Tefferi A. Primary myelofibrosis: 2012 update on diagnosis, risk stratification, and management. Am J Hematol. 2011;86(12):1017–26.

Specific Conditions

Polycythemia Vera

- Epidemiology, etiology, and pathophysiology
  - Increasing frequency with age.
  - Prevalence near 2/100,000 overall (higher in older populations).
  - Occurs in men more than women.
  - Clonal proliferation of all 3 cell lines, most severely affecting erythroid lineage.
  - *JAK2* mutation present in 95% of cases.
  - Increased RBC mass causes hyperviscosity and propensity to thrombosis.
- Presentation: largely related to hyperviscosity.
- Thrombosis
  - Related to hyperviscosity and platelet dysfunction
  - May be arterial or venous
  - Most common complication
  - Leading cause of mortality
  - Includes hepatic vein thrombosis (Budd-Chiari) in up to 10% of cases as well as other more common sites

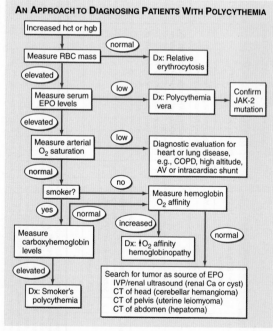

Figure 7-6 An approach to the differential diagnosis of patients with an elevated hemoglobin (possible polycythemia). AV, atrioventricular; COPD, chronic obstructive pulmonary disease; CT, computed tomography; EPO, erythropoietin; hct, hematocrit; IVP, intravenous pyelogram; RBC, red blood cell. (From Longo DL, et al., eds. *Harrison's Principles of Internal Medicine.* 18th ed. New York: McGraw-Hill; 2011.)

TABLE 7-14. CAUSES OF ERYTHROCYTOSIS

Relative Erythrocytosis

Hemoconcentration secondary to dehydration, diuretics, ethanol abuse, androgens or tobacco abuse

Absolute Erythrocytosis

Hypoxia
Carbon monoxide intoxication
High oxygen-affinity hemoglobin
High altitude
Pulmonary disease
Right-to-left cardiac or vascular shunts
Sleep apnea syndrome
Hepatopulmonary syndrome

Renal Disease
Renal artery stenosis
Focal sclerosing or membranous glomerulonephritis
Postrenal transplantation
Renal cysts
Bartter syndrome

Tumors
Hypernephroma
Hepatoma
Cerebellar hemangioblastoma
Uterine myoma
Adrenal tumors
Meningioma
Pheochromocytoma

Drugs
Androgens
Recombinant erythropoietin

Familial (with normal hemoglobin function)
Erythropoietin receptor mutation
VHL mutations (Chuvash polycythemia)
2,3-BPG mutation

Polycythemia Vera

2,3-BPG, 2,3-bisphosphoglycerate; VHL, von Hippel-Lindau.
From Longo DL, et al., eds. *Harrison's Principles of Internal Medicine*. 18th ed. New York: McGraw-Hill; 2012:899.

MEDICAL SPECIALTIES

- Headache
- Dizziness
- Blurred vision
- Epistaxis and other bleeding (also related to platelet dysfunction)
- Pruritus, particularly after warm shower
- Peptic ulcer disease
- Erythromelalgia (painful erythema in the extremities)
- Splenomegaly in majority of cases
- Diagnosis (Figure 7-6)
  - Elevated Hb/Hct: Defined as Hct over 54% in men and 51% in women. Alone, nonspecific (Table 7-14).
  - MCV low or low normal.
  - May have thrombocytosis (>50% of patients) and leukocytosis (>60%) as well.
  - Peripheral smear usually demonstrates normal cellular morphology.
  - EPO level low.
  - RBC mass elevated (no longer frequently measured).
  - *JAK2* mutation.
  - Hypercellular bone marrow (also not frequently used for diagnosis) with decreased iron stores.
  - Vitamin B_{12} levels may be high related to transcobalamin III from WBCs.
  - Hyperuricemia from increased cell turnover.
- Management
  - Treatment of choice is phlebotomy.
    - Target Hct less than 45% in men, less than 42% in women
    - May need weekly phlebotomy at first
    - Will induce iron deficiency, but avoid supplementation
  - Hydroxyurea for those with poor venous access or other problems with phlebotomy. Other targets of therapy include platelet count less than 500,000 per microliter.

TABLE 7-15. CAUSES OF THROMBOCYTOSIS

Tissue inflammation: collagen vascular disease, inflammatory bowel disease	Hemorrhage
Malignancy	Iron deficiency anemia
Infection	Surgery
Myeloproliferative disorders: polycythemia vera, primary myelofibrosis, essential thrombocytosis, chronic myelogenous leukemia	Rebound: Correction of vitamin B_{12} or folate deficiency, post-ethanol abuse
Myelodysplastic disorders: 5q-syndrome, idiopathic refractory sideroblastic anemia	Hemolysis
Postsplenectomy or hyposplenism	Familial: Thrombopoietin overproduction, constitutive
	Mpl activation

From Longo DL, et al., eds. *Harrison's Principles of Internal Medicine.* 18th ed. New York: McGraw-Hill; 2012:903.

- Anagrelide is another alternative.
- Emerging role for peginterferon alfa-2a.
- Avoid alkylating agents as may lead to leukemic conversion.
- Young patients with appropriate donors may undergo curative allogenic bone marrow transplant.
- Aspirin (ASA) 81 mg for all patients.
- Allopurinol for hyperuricemia.
- Antihistamines for pruritus.
- Prognosis
  - CML or primary myelofibrosis evolves in some patients.
  - AML develops in 5% of patients.
  - Still, thrombosis most common cause of death.
  - Survival near 15 years or more (data varies).

Essential Thrombocytosis
- Epidemiology, etiology, and pathophysiology (Table 7-15)
  - Cause unknown.
  - Clonal stem cell disorder causing increased megakaryocytes in bone marrow result in peripheral thrombocytosis.
  - *JAK2* mutation likely plays a role here as well; present in 50% of patients.
  - Mutation in MPL (thrombopoietin receptor) present in 4% and likely also plays a role.
  - Incidence 1 to 2/100,000.
  - Median age of onset 50 to 60 years.
  - More common in women than in men.
- Presentation
  - Typically discovered incidentally on CBC
  - Thrombosis
    - Major cause of morbidity and mortality
    - Arterial more than venous; atypical venous sites such as hepatic veins
  - Erythromelalgia
  - Hemorrhage
    - Mucosal and central nervous system (CNS)
    - Related to qualitative platelet defect and acquired von Willebrand disease
  - Splenomegaly: submassive; 10% of patients

TABLE 7-16. RISK STRATIFICATION FOR PATIENTS WITH ESSENTIAL THROMBOCYTHEMIA

	No High-Risk Features	
High Risk	**Low Risk**	**Intermediate Risk**
Age >60 years	Age <40 years	Age 40–60 years
Prior thrombosis		
Platelets >1500 × 10⁹/L		

From Lichtman MA, Kipps TJ, Uri Seligsohn U, et al. *Williams Hematology*. 8th ed. New York: McGraw-Hill; 2010.

- Diagnosis
  - CBC showing elevated platelet level (may be more than 2×10^6) and often leukocytosis. Hct normal.
  - Peripheral smear shows normal RBCs, normal and giant platelets, and immature myeloid forms.
  - Bone marrow with increased megakaryocytes:
    - Philadelphia chromosome absent (distinguishes from CML). Follow up with fluorescence in situ hybridization for bcr-abl chromosome translocation as this may be present in absence of Philadelphia chromosome.
    - May be difficult to aspirate because of hypercellularity.
- Management
  - Partially dependent on risk of thrombosis (Table 7-16).
  - Most patients should receive ASA 81–100 mg unless contraindicated. Can increase risk of hemorrhage.
  - Bone marrow suppressive therapy indicated for patients at high risk of thrombus.
    - Hydroxyurea to 0.5 to 2 g/day to keep platelet count less than 500,000 per microliter
    - Anagrelide may be added if hydroxyurea yields anemia with suboptimal platelet response.
  - Emerging role for peginterferon alfa-2a.
  - For severe bleeding, plateletpheresis can lower counts rapidly but is rarely used.
  - Aminocaproic acid can be given perioperatively to reduce risk of hemorrhage.
- Prognosis
  - Attempts to define risk factors for complications have been variably successful (Table 7-17).
  - Appears not to shorten overall survival.
  - Risk of progression to myelofibrosis is 10% to 15%.
  - Risk of progression to AML is 1% to 5%.

Primary Myelofibrosis
- Epidemiology, etiology, and pathophysiology
  - Also known as agnogenic myeloid metaplasia.
  - Transformation of a multipotent hematopoietic stem cell.
  - Increased release of platelet-derived growth factor leading to marrow fibrosis.
  - Liver, spleen, lymph nodes become sites of extramedullary hematopoiesis.
  - *JAK2* mutations again appear to play some role.
  - Affects adults, usually older than 50 years of age.
  - Incidence 0.5 to 1.5/100,000
  - Occurs in men more than women.
- Presentation
  - Fatigue caused by anemia.
  - Abdominal fullness caused by splenomegaly.
  - Extramedullary hematopoiesis may lead to portal hypertension, bone pain, and transverse myelitis.
  - With progressive disease, bleeding may ensue.

TABLE 7-17. RISK FACTORS FOR COMPLICATIONS IN ESSENTIAL THROMBOCYTHEMIA

Thrombosis	Hemorrhage	Myelofibrotic Transformation	Acute Myeloid Leukemia
Age >60 years	Marrow fibrosis[b]	Disease duration	Disease duration
Prior thrombosis		Anagrelide therapy[c]	Genotoxic therapy
Cardiovascular risk[a]		Marrow fibrosis[b]	Use of >1 cytoreductive agent
Leukocytosis[b]			
Marrow fibrosis[b]			
JAK2 V617F mutation[d]			

[a]Diabetes, hypertension, hypercholesterolemia, or tobacco use.
[b]At diagnosis.
[c]Compared to hydroxyurea.
[d]Venous thrombosis and total thrombotic events.
From Lichtman MA, Kipps TJ, Uri Seligsohn U, et al. *Williams Hematology*. 8th ed. New York: McGraw-Hill; 2010.

- Diagnosis
  - Must distinguish from other causes of myelofibrosis (Table 7-18).
  - CBC usually shows anemia (normocytic, normochromic) with normal to elevated WBC and platelet levels.
  - Pancytopenia occurs in 10% of patients.
  - May have positive antinuclear antibody and rheumatoid factors.

TABLE 7-18. DISORDERS CAUSING MYELOFIBROSIS

Malignant	Nonmalignant
Acute leukemia (lymphocytic, myelogenous, megakaryocytic)	HIV infection
	Hyperparathyroidism
Chronic myelogenous leukemia	Renal osteodystrophy
Hairy cell leukemia	Systemic lupus erythematosus
Hodgkin disease	Tuberculosis
Idiopathic myelofibrosis	Vitamin D deficiency
Lymphoma	Thorium dioxide exposure
Multiple myeloma	Gray platelet syndrome
Myelodysplasia	
Metastatic carcinoma	
Polycythemia vera	
Systemic mastocytosis	

HIV, human immunodeficiency virus.
From Longo DL, et al., eds. *Harrison's Principles of Internal Medicine*. 18th ed. New York: McGraw-Hill; 2012:901.

TABLE 7-19. RISK STRATIFICATION FOR PRIMARY MYELOFIBROSIS

Risk Factors	Frequency of Occurrence (%)
Age >65 years	45
Constitutional symptoms	26
Hemoglobin <10 g/dL	35
WBC >25 × 109/L	10
Blood blasts >10%	36

Risk Groups	No. of Factors	Proportion of Patients (%)	Median Survival (years)
Low	0	22	11
Intermediate-1	1	29	8
Intermediate-2	2	28	4
High	≥3	21	2

WBC, white blood cell count.
From Cervantes F, et al. *Blood.* 2009;113:2895.

- Peripheral smear: tear drops, nucleated RBCs. Also myelocytes, promyelocytes, and myeloblasts are possible.
- Increased CD43+ cells.
- 7. Alkaline phosphatase, LDH, and reticulocyte levels may be elevated.
- Hepatosplenomegaly: likely massive splenomegaly.
- "Dry tap": inability to aspirate bone marrow because of fibrosis.
- Sclerosis of bones visible on x-ray.
- Management [24]
  - Ranges from observation to drug therapy to allogenic stem cell transplant (curative) depending on risk stratification (Table 7-19).
  - Low or intermediate risk: grade 1 disease
    - Transfusional support
    - Thalidomide plus prednisone or androgen (danazol)
    - Hydroxyurea, target dose 1500 mg, for splenomegaly
  - Intermediate risk: grade 2 or high-risk disease
    - Bone marrow transplant
    - Symptomatic therapy
- Prognosis (see Table 7-19)
  - Dependent on risk category
  - Median survival from diagnosis is 5 years
  - In 10% of patients transforms to AML

CML (see Leukemias)

HYPERCOAGULABLE DISORDERS

Can be split into disorders that cause mostly venous thrombi and those that cause venous and arterial thrombi.

- Venous hypercoagulable disorders include:
  - Factor V Leiden mutation
  - Prothrombin gene mutation

- Protein C deficiency
- Protein S deficiency
- Dysfibrinogenemia

Factor V Leiden Mutation

- Most common cause of inherited thrombophilia, risk of venous thrombosis increased in patients on oral contraceptives. Codon mutation leads to an amino acid substitution rendering factor V resistant to cleavage by activated protein C.
- Screen with an activated protein C resistance test, which if positive, should trigger factor V Leiden mutation testing.

Prothrombin Gene Mutation

- Prothrombin G20210A consists of a mutation in a codon that decreases the rate of breakdown of prothrombin.
- Polymerase chain reaction testing can detect the presence of the mutation at the DNA level.

Protein C Deficiency

- Inherited type I deficiency consists of decreased levels of protein C.
- Inherited type II deficiency consists of normal levels but decreased functional activity of protein C.
- Acquired protein C deficiency can be seen in liver disease, sepsis, disseminated intravascular coagulation (DIC), acute respiratory distress syndrome, and secondary to renal losses caused by the nephrotic syndrome.
- Coumadin skin necrosis can occur in patients with protein C deficiency as warfarin (Coumadin) can inhibit protein C faster than factor VII. Bridging for 24 hours with heparin and low-molecular-weight heparin (LMWH) can avoid the problem.

Protein S Deficiency

- Inherited type I deficiency consists of decreased levels of protein S.
- Inherited type II deficiency consists of normal levels but decreased functional activity of protein S.
- Acquired protein S deficiency can be seen in DIC, HIV, the nephrotic syndrome, and liver disease.

Antithrombin Deficiency

- Inherited type I deficiency consists of decreased levels of antithrombin.
- Inherited type II deficiency consists of normal levels but decreased functional activity of antithrombin.
- Acquired deficiency can be seen in DIC, liver disease, and the nephrotic syndrome.

Testing and Treatment of Venous Hypercoagulable States

- Testing should be held in the acute state and for 2 weeks after completion of treatment as levels and functional assays can be affected by treatment or venous thromboembolic disease.
- The only exceptions are genetic testing for factor V Leiden mutation and the prothrombin gene mutation, which can be done at any point.
- Treatment consists of unfractionated heparin and LMWH or fondaparinux followed by warfarin (Coumadin) with a target INR of 2 to 3.

Antiphospholipid Antibody (APL-Ab) Syndrome

- Syndrome causes venous and arterial thrombi.

Clinical Manifestations

- Deep vein thrombosis, pulmonary embolism, stroke, and pregnancy loss because of placental insufficiency.

- Hematologic abnormalities include thrombocytopenia and a thrombotic microangiopathy.
- The most common skin manifestation is livedo reticularis.
- Rarely catastrophic, APL-Ab syndrome can occur with thrombi in multiple organ systems.

Diagnostic Criteria

- Two major components are needed:
  - Occurrence of either vascular thrombi or pregnancy morbidity
  - Occurrence of at least one characteristic antibody confirmed again on repeat testing at least 12 weeks apart
- Characteristic antibodies include lupus anticoagulant, anticardiolipin (IgG or IgM) or anti-β_2-glycoprotein (IgG or IgM).

Laboratory Findings

- Thrombocytopenia and a prolonged prothrombin time (PT) or partial prothrombin time (PTT) can alert to the possibility of APL-Ab syndrome.
- APL antibodies interact with the phospholipid matrix used in testing for PT and PTT and thus can prolong both in vitro whereas APL antibodies cause a hypercoagulable state in vivo.
- Mixing studies for coagulation panels including the patient's plasma and normal plasma should be done to differentiate between factor deficiency, which corrects with mixing, and the presence of an APL antibody, which does not correct with mixing.

Treatment

- Unfractionated heparin or LMWH or fondaparinux followed by warfarin (Coumadin) with a target INR of 2 to 3.

TTP and Hemolytic Uremic Syndrome (HUS)

- TTP and HUS represent a spectrum.
- TTP is seen more often in adults and is more often associated with CNS disease, whereas HUS is more commonly seen in children and associated with more severe renal failure as well as diarrhea from *Escherichia coli* O157H7.
- The classical pentad below is rarely seen:
  - CNS changes
  - Renal dysfunction
  - Microangiopathic hemolytic anemia
  - Fever
  - Thrombocytopenia
- TTP and HUS should be considered in any patient with thrombocytopenia and a microangiopathic hemolytic anemia.

Clinical Manifestations

- Fatigue, malaise, and a wide spectrum of CNS complaints can be seen, including confusion and headache most commonly, but also more rarely transient ischemic attack, stroke, grand mal seizures, and coma.

Physical Examination Findings

- Include fever, purpura, and focal neurologic findings

Laboratory Findings

- Evidence of hemolysis such as an elevated LDH, low haptoglobin, elevated indirect and total bilirubin.
- Evidence of a microangiopathic hemolytic anemia on peripheral smear with a schistocyte count greater than 1%, RBC fragments, and thrombocytopenia.
- In contrast to DIC , TTP and HUS presents with normal PT and PTT.
- Evidence of renal dysfunction can also be seen especially in HUS and quinine-related TTP.

Associated Conditions

- Causative meds include mitomycin, gemcitabine, cyclosporine, clopidogrel, ticlopidine, and quinine.
- Underlying causative systemic disorders include *E. coli* O157H7, HIV, pregnancy, and advanced malignancies.

Idiopathic TTP

- Idiopathic TTP is associated with either a congenital marked deficiency of *ADAMTS13* or antibodies directed to it. *ADAMTS13* is a cleaving protease that when deficient leads to the accumulation of large von Willebrand factor (VWF) multimers that activate TTP.
- Testing for *ADAMTS13* has poor sensitivity and specificity. Results of the test take time to return and should not affect the decision to start treatment, which should not be delayed.

Treatment

- Transfusing platelets should be done only in the presence of bleeding or in preparation for invasive procedures.
- Plasma exchange should be initiated emergently if TTP and HUS are suspected as it can be lifesaving.
- Poorly responsive or refractory patients can be treated by increasing the frequency of plasma exchange as well as adding corticosteroids, rituximab, or cyclosporine.

Immune (Idiopathic) Thrombocytopenic Purpura (ITP)

- Defined as thrombocytopenia caused by an autoimmune process with IgG antibody production against platelet membrane glycoproteins especially glycoproteins II b and III a (GPIIb/IIIa).
- Thrombocytopenia must be isolated; in the presence of blood loss, can have a concomitant anemia.
- Clinical presentation consists commonly of epistaxis, gingival bleeding, or menorrhagia and more rarely GI bleeding or hematuria. Intracerebral hemorrhage is exceedingly rare but potentially fatal.
- Physical examination findings include petechiae, purpura, and bruising. Purpura is asymptomatic and nonpalpable in contrast to vasculitis.
- ITP is a diagnosis of exclusion. Drug-related thrombocytopenia (heparin, co-trimoxazole [Bactrim], histamine-2 blockers, antibiotics) as well as infections (HIV, hepatitis C virus), hypersplenism, myelodysplasia, and pseudothrombocytopenia must be excluded.
- Autoantibody testing lacks sensitivity and specificity to make the diagnosis.
- Bone marrow biopsy is not necessary except when there are abnormalities in 2 bone marrow cell lines or if ITP is a new diagnosis in an older patient.
- Treatment should be initiated for platelets less than 30,000 in adults because of the variable course in that population. Treatment should also be initiated for a platelet count less than 10,000/microliter.
- First-line treatment consists of 1 mg/kg prednisone with taper after several weeks. Second-line treatment consists of splenectomy, IVIG, or anti-D Ig in patients who are D positive and have a spleen. Rituximab and thrombopoietin agonists are third-line treatments.

TRANSFUSION AND BLOOD PRODUCTS

- Fresh frozen plasma (FFP):
  - Preparation:
    - Derived most often from single units of whole blood.
    - Acellular.
    - Frozen within 8 hours of collection
    - Usable for 1 year.
    - Can be transfused up to 5 days after being thawed, if kept in fridge.
    - Approximately 250 cc per unit.
    - Needs ABO compatibility, but not cross-matching and Rh typing.
  - Ingredients:
    - Contains all coagulation factors in the original unit of blood.
  - Indications:
    - Vitamin K deficiency
    - Liver failure
    - Dilutional coagulopathy caused by massive transfusion

- Inherited factor XI deficiency
- Warfarin overdose
- Not for treatment of single-factor deficiencies or as a volume expander.
- Not for minimally elevated INR (eg, <1.6).
  - Dosing:
    - No universal dosing guideline available.
    - We recommend using the following formula:

$$\text{INR before 1 FFP} - \text{INR after 1 FFP} = 0.6 \times \text{INR before FFP} - 0.7$$

  - Product-specific risks of transfusion (see section on transfusion reactions for more details):
    - No risk of transmitting intracellular viruses because FFP is acellular.
    - Risk of volume overload.
- Cryoprecipitate:
  - Preparation:
    - Precipitate from FFP thawed at 4°C (39.2°F).
    - One bag of cryoprecipitate is derived from 1 unit of FFP.
    - 10–15 cc per unit.
  - Ingredients:
    - Contains all of factors VIII, XIII, fibrinogen (200 mg per unit), fibronectin, and VWF that exist in 1 unit of FFP.
  - Indications:
    - von Willebrand disease
    - Uremic bleeding
    - Deficiencies of fibrinogen and factor XIII
    - Not recommended for treatment of hemophilia A
  - Dosing:
    - Ten bags of cryoglobulin increases the fibrinogen by 70 mg/dL in a 70-kg recipient.
  - Product-specific risks of transfusion:
    - Same infection risk as with 1 unit of FFP.
- Platelets:
  - Preparation:
    - Two ways to prepare:
      - Pooled from whole blood: multiple donors required.
      - Apheresis: single donor.
    - ABO compatibility preferred.
    - Frequently leukoreduced and irradiated.
  - Ingredients:
    - Each apheresis unit is equivalent to 6 units of whole blood-derived platelets.
    - Slightly cellular (which may make RBC transfusion difficult in future by sensitization) and with some plasma.
  - Indications:
    - Platelet level less than 10,000 per microliter for all platelet
    - Platelet level less than 20,000 with active infection
    - Platelet level less than 50,000 with active bleeding, invasive procedure, or qualitative intrinsic platelet disorder
    - Platelet level less than 100,000 with CNS injury or procedure
    - Platelet level more than 100,000 with active bleeding and platelet dysfunction (congenital, aspirin use, uremia)
    - Not recommended in TTP, HUS, heparin-induced thrombocytopenia, and DIC (unless life-threatening hemorrhage).
    - Ineffective if rapid platelet destruction:
      - Sepsis
      - Hyperthermia

- Hypersplenism
- Drug-induced thrombocytopenia
- Alloantibodies against platelets
- Dosing:
  - One whole-blood derived unit increases platelet level by 5,000 to 10,000
  - One apheresis unit increases platelet level by 30,000 1 hour posttransfusion
  - Back to baseline after 72 hours
- Product-specific risks of transfusion:
  - If platelet destruction caused by alloantibodies, use single donor human leukocyte antigen (HLA)-matched platelets.
  - Risk of infection lower with apheresis platelets.
  - Leukoreduction minimizes the risks of:
    - Cytomegalovirus transmission
    - HLA alloimmunization
    - Febrile reactions
    - Immunomodulation
    - Lung injury
  - Transfusion-associated graft-versus-host disease: minimized by irradiation.
- Transfusion-related reactions:
  - Febrile nonhemolytic reaction:
    - Most common reaction
    - Posttransfusion 1 to 6 hours
    - With platelet and packed RBC transfusion
    - Etiology:
      - Caused by cytokines generated during storage of products
    - Treatment:
      - Benign
      - Stop transfusion and determine it is not a hemolytic reaction
      - Antipyretics
      - Meperidine if severe rigors
      - No evidence for prophylactic antihistamine or acetaminophen.
- Acute hemolytic reaction:
  - Diagnosis:
    - Classic but rare triad: fever, flank pain, hemoglobinuria
    - Pink plasma
    - Direct Coombs test positive
    - Check direct Coombs test and plasma-free Hb from the other arm
    - Type and cross match from the other arm
    - Check urinalysis
  - Etiology
    - ABO incompatibility
  - Treatment:
    - Medical emergency
    - Stop transfusion
    - Check airway, breathing, circulation
    - Normal saline 100 to 200 cc/h
- Delayed hemolytic reaction:
  - Posttransfusion 2 to 10 days
  - Etiology:
    - Anamnestic antibody production
    - Antibodies in Kidd blood group and Rh system
    - Extravascular hemolysis
  - Diagnosis:
    - New positive direct Coombs or suspicious antibodies

- Anaphylactic reaction:
  - Seconds to minutes from transfusion initiation
  - Typical anaphylaxis
  - Treatment:
    - Stop transfusion
    - Check airway, breathing, circulation
    - Fluid resuscitation
    - Epinephrine intramuscularly 0.3 mL of 1:1000 solution
- Urticarial reactions:
  - Etiology:
    - Allergenic substances in donor plasma
  - Treatment:
    - Stop transfusion
    - If severe: diphenhydramine 25 to 50 mg orally or IV
    - Continue transfusion once symptoms improved.
- Hypotensive reaction:
  - Minutes from onset of transfusion
  - Most common with platelet transfusion
  - Etiology:
    - Mediated by bradykinin
    - Treatment: Stop transfusion.
- Transfusion-related acute lung injury:
  - During or within 6 hours of transfusion
  - Possible with any product
  - Etiology:
    - Unknown
  - Diagnosis:
    - Acute respiratory distress syndrome picture
    - Sudden onset respiratory distress
    - Noncardiogenic pulmonary edema
  - Treatment:
    - Supportive
    - No further plasma-containing product from the implicated donor
- Posttransfusion purpura:
  - Posttransfusion 5 to 10 days
  - Usually in women sensitized in pregnancy
  - Severe
  - Etiology:
    - Alloantibody against human platelet antigen-1a
  - Treatment:
    - IVIG

REFERENCES

1. Provan, Lancet 2000; Alleyne, Am J of Med, 2003; Haematology ASH Educ Prog 2003
2. Andrews, NEJM 1999
3. CMDT; Williams Hematology
4. CMDT
5. Kaferle, Am Fam Phys 2009; CMDT; Harrison's Online
6. Provan, Lancet 2000; CMDT; Harrison's Online
7. Provan, Lancet 2000; CMDT
8. Harrison's Online, Williams Hematology
9. Harrisons Online
10. Stuart, Lancet 2004; Steinberg, NEJM 1999
11. Castro, Blood 1994

12. Adams, NEJM 1998
13. Gladwin, NEJM 2004
14. Klings ES, Wyszynski DF, Nolan VG, Steinberg MH. Abnormal pulmonary function in adults with sickle cell anemia. Am J Respir Crit Care Med 2006; 173:1264.
15. Cochrane Database 2006, 2007;
16. Gladwin, NEJM 2008
17. Adams, NEJM 1998; Adams NEJM, 2010
18. Brawley, Ann Int Med 2008
19. Lottenberg, Hematology 2005
20. Platt, NEJM 2008
21. Lottenberg, Hematology 2005; Josephson, Transfusion Medicine Reviews 2007
22. Adams, NEJM 2005
23. CMDT; Harrison's Online; Williams Hematology Online
24. Tefferi, Am J or Hematology 2011

CHAPTER 8

Infectious Diseases

Stephanie B. Troy, Catherine J. Derber, L. Beth Gadkowski, Ronald W. Flenner, and Edward C. Oldfield

INFECTIOUS DISEASES: GENERAL PRINCIPLES

History, Physical, and Diagnostic Tests

History: In addition to the standard history of present illness, the following information is important:

- *Symptoms suggesting systemic infection*: fever (quality, timing, duration), chills, sweats, myalgias, arthralgias, fatigue, decreased appetite, weight loss, mental status changes.
- *Localizing symptoms*: pain anywhere, headache, vision changes, neck stiffness, sinus symptoms, sore throat, cough (productive or nonproductive), dyspnea, abdominal pain (location and quality), diarrhea (watery, black, and/or bloody), nausea and vomiting, pelvic pain, dysuria, urinary frequency, urethral and vaginal discharge, penile and vaginal lesions, rash, ulcer.
- *Immunocompromising factors*: human immunodeficiency virus (HIV) (CD4 count), congenital immunodeficiency, history of transplant, cancer (currently undergoing chemotherapy), diabetes, rheumatologic/inflammatory disease requiring immunosuppressive drugs (steroids, tumor necrosis factor [TNF] inhibitors, etc.).
- *Prosthetic material in the body*: central lines, dialysis catheter, arteriovenous graft, inferior vena cava filter, prosthetic heart valve, pacemaker, automatic implantable cardioverter-defibrillator (AICD), prosthetic joint, surgical screws and rods, ventricle-to-peritoneal-cavity shunt.
- *Exposure history*: any travel in the past 2 years (location, urban or rural, diet while traveling), pets and animal exposure, insect bites (ticks, mosquitos), recreational activities (gardening, camping, hunting, swimming in fresh or salt water), dietary habits (unpasteurized milk, source of food consumed), occupational exposures, household contacts (are there young children in the house?), sick contacts, recent antibiotics, history of drug abuse (history of intravenous [IV] drug use?).
- *Sexual history*: sex with men or women, protection used, number of partners (were partners known well by patient?), type of sex (vaginal, anal, oral), history of sexually transmitted diseases (STDs).
- *Allergy history*: If antibiotic allergy reported, note reaction experienced with offending drug.

Physical examination: In addition to the standard physical examination, the following are important to note:

- Signs that may indicate HIV or acquired immunodeficiency syndrome (AIDS): wasting, thrush, lymphadenopathy (cervical, axillary, and inguinal), skin lesions (molluscum-like lesions, seborrheic dermatitis, herpetic outbreaks, papular eruptions, vascular or bruiselike lesions).
- Portals of entry for infection: poor dentition; onychomycosis; lines, catheters, tubes (when were they placed?); areas of skin breakdown (decubitus ulcers).
- Signs indicative of specific infections: (See sections on specific infections below).

Diagnostic tests: **Localizing symptoms and signs should direct the diagnostic workup** (See sections on specific infections below). In hospitalized patients suspected of having infection without a known source, the following can be ordered as a start:

- Complete blood count with manual differential
- Comprehensive metabolic panel
- Urinalysis and urine culture
- Blood cultures (2 sets)
- Chest x-ray

TABLE 8-1. STERILE VERSUS NONSTERILE SITES

Sterile Sites	Nonsterile Sites
Blood	Respiratory secretions
Bone marrow	Throat swabs
Cerebrospinal fluid	Wound and ulcer swabs
Pericardial fluid	Genital swabs
Pleural fluid	Urine in the presence of a Foley catheter
Peritoneal fluid	Any normally sterile site connected to the environment by a tube or catheter
Joint fluid	
Urine in the absence of a Foley catheter	Stool
Unexposed bone and tissue	

INFECTIOUS DISEASES: GENERAL PRINCIPLES—CULTURES AND GRAM STAINS

If possible, always obtain cultures prior to starting antibiotics.

- Positive cultures from sterile sites that are properly collected usually indicate infection.
  - Improperly collected samples obtained percutaneously can be contaminated by common skin flora-like coagulase-negative staphylococcus and bacillus.
    - Order blood cultures in duplicate sets (this increases the yield of true pathogens, and contamination is less likely if the same organism grows from both sets).
    - Rarely, media used in the microbiology laboratory can be contaminated.
- Positive cultures from nonsterile sites *do not* indicate infection unless there are clinical symptoms and signs of infection (positive cultures from nonsterile sites may equal colonization) (Table 8-1).

Gram stains from preliminary cultures can help guide antibiotic therapy. In general:

- Gram-positive cocci
  - Clusters: *Staphylococcus* (*Staphylococcus aureus* or coagulase negative staphylococcus)
  - Pairs or chains: *Streptococcus* or *Enterococcus*
    - α-hemolytic: *Streptococcus pneumoniae* and *Streptococcus viridans*
    - β-hemolytic: group A (*Streptococcus pyogenes*) and group B streptococci
    - γ-hemolytic: *Enterococcus*
- Gram-negative cocci: *Neisseria*, *Moraxella*, or *Acinetobacter* (pleomorphic)
- Gram-positive rods:
  - Box-car shaped: *Clostridium*, *Bacillus*, or *Lactobacillus*
  - Small, coccobacilli: *Listeria*
  - Branched: *Actinomyces* or *Nocardia*
- Gram-negative rods (GNRs):
  - Lactose-fermenting GNR: enteric organisms like *Escherichia coli*, *Klebsiella*, *Enterobacter*, and *Citrobacter* (not pseudomonas)
  - Nonlactose-fermenting GNR: *Pseudomonas*, *Acinetobacter*, *Proteus* (*Amoeba*), *Stenotrophomonas*, *Serratia*, *Salmonella*, *Shigella*
  - Small coccobacilli: *Haemophilus*, *Brucella*, or *Acinetobacter*
- Yeast: *Candida*

While anaerobes grow better in anaerobic culture and aerobes grow better in aerobic culture, it is possible for aerobes and anaerobes to grow on either aerobic or anaerobic culture

INFECTIOUS DISEASES: GENERAL PRINCIPLES—ANTIBIOTIC CHOICE

Factors that influence antibiotic choice:

- Causative pathogen
  - For empiric treatment, cover most likely pathogens at source or site of infection
    - Oropharynx: streptococci and anaerobes

TABLE 8-2. BACTERICIDAL VERSUS BACTERIOSTATIC DRUGS

Bactericidal	Bacteriostatic
β-lactams[a] (penicillins, cephalosporins, carbapenems, aztreonam)	Macrolides (eg, azithromycin)
	Tetracyclines
Aminoglycosides	Tigecycline
Trimethoprim, sulfa	Clindamycin
Vancomycin[a]	Linezolid (except cidal against streptococci)
Quinupristin, dalfopristin	
Daptomycin	
Fluoroquinolones	
Metronidazole	

[a]Penicillins or vancomycin are bactericidal for enterococcus only in combination with an aminoglycoside.

- Skin (nondiabetics): *Staphylococcus*, especially methicillin-resistant *S. aureus* (MRSA); and *Streptococcus*
- Osteomyelitis (hematogenous spread): often *S. aureus*
- Gastrointestinal (GI) tract: enteric GNRs and anaerobes
- Urinary tract infections: enteric GNRs
- Narrow coverage when pathogen is identified
- Broad coverage does not offer better coverage
  - Nafcillin and cefazolin are superior to vancomycin for methicillin-susceptible *S. aureus* (MSSA)
  - When susceptible, ampicillin is the best treatment for *Enterococcus*
- Broad coverage can lead to antibiotic resistance and *Clostridium difficile* infection.
- Site of infection
  - Not all antibiotics work in or reach all places. For example:
    - Moxifloxacin, tigecycline, and all antifungals except fluconazole do not achieve adequate urine levels.
    - Daptomycin is inactivated by surfactant in the lungs.
    - Nitrofurantoin can only be used for simple urinary tract infections (UTIs) (does not work in tissue).
    - Aminoglycosides have poor tissue penetration (except for the renal cortex).
- Severity of infection
  - IV antibiotics are preferred for severe infections (septic shock, meningitis, endocarditis, osteomyelitis) and when ability to absorb orally (PO) is in question.
  - Bactericidal antibiotics are preferred for bacteremia in a neutropenic host, meningitis, and endocarditis (Table 8-2).
- Drug allergies and interactions
  - A true penicillin allergy has 4% to 10% cross-reactivity with cephalosporins and 1% to 9% cross-reactivity with carbapenems (negligible cross-reactivity with aztreonam). If needed, desensitization can be done in the intensive care unit (ICU) for an immunoglobulin E (IgE)-mediated allergy.
  - Many antimicrobials interact with other drugs the patient may need (rifamycins, fluoroquinolones, azoles, macrolides, and protease inhibitors are the worst offenders (see http://accessmedicine.com/content.aspx?aID=9092608&searchStr=drug+interactions).
- Renal and hepatic function
  - Trimethoprim sulfa, amphotericin, cidofovir, and aminoglycosides can cause renal impairment and should be avoided in patients with renal disease.
  - Nitrofurantoin is ineffective if creatinine clearance is less than 50 mL/min.
  - Many drugs need dose adjustment for renal dysfunction (see www.globalrph.com).
  - A number of drugs need dose adjustment or avoidance for hepatic dysfunction (for example, isoniazid [INH], rifampin, ceftriaxone, nafcillin, clindamycin, metronidazole).

TABLE 8-3. COMMON RESISTANT BACTERIA AND ANTIBIOTICS THAT MAY BE EFFECTIVE AGAINST THEM

MRSA	Pseudomonas Aeruginosa	VRE
Vancomycin	Piperacillin	Daptomycin
Daptomycin	Piperacillin-tazobactam	Linezolid
Linezolid (IV or PO)	Ticarcillin	Tigecycline
Tigecycline	Ticarcillin-clavulanic acid	Quinupristin-dalfopristin (only *Enterococcus faecium*, not *E. faecalis*)
Quinupristin-dalfopristin	Carbapenems except ertapenem (imipenem, meropenem, and doripenem)	Ceftobiprole (only *E. faecalis*, not *E. faecium*)
Fifth-generation cephalosporins (ceftobiprole and ceftaroline)	Aztreonam	When susceptible, ampicillin or penicillin ± an aminoglycoside is the treatment of choice.
Telavancin	Ceftazidime	
For community-acquired MRSA, the following might also work:	Cefepime	Alternate, less trusted agents: tetracyclines and chloramphenicol.
tetracyclines (IV or PO), trimethoprim sulfa (IV or PO), clindamycin (IV or PO)	Ceftobiprole	
	Ciprofloxacin (IV or PO)	
	Levofloxacin (IV or PO)	
	Aminoglycosides	
	Colistin	

IV, intravenous; MRSA, methicillin-resistant *Staphylococcus aureus*; PO, oral; VRE, vancomycin-resistant *Enterococcus*.

- Logistics and preparation for discharge
  - Sometimes IV antibiotics can be transitioned to oral after the patient improves (not with endocarditis or meningitis).
    - Oral fluoroquinolones and linezolid have excellent bioavailability.
  - Infusion centers often only provide IV antibiotics that are given once (or at most twice) daily.
    - Daptomycin, ertapenem, and ceftriaxone (nonmeningitis dosing) are given daily.
  - For hemodialysis, antibiotics that can be dosed with or after dialysis; without additional doses are preferable (vancomycin, cefazolin, ceftazidime, cefepime, ampicillin and sulbactam [Unasyn], fluconazole, daptomycin, and the aminoglycosides)
  - See Table 8-3 for antibiotics that are often effective for common resistant bacteria (always check the susceptibilities of the specific organism when they are available)

CENTRAL NERVOUS SYSTEM (CNS) INFECTIONS: MENINGITIS, ENCEPHALITIS, AND BRAIN ABSCESS

- Meningitis: inflammation of the meninges surrounding the brain and the spinal cord
- Encephalitis: inflammation of the brain
- Brain abscess: localized collection of pus within the brain parenchyma

There is frequently overlap (meningoencephalitis, brain abscess with meningitis, etc.).

- Common complaints and review of systems
  - Meningitis: the classic triad of fever, neck stiffness, and altered mental status; headache; photophobia; focal neurologic deficits; seizures; lethargy
  - Encephalitis: altered mental status, seizures, focal neurologic deficits, fever, headache
  - Brain abscess: headache; fever; focal neurologic deficits; seizures; neck stiffness; lethargy; nausea and vomiting; prior ear, sinus, dental infection (if direct spread); symptoms of infection elsewhere in the body (if hematogenous spread)
- Physical examination
  - Signs suggestive of meningitis in particular
    - Nuchal rigidity: inability or reluctance to touch chin to chest
      - Brudzinski's sign: spontaneous flexion of hips with passive neck flexion
      - Kernig's sign: reluctance to fully extend knee when hip is flexed 90 degrees

TABLE 8-4. EXPECTED CEREBRAL SPINAL FLUID FINDINGS[a]

	Bacterial Meningitis	Fungal or TB Meningitis	Viral Meningitis or Encephalitis
WBC count	25–10,000 (usually >1000)	10–500	10–500
Predominant cells	Neutrophils	Lymphocytes	Lymphocytes
Glucose	Usually low	Often low	Rarely low
Protein	Elevated	Moderately elevated (<500)	Normal to slightly elevated
Opening pressure	Usually elevated	Often elevated	Rarely elevated

TB, tuberculous; WBC, white blood cell.
[a]Exceptions are possible.

- Jolt accentuation of headache: worsening of headache by horizontal rotation of the head 2 to 3 times per second
- Signs suggestive of brain abscess in particular
  - Papilledema
  - If direct spread: sinus pain; poor dentition; or ear pain, drainage, dysfunction
  - If hematogenous spread: signs of infection elsewhere in the body (particularly lung infection in immunocompromised hosts or endocarditis)
- Signs suggestive of CNS infection in general
  - Focal neurologic deficits (cranial nerve palsies, hemiparesis, etc.)
  - Altered mental status (disorientation to obtundation)
  - Fever
- Diagnostic tests
  - *Lumbar puncture* (LP) with opening pressure: cerebral spinal fluid (CSF) should be sent for cell count and differential, protein, glucose, Gram stain, and culture (and other tests based on risk factors) (Table 8-4)
    - Red blood cells and protein are often increased in herpes simplex virus (HSV) encephalitis.
    - Eosinophilia may be present in fungal, tuberculosus (TB), or parasitic meningitis
  - Other CSF tests:
    - If encephalitis is suspected, always check a CSF HSV polymerase chain reaction (PCR)
    - If CSF analysis suggests fungal or TB meningitis, check CSF fungal and acid-fast bacillus (AFB) cultures, CSF mycobacterium tuberculosis PCR (~50% sensitivity), CSF VDRL, CSF and serum cryptococcal antigen, and (depending on residence and travel history) CSF and serum coccidioides immunodiffusion and complement fixation antibodies and/or CSF and urine histoplasma antigen.
    - If TB meningitis is suspected, yield increases with 3 consecutive daily large volume LPs with 10- to 15-mL CSF sent each tap for AFB smear and culture.
    - If viral meningitis is suspected, check a CSF enteroviral PCR.
- Brain imaging
  - In patients with certain risk factors (age ≥60 years, history of CNS disease, immunosuppressed state, seizure within the last week, papilledema, altered mental status, or focal neurologic deficits), a head computed tomography (CT) should be obtained prior to LP to rule out increased intracranial pressure (LP poses slight risk of brain herniation in the presence of increased intracranial pressure). In these cases, do not wait for LP to start antibiotics if meningitis is suspected.
  - Otherwise, brain magnetic resonance imaging (MRI) is more sensitive and specific than a head CT.
- Blood cultures (obtain prior to antibiotics)

TABLE 8-5. EMPIRIC INTRAVENOUS TREATMENT FOR BACTERIAL MENINGITIS

Patient Age	1 month–50 years old	>50 years old	Special circumstances: trauma or neurosurgery
Treatment	Vancomycin 1 g q 12 h + ceftriaxone 2 g IV every 12 h	Vancomycin + ceftriaxone + ampicillin 2 g every 4 h	Vancomycin + (cefepime, ceftazidime, or meropenem, all 2 g IV every 8 h)

- Common etiologies
  - Acute bacterial meningitis:
    - *S. pneumoniae* and *Neisseria meningitidis*
    - If patient is older than 50 years of age, *S. pneumoniae, N. meningitidis,* and *Listeria monocytogenes* and aerobic GNRs
    - If head trauma or postneurosurgery: Streptococci, staphylococci, *Haemophilus influenzae,* aerobic GNRs (including pseudomonas), and *Propionibacterium*
  - Nonbacterial meningitis: viruses (enterovirus, primary HIV), tuberculosis, fungi (*Cryptococcus, Coccidioides, Histoplasma*), syphilis, parasites (neurocysticercosis), parameningeal infection, malignancy.
  - Encephalitis: usually viral (HSV 5%–10% of all cases), but etiology not found in more than 60% of cases.
  - Brain abscess:
    - Streptococci (70% of all cases), enteric GNRs, anaerobes, *S. aureus* (10%–20% of all cases, usually associated with trauma or endocarditis)
    - Numerous etiologies in immunocompromised hosts (fungi, nocardia, toxoplasma, etc.)
- Triage and prognosis:
  - Many CNS infections (like bacterial meningitis and brain abscess) can be rapidly fatal or have severe neurologic sequelae (HSV encephalitis) without prompt treatment.
  - Start patients presenting with suspected meningitis on empiric IV antibiotic treatment for bacterial meningitis as soon as possible (prior to LP if delayed for CT).
  - Consult neurosurgery for brain abscesses for possible drainage and/or biopsy.
- Treatment:
  - Empiric adult IV treatment for bacterial meningitis (narrow once pathogen identified) (Table 8-5)
    - Adjunctive dexamethasone (0.15 mg/kg every 6 h × 2–4 days starting with first dose of antibiotics); recommended if pneumococcal meningitis is suspected.
    - Also include ampicillin in immunocompromised patients younger than 50 years of age.
  - Empiric treatment for suspected tuberculous meningitis
    - Isoniazid plus rifampin plus ethambutol plus pyrazinamide plus adjunctive steroids (dexamethasone 10 mg/day or prednisone 60 mg/day)
  - Empiric treatment for encephalitis (until HSV encephalitis is ruled out)
    - Acyclovir 10 mg/kg IV every 8 h
  - Empiric IV treatment for bacterial brain abscess (narrow once pathogen identified) (Table 8-6)
    - If abscess is larger than 2.5 cm or patient is neurologically unstable, perform surgical drainage.
- Pearls and pitfalls
  - Temporal lobe involvement is highly indicative of HSV encephalitis.
  - When usual diagnostic methods fail, meningeal biopsy in the presence of meningeal enhancement on MRI has a diagnostic yield approximately 80%.
  - Infectious diseases consultation is indicated with most CNS infections.
- Links to guidelines:http://www.idsociety.org/uploadedFiles/IDSA/Guidelines-Patient_ Care/PDF_Library/Bacterial%20Meningitis(1).pdf and http://www.idsociety.org/ uploadedFiles/IDSA/Guidelines-Patient_Care/PDF_Library/Encephalitis.pdf

TABLE 8-6. EMPIRIC TREATMENT FOR BACTERIAL BRAIN ABSCESS

Risk Factor	Treatment
Sinusitis/mastoiditis/otitis media	Vancomycin 15 mg/kg IV q8-12h (goal through 15–20) + cefepime 2g IV q8h plus metronidazole 7.5 mg/kg q6h
Dental infection	Ceftriaxone 2g IV q12h + metronidazole
Trauma/neurosurgery	Vancomycin + meropenem 2g IV q8h
Lung abscess/empyema	Meropenem + trimethoprim-sulfamethoxazole (15 mg/kg/day TMP divided in 2–4 doses)
Bacterial endocarditis	Vancomycin + gentamicin 1 mg/kg every 8 h
Unknown	Vancomycin + meropenem

TMP, trimethoprim.

PNEUMONIA

- Pneumonia: infection of the lung parenchyma diagnosed by a new or progressive radiographic lung infiltrate plus suggestive clinical features (fever, leukocytosis or leukopenia, cough, pleuritic chest pain, and/or sputum production)
- Community-acquired pneumonia (CAP): pneumonia acquired in the community
- Hospital-acquired pneumonia (HAP): pneumonia beginning 48 hours or more after hospital admission (for ventilator-associated and health care-associated pneumonia, use HAP treatment).
- Common complaints and review of systems
  - Cough, fever, chills, pleuritic chest pain, dyspnea, sputum production, nausea and vomiting, and diarrhea
  - In ventilated patients: fever, decreased oxygenation, and increased purulent respiratory secretions
- Physical examination: fever (80%), tachypnea, tachycardia, audible rales on lung auscultation
- Diagnostic tests
  - Chest x-ray (if negative but clinically suspect pneumonia, repeat in 24–48 hours)

TABLE 8-7. PNEUMONIA COMMON ETIOLOGIES

CAP: outpatient and inpatient non-ICU	*Streptococcus pneumoniae, Mycoplasma pneumoniae, Chlamydia pneumoniae, Haemophilus influenzae, Legionella,* respiratory viruses
CAP-ICU	Above plus *Staphylococcus aureus* (MRSA) and gram-negative rods
Early onset HAP (within 4 days of admission)	*S. pneumoniae, H. influenzae, S. aureus* (MSSA), gram-negative rods (*Escherichia coli, Klebsiella, Enterobacter, Proteus,* or serratia)
Late-onset HAP (at least 5 days after admission) or risk factors for multidrug-resistant organisms	Pathogens listed above for early onset HAP plus *Pseudomonas aeruginosa,* ESBL+ *Klebsiella pneumoniae, Acinetobacter,* MRSA, and *Legionella pneumophila*

CAP, community-acquired pneumonia; ESBL, extended-spectrum β-lactamase; HAP, hospital-acquired pneumonia; ICU, intensive care unit; MRSA, methicillin-resistant *Staphylococcus aureus*; MSSA, methicillin-susceptible *Staphylococcus aureus*.

TABLE 8-8.　CURB-65

CURB-65 score	0	1	2	3	4	5
30-day mortality	0.7%	2.1%	9.2%	14.5%	40%	57%

- Sputum Gram stain and culture before antibiotics (<25 squamous epithelial cells on Gram stain and positive polymorphonuclear leukocytes indicate a "good" sputum sample)
- Blood cultures before antibiotics (particularly in severe CAP and ventilated patients)
- Complete blood count (CBC), basic metabolic panel, and liver function tests (to determine severity of disease)
- Arterial blood gas test in severe CAP or HAP
- Diagnostic thoracentesis with Gram stain and culture if pleural effusion is greater than 5 cm
- Consider *Legionella* and/or pneumococcal urine antigen tests
- Consider rapid influenza test in the appropriate season
- Consider chest CT and/or bronchoscopy if no clinical improvement within 72 hours
- Common Etiologies (Table 8-7)
- Triage and prognosis
  - For CAP, a CURB-65 score can triage who needs to be admitted (>1 factor) and who should be considered for ICU care (>2 factors). CURB criteria: **c**onfusion of new onset, **u**remia (blood urea nitrogen level >20 mg/dL), **r**espiratory rate 30 breaths/min or more, low **b**lood pressure (systolic <90 mm Hg or diastolic ≤60 mm Hg), and age **65** years or older (Table 8-8).
  - Criteria for severe pneumonia requiring ICU admission include at least 1 major criteria or 3 minor criteria (Table 8-9).
- Treatment: empiric treatment (Table 8-10)
  - For CAP ICU patients with bronchiectasis, recent antibiotics, or chronic obstructive pulmonary disease, use late onset HAP treatment (but include a fluoroquinolone or add azithromycin).
  - Antibiotics should be given within 6 hours of presentation of symptoms or suspected pneumonia.
  - Tailor therapy to pathogen if identified.
  - Duration of treatment: minimum of 5 days for CAP and 7 days for HAP (14 days if caused by *Pseudomonas* or *Acinetobacter*)

TABLE 8-9.　CRITERIA FOR SEVERE PNEUMONIA REQUIRING INTENSIVE CARE UNIT ADMISSION

Major Criteria	Minor Criteria
Need for mechanical ventilation	Respiratory rate ≥30 breaths/min
Pressor requirement	PaO₂/FiO₂ ≤250
	Multilobar infiltrates
	Confusion and disorientation
	Uremia (BUN ≥20 mg/dL)
	Leukopenia (WBC <4000 cells/mm³)
	Thrombocytopenia (platelets <100,000 cells/mm³)
	Hypothermia (core temperature <36°C [96.8°F])
	Hypotension requiring fluid resuscitation

BUN, blood urea nitrogen; FiO₂, fraction of inspired oxygen; PaO₂, partial pressure of alveolar oxygen; WBC, white blood cell count.

TABLE 8-10. SEVERE PNEUMONIA EMPIRIC TREATMENT

CAP: non-ICU inpatient	Moxifloxacin 400 mg, levofloxacin 750 mg, or gemifloxacin 320 mg daily **OR**
	Ceftriaxone 1 g daily (or ertapenem, ceftaroline, cefotaxime, or ampicillin and sulbactam [Unasyn]) plus azithromycin 500 mg daily
CAP: ICU	Vancomycin 1 g IV every 12 h or linezolid 600 mg every 12 h **PLUS** ceftriaxone, ertapenem, ceftaroline, cefotaxime, or ampicillin and sulbactam (Unasyn) **PLUS** moxifloxacin, levofloxacin, gemifloxacin, or azithromycin
HAP: early onset	Ceftriaxone, moxifloxacin, levofloxacin, ciprofloxacin 400 mg IV every 8 h, ampicillin and sulbactam (Unasyn), or ertapenem
HAP: late onset or risk for MDR pathogen	Vancomycin or linezolid **PLUS** cefepime 2 g every 12 h, ceftazidime 2 g every 8 h, imipenem 500 mg every 6 h, meropenem 1 g every 8 h, doripenem 500 mg every 8 h, or piperacillin and tazobactam (Zosyn) 4.5 g every 6 h **PLUS** levofloxacin, ciprofloxacin, gentamicin 5–7 mg/kg/day, tobramycin 5–7 mg/kg/day, or amikacin 15 mg/kg/day

CAP, community-acquired pneumonia; HAP, hospital-acquired pneumonia; ICU, intensive care unit; MDR, multidrug-resistant.

- Pearls and pitfalls
  - Positive respiratory culture does not indicate pneumonia without radiographic or clinical signs of pneumonia.
- Links to guidelines: http://www.idsociety.org/uploadedFiles/IDSA/Guidelines-Patient_Care/PDF_Library/CAP%20in%20Adults.pdf and http://www.idsociety.org/uploadedFiles/IDSA/Guidelines-Patient_Care/PDF_Library/HAP.pdf.

BACTEREMIA: INFECTIVE ENDOCARDITIS AND LINE INFECTIONS

- Bacteremia: the presence of bacteria in the blood. This can be transient (resolves without treatment) or indicative of the following infections:
  - Infective endocarditis: infection of the endocardium, particularly the heart valves
  - Line infection: infection of an intravascular (usually central venous) catheter
  - Other intravascular infection (infected vascular graft, pacer wire, clot, etc.)
  - Serious infection elsewhere in the body (UTI, pneumonia, abscess, ulcer, etc.)

Infective Endocarditis (IE)

- Common complaints and review of systems
  - Fever, chills, sweats, weight loss, malaise, myalgias and arthralgias, back pain.
  - In more advanced IE, symptoms caused by septic emboli (cough and pleuritic chest pain in right-sided IE; altered mental status, seizures, and symptoms of stroke with left-sided IE).
  - Presence of IE predisposing condition: injection drug use, prosthetic heart valves, structural heart disease, history of endocarditis, recent intravascular invasive procedure or line infection, or hemodialysis.
- Physical examination: fever, heart murmur (especially new or worsened), splenomegaly, clubbing, focal neurologic deficits, with or without the following peripheral manifestations:
  - Osler nodes: painful nodules on the fingers and toes
  - Splinter hemorrhages: linear reddish-brown lesions in the nail bed
  - Janeway lesions: nonpainful, blanching, erythematous macules on the palms and soles
  - Roth spots: hemorrhagic lesions of the retina
- Diagnosis and diagnostic tests: Duke Modified Criteria (Table 8-11)
  - Definite IE: 2 major criteria, 1 major and 3 minor criteria, or 5 minor criteria
  - Possible IE: 1 major and 1 minor criteria or 3 minor criteria

TABLE 8-11. DUKE MODIFIED CRITERIA

Major Criteria	Minor Criteria
1. *Blood culture positive for IE* Viridans streptococci, *Streptococcus bovis*, HACEK group, *Staphylococcus aureus*, or *Enterococcus* in 2 separate blood cultures in the absence of a first-degree focus. Microorganism consistent with IE from persistently positive blood cultures (2 cultures >12 h apart or ≥3 cultures 1 h apart) *Coxiella burnetii* single positive blood culture or antiphase 1 IgG antibody titer >1:800 2. *Echocardiogram positive for IE*	1. IE predisposing condition 2. Temperature >38°C (100.4°F) 3. Vascular phenomena: arterial emboli, septic pulmonary infarcts, mycotic aneurysm, intracranial hemorrhage, conjunctival hemorrhages, and Janeway lesions 4. Immunologic phenomena: glomerulonephritis, Osler nodes, Roth spots, positive rheumatoid factor 5. Microbiologic evidence: positive blood culture that does not meet major criterion or serologic evidence of infection with organisms consistent with IE.

HACEK, *Haemophilus* spp., *Actinobacillus actinomycetemcomitans, Cardiobacterium hominis, Eikenella corrodens*, and *Kingella kingae*; IE, infective endocarditis; IgG, immunoglobulin G.

- Transthoracic echocardiography is recommended as first test over transesophageal echocardiography (TEE) unless the patient has prosthetic valves, AICD, "possible IE" by clinical criteria alone, or suspected perivalvular abscess.
- Electrocardiogram to look for conduction abnormalities suggesting perivalvular extension.
- Although not formally part of Duke criteria, elevated erythrocyte sedimentation rate and C-reactive protein and microscopic hematuria also support IE.
- Common etiologies
  - Typical organisms: Viridans group streptococci, *Streptococcus bovis*, staphylococci, enterococci, and the HACEK group (*Haemophilus parainfluenzae, Haemophilus aphrophilus, Haemophilus paraphrophilus, H. influenzae, Actinobacillus actinomycetemcomitans, Cardiobacterium hominis, Eikenella corrodens, Kingella kingae*, and *Kingella dentrificans*)
  - Less frequent but still consistent organisms: salmonellae, *E. coli, Serratia, Proteus, Klebsiella, Pseudomonas, Neisseria, Moraxella, Bartonella, Coxiella burnetii, Chlamydia, Brucella, Legionella, Tropheryma whippleii, Candida*, and *Aspergillus*.
- Triage and prognosis: features that suggest need for surgical intervention:
  - Vegetations at high risk for embolization (embolic events during first 2 weeks therapy, >10 mm anterior mitral vegetation, increase in size on therapy).
  - Valvular dysfunction (acute aortic or mitral insufficiency, heart failure, valve perforation or rupture).
  - Perivalvular extension (valvular dehiscence, rupture, or fistula, new heart block, large abscess or enlarging abscess on therapy).
- Treatment for native and prosthetic valve IE (Table 8-12).
- Pearls and pitfalls
  - Once daily dosing of aminoglycosides cannot be used for enterococcal endocarditis.
- Links to guidelines: http://www.idsociety.org/uploadedFiles/IDSA/Guidelines-Patient_Care/PDF_Library/Endocarditis%20Management.pdf.

Line Infections

- Common complaints and review of systems: fever, chills, inflammation and purulence at the catheter insertion site (often not present), catheter dysfunction, altered mental status
- Physical examination: fever, inflammation and purulence at the catheter insertion site, hemodynamic instability.
- Diagnostic tests: diagnosis of catheter-related bloodstream infection requires either:
  - Same organism to grow from percutaneous blood culture and catheter tip culture

TABLE 8-12. INFECTIVE ENDOCARDITIS VALVE TREATMENT

Streptococcus bovis and *Viridans* spp., PCN-susceptible (MIC ≤0.12 μg/mL)	**NV:** PCN-G 2–3 million units every 4 h or ceftriaxone 2 g daily × 4 wk (alone) or × 2 wk (if + gentamicin 1 mg/kg q 8 h × 2 wk) OR vancomycin 15 mg/kg every 12 h × 4 wk **PV:** PCN-G 4 million units every 4 h (or ceftriaxone) × 6 wk ± gentamicin × 2 wk OR Vancomycin × 6 wk
S. bovis and viridans, PCN-resistant (MIC >0.12 μg/mL)	**NV:** PCN-G 4 million units every 4 h (or ceftriaxone) × 4 wk + gentamicin × 2 wk OR vancomycin × 4 wk **PV:** PCN-G (or ceftriaxone) × 6 wk + gentamicin × 6 wk OR vancomycin × 6 wk
MSSA	**NV:** Nafcillin 2 g every 4 h (or cefazolin 2 g every 8 h) × 6 wk ± gentamicin × 3–5 days **PV:** Nafcillin + rifampin 300 mg every 8 h × ≥6 wk + gentamicin × 2 wk
MRSA	**NV:** Vancomycin × 6 wk **PV:** Vancomycin + rifampin × ≥6 wk + gentamicin × 2 wk
Enterococcus, pan-susceptible	Ampicillin 2 g every 4 h (or PCN-G 3–5 million units every 4 h) + gentamicin × 4–6 wk OR vancomycin + gentamicin × 6 wk
Enterococcus, PCN-resistant only	Vancomycin + gentamicin × 6 weeks
VRE (and PCN-resistant)	***Enterococcus faecium:*** Linezolid 600 mg every 12 h or quinupristin-dalfopristin 8.5 mg/kg every 8 h × ≥8 wk (alternative: daptomycin) ***Enterococcus faecalis:*** Imipenem/cilastin 500 mg every 6 h (or ceftriaxone 2 g every 12 h) + ampicillin × ≥8 wk
HACEK group	Ceftriaxone 2 g every 24 h or ampicillin-sulbactam 3 g every 6 h or ciprofloxacin 400 mg IV every 12 h × 4 wk

HACEK, *Haemophilus* spp., *Actinobacillus actinomycetemcomitans, Cardiobacterium hominis, Eikenella corrodens,* and *Kingella kingae*; MIC, minimal inhibitory concentration; MRSA, methicillin-resistant *Staphylococcus aureus*; MSSA, methicillin-susceptible *Staphylococcus aureus*; NV, native valve; PCN, penicillin; PV, prosthetic valve; VRE, vancomycin-resistant *Enterococcus*.

MEDICAL SPECIALTIES

- Same organism to grow from blood collected from catheter hub and from peripheral vein, and colony count either threefold higher or positive culture 2 hours or more earlier from catheter hub.
  - If exudate at catheter insertion site, swab drainage and send for Gram stain and culture.
  - Repeat blood cultures until negative
- Common etiologies: coagulase-negative staphylococci, *S. aureus, Candida,* enteric gram-negative rods, and *Pseudomonas aeruginosa*
- Triage and prognosis: Catheter retention therapy should *not* be attempted if:
  - Signs of exit site or tunnel infection
  - Complications such as sepsis, suppurative thrombophlebitis, or endocarditis
  - Persistent positive blood cultures despite more than 72 h of appropriate antimicrobials
  - Infection with *S. aureus, Pseudomonas, Bacillus, Micrococcus, Propionibacteria,* fungi (including candida), or mycobacteria
- Treatment
  - When catheter retention is attempted, combined systemic antimicrobial therapy and antibiotic lock therapy for 7 to 14 days.
  - When catheter is removed, duration of systemic antimicrobials varies by organism.

- Pearls and pitfalls
  - With catheter retention, obtain a repeat blood culture 1 week after antibiotic course.
  - Give 6 weeks of antimicrobials when blood cultures remain positive more than 72 hours after catheter removal (or with suppurative thrombophlebitis or endocarditis)
  - With *S. aureus*, TEE to rule out endocarditis or 4 to 6 weeks antibiotics
- Link to guidelines: http://www.idsociety.org/uploadedFiles/IDSA/Guidelines-Patient_Care/PDF_Library/Management%20IV%20Cath.pdf

COMPLICATED INTRAABDOMINAL INFECTIONS AND *C. DIFFICILE* INFECTION

Complicated Intraabdominal Infections (CIAI)

CIAI are infections that extend beyond the hollow viscus of the GI tract into the peritoneal space, with associated abscess or peritonitis.

- Common complaints and review of systems: acute abdominal pain, fever, anorexia, nausea and vomiting, bloating, and obstipation.
- Physical examination: fever, abdominal tenderness (positive rebound), tachycardia, tachypnea.
- Diagnostic tests:
  - CT abdomen and pelvis if not undergoing immediate surgical laparotomy.
  - Blood cultures if septic or immunocompromised (seldom useful otherwise).
  - Cultures (aerobic and anaerobic) from intraabdominal site of infection.
- Common etiologies: coliforms (enteric GNRs), anaerobes (especially *Bacteroides fragilis*), and/or *Candida*.
- Triage and prognosis:
  - Antibiotics within 1 h with septic shock and within 8 h without septic shock.
  - STAT surgical consult to determine best method of source control (percutaneous drainage by interventional radiology versus surgical intervention).
- Treatment: Suggestions for Initial Empiric Therapy (Table 8-13)
- Add antifungal therapy if *Candida* grows from intraabdominal cultures
- Use past culture results to tailor therapy if history of multidrug-resistant pathogens.
- Narrow coverage once culture results are back (if cultures taken prior to antibiotics)
- With adequate source control (surgery), antibiotics can be limited to 4 to 7 days.

TABLE 8-13. EMPIRIC THERAPY FOR COMPLICATED INTRAABDOMINAL INFECTIONS

Community-acquired CIAI, mild-to-moderate severity	Ertapenem 1 g daily, moxifloxacin 400 mg daily, tigecycline 100 mg × 1 then 50 mg daily, or piperacillin and tazobactam (Zosyn) 3.375 g every 6 h **OR** metronidazole 500 mg every 6 h + ceftriaxone 2 g daily, cefotaxime 2 g every 8 h, ciprofloxacin 400 mg IV every 12 h, or levofloxacin 750 mg daily
Community-acquired CIAI, high severity	Imipenem 500 mg every 6 h, meropenem 1 g every 8 h, doripenem 500 mg every 8 h, or piperacillin and tazobactam (Zosyn) **OR** metronidazole + cefepime 2 g every 12 h, ceftazidime 2 g every 8 h, ciprofloxacin, or levofloxacin
Health care-associated CIAI	Imipenem, meropenem, doripenem, or piperacillin and tazobactam (Zosyn) ± vancomycin 1 g every 12 h (if MRSA colonized); ceftazidime or cefepime + metronidazole can be used if resistant GNRs <20% in community

CIAI, complicated intraabdominal infections; GNR, gram-negative rod; IV, intravenous; MRSA, methicillin-resistant *Staphylococcus aureus*.

- Pearls and pitfalls
  - Consider CIAI in patients with obtundation, old age, spinal cord injury, or immunosuppression who have clinical signs of infection but no known source.
- Link to guidelines: http://www.idsociety.org/uploadedFiles/IDSA/Guidelines-Patient_Care/PDF_Library/intraabdominal%20Infectin.pdf.

C. difficile Colitis

- Presence of symptoms (usually diarrhea) plus pseudomembranous colitis on colonoscopy or a stool test positive for *C. difficile* or *C. difficile* toxins.
- Common complaints and review of systems: watery diarrhea (≥3 loose stools within 24 h), history of antibiotic use or chemotherapy in the past 8 weeks, fever, abdominal cramping and pain, nausea, anorexia, malaise.
- Physical examination: fever, abdominal tenderness, abdominal distension, shock (in severe cases).
- Diagnostic tests:
  - Leukocytosis (15,000/μL on average, but can be higher than 40,000/μL)
  - Stool testing for *C. difficile*:
    - Stool culture is the most sensitive but is too slow for clinical practice.
    - Enzyme immunoassay (EIA) for *C. difficile* toxins A and B is rapid but less sensitive than culture.
    - PCR is rapid, sensitive, and specific and the ideal modality if offered.
    - If test is negative, repeat testing more frequently than every 7 days is of limited value.
    - Test of cure not recommended (test may stay positive even if clinically cured).
  - Colonoscopy and sigmoidoscopy to detect pseudomembranes (sensitivity ~50%).
  - In severe cases, abdominal plain films can detect toxic megacolon.
  - Abdominal CT can show colonic wall thickening.
- Common etiologies: In general, asymptomatic *C. difficile* colonization (or recent *C. difficile* acquisition through the fecal-oral route) plus recent antibiotics (which suppress the normal gut flora, allowing *C. difficile* to multiply and create toxins).
- Triage and prognosis: Severe *C. difficile* can cause a fulminant colitis with toxic megacolon, bowel perforation, shock, and/or death.
- Treatment:
  - Discontinue inciting antibiotics as soon as possible.
  - For mild-to-moderate *C. difficile*: metronidazole 500 mg orally every 8 h over 10 to 14 days.
  - For severe *C. difficile* (leukocytosis ≥15,000/μL or creatinine 1.5 × baseline): vancomycin 125 mg orally four times daily over 10 to 14 days.
  - For severe *C. difficile* with complications (shock, ileus, megacolon): vancomycin 500 mg orally four times daily plus IV metronidazole 500 mg every 8 h with or without vancomycin 500 mg/100 mL saline as retention enema every 6 h with or without colectomy.
  - For recurrence, same treatment for first recurrence, then switch to oral vancomycin. Dose tapering or pulse dosing might help prevent additional recurrences. Stool transplants are the most effective treatment in the setting of multiple recurrences.
- Pearls and pitfalls
  - Consider *C. difficile* in any patient on antibiotics with diarrhea and unexplained leukocytosis.
  - When a patient is on narcotics (causing constipation) or has severe colitis, *C. difficile* can present without diarrhea (suspect if abdominal pain and tenderness and high-dose narcotics).
  - Hand hygiene to prevent spread (use soap and water as alcohol-based gels and foams are ineffective).
  - Vancomycin given IV does *not* treat *C. difficile*. However, the IV preparation of vancomycin given orally is *much* cheaper than vancomycin pills and equally efficacious.
  - Recurrent *C. difficile* is common after treatment as nothing kills the spore form of *C. difficile*.
- Link to guidelines: http://www.idsociety.org/uploadedFiles/IDSA/Guidelines-Patient_Care/PDF_Library/cdiff2010a.pdf.

URINARY TRACT INFECTIONS

UTIs include cystitis (bladder infection) and pyelonephritis (kidney infection).

- Complicated UTI: UTI associated with underlying condition that increases risk of treatment failure (male sex, history of pyelonephritis, renal failure, urinary tract obstruction or anatomic abnormality, presence of urinary catheter or stent, pregnancy, or immunosuppression)
- Catheter-associated UTI: indwelling urethral or suprapubic catheter and symptoms or signs of UTI with no other source of infection along with 10^3 or more colony-forming units per mL of 1 or more bacterial species in urine collected within 48 h after urinary catheter removal.
- Common complaints and review of systems:
  - Dysuria, urinary frequency, urgency, suprapubic pain, hematuria, fevers, chills, confusion, malaise, flank pain (indicates pyelonephritis), and nausea and vomiting.
  - In elderly, only symptom might be confusion.
- Physical examination: fever, suprapubic or costovertebral angle tenderness, altered mental status.
- Diagnostic tests:
  - Urinalysis and urine culture (preferably from clean catch, straight cath, or if catheter in place, freshly replaced catheter)
  - Blood cultures (if fever or signs of sepsis)
  - CT abdomen and pelvis (contrast not needed to detect most upper tract infections or abnormalities) if symptoms persist 2 to 3 days after starting antibiotics (to look for perinephric abscess needing drainage), or if clinical suspicion of pyelonephritis or obstruction.
- Common etiologies:
  - Uncomplicated UTI: *E. coli* (~80%), other enteric GNRs (*Klebsiella*, *Proteus*), and *Staphylococcus saprophyticus*.
  - Complicated UTI: above organisms plus *Pseudomonas*, *Serratia*, Providencia, enterococci, staphylococci, and fungi
- Triage and prognosis: ranges from asymptomatic to urosepsis and death.
- Treatment: empiric and suggested durations (Table 8-14).
  - Use culture data to tailor the antibiotics once available.
  - Oral β-lactams are inferior to trimethoprim-sulfamethoxazole (TMP-SMX) and fluoroquinolones for pyelonephritis.
  - Renal or perinephric abscesses larger than 5 cm require drainage.

TABLE 8-14. URINARY TRACT INFECTION EMPIRIC TREATMENT

Uncomplicated cystitis	Nitrofurantoin 100 mg PO BID × 5 days or TMP-SMX DS PO BID × 3 days (if local resistance <20%) or fosfomycin 3 g PO × 1. Alternatives: ciprofloxacin 500 mg BID or levofloxacin 750 mg daily × 3 days or amoxicillin and clavulanate (Augmentin) or cefpodoxime × 3–7 days.
Uncomplicated pyelonephritis	Cipro or levofloxacin × 7 days (if local resistance <10%) or TMP-SMX × 14 days (if pathogen susceptible) ± ceftriaxone 1 g or aminoglycoside 24 h dose × 1. *If severe:* IV aminoglycoside ± ampicillin, or ceftriaxone, cefepime, piperacillin and tazobactam (Zosyn), or carbapenem × 10–14 days (transition to PO if improved and pathogen susceptible).
Complicated UTI	14–21 days of ampicillin + gentamicin, piperacillin and tazobactam (Zosyn), cefepime, carbapenem, ciprofloxacin, or levofloxacin (can transition to PO if improved).
CAUTI	Remove or replace catheter. Antibiotics × 7 days, or 10–14 days if delayed response.

BID, twice daily; CAUTI, catheter-associated urinary tract infection; PO, orally; TMP-SMX, trimethoprim-sulfamethoxazole.

- Pearls and pitfalls
  - In catheterized patients, pyuria (or positive urine culture) is not diagnostic of a UTI, but no pyuria suggests no UTI.
  - Moxifloxacin should not be used for a UTI (inadequate urine levels).
  - Nitrofurantoin should only be used for uncomplicated cystitis (inadequate tissue levels).
- Links to guidelines:
  - http://www.idsociety.org/uploadedFiles/IDSA/Guidelines-Patient_Care/PDF_Library/Comp%20UTI.pdf
  - http://www.idsociety.org/uploadedFiles/IDSA/Guidelines-Patient_Care/PDF_Library/Uncomp%20UTI.pdf

SEXUALLY TRANSMITTED DISEASES: URETHRITIS, CERVICITIS, AND SYPHILIS

A good sexual history (sex with men, women, or both; vaginal, anal, and/or oral; number of partners; frequency of condom use; history of STDs; partners' history of STDs) is paramount.

Urethritis and Cervicitis

- Definition: urethral or cervical inflammation from infectious or noninfectious causes.
- Common complaints and review of systems: urethral or cervical discharge, dysuria, urethral pruritus, abnormal vaginal bleeding, lower abdominal pain, dyspareunia
- Physical examination: genital examination
  - Men: mucopurulent or purulent urethral discharge, testicular examination to look for epididymitis (unilateral testicular pain and swelling)
  - Women: pelvic examination (cervicitis indicated by either mucopurulent or purulent endocervical discharge or endocervical bleeding with gentle passage of cotton swab. (Erosive cervicitis indicates HSV; strawberry cervix indicates trichomonas), bimanual examination to look for pelvic inflammatory disease, abdominal tenderness
- Diagnostic tests:
  - Urinalysis on first-void urine: positive leukocyte esterase or at least 10 white blood cells per high-power field (WBC/hpf) on microscopy indicates urethritis.
  - Gram stain of urethral secretions (≥5 WBC/hpf indicates urethritis; Gram stain showing diplococci indicates gonorrhea)
  - Urethritis can also be confirmed by mucopurulent or purulent urethral discharge on examination.
  - Wet mount of cervical secretions showing many leukocytes indicates cervicitis
  - *Neisseria gonorrhea* and *Chlamydia trachomatis* nucleic acid amplification testing (NAAT) on urine, cervical secretions, or urethral secretions (highly sensitive and specific).
  - Depending on sexual history, pharyngeal and rectal *N. gonorrhea* and *C. trachomatis* NAAT
- Common etiologies:
  - Urethritis: predominantly *N. gonorrhea* and *C. trachomatis*; also *Ureaplasma urealyticum*, *Mycoplasma genitalium*, *Trichomonas vaginalis*, HSV, adenovirus, or enteric pathogens (if anal sex).
  - Cervicitis: predominantly *N. gonorrhea* and *C. trachomatis*; also *M. genitalium*, trichomonas, HSV
- Triage and prognosis
  - *N. gonorrhea* and *C. trachomatis* infections can lead to epididymitis, pelvic inflammatory disease (10%–40% untreated cases), urethral strictures, infertility, proctitis (if anal sex), pharyngitis (if oral sex, mainly *N. gonorrhea*), prostatitis, conjunctivitis, perinatal infections, and spread to partners.
  - *N. gonorrhea* causes disseminated infection (arthritis with or without rash) in 0.5% to 3% of cases.
  - *C. trachomatis* causes Reiter syndrome (urethritis, arthritis, and uveitis) in 1% to 2% cases.
- Treatment (for urethritis and cervicitis)
  - Azithromycin 1 g PO, single dose or doxycycline 100 mg PO twice daily (BID) over 7 days **AND** ceftriaxone 250 mg intramuscularly (IM), single dose

- If not *N. gonorrhea* and initial treatment fails give metronidazole or tinidazole 2 g PO, single dose (for *Trichomonas*) and azithromycin 1 g PO, single dose if not previously given (for *Mycoplasma* and *U. urealyticum*)
- Advise patient to abstain from sex for 1 week after treatment.
- Pearls and pitfalls
  - *N. gonorrhea* and *C. trachomatis* infections are often asymptomatic; screen in high-risk patients.
  - With documented urethritis, always treat for both *N. gonorrhea* and *C. trachomatis* (11%–50% coinfection rate) immediately (before *N. gonorrhea* and *C. trachomatis* NAAT results are back).
  - Anyone with *N. gonorrhea* or *C. trachomatis* should be tested for other STDs (HIV, syphilis, bacterial vaginitis in women)

Syphilis

- Known as "the great imitator"; systemic disease caused by *Treponema pallidum.*
- Common complaints, review of systems, and physical examination:
  - Primary syphilis: ulcer or chancre at the infection site (genitals, oropharynx, rectum)
  - Secondary syphilis: skin rash, mucocutaneous lesions, lymphadenopathy, fever, malaise, anorexia
  - Tertiary syphilis:
    - Neurosyphilis: cranial nerve dysfunction, meningitis, stroke, altered mental status, loss of vibration sense, tabes dorsalis, auditory or ophthalmologic abnormalities
    - Gummas: ulcers or heaped up granulomatous lesions anywhere on the body
    - Aortitis or aortic aneurysm: new murmur or signs of left heart failure
  - Latent syphilis: by definition, asymptomatic
- Diagnostic tests
  - Darkfield examination of tissue and exudate is definitive but rarely available
  - Serologic tests: need to confirm nontreponemal tests (VDRL and rapid plasma reagin [RPR] with treponemal tests (EIAs, fluorescein treponemal antibody absorbed [FTA-ABS], and *Treponema pallidum* particle agglutination assay) to avoid false-positive results, and visa versa.
    - Nontreponemal tests provide quantitative titers that should be followed to determine treatment response.
    - Treponemal tests (and sometimes nontreponemal tests) can stay positive for life.
  - LP if neurosyphilis suspected (neurosyphilis suggested if elevated CSF protein or white count or positive CSF VDRL [insensitive but specific]; CSF FTA-ABS is highly sensitive but nonspecific and so can be used to rule out if negative).
- Triage and prognosis: always treat syphilis to avoid late complications (tertiary syphilis).
- Treatment
  - Primary, secondary, and early latent (<1 yr): IM benzathine penicillin G 2.4 million units, single dose (if penicillin allergy, doxycycline 100 mg PO BID × 14 days).
  - Late latent or latent of unknown duration or gummas alone: IM penicillin G 2.4 million units every week for 3 weeks (if penicillin allergy, doxycycline 100 mg PO BID × 28 days).
  - Neurosyphilis or cardiovascular syphilis: aqueous penicillin G 18 to 24 million units IV daily, divided every 4 h or by continuous infusion, over 10 to 14 days. If penicillin allergy, desensitize.
- Pearls and pitfalls
  - HIV and syphilis have high coinfection rates; always test one if positive for the other.
  - In HIV-infected patients, CD4 count less than 350 cells/mm^3 and RPR of 1:32 or greater suggests neurosyphilis (consider LP)
  - If RPR does not drop fourfold 6 to 12 months after treatment, consider retreatment and LP.
- Links to guidelines: http://www.cdc.gov/std/treatment/2010/STD-Treatment-2010-RR5912.pdf

OSTEOMYELITIS AND SEPTIC ARTHRITIS

Osteomyelitis (OM)

OM is a bone infection caused by hematogenous seeding, contiguous spread, or direct inoculation (trauma or surgery) of microorganisms.

- Common complaints and review of systems: usually just dull pain at involved site. Rarely, local findings (warmth, redness, and swelling), fever, or rigors. If contiguous spread, may be associated with skin ulcer.
- Physical examination: possibly fever, tenderness at involved site, erythema, swelling, warmth, draining sinus tract (if chronic). If diabetic ulcer is present, probing to bone is diagnostic.
- Diagnostic tests:
  - Imaging (not necessary in diabetic ulcers if can probe to bone):
    - X-ray (low sensitivity for early OM, but diagnostic if positive)
    - MRI: 95% sensitive (Can do nuclear study if metal hardware precludes MRI)
  - Bone biopsy (sent for aerobic, anaerobic, mycobacterial and fungal cultures and histopathology) can identify causative pathogen and aid in diagnosis when questionable.
    - Ideally patient should be off antibiotics 48 to 72 h prior for better yield.
    - Open biopsy is more sensitive than percutaneous needle biopsy.
  - C-reactive protein (CRP) with or without erythrocyte sedimentation rate (often elevated, and useful to follow through treatment).
  - Blood cultures (if positive for likely organism, can be used in lieu of bone biopsy).
- Common etiologies:
  - Predisposing factors include diabetes, vasculopathy, invasive procedure, and IV drug use.
  - With hematogenous seeding, usually single infecting organism; with contiguous spread or direct inoculation, usually polymicrobial.
  - Organisms: most often (>50%) *S. aureus*, particularly if hematogenous spread, but many organisms possible.
- Triage and prognosis:
  - Surgical debridement may be necessary, especially with advanced OM.
  - If any hardware is present, it should be removed if possible.
  - With overlying wound or ulcer, wound closure necessary for cure.
- Treatment should be culture directed.
- MSSA: nafcillin 2 g IV every 4 h or cefazolin 2 g IV every 8 h.
- MRSA: vancomycin 15 mg/kg every 12 h with or without rifampin 300 PO BID if susceptible.
- Duration: 8 or more weeks for MRSA, 6 or more weeks for MSSA and most other bacteria (longer for mycobacteria, fungi, and slow-growing bacteria like *Brucella*). If infected bone is all removed, shorter course may be sufficient (1–2 wk).
- IV therapy for full course is generally preferred (but fluoroquinolones have excellent bone penetration and bioavailability and can be given oral or IV for susceptible GNRs).
- If empiric therapy is necessary, vancomycin alone (if hematogenous), vancomycin plus gram-negative coverage (if contiguous, nondiabetic), vancomycin plus gram-negative coverage plus anaerobic coverage (if contiguous and diabetic or vascular insufficiency).
- Pearls and pitfalls
  - A wound culture is not sufficient to determine the etiologic pathogen for contiguous OM (the bacteria infecting the bone can be different than bacteria in the wound).
- Links to guidelines: Infectious Diseases Society of America (IDSA) OM guidelines at www.idsociety.org/Organ_System/.

Septic Arthritis

- Joint infection caused by hematogenous seeding (most common route), contiguous spread, or direct inoculation (trauma or surgery) of microorganisms.
- Common complaints, review of systems, and physical examination: joint pain, swelling, warmth, and decreased range of motion (knee ~50%; usually monoarticular) with or without fever and malaise.

TABLE 8-15. SEPTIC ARTHRITIS TREATMENT

Gram Stain	Treatment
GPCs	Vancomycin 15 mg/kg IV every 12 h
GNCs	Ceftriaxone 1 g every 24 h
GNRs	Ceftazidime 2 g every 8 h, cefepime 2 g every 12 h, piperacillin and tazobactam (Zosyn) 4.5 g every 6 h, or antipseudomonal carbapenem (can use aztreonam or fluoroquinolone if PCN or cephalosporin allergy)
Negative	Vancomycin + ceftazidime

GNC, gram-negative cocci; GNR, gram-negative rod; GPC, gram-positive cocci; IV, intravenous; PCN, penicillin.

- Diagnostic tests:
  - Joint fluid sent for cell count and differential (usually >50 K with neutrophilic predominance), Gram stain, culture (80%–90% sensitivity unless gonococcal infection), and crystal examination (to rule out gout and pseudogout).
  - Blood cultures (if sent before antibiotics, positive in ~50% cases).
  - Joint radiographs are useful to determine extent of disease (check for OM) and as baseline.
  - If joint cultures nonrevealing, consider gonorrhea urine NAAT and Lyme serology.
- Common etiologies:
  - Predisposing factors: arthritis, advanced age, diabetes mellitus, sickle cell disease, malignancy, immunosuppression, indwelling catheter, endocarditis, IV drug use, prosthetic joint, recent joint surgery or joint injection.
  - Pathologic organism (usually just one): usually *S. aureus*, often streptococci, *N. gonorrhea* (with sexual risk factors), or GNRs. Rarely mycobacteria, fungi, Lyme disease, tick-borne infections, or viruses.
- Triage and prognosis: surgical drainage and washout usually required (with removal of prosthesis if prosthetic joint infection); 50% of patients have decreased joint function after infection.
- Treatment: surgical drainage and antibiotics (Table 8-15).
  - Narrow treatment when cultures are available.
  - Duration: typically 4 weeks. 6 weeks if OM suspected or prosthetic joint.
- Pearls and pitfalls
  - Suspect endocarditis with septic arthritis caused by *S. aureus*, *Streptococcus*, or *Enterococcus* and no obvious predisposing factor.

SKIN AND SOFT TISSUE INFECTIONS

- Include *cellulitis* (infection of the skin and subcutaneous fat), *necrotizing fasciitis* (severe, rapidly-spreading bacterial infection of the subcutaneous tissue), myonecrosis (severe, rapidly-progressing muscle infection usually due to *Clostridium* spp.)
- Common complaints, review of systems, and physical examination:
  - Cellulitis: area of skin erythema, edema, warmth, and tenderness. Fever, hypothermia, hypotension, and tachycardia suggest more severe infection.
  - Necrotizing fasciitis: severe pain out of proportion to examination with or without fever, rapidly progressing to skin crepitus, anesthesia, necrosis, and sloughing, woody edema, and/or violaceous bullae plus altered mental status, lethargy, shock.
  - Myonecrosis: increasingly severe pain at injury site, darkly erythematous and tender skin, violaceous bullae, skin crepitus, tachycardia, fever, diaphoresis, shock.
- Diagnostic tests:
  - If fever, hypothermia, hypotension, or tachycardia present, obtain blood cultures, CBC with differential, CRP, creatine phosphokinase, and chemistry panel.
  - STAT surgical exploration if there is any suspicion for necrotizing fasciitis or myonecrosis with tissue sent for Gram stain and culture (do not wait for imaging).

TABLE 8-16. SKIN AND SOFT TISSUE INFECTIONS CAUSES

Dog and cat bites	*Pasteurella*, *Staphylococcus aureus*, streptococci, *Capnocytophaga*, anaerobes
Human bites	*S. aureus*, streptococci, *Eikenella*, anaerobes
Water exposure	*Aeromonas hydrophila* (fresh) and *Vibrio vulnificus* (salt)
Animal contact	*Erysipelothrix rhusiopathiae*
Penetrating injury	*Pseudomonas aeruginosa* (also "hot-tub folliculitis")
Immunocompromised	Multiple pathogens. Consider fungi.
Diabetic foot ulcers	Mixed aerobic and anaerobic

- For cellulitis, low (~25%) yield for punch biopsy and needle aspiration cultures, but consider punch biopsy in immunocompromised hosts to look for unusual pathogens.
- Imaging can be useful to exclude occult abscess if slow response to therapy.
- Common etiologies:
  - Predisposing factors: breaches to the skin (IV drug use, toe web intertrigo), diabetes mellitus, peripheral vascular disease, lymphatic obstruction (eg, after lymph node dissection), skin inflammation.
  - Microbiology:
    - Cellulitis: primarily *S. aureus* (if purulent, or associated with abscess) and Streptococcus (if nonpurulent), but multiple etiologies (Table 8-16).
    - Necrotizing fasciitis
      - Type I: Polymicrobial (abdominal surgery, decubitus ulcer and perianal abscess, IV drug abuse, vulvovaginal origin)
      - Type II: *S. pyogenes* (a.k.a. group A *Streptococcus*, although MRSA has been reported)
    - Myonecrosis: Usually clostridial species (after crush injuries or penetrating trauma, or GI malignancy with neutropenia ["gas gangrene"]), or in association with necrotizing fasciitis. If fresh water exposure, consider *A. hydrophila*.
    - Skin abscess: usually *S. aureus*; mixed if perirectal, perioral, or perivaginal.
- Triage and prognosis:
  - Necrotizing fasciitis and myonecrosis are surgical emergencies (~25% mortality) and often require ICU stays with IV fluids with and without pressors.
  - For cellulitis, consider hospitalization if hypotensive, increased creatinine, low serum bicarbonate level, creatine phosphokinase two- to threefold normal, marked left shift, or CRP higher than 13 mg/L.
- Treatment: empiric therapy in the absence of unusual risk factors (Table 8-17).
  - Tailor therapy based on culture data if available.
  - Can transition to oral therapy when stable.
  - Duration: 7 to 14 days (cellulitis), 3 days after fever resolved and surgical debridement no longer necessary (necrotizing fasciitis).
- Pearls and pitfalls
  - Consider tularemia, anthrax, or plague with ulcers or eschar and lymphadenopathy and animal contact (also potential bioterrorism agents).
  - Cultures of skin swabs are useless; even without infection, the skin is not a sterile site.
- Links to guidelines:
  - http://www.idsociety.org/uploadedFiles/IDSA/Guidelines-Patient_Care/PDF_Library/Skin%20and%20Soft%20Tissue.pdf
  - http://www.idsociety.org/uploadedFiles/IDSA/Guidelines-Patient_Care/PDF_Library/MRSA.pdf

TABLE 8-17. SKIN AND SOFT TISSUE INFECTIONS TREATMENT

Cellulitis: outpatient	Clindamycin 300--450 mg po tid or linezolid 600 mg every 12 h alone **OR** TMP-SMX 1–2 tablets PO BID or doxycycline 100 mg BID **PLUS** amoxicillin 500 mg PO TID
Cellulitis: inpatient	Vancomycin 15 mg/kg IV every 12 h, linezolid, daptomycin 4 mg/kg daily, telavancin 10 mg/kg daily, or clindamycin 600 mg IV every 8 h
Cellulitis and diabetic foot	If severe: vancomycin, linezolid, or daptomycin PLUS a carbapenem
Cellulitis and animal bite	Ampicillin and sulbactam (Unasyn) 1.5 g IV every 6 h or ertapenem 1 g IV daily (inpatient) or amoxicillin and clavulanate (Augmentin) 875/125 mg PO BID (outpatient)
Necrotizing fasciitis type I (polymicrobial)	Surgical debridement + a carbapenem alone OR piperacillin and tazobactam (Zosyn) 3.375 g every 6–8 h or ampicillin and sulbactam (Unasyn) 3 g IV every 6 h + clindamycin IV + ciprofloxacin mg 400 IV BID
Necrotizing fasciitis type II (GAS, MRSA)	Surgical debridement + penicillin 4 million U IV every 4 h + clindamycin IV + (vancomycin or linezolid or daptomycin)
Clostridial myonecrosis	Surgical debridement + penicillin IV + clindamycin IV

BID, twice daily; GAS, group A Streptococcus; IV, intravenous; MRSA, methicillin-resistant *Staphylococcus aureus*; PO, orally; TID, thrice daily; TMP-SMX, trimethoprim-sulfamethoxazole.

TUBERCULOSIS AND ATYPICAL MYCOBACTERIA

Tuberculosis (TB)

- Pulmonary or extrapulmonary disease caused by organisms in the *Mycobacterium tuberculosis* complex.
  - Pulmonary disease: most common manifestation of TB.
  - Extrapulmonary disease: includes lymphadenopathy, skeletal, meningitis, pleural, miliary disease. More common in HIV-positive patients.
- Common complaints and review of systems:
  - Pulmonary disease: cough lasting more than 3 weeks, fever, night sweats, weight loss, anorexia.
  - Extrapulmonary disease: dependent on location.
    - Lymphadenopathy: painless swelling of one or more lymph nodes, usually in posterior or anterior cervical chain, or supraclavicular fossa.
    - Skeletal: pain at site of lesion, swelling in involved joint.
    - Meningitis: headache, decreased level of consciousness, neck stiffness.
- Physical examination: fever, cachexia, adventitious sounds on lung examination.
- Diagnostic tests:
  - Sputum smear for AFB and culture: obtain one specimen every 8 hours over a 24-hour period (3 specimens) to evaluate for infectiousness.
    - If high suspicion for TB and patient cannot cough, may need induced sputum or bronchoscopy.
  - Nucleic acid amplification should be performed on at least 1 respiratory specimen from patients with signs and symptoms of pulmonary TB.
  - Chest x-ray: infiltrates usually involving the apical and posterior segments of the upper lobes or superior segment of lower lobes, cavitation.
    - In HIV-positive patients with low CD4 count, chest x-ray findings may be atypical.
  - Tuberculin skin test may support diagnosis of TB if positive. See guidelines for interpretation of tuberculin skin test (www.atsjournals.org).
  - Interferon-γ release assay may support diagnosis of TB if positive.

TABLE 8-18. TUBERCULOSIS TREATMENT

Initiation phase (8 weeks)	Isoniazid 5 mg/kg daily (300 mg), rifampin 10 mg/kg daily (600 mg), pyrazinamide 15–30 mg/kg daily, and ethambutol 15–20 mg/kg daily (see guidelines for dosage range)
Continuation phase (18 weeks)	Isoniazid 15 mg/kg (900 mg) twice weekly and rifampin 10 mg/kg (600 mg) twice weekly (if isolate is susceptible)

- Common etiologies:
  - Predisposing factors: HIV infection; exposure to known TB case in prior 2 years; use of TNF-α inhibitors, steroids or other immunosuppressive agents; foreign-born from TB endemic countries; diabetes; IV drug or crack cocaine use; history of incarceration; homeless.
- Triage and prognosis:
  - TB is spread by airborne transmission: Place pulmonary TB suspects on airborne precautions in a negative-pressure room until 3 AFB sputum smears are negative.
- Treatment:
  - **Decision to initiate and continue treatment should be done in conjunction with infectious diseases or pulmonary specialist (Table 8-18).**
  - Duration of therapy for drug-susceptible pulmonary disease is usually 6 months.
  - Treatment duration may be prolonged if patient remains smear or culture-positive, or if disease in specific extrapulmonary sites (skeletal TB: treat for 6–9 months; meningitis TB: treat for 9–12 months).
  - TB is a reportable disease: Treatment for TB should be given via directly observed therapy in conjunction with local health department.
- Pearls and pitfalls
  - A high suspicion for TB is necessary in patients with risk factors.
  - Fluoroquinolones are active against TB:
    - Use caution in prescribing fluoroquinolones to treat suspected CAP in patient who may be at high risk for having TB.
    - Patients with recurrent CAP that improves with use of fluoroquinolones should be evaluated for TB.
    - Recent fluoroquinolone use may render AFB cultures negative.
  - Obtain HIV test on all TB suspects if status is unknown.
  - Patients with extrapulmonary TB need to be evaluated for pulmonary TB.
  - Rifampin, isoniazid, and pyrazinamide are potentially hepatotoxic: Monitor liver function tests.
  - Ethambutol may cause optic neuritis: Monitor visual acuity and color vision.
  - Culture is the gold standard for TB diagnosis but may take as long as 8 weeks to grow.
  - Drug susceptibilities should be done on all isolates.
- Links to guidelines: http://www.idsociety.org/uploadedFiles/IDSA/Guidelines Patient_Care/PDF_Library/TB.pdf.

Nontuberculous (Atypical) Mycobacteria (NTM)

- Pulmonary, lymphatic, skin and soft tissue or disseminated diseases caused by mycobacterial species that are widely found in the environment.
- Common complaints and review of systems:
  - Pulmonary disease: chronic or recurring cough, sputum production, weight loss, fatigue, malaise, dyspnea, fever, hemoptysis.
  - Lymphatic disease: enlarged lymph nodes in head and neck; mostly seen in children or HIV-positive adults.
  - Skin and soft tissue disease: nonhealing skin lesions present for longer than 1 month.
  - Disseminated disease: Majority is seen in advanced HIV with CD4 less than 50 cells/mm^3; fever, night sweats, weight loss, abdominal pain, diarrhea.

MEDICAL SPECIALTIES

TABLE 8-19. NONTUBERCULOUS MYCOBACTERIA CAUSES

Pulmonary disease	*Mycobacterium avium* complex
	Mycobacterium kansasii
	Mycobacterium abscessus
Lymphadenitis	*M. avium* complex
Skin, soft tissue, and bone disease	*Mycobacterium chelonae/abscessus* group
	Mycobacterium fortuitum
	Mycobacterium marinum
Disseminated disease	*M. avium* complex
Specimen contaminant	*Mycobacterium gordonae*
	Mycobacterium terrae complex

- Physical examination:
  - Pulmonary disease: rhonchi, crackles, wheezes on lung examination. Postmenopausal women affected by disease may have thin body habitus and may additionally have scoliosis, pectus excavatum, and mitral valve prolapse.
  - Lymphatic disease: Enlarged, nontender unilateral lymph nodes in the head and neck region. Systemic symptoms are largely absent.
  - Skin and soft tissue disease: papules, plaques, pustules or nodules.
  - Disseminated disease: nonspecific but may include fever, abdominal tenderness, hepatosplenomegaly.
- Diagnostic tests:
  - Pulmonary disease: Chest radiograph or high-resolution CT scan, three or more sputum specimens for AFB smear and culture.
  - Lymphatic disease: Fine-needle aspiration or incision and drainage of involved lymph nodes with tissue sent for pathology and culture.
  - Skin and soft tissue disease: Biopsy of lesion sent for pathology and AFB culture.
  - Disseminated disease: Blood cultures for AFB, biopsy and culture of bone marrow, lymph node or liver.
- Common etiologies (Table 8-19).
  - Predisposing factors:
    - *Mycobacterium marinum* skin infection: fresh- and saltwater exposure
    - *Mycobacterium chelonae/abscessus* group *or Mycobacterium fortuitum* skin infection: exposure to footbaths
- Triage and prognosis: NTM are not communicable from one patient to another.
- Treatment: Dependent on organism, location of disease, and clinical suspicion for true disease. Treatment should be done in conjunction with a pulmonary or infectious diseases specialist. Please see attached guidelines for treatment recommendations. http://www.cdc.gov/mmwr/preview/mmwrhtml/rr5211a1.htm
- Pearls and pitfalls:
  - NTM is ubiquitous in the environment; need to know the context to accurately assess whether the culture result is clinically significant.
  - Because of this, more than one culture-positive specimen for NTM is necessary for diagnostic purposes in pulmonary disease.
  - The majority of patients with suspected NTM disease should not be treated until organism is identified in order to prescribe appropriate therapy.
- Links to guidelines: http://www.idsociety.org/uploadedFiles/IDSA/Guidelines-Patient_Care/PDF_Library/NTM%20Disease.pdf.

FUNGI

- *Yeasts:* Candida species, *Cryptococcus* species, *Malassezia furfur*
- *Dimorphic fungi* (yeast at body temperature, mold at room temperature): blastomycosis, coccidioidomycosis, histoplasmosis, paracoccidioidomycosis, *Penicillium marneffei*, sporotrichosis

- **Molds:** *Aspergillus*, dematiaceous fungi, *Fusarium*, *Scedosporium*, Zygomycetes (*Mucor*, *Rhizopus*)

Yeasts

Candida Species

- Clinical syndromes
  - Mucocutaneous (thrush, esophagitis, vulvovaginitis)
  - Invasive (candidemia [blood stream infection], endophthalmitis, endocarditis, osteomyelitis, hepatosplenic candidiasis, other intraabdominal infections)
- Diagnostic tests: varied based on location
  - Routine cultures (fungal cultures not necessary) and/or pathology.
  - Mucocutaneous infections (thrush, esophagitis, vulvovaginitis): diagnosed clinically by characteristic appearance on examination or endoscopy (cultures can be confirmatory).
  - Consider abdominal imaging in neutropenic patients with candidemia.
- Common etiologies:
  - Risk factors for candidemia include recent broad-spectrum antibiotics, indwelling lines and devices, recent surgery, abdominal pathology, total parenteral nutrition, and immunosuppression.
  - Species prevalence varies by health care facility, but in general: *Candida albicans* is more prevalent than *Candida glabrata*, *Candida parapsilosis* is more prevalent than *Candida krusei*, *Candida lusitaniae*, other *Candida* isolates.
- Triage and prognosis: invasive infections such as candidemia must be treated promptly.
- Treatment:
  - Mucocutaneous infections: fluconazole (oral or IV).
  - Invasive infections (candidemia, osteomyelitis, peritonitis, etc.):
    - Echinocandin (transition to fluconazole if not *C. glabrata* or *C. krusei*).
    - For candidemia: remove indwelling lines, obtain dilated funduscopic examination to rule out endophthalmitis, and treat at least 2 weeks from first negative blood cultures.
    - Infectious disease consult is warranted for any invasive candidal infection.
- Pearls and pitfalls
  - *Candida* in sputum is almost always a colonizer and does not require treatment unless patient is extremely immunocompromised (stem cell transplant recipient, etc.).
  - *Candida* in urine is often a colonizer and often does not require treatment:
    - Changing Foley catheter can often clear candiduria.
    - Treat only if symptomatic, undergoing urologic procedure, or immunocompromised (fluconazole only antifungal with good urine penetration).
- Links to guidelines: http://www.idsociety.org/uploadedFiles/IDSA/Guidelines-Patient_ Care/PDF_Library/Candidiasis.pdf

Cryptococcal Species

Refer to section XVII. HIV and Common Opportunistic Infections for HIV-associated cryptococcal meningitis.

- *Cryptococcus gattii* is increasingly seen in immunocompetent hosts and is associated with more severe CNS disease and more CNS complications (such as cryptococcomas). Reported in the Pacific Northwest and British Columbia.
- Treatment regimens for immunocompetent individuals with CNS *Cryptococcus* are similar to those used in immunocompromised patients but with longer (≥4 wk) induction course.
- Links to guidelines: http://www.idsociety.org/uploadedFiles/IDSA/Guidelines-Patient_ Care/PDF_Library/Cryptococcal.pdf.

Dimorphic Fungi (Table 8-20)

- Links to guidelines:
  - Blastomycosis: http://www.idsociety.org/uploadedFiles/IDSA/Guidelines-Patient_Care/ PDF_Library/Blastomycosis.pdf
  - Coccidioidomycosis: http://www.idsociety.org/uploadedFiles/IDSA/Guidelines-Patient_ Care/PDF_Library/Coccidioidomycosis.pdf

TABLE 8-20. DIMORPHIC FUNGI

	Clinical Syndromes	Endemic Regions	Diagnostic Tests	Treatment
Blastomyces dermatitidis	Mostly pulmonary disease Extrapulmonary in 25%–40%: cutaneous, prostate, bone, CNS	Midwest or southeast United States (Mississippi River, Ohio River, Great Lakes)	Fungal cultures and biopsies (broad-based budding)	Amphotericin B or itraconazole (consider voriconazole if CNS disease)
Coccidioides immitis	Usually self-limited pulmonary disease <5% extrapulmonary disease (skin, bone, CNS)	Southwest United States (Arizona, central valley of California, and southwest Texas) and regions of Mexico	Serum or CSF serologic tests (complement fixation titer >1:16 suggests dissemination) Fungal cultures and biopsies (large spherules with endospores)	Fluconazole or amphotericin B (lifelong therapy is required for meningitis)
Histoplasma capsulatum	Usually self-limited pulmonary disease Complications of pulmonary disease (mediastinal fibrosis, pericarditis, arthritis, erythema nodosum) Extrapulmonary disease primarily in immunocompromised (bone marrow; CNS; GI; cutaneous)	Ohio and Mississippi River valleys (bat exposures and spelunkers)	Urine Histoplasma Ag-fungal cultures and biopsies	Amphotericin B or itraconazole
Paracoccidioides brasiliensis	Pulmonary Mucus membrane Disseminated disease (CNS, bone, skin)	Forests in Central and South America	Fungal cultures and biopsies ("pilot wheel")	Itraconazole (Amphotericin B in severe cases)
Penicillium marneffei	Pulmonary, cutaneous, and/or CNS	Southeast Asia (primarily AIDS patients)	Fungal culture and biopsies	Amphotericin B or itraconazole
Sporothrix schenckii	Cutaneous inoculation during gardening or farming leads to lymphatic spread Spread to bone in immunocompromised patients Rare: pulmonary or disseminated disease	Worldwide (decaying vegetation; gardeners)	Fungal cultures and biopsies (cigar-shaped budding yeast)	Itraconazole (Amphotericin B in severe cases)

AIDS, acquired immunodeficiency syndrome; CNS, central nervous system; GI, gastrointestinal.

- Histoplasmosis:http://www.idsociety.org/uploadedFiles/IDSA/Guidelines-Patient_Care/PDF_Library/Histoplasmosis.pdf
- Sporotrichosis:http://www.idsociety.org/uploadedFiles/IDSA/Guidelines-Patient_Care/PDF_Library/Sporotrichosis.pdf

Invasive Molds

- Clinical syndromes: sinusitis (particularly *Aspergillus* and Zygomycetes), infected wounds, pulmonary infections, disseminated disease in immunocompromised (often to brain).
  - Suspect invasive fungal sinusitis if fever, facial pain, and sinus complaints in immunocompromised or diabetic patients.
  - In immunosuppressed patients, fever may be the only clue to invasive fungal infections.
  - Fusarium infections may present with tender, erythematous nodules.
  - Infections are often angioinvasive (necrotic areas on nasal endoscopy with sinusitis, hemoptysis with pulmonary disease).
- Diagnostic tests:
  - Biopsies and fungal cultures
    - Aspergillosis and *Fusarium*: acute-angle branching, septate.
    - Dematiaceous fungi: pigmented
    - Zygomycetes: wide, nonseptate
    - **Histopathology has high frequency (~30%) of misidentifying fungi; need cultures to distinguish.**
  - Serologic testing:
    - $(1,3)$-β-D-glucan test: not specific (positive in many fungal infections, except *Cryptococcus* and Zygomycetes)
    - Galactomannan assay: specific to aspergillosis and *Penicillium* infections, but piperacillin and tazobactam (Zosyn) can cause false-positive results.
  - Chest CT for pulmonary infection ("halo sign")
  - Sinus CT (and STAT ear, nose, and throat exploration) for invasive sinus disease
  - Brain imaging with sinopulmonary disease to rule out CNS involvement
  - Fungal blood cultures: low yield, but may be positive with Fusarium
- Common etiologies: Risk factors include immunosuppression (steroids, transplant recipients, hematologic malignancies), prolonged neutropenia, poorly-controlled diabetes, iron overload, and burn wounds.
- Triage and prognosis: Poor prognosis. STAT antifungals (and STAT surgical debridement for sinusitis and wound infections).
- Treatment:
  - Amphotericin B has broadest antifungal coverage, although some fungi may be resistant (*Scedosporium* and *Aspergillus terreus*). **Always give amphotericin if Zygomycetes infection is suspected, such as with invasive fungal sinusitis.**
  - Voriconazole recommended for invasive aspergillosis (IV or oral).
  - Posaconazole has broad coverage but can only be given orally (best absorption if with full meal) and may take a week to reach steady state.
  - Caspofungin has some activity against *Aspergillus* species, but is not a first-line treatment.
- Pearls and pitfalls:
  - Drug interactions are common, particularly with azoles.
  - Amphotericin B has high risk of nephrotoxicity (less with liposomal formulations); hydrate with IV fluids and replete electrolytes when using.
  - Antifungal susceptibility testing must be specifically requested (isolates are often sent to a reference laboratory).
- Link to guidelines: http://www.idsociety.org/uploadedFiles/IDSA/Guidelines-Patient_Care/PDF_Library/Aspergillosis.pdf.

TICK-BORNE DISEASES

Rocky Mountain Spotted Fever

- Disseminated infection with *Rickettsia rickettsia* transmitted via tick bite (incubation period 2–14 days).

- Common complaints and review of systems: rash, fever, headache, malaise, myalgias, nausea, abdominal pain (mimicking appendicitis and cholecystitis), bloodshot eyes.
- Physical examination: macular petechial rash that starts on ankles and wrists and spreads to trunk in 90%, conjunctivitis, funduscopic hemorrhages, fever.
- Diagnostic tests: presumptive diagnosis based on epidemiology and clinical manifestations
  - Skin biopsy with immunofluorescence staining (high specificity, 70% sensitivity, but sensitivity decreases rapidly after treatment started).
  - Serology can provide a retrospective diagnosis (acute and convalescent serum).
  - Often associated with thrombocytopenia, transaminitis, hyponatremia, azotemia and acute renal failure, and increased prothrombin time and partial prothrombin time.
- Common etiologies:
  - Primary vectors: the dog tick (*Dermacentor variabilis*) in the South and the wood tick (*Dermacentor andersoni*) in the West.
  - Geographic range: most common in southeastern United States, but throughout North and South America.
  - Occurs primarily in late spring and summer.
- Triage and prognosis: can be lethal. When in doubt, treat (do not wait for diagnostic tests).
- Treatment: doxycycline 100 mg PO BID × 7 days (or 3 days after fever resolved). Can use chloramphenicol in pregnant women.
- Pearls and pitfalls: often mistaken for viral syndrome, drug allergy, or meningococcemia.

Lyme Disease

- Disseminated infection with *Borrelia burgdorferi* transmitted by the Ixodes tick. (most common insect-borne disease in the United States).
- Common complaints, review of systems, and physical examination:
  - Primary disease: erythema migrans (painless macular expanding skin lesion with central clearing 1 month after tick bite).
  - Secondary disease: headache, cranial nerve deficits (Bell palsy), irregular heart beat, peripheral neuritis, with or without multiple erythema migrans lesions.
  - Tertiary disease (months to years after primary disease): migrating arthritis and arthralgias; encephalopathy with mood, cognitive, and sleep disorders; fibromyalgia-like or chronic fatigue-like syndrome.
- Diagnostic tests:
  - If erythema migrans present, can diagnose clinically.
  - In absence of erythema migrans, clinical syndrome and positive serology for diagnosis:
    - Immunoglobulin G (IgG) and immunoglobulin M (IgM) by enzyme-linked immunosorbent assay (ELISA) for screening (IgG turns positive 6 weeks after infection).
    - Western blot: 2:3 positive bands for IgM and 5:10 positive bands for IgG.
    - Positive ELISA must be confirmed with Western blot; negative ELISA excludes diagnosis unless early disease (within 6 weeks of infection).
- Common etiologies: bite of the Ixodes tick (must attach for 36–48 hours to transmit the spirochete).
- Triage and prognosis: given propensity to cause chronic infection, always treat Lyme disease.
- Treatment:
  - Early Lyme (erythema migrans): doxycycline 100 mg PO BID, amoxicillin 500 mg PO 3 times daily (TID), or cefuroxime 500 mg BID over 14 days.
  - Primary heart block with normal PR interval or cranial nerve palsy: doxycycline or amoxicillin PO or ceftriaxone 2 g IV daily over 14 to 21 days.
  - Secondary or more heart block or meningitis: ceftriaxone 2 g IV daily or penicillin G 3 to 4 million units every 4 h over 14 to 28 days (hospitalization and cardiac monitoring and/or temporary pacemaker recommended for carditis with symptoms or advanced heart block).
  - Chronic arthritis: doxycycline, amoxicillin, or cefuroxime PO for 28 to 56 days.
  - Prophylaxis (engorged tick, endemic area): doxycycline 200 mg, 1 dose.

- Pearls and pitfalls
  - If untreated, can survive for years in the joint fluid, CNS, and skin.
  - Ixodes ticks can also transmit *Anaplasma phagocytophilum* (ehrlichiosis) and *Babesia microti* (babesiosis), and patients may be infected with all three concurrently (doxycycline will treat both Lyme and ehrlichiosis but not babesiosis).
  - Antibiotic therapy is not indicated for post-Lyme syndrome (>6 months of symptoms despite appropriate treatment).
  - Links to guidelines:
    - http://www.idsociety.org/uploadedFiles/IDSA/Guidelines-Patient_Care/PDF_Library/ Lyme%20Disease.pdf
    - http://www.idsociety.org/uploadedFiles/IDSA/Guidelines-Patient_Care/PDF_Library/ Nervous%20System%20Lyme%20Disease.pdf

Ehrlichiosis

- Disseminated infection with *Ehrlichia chaffeensis* (human monocytic ehrlichiosis or HME) or *A. phagocytophilum* (human granulocytic anaplasmosis or HGA).
  - Common complaints and review of systems: gradual onset of fever, chills, headache, myalgias, anorexia, nausea, cough, and malaise. Rarely, altered mentation or stiff neck.
  - Physical examination: macular, petechial rash (30%–40% with HME, 2%–11% with HGA), fever.
  - Diagnostic tests: diagnosis is usually presumptive.
    - Serology can provide a retrospective diagnosis.
    - Morulae (intracytoplasmic inclusion) in peripheral blood smears (HGA > HME).
    - Often associated with thrombocytopenia, leukopenia, and moderate transaminitis.
- Common etiologies
  - HME: Lone star tick found on whitetail deer in Southeastern United States.
  - HGA: Ixodes tick found in California, Connecticut, Florida, Massachusetts, Minnesota, New York, and Wisconsin.
  - Incubation period is 5 to 21 days from tick bite.
  - HGA is infrequent in children.
- Triage and prognosis: Often resolves without treatment, but rarely can be fatal (treat all suspected cases that are symptomatic).
- Treatment: doxycycline 100 mg PO BID over 7 to 14 days.
- Pearls and pitfalls: Differential diagnosis includes Rocky Mountain Spotted Fever, Lyme disease, and viral illnesses.

EVALUATION OF FEBRILE ILLNESS IN TRAVELERS

Travel history is essential:

- Country, rural exposure
- Fresh water exposure (schistosomiasis, leptospirosis)
- Sexual activities
- Local medical care, including injections and surgeries
- History of malaria chemoprophylaxis (but does not exclude malaria)

Focus on infections that can be:

- Rapidly progressive (malaria, especially *Plasmodium falciparum*)
- Treatable (enteric fever [*Salmonella typhi* and *Salmonella paratyphi*], malaria, rickettsial infections and leptospirosis)
- Common complaints (Table 8-21): **Fever**
  - Persistent fever with a diagnosis of malaria made in a developing country despite adequate treatment: may not be malaria; up to 75% of positive malaria smears in some developing countries are false-positive results.
- Diagnosis:
  - Incubation periods can exclude certain diagnoses: Fever onset less than 6 days after arrival in a malarious area excludes malaria, fever onset more than 14 days after leaving an endemic area excludes dengue, chikungunya and hemorrhagic fevers (Lassa, Ebola).

TABLE 8-21. FEBRILE ILLNESS IN TRAVELERS

Presents >6 wk after travel	*Plasmodium vivax* malaria, tuberculosis, amoebic liver abscess
With rash	Dengue, chikungunya, rickettsial infections, measles
With altered mental status	Viral encephalitis (Japanese B and others), bacterial meningitis, African trypanosomiasis
With abdominal pain	Enteric fever, amoebic liver abscess
With eosinophilia	Acute schistosomiasis, hookworm, *Strongyloides*, filariasis, visceral larva migrans (toxocariasis)
With decreased or normal WBC count	Dengue, malaria, rickettsial infections, enteric fever
With thrombocytopenia	Malaria, dengue, rickettsial infections
With arthralgias and arthritis	Chikungunya

WBC, white blood cell.

- Geographic clues (Table 8-22): Refer to Centers for Disease Control and Prevention (CDC) Yellow Book for country-specific information at wwwnc.cdc.gov/travel/page/yellowbook-2012-home.htm.
- Common etiologies:
  - Malaria: most common febrile infection from sub-Saharan Africa, especially West Africa. Highest risk among expatriates, those visiting friends and relatives, and foreign visitors and migrants. Decreased platelet count and low or normal WBC count are typical; rash and lymphadenopathy are very rare.
  - Dengue: high fever, severe myalgias ("breakbone fever"), headache (retroorbital), leukopenia, thrombocytopenia, rash occurring at the end of the fever. Current outbreaks can be found at: http://healthmap.org/dengue.
  - Chikungunya: similar to dengue with arthralgias or arthritis.
  - Enteric fever: most common in South Central Asia. Typical stairstep fever increasing daily with temperatures persistently elevated, constipation occurs more often than diarrhea, abdominal pain, headache, lassitude.
  - Rickettsial infection: most common in sub-Saharan Africa. fever, myalgias, severe headaches, normal or decreased WBC count, decreased platelets. May have history of tick bite or eschar at site of bite. Macular papular rash which may become petechial.

TABLE 8-22. FEBRILE ILLNESS BY REGION

Sub-Saharan Africa	Malaria (*Plasmodium falciparum*). Less common: tick-borne rickettsioses, acute schistosomiasis, African trypanosomiasis
South Central Asia	Malaria (especially *Plasmodium vivax*), dengue, enteric fever, chikungunya
Southeast Asia	Dengue and malaria (especially *P. vivax*). Less common: chikungunya, leptospirosis
Central America	Dengue and malaria (*P. vivax*, especially Honduras, Mexico). Less common: leptospirosis, histoplasmosis
Caribbean	Dengue, malaria (*P. vivax*; Haiti, *P. falciparum*)
South America	Dengue, malaria (*P. vivax*). Less common: bartonellosis, leptospirosis

- Empiric treatment

Malaria

- May be needed in the absence of rapid, reliable diagnostic capability.
- Guidelines for malaria treatment are available at http://www.cdc.gov/malaria/diagnosis_treatment/treatment.html.
- Treatment advice is also available from the CDC Malaria Branch at 770-488-7788 Monday-Friday 08:00 to 16:30 and toll free at 855–856-4713.
- After-hours advice: CDC Emergency Ops Center at 770-488-7100.

Enteric Fever

- Quinolone (ciprofloxacin, levofloxacin).
- Increasing quinolone resistance in Indian subcontinent and Southeast Asia, consider ceftriaxone or azithromycin.

Rickettsial Disease

- Doxycycline 100 mg BID

Leptospirosis

- Ceftriaxone 1 g daily or penicillin G 1.5 million units every 6 h or doxycycline 200 mg daily for 7 days
- Pearls and pitfalls: A missed diagnosis and delayed treatment of malaria has the highest risk for a severe, preventable adverse outcome.
  - The old adage that fever in a traveler to a malarious area should be considered malaria until proven otherwise should guide the evaluation of febrile travelers.
  - Travelers with malaria may be afebrile at the time of evaluation (10%–40%), but will usually give a history of chills. Fever that recurs in a regular 48- to 72-hour pattern is essentially pathognomonic of malaria.
  - Remember that common causes of fevers in travelers are not necessarily exotic imported infections, but may be common community acquired infections (pneumonia, pyelonephritis).

INFECTIONS IN THE TRANSPLANT OR NEUTROPENIC PATIENT (TABLE 8-23)

- Fever: isolated oral temperature 38.3°C (101°F) or higher, or temperature 38.0°C (100.4°F) or higher for more than 1 hour

TABLE 8-23. INFECTIONS IN THE TRANSPLANT OR NEUTROPENIC PATIENT

<1 month	1–6 months	>6 months
· Infections related to surgery or graft injuries · Nosocomial infections · Recipient-derived infections related to colonization with fungal or multidrug resistant pathogens · Donor-derived infections	· *If no PCP prophylaxis with TMP-SMX:* Pneumocystis, Toxoplasmosis, Nocardia, Listeria · *If no antiviral prophylaxis with valganciclovir:* herpes viruses (HSV, VZV, CMV, EBV) · Polyomavirus hominis 1 (BKV) (nephropathy) · Others: Cryptococcal infection, viral hepatitis, strongyloides, leishmania, *Trypanosoma cruzi*	· Community-acquired infections · Fungal infections · Nocardia · Rhodococcus · Late viral infections (CMV, viral hepatitis, HSV, JC polyomavirus, PML) · Viral associated malignancies: skin cancers, lymphoma (PTLD)

BKV, BK virus; CMV, cytomegalovirus; EBV, Epstein-Barr virus; HSV, herpes simplex virus; PCP, *Pneumocystis jiroveci* pneumonia; PML, progressive multifocal leukoencephalopathy; PTLD, posttransplantation lymphoproliferative disease; TMP-SMX, trimethoprim-sulfamethoxazole; VZV, varicella-zoster virus.
Chart adapted from Infection in solid-organ transplant recipients. Fishman JA, *N Engl J Med.* 2007 Dec 20;357(25):2601-14.

- Neutropenia: absolute neutrophil count (ANC) less than 500 cells/mm^3 or ANC expected to decrease to less than 500 cells/mm^3 over next 48 hours. Patients with "functional neutropenia" should be considered at risk for infection despite a normal neutrophil count.

Always review prior culture data (eg, Is there history of multidrug-resistant pathogens?) and whether the patient has been on any prophylactic antimicrobials (changes spectrum of possible pathogens).

In transplant recipients, the serostatus of the donor is important in establishing risk of certain viral infections, particularly cytomegalovirus (CMV).

- Common complaints, review of systems, and physical examination:
  - Fever may be the only finding in infected, immunosuppressed patients.
  - GI mucositis: sore throat, difficulty swallowing, diarrhea, abdominal pain.
  - Avoid rectal examination in neutropenic patients.
  - CMV syndrome: fever, generalized weakness, body aches, pancytopenia.
- Diagnostic tests:
  - Always include a differential with the CBC. Note that WBCs may be absent from urinalysis and CSF studies in neutropenic patients.
  - Blood cultures *prior* to starting antibiotics—one from each central line port and one peripheral.
  - Consider respiratory viral PCR samples (nasopharyngeal, bronchoalveolar lavage) in patients with pulmonary symptoms.
  - In patients at risk for invasive fungal infections:
    - CT sinus and chest: "halo sign" or cavitary lesions during periods of neutropenia, and air-crescent sign during recovery.
      - Fungal diagnostic assays: (1,3)-β-D-glucan test (detects most fungal pathogens except Zygomycetes and *Cryptococcus* species) or galactomannan assay (detects only *Aspergillus* species and *Penicillium* species). False positives with galactomannan assay with concurrent use of β-lactam and β-lactamase combinations.
  - CT abdomen and pelvis to evaluate for necrotizing enterocolitis in patients with abdominal pain or diarrhea.
  - In transplant recipients at risk for CMV infection, check serum CMV DNA PCR. Assay can be negative in CMV infection of the CNS or GI system, and invasive testing (LP, endoscopy) may be necessary for diagnosis.
- Common etiologies:
  - Nosocomial infections: pneumonias; sepsis related to central lines, Foley catheters, or other indwelling devices.
  - In neutropenic patients with mucositis: bacteremia from oral flora; intraabdominal infections.
  - Oral ulcerations or odynophagia may be from *Candida*, HSV, or CMV.
  - Diarrhea may be from CMV or *C. difficile* infection.
  - Atypical pneumonia presentations: viral, *Pneumocystis jiroveci* pneumonia (PCP), atypical mycobacteria, invasive fungal, nocardia, noninfectious.
  - Patients with 2 weeks or longer of neutropenia are at risk for invasive fungal infections.
  - Infections in solid organ transplant recipients are determined by date from transplant. Risk of infection decreases at 6 months posttransplant. The clock resets if transplant recipient is treated for any rejection.
- Triage and prognosis:
  - Neutropenic patients can be stratified as:
    - High-risk:
      - Profound neutropenia (ANC ≤100 cells/mm^3) expected to persist for 7 or more days.
      - Presence of medical comorbidities (mucositis, hemodynamic instability, neurologic symptoms, new pulmonary infiltrate).
      - Hepatic (transaminases >5x upper limits of normal [ULN]) or renal insufficiency (creatinine clearance <30 mL/min).
    - Low-risk: neutropenia expected to resolve within 7 days and no associated medical comorbidities.

TABLE 8-24. PROPHYLACTIC AGENTS FOR THE TRANSPLANT OR NEUTROPENIC PATIENT

Prophylaxis	Clinical Scenario
G-CSF	Anticipated risk for fever and neutropenia is ≥20%
Posaconazole	High risk for *Aspergillus* infections (prolonged neutropenia)
Fluconazole, voriconazole, echinocandin	High risk for invasive *Candida* infections (hematologic malignancies, HSCT recipients)
Acyclovir or ganciclovir	HSV-seropositive individuals; ganciclovir also covers CMV and HHV-6
Fluoroquinolone (levofloxacin or ciprofloxacin)	Prolonged, profound neutropenia (ANC ≤100 for >7 days)

ANC, absolute neutrophil count; CMV, cytomegalovirus; G-CSF, granulocyte colony-stimulating factor; HHV, human herpesvirus; HSCT, hematopoietic stem-cell transplant; HSV, herpes simplex virus.

- Treatment:
  - In documented infections, treatment decisions should be guided by the individual diagnosis.
  - In high-risk neutropenic patients with fever and no known source of infection:
    - Monotherapy with an antipseudomonal agent (cefepime, piperacillin-tazobactam, or carbapenem) is warranted. Addition of a second agent (aminoglycosides or fluoroquinolones) may be used if high suspicion for multidrug resistance.
    - Treatment directed toward gram-positive pathogens (IV vancomycin, daptomycin, linezolid) should be added if any concern for catheter-related infections, soft tissue infection, pneumonia, or for any hemodynamic instability. Stop if cultures negative for gram-positive pathogen at 48 hours.
    - Consider the addition of antifungals (echinocandin, Amphotericin B, voriconazole) for high-risk patients with persistent fever despite 4 to 7 days of antibiotics.
    - If no documented infection is found, continue antibiotics until patient has been afebrile for at least 48 hours and neutrophil count is increasing beyond 500 cells/mm^3.
- Prophylactic agents (Table 8-24):
- Pearls and pitfalls
  - Most cases of neutropenic fever have no documented source of infection.
  - Fever may have a noninfectious etiology, including transplant rejection.
  - Toxicities of immunosuppressants may mimic infection (eg, sirolimus-induced pneumonitis can look like PCP or viral pneumonia on imaging).
  - Reducing immunosuppression is often a necessary adjunct to treating transplant-related infections.
- Link to guidelines:
  - http://www.idsociety.org/uploadedFiles/IDSA/Guidelines-Patient_Care/PDF_Library/FN.pdf
  - http://www.idsociety.org/uploadedFiles/IDSA/Guidelines-Patient_Care/PDF_Library/OI.pdf.

HIV AND COMMON OPPORTUNISTIC INFECTIONS

- Opportunistic infections (OIs): infections that are more frequent or more severe because of HIV-associated immunosuppression.
- AIDS: HIV infection *plus* history of CD4 count less than 200 cells/mm^3 or AIDS indicator condition (listed below):
  - Candidiasis of esophagus, trachea, bronchi, or lungs
  - Invasive cervical cancer

- Extrapulmonary coccidioidomycosis, cryptococcosis, or histoplasmosis
- Cryptosporidiosis or isosporosis with diarrhea longer than 1 month
- Cytomegalovirus infection of any organ other than liver, spleen, or lymph nodes
- Herpes simplex infection with ulcer longer than 1 month or bronchitis, pneumonitis, or esophagitis
- Disabling HIV-associated dementia
- HIV-associated wasting (involuntary >10% weight loss plus chronic diarrhea or weakness)
- Kaposi sarcoma
- CNS or non-Hodgkin B cell lymphoma or immunoblastic sarcoma
- Disseminated *M. tuberculosis*, *Mycobacterium avium*-intracellulare complex (MAC), or *Mycobacterium kansasii*, or pulmonary TB
- Nocardiosis
- PCP
- Recurrent bacterial pneumonia
- Progressive multifocal leukoencephalopathy (PML)
- Recurrent salmonella (nontyphoid) septicemia
- Extraintestinal strongyloidosis
- Toxoplasmosis of internal organ

HIV and AIDS

- Common complaints, review of systems, and physical examination: weight loss, wasting, unexplained fevers, lymphadenopathy, oral thrush, (others based on presence of specific OIs).
- Diagnostic tests:
  - For HIV diagnosis: HIV EIA with confirmatory Western blot if positive; positive rapid tests should be confirmed with EIA and Western blot. Diagnose acute HIV infection (<6–12 weeks) with HIV RNA PCR (serologic tests may be negative).
  - If HIV positive, key tests include: CBC with differential, T cell subsets (CD4 count and percentage), quantitative HIV RNA by PCR, comprehensive metabolic panel (to look for renal or hepatic dysfunction), tests for other STDs (RPR or syphilis EIA, urine *N. gonorrhea* and *C. trachomatis* NAAT), toxoplasma IgG, and hepatitis serologies (A, B, and C).
- Common etiologies: history of unprotected sex (anal, vaginal, or oral), sex with multiple partners, blood transfusion (especially outside of the United States), IV drug abuse, and tattoos. Can also acquire perinatally (although rare in United States with good prenatal care).
- Triage and prognosis: **CD4 count** determines risk for specific OIs and conditions (Table 8-25).

TABLE 8-25. CD4 COUNT IMPLICATIONS FOR HIV AND AIDS PATIENTS

Cells/mm³	Risk
Any	Elevated risk for herpes zoster, TB, skin conditions, bacterial infections (pneumonia, sinusitis)
<500	Cutaneous KS, vaginal candidiasis, idiopathic thrombocytopenic purpura
<200	Thrush, oral hairy leukoplakia, PCP, disseminated histoplasmosis or coccidioidomycosis
<100	Toxoplasmosis, cryptococcal meningitis, primary CNS lymphoma, PML
<50	Disseminated MAC, CMV retinitis or encephalitis, HIV-associated wasting or encephalopathy

CMV, cytogelovirus; CNS, central nervous system; HIV, human immunodeficiency virus; KS, Kaposi sarcoma; MAC, *Mycobacterium avium*-intracellulare complex; PCP, *Pneumocystis jiroveci* pneumonia; PML, progressive multifocal leukoencephalopathy; TB, tuberculosis.

- Treatment:
  - Antiretroviral therapy (ART): combination (usually ≥3 drugs) HIV therapy:
    - Start or change ART in consultation with an infectious disease or HIV specialist.
    - Timing: per guidelines, start ART at CD4 less than 500 cells/mm^3, but consider at any CD4. Can start ART concurrently with OI treatment (with TB and cryptococcal meningitis with elevated intracranial pressure (ICP), delay may be beneficial to prevent immune reconstitution inflammatory syndrome (IRIS).
    - IRIS: an unmasking or worsening of an OI after ART initiation because of an increased inflammatory response from the increased number of CD4 T lymphocytes.
  - OI prophylaxis:
    - CD4 less than 200 cells/mm^3: TMP-SMX 1 tablet PO daily (alternatives: dapsone or atovaquone)
    - CD4 less than 50 cells/mm^3: azithromycin 1200 mg PO weekly
- Pearls and pitfalls
  - Test for glucose-6-phosphate dehydrogenase deficiency before starting dapsone (hemolytic anemia) and human leukocyte antigen (HLA)-B*5701 before starting abacavir (associated with hypersensitivity reaction that can be fatal).
  - Antiretrovirals (particularly ritonavir) interact with a number of other drugs, often requiring dose adjustments.
  - HIV-infected people have much higher incidence of drug allergies and adverse drug reactions (~30% have rash and/or fever with TMP-SMX).
- Links to guidelines: http://aidsinfo.nih.gov/contentfiles/Adult_OI_041009.pdf; http://www.aidsinfo.nih.gov/ContentFiles/AdultandAdolescentGL.pdf

Pneumocystis jiroveci Pneumonia (PCP)

- Common complaints and review of systems: subacute (days to weeks) onset of progressive dyspnea (especially on exertion), fever, nonproductive cough, and chest discomfort.
- Physical examination: fever; tachypnea, tachycardia, and diffuse dry rales on exertion; hypoxemia; decreased oxygen saturation with exertion; oral thrush (common coinfection).
- Diagnostic tests:
  - Histologic stains for PCP from induced sputum (50%–90% sensitivity), bronchoalveolar lavage (90%–99% sensitivity), or lung tissue (95%–100% sensitivity). Try induced sputum first (less invasive).
  - Suggestive tests: lactate dehydrogenase >500 mg/dL and chest x-ray with diffuse, bilateral, symmetrical interstitial infiltrates and/or pneumothorax (may be normal in early disease).
- Risk factors: CD4 less than 200 cells/mm^3 or CD4 percentage less than 14%, nonadherence to PCP prophylaxis, prior PCP, oral thrush, recurrent bacterial pneumonia, elevated HIV viral load.
- Triage and prognosis: 50% survival if hypoxemia requiring mechanical ventilation and ICU.
- Treatment:
  - TMP-SMX: 2 DS tablets PO every 8 h or 5 mg/kg trimethoprim (TMP) component IV every 8 h (if cannot take oral).
  - Alternatives: clindamycin plus primaquine, IV pentamidine, dapsone plus TMP, or atovaquone.
  - Adjunctive steroids if breathing room air, patient's arterial oxygen partial pressure (PaO$_2$) is less than 70 mm Hg or alveolar-arterial A-a gradient is more than 35 mm Hg (prednisone 40 mg PO BID × ≥5 days then taper based on clinical response).
  - Duration: 21 days, then switch to PCP prophylaxis (TMP-SMX 1 tablet daily).
- Pearls and pitfalls
  - If not on steroids, after starting effective treatment, symptoms may worsen over 2 to 3 days, and fever may persist for a week.
  - Organisms persist in clinical specimens for days to weeks after treatment initiated.
- Links to guidelines: http://aidsinfo.nih.gov/contentfiles/Adult_OI_041009.pdf

Cryptococcal Meningitis

- Common complaints and review of systems: subacute onset of fever, malaise, and headache. Less often, neck stiffness and photophobia (~30%), lethargy, or altered mental status. If associated pulmonary infection, may have cough and dyspnea.
- Physical examination: fever, neck stiffness, focal neurologic deficits, altered mentation. If disseminated, may have molluscum-like skin lesions and/or tachypnea.
- Diagnostic tests:
  - CSF analysis: mildly elevated protein, low to normal glucose, usually a lymphocytic pleocytosis (although can have 0 WBCs), elevated opening pressure (75% > 20 cm H_2O), positive India ink stain for yeast (~50% sensitivity).
  - Cryptococcal antigen (CrAg) usually positive in CSF and serum.
  - Blood cultures: up to 75% may grow *Cryptococcus neoformans.*
  - Brain MRI may show cryptococcomas and/or hydrocephalus.
- Risk factors: CD4 less than 100 cells/mm³ (usually CD4 <50 cells/mm³); exposure to pigeons, soil, plants (eucalyptus).
- Triage and prognosis: Cryptococcal meningitis has a high mortality rate; CSF WBC count <20/μL, CSF CrAg more than 1:1024, and abnormal mental status are poor prognostic factors.
- Treatment:
  - At least 2 weeks of induction therapy (IV amphotericin B deoxycholate 0.7–1.0 mg/kg/day or amphotericin B [AmBisome] 3–4 mg/kg/day or amphotericin B [Abelcet] 5 mg/kg/day PLUS flucytosine 25 mg/kg 4 times daily).
  - Followed by at least 8 weeks of consolidation therapy (fluconazole 400 mg daily).
  - Followed by at least 10 months of maintenance therapy (fluconazole 200 mg daily); maintenance therapy can be stopped after 12 months or longer of therapy if on ART and CD4 count is more than 100 cells/mm³ and HIV viral load is undetectable for 3 months.
  - If ICP is 25 cm H_2O or more, relieve ICP by draining CSF until ICP is 20 cm H_2O or less. Then repeat daily LPs until ICP and symptoms are stable for at least 2 days (consider temporary lumbar drain or ventriculostomy if prolonged elevated ICP).
- Pearls and pitfalls
  - Monitor renal function and electrolytes (K, Mg) with amphotericin and lipid formulations; preinfusion with 500 cc normal saline (± KCl) decreased risk of nephrotoxicity.
  - Monitor CBC and flucytosine blood levels (peak should be 30–80 μg/mL) with flucytosine to prevent bone marrow suppression.
  - IRIS after initiation of ART: 30% HIV patients with cryptococcal meningitis.
  - Increased prevalence in sub-Saharan African (fourth highest cause of death from infection).
  - Serum CrAg is a good predictor of who will develop cryptococcal meningitis in patients newly diagnosed with HIV and CD4 is less than 100 cells/mm³. If CrAg is positive, obtain LP. If LP shows no evidence of meningoencephalitis, treat with fluconazole 400 mg daily until CD4 is greater than 100 cells/mm³.
- Links to guidelines: http://www.idsociety.org/uploadedFiles/IDSA/Guidelines-Patient_Care/PDF_Library/Cryptococcal.pdf

Toxoplasma gondii **Encephalitis**

- Common complaints and review of systems: headache, confusion, motor weakness, fever.
- Physical examination: fever, focal neurologic deficits (can progress to seizures, stupor, and coma).
- Diagnostic tests:
  - Brain MRI or CT with ring-enhancing lesions (usually multiple).
  - Serum *T. gondii* IgG (less likely if negative).
  - CSF *T. gondii* PCR (specificity 96%–100%, but sensitivity only 50%).
  - CSF Epstein-Barr virus PCR (if positive, highly suggestive of CNS lymphoma rather than *T. gondii*).

- Risk factors:
  - CD4 less than 100 cells/mm³ (usually CD4 <50 cells/mm³).
  - Usually reactivation of latent tissue cysts, but can be because of primary infection (eating undercooked meat or contact with feces of infected cats).
- Triage and prognosis: if CNS mass lesion, CD4 less than 100 cells/mm³, and toxoplasmosis suspected (especially if positive IgG and not on prophylaxis with TMP-SMX or atovaquone), should be empirically treated for *T. gondii* encephalitis. Monitor clinically and repeat brain imaging in 10 to 14 days, and if no improvement or worsening consider brain biopsy to look for alternate diagnosis.
- Treatment:
  - Initiate 6 weeks or more of acute therapy with pyrimethamine (200 mg PO × 1 then 75 mg/day) + sulfadiazine (1–1.5 g PO every 6 h) + leucovorin (10–25 mg/day); alternatives include clindamycin plus pyrimethamine plus leucovorin, TMP-SMX, pyrimethamine plus azithromycin, pyrimethamine plus atovaquone, or sulfadiazine plus atovaquone.
  - Followed by secondary prophylaxis (until on ART with CD4 ≥200 cells/mm³ for >6 months) with pyrimethamine (25–50 mg/day) plus sulfadiazine (2–4 g/day in 2–4 divided doses) plus leucovorin (10–25 mg/day); alternatives include clindamycin plus pyrimethamine plus leucovorin, atovaquone with or without pyrimethamine and leucovorin, and atovaquone plus sulfadiazine.
- Pearls and pitfalls: primary differential diagnosis is CNS lymphoma, although could be mycobacterial abscess, cryptococcoma, bacterial abscess, or PML.
- Links to guidelines: http://aidsinfo.nih.gov/contentfiles/Adult_OI_041009.pdf

Disseminated MAC

- Common complaints and review of systems: usually disseminated disease with fever, night sweats, weight loss, fatigue, diarrhea, and abdominal pain.
- Physical examination: fever, hepatomegaly, splenomegaly, or lymphadenopathy.
- Diagnostic tests:
  - MAC isolated from AFB cultures of blood, lymph node, bone marrow, or other normally sterile tissue or body fluid (with compatible signs and symptoms) is diagnostic.
  - Suggestive laboratory tests include positive AFB smear and culture of stool, anemia, elevated alkaline phosphatase.
- Risk factors:
  - CD4 less than 50 cells/mm³, plasma HIV more than 100,000 copies/mL, or previous OIs or colonization with MAC.
- Triage and prognosis: associated with increased mortality
- Treatment: 2 or more antimycobacterial drugs (clarithromycin 500 mg PO BID + ethambutol 15 mg/kg/day ± rifabutin 300 mg PO daily) for 12 months or longer. Can substitute azithromycin 500–600 mg PO daily for clarithromycin (~20% deafness with prolonged azithromycin).
- Pearls and pitfalls
  - Hold off on starting ART until after 2 weeks or longer of MAC therapy.
  - Clinical improvement should be seen within 2 to 4 weeks; if not, repeat AFB blood culture to look for ongoing mycobacteremia.
- Links to guidelines: http://aidsinfo.nih.gov/contentfiles/Adult_OI_041009.pdf

MEDICAL SPECIALTIES

CHAPTER 9

Nephrology

James S. Cain

ACUTE RENAL FAILURE (ARF)

Definition

- A sudden loss of renal function measured by:
  - Increase in serum creatinine or reduction in in glomerular filtration rate

Characteristics

- May be nonoliguric
- Occurs commonly during hospitalization
- Usually multifactorial[1]

Diagnostic Workup of ARF

- Complete history is necessary.
  - Past medical history: may identify important risk factors:
    - Diabetes
    - Hypertension
    - Renal disease
    - Recent urologic or gynecologic surgery
  - Family history:
    - Relatives with dialysis
    - Polycystic kidney disease
    - Alport syndrome
    - Diabetes
    - Hypertension
  - Social history:
    - "Ecstasy" use induces syndrome of inappropriate antidiuretic hormone (SIADH).
    - Athletic activity leads to volume depletion, rhabdomyolysis, and hyponatremia.[2,3]
    - History of residence in a chronic care facility identifies patients at risk for volume depletion.
  - Medication history:
    - Diuretics
    - Nonsteroidal anti-inflammatory drugs (NSAIDs) (perhaps not prescribed)
    - Metformin
    - Bactrim
    - Antivirals
    - Cimetidine
    - Aminoglycoside antibiotics
    - Intravenous (IV) contrast agents
    - Calcium supplements, especially when accompanied by vitamin D and thiazide diuretics can cause hypercalcemia and dehydration.[4-6]
    - Lithium may be toxic with acute volume depletion or cause a chronic interstitial disease with diabetes insipidus (DI).
    - A history of bowel preparation for colonoscopy with sodium phosphate containing purgatives (even years in the past) can lead to hyperphosphatemic renal failure.[7,8]
    - Recent chemotherapy can cause hyperuricemia and tumor lysis syndrome[9,10] or cisplatinum toxicity.

- A large list of medications may cause interstitial nephritis.
- Review of systems
  - Previous treatments
  - Polydipsia
  - Polyuria
  - Thirst
  - Environmental exposure and duration (eg, How many miles did you run?)
  - Difficult, excessive or scant urination
  - Change in urinary frequency, color, odor or appearance (blood red, frothy, tea-colored)

Laboratory Investigation

- Urinalysis looking for cells and casts
  - Red blood cell (RBC) casts are indicative of glomerular disease.
  - White blood cells (WBCs) and WBC casts confirm pyelonephritis or interstitial nephritis.
  - Muddy-brown[11,12] or golden granular casts are indicative of acute tubular necrosis (ATN)
  - Antinuclear antibody (ANA)
  - dsDNA
  - C3 and C4
  - Cytoplasmic antineutrophil cytoplasmic antibody (cANCA) and Perinuclear antineutrophil cytoplasmic antibody (pANCA)
  - Antistreptolysin-O (ASO) titer
  - Rheumatoid factor should be performed to help rule out serologically diagnosable glomerulopathies and to determine if renal biopsy will be performed.[13]
  - Serum protein electrophoresis (SPEP), urine protein electrophoresis (UPEP), and glycated hemoglobin to rule out underlying diabetes or paraproteinemias.
  - Urine electrolytes
  - Urea, protein, and creatinine to calculate fractional excretion of sodium (FeNa), transtubular potassium concentration gradient and clearances if they are required.
  - Eosinophils: Hansel's stain[14] is helpful if pyuria is present and interstitial nephritis is suspected. This test should not be requested without a positive LES or microscopic confirming pyuria.

Diagnostic Studies

- Renal ultrasound
- Confirms the presence and location of the kidneys and rules out obstruction, stones, cystic disease and masses.
- An asymmetric renal size may indicate renal artery stenosis (RAS).
- Renal artery Doppler images help identify and localize renal artery disease.

Clinical Presentation Causes of Acute Kidney Injury are Presented in Table 9.1

- Renal azotemia (ineffective renal perfusion)
  - Volume depletion leads to azotemia and if uncorrected leads to tubular necrosis.
  - Sources of volume loss:
    - Blood loss
    - Perspiration
    - Polyuria
    - Diarrhea
    - Gastric suction
    - Fluid losses from burns, wounds or drains
  - Azotemia is attained as the kidneys retain urea in volume depletion.
  - Elderly patients in long-term care facilities who are unable to obtain water at will are at risk for water depletion and prerenal azotemia.
    - This is more often seen during the hot summer months.
    - Water should be provided regularly to avoid this problem as the patients cannot ask for water appropriately.

TABLE 9-1. CAUSES OF ACUTE KIDNEY INJURY

Prerenal	
	Gastrointestinal hemorrhage
	Burns
	Pancreatitis
	Capillary leak
	Diarrhea, vomiting, nasogastric suction, fistula fluid loss Diaphoresis
	Diuretics, nonsteroidal anti-inflammatory drugs
	Congestive heart failure
	Cirrhosis
Parenchymal	
	Ischemia (eg, postoperative acute tubular necrosis)
	Nephrotoxins (eg, radiocontrast agents, aminoglycosides, myoglobin)
	Sepsis
	Acute interstitial nephritis
	Acute glomerulonephritis
	Acute vascular syndrome (eg, bilateral renal artery thromboembolism or dissection)
	Atheroembolic disease Vasculitis
Postrenal	
	Bilateral upper tract obstruction (eg, nephrolithiasis, papillary necrosis) or obstruction of solitary functioning kidney
	Lower tract obstruction (eg, prostatic hypertrophy, urethral stricture, bladder mass or stone, obstructed urinary catheter)

From Taal MW, et al. *Brenner and Rector's The Kidney*. 9th ed. Philadelphia: Saunders; 2012.

- Symptoms:
  - Thirst
  - Weakness
  - Dizziness
  - Fatigue
  - Confusion
  - Disorientation
- Physical findings:
  - Orthostasis
  - Low blood pressure
  - Dry mucous membranes
  - Tachycardia
  - Tenting of the skin
  - Shrunken eyeballs in extreme cases

TABLE 9-2. TESTS TO DIFFERENTIATE PRERENAL FROM INTRINSIC KIDNEY DAMAGE

Test	Prerenal	Renal
Urine Na (mEq/L)	<20	>40
Urine osmolality (mmol/kg H_2O)	>500	<350
Serum BUN/Cr ratio[a]	>20	10–15
Fractional excretion of Na[b]	<1	>2
Fractional excretion of urea (in the case of loop diuretic use)	<30	>50

BUN, blood urea nitrogen; Cr, creatinine.
[a] A BUN/Cr ratio of <10 may occur with rhabdomyolysis because the Cr concentration increases sharply as a result of increased release from necrotic muscle. A low BUN/Cr ratio can also develop in malnourished individuals because of very low BUN.
[b] The fractional excretion of sodium and fractional excretion of urea are often also very low with contrast nephropathy, rhabdomyolysis, acute myeloma kidney, and acute urate nephropathy.
From Taal MW, et al. *Brenner and Rector's The Kidney.* 9th ed. Philadelphia: Saunders; 2012.

- Laboratory findings (Table 9-2):
  - Increased blood urea nitrogen (BUN)-to-creatinine ratio
  - Elevated BUN and creatinine
  - Metabolic alkalosis
  - Concentrated urine specific gravity with a bland microscopic
  - No significant proteinuria or hematuria
  - Hyaline casts may be seen, especially on rehydration
  - Hypokalemia because of aldosterone activity should be present.
  - A low FeNa is characteristic in prerenal states when the kidneys are intact.
    - FeNa greater than 1.0 with renal failure indicates that a prerenal state is not present or is present with acute tubular necrosis or diuretic use.
- Treatment:
  - Volume replacement, usually with normal saline and correction of any underlying metabolic problem
  - Hypercalcemia causes nephrogenic DI with polyuria, volume loss, and a prerenal state.
    - Correction of the volume loss without correcting the elevated calcium will allow recurrence.
    - Likewise for the polyuria induced by lithium toxicity
  - Central DI (lack of antidiuretic hormone [ADH]) presents with polyuria usually hypernatremia and volume depletion unless free access to water is allowed.
    - The urine is not concentrated in DI
  - Congestive heart failure (CHF): Diuretic therapy improves pulmonary edema and reduces peripheral edema while inducing further azotemia, hypokalemia, and alkalosis.
  - Some patients will have improved cardiac output and resolve the azotemia with diuretics alone.
    - Conivaptan has recently been used to relieved fluid overload in CHF to good effect and high potential cost.[15]
    - The use of angiotensin-converting enzyme inhibitors (ACEIs) while beneficial to the cardiac status, reduce glomerular filtration rate (GFR) and in combination with aggressive diuresis and NSAIDs are frequent causes of ARF.[16,17]
    - Progressive loss of cardiac function can reduce renal perfusion and decrease GFR, a trial of pressor agents may improve cardiac output and GFR.
  - Liver disease: induces a state of sodium avidity, fluid retention and azotemia referred to as the hepatorenal syndrome (HRS)
    - HRS can occur in cirrhosis, metastatic disease to the liver and severe hepatitis.

- It is a sign of poor prognosis.[18–21]
- Treatment includes liver transplant, support, sometimes requiring dialysis and octreotide with midodrine or terlipressin.[22–24]
- When diuretics are required in chronic liver disease, the agent of choice is spironolactone[25] because it does not require secretion into the tubule as do the highly protein-bound thiazide and loop diuretics that enter the tubule by secretion and then bind to the Na-K-2-CL transporter in the TALH (furosemide [Lasix], loop diuretics) or the distal tubule NaCL carrier for thiazides.
  - Spironolactone enters the collecting tubule cells from the blood side[25] and does not require ultrafiltration to hit the target.
- Renal Artery Stenosis (RAS) can induce prerenal azotemia and renal failure.[26,27]
  - Prerenal states are in this case accompanied by hypertension as a result of activation of the renin-angiotensin system.
  - The use of ACEIs or angiotensin receptor blockers (ARBs) may induce or exacerbate renal failure in this situation.[17]
  - Removal of the offending medication should improve renal function. ACEI and ARB are the drug of choice in unilateral RAS but are contraindicated in bilateral disease because of the risk of ARF. Shorter acting ACEI with lower doses may be helpful.
  - Nephrosis caused by diabetes mellitus, focal and segmental glomerulosclerosis (FSGS), membranous nephropathy (MN), and nil disease is characterized by high urine protein excretion, low serum albumin and edema. Ineffective intravascular volume may result with azotemia. The treatment of nephrosis with diuresis frequently leads to a prerenal state.[28]
  - All prerenal states lead to increased prostaglandin production as a means to maintain renal blood flow, the use of NSAIDs (which counteract prostaglandins) in this setting further leads to decreased GFR.
  - Other common drugs that impair renal blood flow and mimic prerenal azotemia include iodinated radiographic contrast, cyclosporine, ACEI, ARBs, tacrolimus, and amphotericin.
- Obstructive Uropathy:
  - This set of problems is easily diagnosed via renal ultrasound.
  - Directly managed by relief of the obstruction.
  - Foley catheterization is an excellent first step followed by percutaneous nephrostomy.
  - Stenting past obstructions is also a viable alternative.
  - Bilateral obstruction is necessary to cause renal failure or if only a single functioning organ then on the side of the functioning kidney.
  - Causes:
    - Children: The leading cause of obstructive uropathy is anatomic abnormality, stricture or abnormal posterior urethral valve function.
    - Young adults: Obstructing calculi are most common.
    - Older adults: Carcinomas, retroperitoneal carcinomas and prostatic hypertrophy are more common.
    - The variety of clinical presentation is wide so that any patient presenting with unexplained renal failure needs to have ultrasonography performed.[29]
- Parenchymal Renal Disease:
  - Acute Tubuler Necrosis (ATN)
  - Follows ischemic or toxic insult.
  - Rapid rise in creatinine 1 to 2 mg/dL per day.
  - This definition lacks the nuances of the Risk Injury Failure Loss and End Stage Renal Disease (RIFLE) and Acute Kidney Injury (AKI) schemes but addresses clinical needs well, leaving the criteria score to be settled later.
  - ARF: 50% is thought to be iatrogenic, and in the hospital setting is often multifactorial with underlying diabetic and hypertensive nephropathies exacerbated by medications, hypotension, shock, and sepsis.
  - Knowledge of preexisting renal disease helps predict recovery and prognosis.
  - Renal size
    - Small kidneys: chronic disease
    - Large kidneys: diabetic and paraproteinemic disease

- Other signs of chronic disease include normochromic anemia, low calcium and high phosphate.
- Causes:
  - Extended loss of renal perfusion should be considered first
    - Identical to prerenal azotemia except that tubular cell dysfunction is now obvious with rising creatinine and elevated FeNa.
    - The lack of reversibility with improved renal perfusion is characteristic.
  - Aminoglycosides have been the most common cause of drug-induced ATN
- Medications and toxins
  - Methotrexate, cisplatinum, hemoglobin, and myoglobin
- Laboratory investigation
  - High FeNa
  - High fractional excretion of urea
  - Renal tubular epithelial cells
  - Muddy-brown casts on microscopic examination
- Treatment
  - Remove the offending agent
  - Supportive care
  - Dialysis or continuous renal replacement therapy may be required.
  - Recovery is expected, but preexisting renal disease may lead to end-stage kidney disease.
- Acute interstitial nephritis (AIN):
  - The classic triad of fever, rash, and eosinophiluria[14,30–32] with renal failure was found when methicillin was in clinical use.
  - These findings, while still relevant, are not often seen, calling for a higher index of suspicion[30,33,34] as AIN is estimated to cause 10% to 15% of acute renal failure.
  - Renal biopsy is the only definitive diagnostic test for this disease.
  - Biopsy reveals a dense mononuclear infiltrate of the intertubular space. This infiltrate consists of T cell lymphocytes, although eosinophils, macrophages and neutrophils may also be present.
  - Damage is limited to the tubular structures with vasculature and glomeruli spared.
  - Causes
    - Drugs
      - β-lactam antibiotics
      - Penicillin analogs
      - Cephalosporins
      - Sulfonamides
      - Rifampin
      - NSAIDs
      - Proton pump inhibitors, (omeprazole),
      - Diuretics (thiazides and furosemide [Lasix])
      - Rifampin
      - Gentamicin
      - Ciprofloxacin
      - Vancomycin
      - Acyclovir
      - Erythromycin
      - Azithromycin
      - Tetracyclines
    - Infectious processes include direct renal infection and systemic infections
    - Autoimmune disorders
      - Systemic lupus
      - Sjögren syndrome
      - Sarcoidosis
      - Tubulointerstitial nephritis and uveitis syndrome

MEDICAL SPECIALTIES

- Cryoglobulinemia
- Acute allograft rejection
- Clinical presentation
  - Fever
  - Rash
  - Arthralgias
  - Flank pain
  - Gross hematuria with sterile pyuria.
  - Microscopic hematuria is common.
  - WBC casts are typical
  - RBC casts have rarely been reported.
  - Eosinophilia, greater than 1% with Hansel stain is suggestive of AIN, but is seen in other renal disease.[14,31,32]
  - Proteinuria is mild, serologies remain normal, except that omeprazole, cimetidine, and ciprofloxacin seem able to induce a positive pANCA with AIN, and tubulointerstitial nephritis and uveitis syndrome induces a positive cANCA.
  - FeNa is unreliable. Because the tubular interstitium is involved a variety of acid-base and concentrating defects have been described.
- Rapidly progressive glomerulonephritis (RPGN)
  - Glomerular diseases and vasculitis have many causes.
  - Classified as primary or secondary.
    - Secondary diseases have systemic features.
    - "Systemic" involvement is the rule.
      - A recent discovery of apolipoprotein L1 (*APOL1*) and its connection to trypanosomiasis and African American end-stage renal disease (ESRD) make this primary disease certainly secondary to a nonrenal genetic mutation.
    - A way to organize glomerular and vascular disease is to categorize those diseases that cause RPGN into one group, those that cause chronic renal disease and nephrosis, with or without loss of GFR into another.
  - RPGN has been classified by immunofluorescent microscopy into three types:
    - Antiglomerular basement membrane disease
    - Immune complex disease
    - Pacui immune disease[35-37]
  - All types of RPGN require aggressive diagnostic and therapeutic efforts.
  - These diseases lead to ESRD with high morbidity and mortality.
- Antiglomerular basement membrane disease
  - Type 1 RPGN contains only one disease:
    - Goodpasture syndrome in which immunofluorescent microscopy of renal biopsy reveal linear staining of the glomerular basement membrane (GBM).
    - Goodpasture syndrome consists of the combination of hemoptysis with hematuria.
    - These patients have an antibody that attacks not only the GBM but also the pulmonary alveolar basement membrane leading to hemoptysis.
    - Iron deficiency is a frequent finding, and the urine contains the characteristic RBC casts, hematuria, and low-grade proteinuria.
    - An indirect test for anti-GBM can be done with the patients serum and normal renal tissue, but this test has a high rate of false-negative results.
      - If done and negative, then renal biopsy is indicated. Light microscopy reveals diffuse crescentic glomerulonephritis (GN).
      - Immunofluorescent microscopy will reveal immunoglobulin G (IgG) staining alone GBMs.
    - Two other diseases can cause linear deposition, diabetic nephropathy, and fibrillary GN, neither of which have circulating anti-GBM or crescents.[38,39]
  - Treatment:
    - Treatment is required to avoid ESRD and consists of cyclophosphamide, prednisone, and plasmapheresis daily for 4 to 10 days.
    - Albumin rather than fresh frozen plasma is preferred for replacement fluid. The immunosuppression is continued for 6 to 12 months.

- This aggressive therapy is not needed for patients with ESRD or who lack hemoptysis.
- The risk of immunosuppression outweighs the benefit of continuing. Aggressive therapy is continued for those with positive antineutrophil cytoplasmic antibody (ANCA) and anti-GBM.[40]
- Immune complex GN:
  - General considerations:
    - In these diseases the serologic and renal biopsy findings identify the systemic disease causing the renal problem.
    - The renal biopsy reveals immune complexes on immunofluorescent microscopy that are characteristic of the disease.
    - IgA nephropathy reveals mesangial IgA deposits.
    - Systemic lupus nephritis has subendothelial deposits on biopsy and circulating ANAs.
    - Cryoglobulin-related disease shows circulating cryoglobulins, usually hepatitis C virus (HCV) antigens and intraluminal "thrombi."
    - Poststreptococcal GN reveals ASO titers and subepithelial humps on biopsy.
  - Classification:
    - Poststreptococcal GN
    - IgA nephropathy and Henoch-Schönlein purpura (mesangial proliferative GN)
    - Postinfectious GN (shunt nephritis, subacute bacterial endocarditis, methicillin-resistant *Staphylococcus aureus* infection)
    - Membranoproliferative glomerulonephritis (MPGN) (also hypocomplementemic GN)
      - Type I, found in monoclonal gammopathies
      - Type II, monoclonal gammopathy with rheumatoid factor activity that binds with polyclonal immunoglobulins, found in 75% of HCV-related MPGN
      - Type III, polyclonal gammopathy, seen in HCV-related MPGN
    - Hepatitis B virus (HBV)-related membranous nephropathy
    - Systemic lupus erythematosus
  - Diagnostics:
    - Requires consideration of the underlying disease
    - Any of the preceding diagnoses may be accompanied by such common renal diseases as diabetic or MN.
    - Urinalysis will reveal hematuria and proteinuria in GN.
    - Microscopic examination will confirm glomerular disease if RBC casts are seen.
    - Renal ultrasound will rule out obstruction, stones, cystic disease, and renal tumors.
    - The confirmation of the presence of two normal-sized kidneys rules out obviously chronic renal disease and allows plans for diagnostic biopsy, (contraindicated in solitary kidney).
    - Diagnostic serologies will include ANAs, anti-DNA, complement studies, HBV and HCV, cryoglobulins, ASO, cANCA and pANCA, and anti-GBM.
    - Rheumatoid factor is a useful rapid screen for circulating immune complexes.
    - Renal biopsy should be considered when the diagnosis is elusive, will make a difference in the therapy, and the expertise to obtain and interpret the results are available.[13]
      - The complication rate for renal biopsy is low but should be taken into consideration.[29]
    - In addition to specific immune complex diseases, other renal diseases will be diagnosed via renal biopsy.
      - Rule out diabetes if not previously diagnosed with glycated hemoglobulin and paraproteinemia and most forms of amyloidosis[41] with SPEP, UPEP, and free light-chains studies.
  - Treatment:
    - May include watchful waiting depending on the clinical situation.[42, 43]
    - Strategies for each diagnosis have been worked out.

- Severe disease with renal failure and hemoptysis requires immunosuppression and plasma exchange.
- Immunosuppression and plasma exchange is not started without renal biopsy except in life sparing situations.

- Pauci-immune RPGN:
  - The renal system is highly vascular and can be affected by a number of vascular diseases.
  - Ischemia can be caused by Takayasu arteritis and giant cell arteritis affecting the aorta or renal arteries.
  - Polyarteritis nodosa and Kawasaki disease can affect the medium-sized arteries.
  - Small vessel arteritis such as microscopic polyangiitis, cryoglobulinemic vasculitis, Wegener granulomatosis, and Henoch-Schönlein purpura frequently involve the kidneys and cause GN.
  - Polyarteritis nodosa and Kawasaki disease affect the main visceral arteries alone, sparing capillaries and venules.[44,45]
  - The vasculitides that cause GN are characterized by circulating ANCA antibodies and a paucity of immunofluorescent staining on microscopy.
  - Microscopic polyangiitis has vasculitis without reactive airways disease (RAD) and no granulomas on biopsy
  - Wegener granulomatosis is characterized by granulomas and lack of RAD. Churg-Strauss syndrome has RAD, eosinophilia, and granuloma formation.[46]
  - The glomerular lesions of microscopic polyangiitis, Wegener, and Churg-Strauss are indistinguishable from one another and contain segmental fibrinoid necrosis, crescents and scant immunofluorescent staining.
  - The ANCA test is positive in only 85% of patients with biopsy-positive Wegener and microscopic polyangiitis, and only 50% of patients with Churg-Strauss.[47]
  - There are two major subtypes of ANCA: the cytoplasmic staining cANCA and the perinuclear staining pANCA.
  - The cANCA has been found to be specifically directed against a neutrophil and monocyte proteinase called *proteinase-3* (PR3-ANCA).[48] Most pANCAs are directed against myeloperoxidase (MPO-ANCA).
  - Evidence that ANCAs cause disease is scant but anti-MPO antibodies cause crescentic GN in mice, and in one observational case in humans in which anti-MPO crossed the placenta to induce GN and pulmonary capillaritis in a newborn.
  - Clinical features of systemic vasculitis syndromes:
    - Most patients will have signs of inflammatory disease, fever, arthralgias, myalgia, and weight loss.
    - The large vessel syndromes (giant cell arteritis and Takayasu) will have ischemia in the area the involved artery supplies.
    - Claudication, absent pulses, and bruits are found most frequently in the upper extremities.
    - Renovascular hypertension is found in 40% of patients with Takayasu but rarely in giant cell arteritis.
    - Kawasaki disease and polyarteritis nodosa frequently present as infarction of medium-sized arteries in multiple organs, and laboratory investigation reveals clinically evident organ damage.
      - Kawasaki is most frequently seen in children and affects coronary, axillary, and iliac arteries.
      - Kawasaki is seen with the mucocutaneous lymph node syndrome, which includes fever, lymphadenopathy, mucosal, and cutaneous inflammation.
      - The renal arteries are frequently involved without clinically evident renal disease.
    - Small vessel disease frequently presents with hematuria, proteinuria, and impaired renal function, signs of the glomerular disease.
      - Other presenting features include purpura, abdominal pain, and positive stool guaiac from bowel infarcts. Necrotizing sinusitis and pulmonary hemorrhage can be seen with any of the small vessel vasculitides.
    - Wegener patients may have necrotizing granulomas of the upper and lower respiratory tract; these appear as nodules on chest radiography.

• Churg-Strauss patients have eosinophilia and asthma.
• Diagnosis:
  • PR3-ANCA (cANCA) is positive in 75% of Wegener, 40% of microscopic polyangiitis, 5% of Churg-Strauss, and 25% of renal-limited vasculitis.
  • MPO-ANCA (pANCA) is positive in 20% of Wegener, 50% of microscopic polyangiitis, 40% of Churg-Strauss, and 10% of renal-limited vasculitis. Of patients with anti-GBM disease 25% to 30% are ANCA positive.
  • Renal biopsy is the standard in identifying the correct diagnosis to guide therapy.
• Treatment:
  • Confirmation of glomerular disease leads to treatment identical to that for anti-GBM-related disease.
  • Typically cyclophosphamide and prednisone; the pulmonary renal syndrome indicates the need for plasmapheresis.
  • Streptococcal GN requires supportive care only[49–51] with excellent chances for recovery.

Atheroembolic Renal Disease

• Showers of atheroemboli following cannulation of the aorta.
• Can lead to embolization of arteries downstream.
• Emboli lodge in peripheral arteries; the "blue toe" syndrome occurs.
• When the renal parenchyma is involved varying degrees of acute renal insufficiency result.
• This may be accompanied by livedo reticularis in the skin.
• Hollenhorst plaques may be seen on retinal examination.
• The urinalysis may reveal eosinophiluria.[52]

CHRONIC DISEASES

Nephrosis: Nephrotic Syndrome

• Heavy proteinuria
• Clinical and laboratory findings that accompany it.
• Nephrosis depends on heavy excretion of urinary protein, usually 2.5 to 3 g/24 h.
• Accompanying hypoalbuminemia, hyperlipidemia, and edema.
  • Minimal change (minimal change disease or nil disease)
    • Primarily found in children; 10% of adult nephrotic syndrome is minimal change disease.
    • The most common form of nephrosis
    • Diagnosed on clinical (edema) and basic laboratory observations
    • Treated with empiric steroid therapy with excellent results.
    • Serologies are normal.
    • Recurrent or refractory disease may call for renal biopsy.
    • Biopsy will be normal except for effacement of the foot processes on electron microscopy
  • Membranous nephropathy
    • A disease of middle-aged and older patients
    • Idiopathic in most cases and has no serologic markers.
    • Associated with concomitant diagnosis of carcinomas, successful treatment of which can lead to resolution of the proteinuria.
    • The presence of immune complexes in the kidney suggests an immune complex basis for the disease, but a direct relation between HBV and MN (or other types of glomerular diseases) remains to be proven.
    • Clearance of HBV antigens, either spontaneous or following antiviral treatments results in improvement in proteinuria.
    • Prompt recognition and specific antiviral treatment are critical in managing patients with HBV and renal involvement.
    • Serologies are normal (except in the case of HBV infection), and biopsy is needed to definitively identify this disease.

- Therapy is difficult to justify because of the high rate of spontaneous resolution and is thus reserved for symptomatic patients or those with progressive loss of renal function.
- FSGS and focal glomerular sclerosis:
  - Most commonly diagnosed adult glomerulopathy resulting in nephrosis.
  - Prevalent in African Americans.[53]
  - Associated with an abnormal copy of a gene for *APOL1* that in heterozygotes affords protection from *Trypanosoma brucei*.[54,55]
  - In homozygous it causes FSGS and end-stage kidney disease in patients of African heritage.
  - This pattern of genetic protection and disease is also seen in sickle cell anemia. It appears that the previously identified variant of focal glomerular sclerosis.
  - Human immunodeficiency virus (HIV)-associated nephropathy is also caused by homozygous aberrant *APOL1*.
  - The aberrant *APOL1* gene is reserved to African populations.
  - Renal biopsy reveals focal (not all of the glomeruli are affected) and segmental (not all parts of affected glomeruli are affected) mesangial expansion without increased cellularity.
  - Serologies are negative and clinical presentation is variable. It is important to note that FSGS is a pathologic description that does not identify a specific pathophysiology, thus treatment which works in one group may not be applicable to others.[56]
  - FSGS in whites is more amenable to therapy with encouraging response to steroids alone in many cases.
  - African Americans are resistant to steroids in most cases. The physiology is clearly different; there are several postulated mechanisms for white FSGS.
  - Untreated or in the unresponsive to therapy hypertension, progressive loss of renal function and ESRD result.
  - FSGS recurs in approximately 30% of cases postrenal transplant.
    - This may be because of *APOL1* as homozygous donors have recurrent FSGS. Donors should be screened to prevent donation of homozygous *APOL1* kidneys.[57]
  - Clinical management includes:
    - Blood pressure control with ACEI and/or ARBs when tolerated.
    - Diuretics
    - Sodium restriction with preparation for dialysis when appropriate.
- Diabetic nephropathy:
  - Diabetic nephropathy develops in 25% to 35% of diabetics usually after 5 to 15 years.
  - Begins as microalbuminuria and progresses to renal failure.
  - African Americans are especially prone to develop renal disease from diabetes.
  - All diabetics are at risk to develop renal disease.
  - Risks
    - Glycemic control
    - Weight control
    - Blood pressure control.
    - Use of ACEIs and ARBs have been shown to reduce the proteinuria and prolong renal survival in diabetes.
- Renal Artery Stenosis (RAS):
  - RAS is common in the mature population.
  - Best managed medically unless uncontrolled hypertension or progressive loss of renal function.[37–39]
  - ACEIs are especially useful in unilateral RAS.[44]
    - Contraindicated in bilateral disease.
    - Stenosis of a unilateral kidney where the renin-supported hypertension supports necessary renal blood flow.
    - The sudden loss of GFR after initiation of ACEI or ARB should prompt review of renal vascular studies to see if RAS is present.
  - Young women with hypertension should be screened for the presence of RAS as this disease in common in them.[45,46]

- Dysproteinemias:
  - Abnormal production of immunoglobulin fragments results in several renal diseases both glomerular and tubular.
  - These are most frequently light-chain related but heavy-chain deposition is also seen.
  - Bence Jones protein was first described in 1847.
    - This protein has subsequently been identified as immunoglobulin light chains.
    - Renal involvement in the light chain-associated diseases multiple myeloma, amyloidosis (AL), and monoclonal immune deposition disease is common, and differential diagnosis usually requires renal biopsy.
    - In the evaluation of acute or chronic renal failure these diseases may exacerbate a minor renal insult into renal failure, or they may be the only cause of renal failure.
    - They may be undiagnosed prior to nephrology consultation and must be sought and ruled out in the course of every renal workup for failure.
    - Sources of monoclonal light chains include myeloma; A1 type AL; light-chain deposition disease; Waldenstrom macroglobulinemia; monoclonal gammopathy of undetermined significance; polyneuropathy, organomegaly, endocrinopathy, M protein, and skin changes syndrome; heavy-chain disease, lymphoproliferative disorders.
  - Diseases causes by these abnormal proteins include
    - *Glomerular disease*
      - Monoclonal light-chain and light- and heavy-chain deposition disease
      - May be discovered during workup for ARF or proteinuria.
      - SPEP and UPEP are helpful, but only 73% of patients were positive with this screen.
      - 100% of free light-chain assays were positive. Both tests are likely required.
    - *Al type AL* [58]
      - Usually multiorgan in nature
      - Discovered in the evaluation of cardiac or renal disease
      - Presents as proteinuria, edema, and hypotension
    - *Cryoglobulinemia*
      - Highly associated with active HCV.
      - The renal disease responds to the treatment available for the viral infection.
      - This can present as membranoproliferative GN.
    - *Tubulointerstitial lesion*
      - Cast nephropathy (myeloma kidney) is the classic presentation of dysproteinemic renal disease.
      - On biopsy, the renal tubules are filled with glassy eosin-staining casts.
      - Frequently causes ESRD; renal recovery is rare.
    - *Fanconi syndrome*
      - Light chains are unique to each patient.
      - Some light chains do not form casts or cause renal insufficiency but harm tubular function as they are absorbed and metabolized primarily in the proximal tubule.
      - The tubular dysfunction can result in acidosis, phosphate, protein, and glucose loss.
    - *ATN:*
      - The kidney is more sensitive to toxic and ischemic insults if myeloma or toxic light-chain proteins are present.
      - Therapy should be supportive with oncology consultation to ascertain the proper course for the monoclonal treatment.
    - *Hyperviscosity syndrome:*
      - Occur with high concentrations of immunoglobulins.
      - More often seen in Waldenstrom macroglobulinemia, which has fewer renal issues because of the inability to easily filter the IgM across the basement membrane.
      - Treatment may include plasma exchange in addition to chemotherapy.
      - Treatment is guided by both total protein concentrations and plasma viscosity.
    - *Neoplastic cell infiltration:*
      - Kidney involvement is frequent in hematologic malignancies.
      - Associated with adverse outcomes and treatment difficulties.
      - It can affect every area of the renal parenchyma.

- Thrombotic microangiopathies:
  - Thrombotic thrombocytopenic purpura (TTP):
    - A complex syndrome which seems to be caused by reduced activity of the von Willebrand factor (vWF)-cleaving protein.
    - This inactivity can be inherited or acquired via antibodies.
    - Hemolytic uremic syndrome (HUS) is primarily a kidney disease and TTP also develops in the kidney and at neurologic sites.
    - In HUS, thrombi formation is likely caused by a deregulated complement activation and inappropriate platelet activity.
    - In TTP, thrombi formation occurs because of inappropriate processing of released multimers of vWF.[59]
    - TTP may come to the attention of nephrology through request for plasma exchange, which is frequently performed by nephrologists, or in the course of differentiating TTP from the similar HUS.
    - Treatment requires a series of plasma exchanges although new therapies are being considered.[60]
- Hemolytic Uremic Syndrome (HUS):
  - Once thought to be physiologically identical to TTP, this entity has two major forms.
    - Diarrheal form, also called "typical HUS"[61,62]
    - Nondiarrheal form referred to as "atypical HUS"[63–65]
  - It presents as microangiopathic hemolytic anemia, thrombocytopenia, and kidney disease.
  - The typical form presents in the aftermath of an enteropathic bacterial infection (*Escherichia coli* O157:7) producing diarrhea and severe illness.
  - Other organisms can also cause the problem (*Shigella, Salmonella, Campylobacter, Yersinia*) but not as often.
  - Food-borne exposure can cause an epidemic presentation and children present after contact with animals at zoos and state fairs. Renal failure is less often seen in children.
- The antiphospholipid syndrome (APS):
  - This syndrome is caused by antibodies to cardiolipin; this was the antigen used in the original Venereal Disease Research Laboratory (VDRL) test for syphilis.
  - A false-positive VDRL test identifies these antibodies.
  - Additionally, antibodies to β_2-GP1 (a phospholipid binding protein) and abnormal clotting studies help to identify these patients.
  - It may be seen alone or as part of the spectrum of lupus erythematosus.
  - Renal involvement is mild unless TTP is present, ESRD may result.
  - The clinical syndromes of renal involvement in APS includes renal artery stenosis, arterial hypertension, APS nephropathy—with variable degrees of severity—extension and chronic microangiopathy, renal vein thrombosis, renal[66] failure, and allograft vascular thrombosis.
  - Clinical symptoms of APS includes hypertension, nephritic or nephrotic syndrome, acute renal insufficiency, chronic kidney disease, and reduced survival of renal allografts.
  - Anticoagulation is the primary therapy,[67,68] although dialysis, steroids and plasma exchange may be needed in difficult cases.
- Scleroderma renal crisis:
  - Scleroderma is caused by thickened arteries, most often the arcuate and interlobular arteries with arterioles involved less often.
  - A concentric appearing proliferation of the intima produces an "onion skin" effect in the artery walls.
  - The glomeruli are ischemic.[69]
  - Clinically, patients with other systemic sclerosis are at risk for scleroderma renal crisis, characterized by new and severe hypertension or rapidly progressive renal failure, is seen in 10% of patient.
  - Patients with diffuse systemic sclerosis have a 25% risk of scleroderma renal crisis. Patients with the CREST (calcinosis, Raynaud phenomenon, esophageal motility disorders, sclerodactyly, and telangiectasia) syndrome have only 1% chance of developing scleroderma renal crisis.

- Presentation is hypertension in a patient with systemic sclerosis, accompanied by microangiopathic hemolytic anemia.
- Treatment is ACEI, stopping ACEI for fear of lowering GFR is contraindicated, while the additive value of ARBs is unclear and the combination of the two may hasten renal failure.[70]
- Renal crisis is a rare manifestation of scleroderma that mainly affects patients with diffuse involvement of the disease in the early stages. These patients have a poor prognosis despite treatment with ACEIs.

ACID BASE

Metabolic Acidosis

- Commonly comes to clinical attention via low bicarbonate on routine chemistry testing.
- Occurs as metabolic acidosis or compensation for respiratory alkalosis.
  - Respiratory alkalosis can be ruled out on clinical grounds or with arterial blood gases.
- After identifying metabolic acidosis, the anion gap helps to identify the cause of the problem.

Anion Gap Metabolic Acidosis

- Anion gap acidosis results from the addition of organic acids.
  - Organic acids are not usually measured.
  - They are detected as imbalance in the electrical charges of the routinely monitored electrolytes.
  - Anion gap (AG) = $[Na] - ([Cl] + [HCO_3])$, normal is 12 mEq/L ± 2 mEq/L.
  - Common sources of organic acids include diabetic ketoacidosis where β-hydroxybutyric acid[71] and acetoacetate are made in excess in response to inadequate insulin. Without insulin to allow glucose to enter cells, energy production is shifted to obtaining energy from fat stores.
  - The largest contribution to the population of anions is normally albumin.
    - Abnormally low albumin levels reduce the expected anion gap and must be adjusted up or down.
    - For each 1 g/dL drop in albumin the expected anion gap is decreased by 2.5, so that a modified formula for AG should read AG = AG + 2.5 × (4-serum albumin).
- A helpful mnemonic for the differential diagnosis is **MUDPILES.**
  - **M = Methanol intoxication**
    - Alcohol is transformed to formic acid.
    - Optic inflammation and blindness may result.
    - This has been reported as a result of improperly prepared moonshine.
    - Treatment of methanol ingestion is with dialysis, alcohol infusion, and fomepizole.[72]
    - "Since the clinical signs and symptoms associated with ethylene glycol and methanol poisoning are nonspecific, it is important for the medical community to consider these toxicities given that early treatment prevents death. The hallmark of toxic alcohol poisoning is a combination of a high anion gap metabolic acidosis and osmolar gap."[73]
  - **M = Metformin toxicity**
    - Presents with an anion gap acidosis, usually lactic acidosis and is accompanied by renal failure.[74]
  - **M = Methylmalonic aciduria**
    - An inborn error of metabolism that features repeated metabolic crises with anion gap acidosis[75,76] and high methylmalonic acid levels.
    - It is suspected if other causes of anion gap acidosis have been ruled out.
    - If the patient survives, chronic renal failure becomes a problem.
    - The disease is rare but treatable with vitamin B_{12} and carnitine supplementation. Renal transplantation is curative.
  - **U = uremia**
    - Severely uremic patients cannot excrete PO_4 and SO_4.

- Treatment is to relieve the renal failure:
  - Dialysis treats the acidosis by adding bicarbonate during the process.
  - Patients with chronic renal failure can present with a nongap acidosis also.
- **D = Diabetic ketoacidosis**
  - Creation and retention of acetoacetate and β-hydroxybutyric acid.
  - Treatment for diabetic ketoacidosis is IV insulin, with normal renal function the organic acids will either be excreted or metabolized into bicarbonate.
- **P = Paraldehyde**[77] (no longer in use), and **phenformin** (no longer in use), the agent **propylene glycol** is a commonly used solvent for IV medications and has been reported to cause anion gap acidosis.
  - The medications most often involved are benzodiazepines but other medications are delivered dissolved in this vehicle.
  - Propylene glycol is metabolized into lactic acid.
  - The patients present as other alcohol toxicities with both an anion and an osmolar gap; discontinuation of the medication leads to resolution.[78]
- **I = does not stand for Isopropyl Alcohol which produces ketonuria**[79] **without acidosis, one may be reminded that isoniazid (INH) overdose produces seizures with lactic acidosis.**
  - Treatment for INH overdose will include vitamin B_6 supplementation and control of seizure disorder.
- **L = Lactic acid**
  - Results from anaerobic metabolism
  - Seen in shock, sepsis, and conditions where oxygen delivery is impaired.
  - Treatment if of the underlying cause of shock and tissue underperfusion.
  - Renal replacement may be required, especially if renal failure is present.
  - In this case the dialysate and convectate will deliver bicarbonate to correct the pH, but not the underlying cause of the acid production.[80]
- **L = Liver failure**
  - Patients being treated with infusions of citric acid, in the performance of continuous renal replacement therapy
  - Plasma exchange using citrate as a regional anticoagulant.
  - If the liver disease prevents metabolism of the citric acid then the citric acid will cause an anion gap acidosis.
  - Treatment is to stop the citric acid and consider anticoagulant free dialysis (in liver disease likely the best option) or systemic anticoagulation.[81,82]
- **E = Ethylene glycol**
  - Ethylene glycol is the active ingredient in automotive antifreeze
  - It is an alcohol and ingestion (as a suicidal gesture or ethanol substitute) results in the production of glycolic acid, which is then further metabolized into oxalic acid.
  - The characteristic envelope-shaped urinary crystals are seen in abundance if the victim is nonoliguric.
  - They may play a role in the ARF by blocking renal tubules.
  - Urinalysis clues to the diagnosis:
    - Glow of urine with fluorescein under a Wood lamp.
      - Fluorescein is added to the ethylene glycol during manufacturing of antifreeze.
      - Note that the plastic urine container attached to a Foley catheter may glow also, this test may need to be done in glass containers.
      - A recent report relates a student ingesting computer coolant containing ethylene glycol and suffering acute renal failure.
  - Treatment is ethanol infusion[83–85] to competitively inhibit alcohol dehydrogenase slowing the production of the toxins and allowing time for the liver to metabolize the ethylene glycol.
  - A direct inhibitor of alcohol dehydrogenase (fomepizole) is available and has eliminated the need for ethanol administration.
  - The use of dialysis is almost always indicated, if this is the case and ethanol is used to block alcohol dehydrogenase then the dose of ethanol will need to be adjusted for removal by dialysis.

- To simplify this process, addition of alcohol directly to the dialysate allows stable alcohol levels in these cases. The alcohol infusion or ingestion will need to be restarted after dialysis is completed.
- **E = Ethanol**
  - Leads to intoxication and malnutrition; the infrequent result is alcoholic ketoacidosis.[86,87]
- **S = Starvation**
  - Ketone bodies in the manner of insulin deficiency, but in this case because of the absence of glucose.[88]
  - Seen most often in impaired prehospital patients but also seen in NPO[89,90] inpatients.
- **S = Salicylate toxicity**[91]
  - Aspirin induced an anion gap, lactic acidosis, and ketoacidosis simultaneous with a respiratory alkalosis.[91]
  - Treatment is supportive, alkalinization is helpful, and dialysis is indicated for salicylate levels greater than 100 mg/dL , altered mental status, renal failure interfering with drug clearance, and volume overload interfering with bicarbonate administration.

Nonanion Gap Metabolic Acidosis

- In patients with acidosis and a normal anion gap, the diagnosis is referred to as a nongap, normal anion gap, or hyperchloremic acidosis.
- The physiology is loss of bicarbonate from, or addition of acid (H^+) to the system.
- The possible cause list is short, and the primary cause is frequently renal tubular acidosis.
- Most of these diagnoses can be eliminated by inspection.
- Renal tubular acidosis is the most frequent cause of nonanion gap acidosis.
- Treatment is to supplement with oral bicarbonate or citrate.
- A useful mnemonic is **HARDUP**
- **H = H^+**
  - Hydrogen ions added to the system via hydrochloride infusions or hyperalimentation, (amino acids).
  - Hypervolemia with rapid infusion of saline will dilute the bicarbonate concentration giving the appearance of a nongap acidosis.
- **A = Adrenal insufficiency**
  - Inability to make or use aldosterone, adding H^+ to the patient's system
- **R = Renal tubular acidosis**
  - Bicarbonate loss (type II) or
  - Inability to excrete H^+ (types I and IV)
- **D = Diarrhea**
  - Leads to bicarbonate loss
- **U = Ureteral diversion**
  - Inability to excrete H^+
  - Ammonium ($NH4^+$) is impermeable to the renal tubule but not to the gut
  - Ureters were formerly drained to the colon in cases of cystectomy leading to severe NH4 absorption and acidosis.
    - This procedure is not often performed.
- **P = Pancreatic diversions**
  - Bicarbonate loss, via pancreatic fluids and pancreatic transplants in which the exocrine pancreatic fluids are drained to the bladder.
  - This result is high urine bicarbonate, high urine pH, continuous bicarb loss and resulting acidosis and pneumaturia, as the NH4 reacts with bicarbonate to produce CO_2.

Metabolic Alkalosis (Table 9-3)

- Metabolic alkalosis is characterized by a rise in pH and bicarbonate concentration.
- The bicarbonate is increased either by addition of bicarbonate to the system from external sources, or from internal generation or from the loss of hydrogen ion.
- Metabolic alkalosis is a primary pathophysiologic event characterized by the gain of bicarbonate or the loss of nonvolatile acid from extracellular fluid.

TABLE 9-3. CAUSES OF METABOLIC ALKALOSIS

Exogenous alkali loads	· Alkali administration · Milk alkali syndrome · Crack cocaine in ESRD · Baking soda pica · Bicarbonate precursors (citrate, acetate)
ECV contraction, K deficiency, hyperaldosteronism states	*GI origin:* · Vomiting · Gastric suction · Congenital chloridorrhea · Villous adenoma · sodium polystyrene sulfonate (Kayexalate) with oral antacids · Cystic fibrosis with volume depletion *Renal origin:* · Thiazides and loop diuretics · Edematous states · Posthypercapnic state · Hypercalcemia hypoparathyroidism · Recovery from lactic or ketoacidosis · Nonresorbable anions (penicillins) · Mg deficiency · K deficiency · Bartter syndrome · Gitelman syndrome · Carbohydrate refeeding following starvation
ECV expansion with hypertension, low K, and high aldosterone	*With high renin:* · RAS · Accelerated hypertension · Renin secreting tumor · Estrogen therapy *With low renin:* · Primary aldosteronism · Adenoma · Hyperplasia · Carcinoma · Glucocorticoid suppressible · Adrenal enzymatic defects · 11-β-hydrolase deficiency (see licorice below) · 17-α-hydrolase deficiency · Cushing syndrome or disease · Ectopic corticotropin · Adrenal carcinoma · Adrenal adenoma · Primary pituitary · Licorice (glycyrrhetinic acid, glycyrrhizic acid) is found in both candy and chewing tobacco products, the inhibition of 11-β-hydroxysteroid dehydrogenase allows stimulation of the mineralocorticoid receptor by glucocorticoids with a resultant hypertension, metabolic alkalosis, and hypokalemia. Aldosterone levels are low. · Carbenoxolone · Lydia Pinkham tablets

ECV, extracellular fluid volume; ESRD, end-stage renal disease; GI, gastrointestinal; K, potassium.

- The kidney preserves normal acid-base balance by two mechanisms: bicarbonate reclamation mainly in the proximal tubule and bicarbonate generation predominantly in the distal nephron.
  - Bicarbonate reclamation is mediated mainly by a Na-H antiporter and to a smaller extent by the H-adenosine triphosphatase (ATPase).
- The principal factors affecting bicarbonate reabsorption include effective arterial blood volume, GFR, chloride, and potassium.
- Bicarbonate regeneration is primarily affected by distal sodium delivery and reabsorption, aldosterone, arterial pH, and arterial pCO_2.
- To generate metabolic alkalosis, either a gain of base or a loss of acid, must occur.[92]
- The kidneys usually can excrete bicarbonate to maintain the internal milieu, metabolic alkalosis occurs when they are unable, because of reduced GFR, volume contraction,[93] low chloride, or hypokalemia, to excrete enough bicarbonate. Bicarbonate is retained under this condition.
- The hospital-acquired metabolic alkalosis can be diagnosed from the bedside in most cases, regional anticoagulation with dialysis procedures[94] or plasma exchange is a common source of citrate-induced alkalosis.
  - Blood bank products are anticoagulated with citrate also.
  - A bulging urine bag indicates the presence of diuresis and volume contraction.
- Gastric suction will result in loss of hydrogen ions.
- A dangerous drug combination to avoid is the concomitant use of sodium polystyrene sulfonate (Kayexalate) with aluminum hydroxide antacids, the resulting exchange of sodium for aluminum results in the formation of sodium hydroxide (NaOH) with potentially disastrous results.
- The diagnostic workup for metabolic alkalosis starts with urinary chloride measurement (sodium excretion may be increased by $NaCO_3$ excretion, particularly in a resolving alkalosis)
- If the urinary chloride is less than 10 mEq/L and the patient is normotensive
  - Vomiting, gastrointestinal (GI) suction, diuretics, potassium deficiency, posthypercapnia are likely causes.
- If the patient is hypertensive then Liddle syndrome is likely.
- If the urinary chloride is >15 mEq/L and the patient is hypertensive, primary aldosteronism, Cushing syndrome, RAS or renal failure plus alkali therapy are the answer.
- If the patient is not hypertensive, then magnesium deficiency, severe potassium depletion, diuretic therapy, Bartter syndrome or Gitelman syndrome are present.
- Liddle syndrome:
  - Autosomal dominant
  - Results from the inability of the collecting duct to stop reabsorbing sodium.[95,96]
  - Alkalosis, hypokalemia, and hypertension result.
- Bartter syndrome:
  - Autosomal recessive
  - Seen in consanguineous families
  - Defect in the thick ascending limb (TAL) of the loop of Henle in which the Na-K-2-Cl cotransporter is defective.
    - This causes a clinical situation similar to continuous use of a loop diuretic.
    - The gene has been identified as *NKCC2*, other genes have been described.
  - This disorder must be distinguished from diuretic abuse, laxative abuse, and surreptitious vomiting.
    - A low urinary chloride will help here, as in Bartter the urinary chloride would be normal or high.
    - Most patients have hypercalciuria and normal magnesium levels in contrast to patients with Gitelman syndrome.
  - The syndrome causes juxtaglomerular apparatus hypertrophy, because of chronic hyperreninemic hyperaldosteronism from volume contraction.
  - Overproduction of prostaglandins to preserve renal blood flow leads to use of NSAIDs in conjunction with potassium repletion, spironolactone, ACEI, propranolol, and amiloride.
  - Magnesium repletion is also frequently required.[97]

- Gitelman syndrome:
  - Similar to Bartter: both have autosomal recessive chloride- resistant metabolic alkalosis with low potassium, low blood pressure, volume depletion, hyperreninemic hyperaldosteronism with juxtaglomerular apparatus hyperplasia.
  - Gitelman syndrome patients have persistent hypocalciuria and frequently hypomagnesemia.
  - This presentation mimics the use of thiazide diuretics.
  - The gene that codes for the sodium chloride cotransporter that is the target of thiazide diuretics, SLC12A3, has been identified as having numerous missense mutations in these patients.
  - These patients tend to have salt craving, complain of leg cramps, and have more symptoms during menses.
  - Treatment is by potassium and magnesium repletion and mirrors the therapy in Bartter except that ACEI use may cause frank hypotension.[98]

ELECTROLYTE DISORDERS

Sodium Disorders

- Hyponatremia usually results from the inability to excrete excess water.
- It is a common hospital problem and related to considerable morbidity.[99]
- Loss of sodium is another potential cause of hyponatremia.
- Because sodium is the major extracellular osmole this condition also causes hypoosmolality.
- Serum osmolality should be measured by freezing point depression, it can be estimated by the formula

$$\text{Osmolality} + [(2\ Na) + (\text{glucose}/18) + (\text{BUN}/2.8)]$$

- The initial evaluation of hyponatremia is to measure the serum osmolality.
- High serum osmolality indicates that an osmole is present (usually glucose) causing dilution of the sodium concentration.
- A normal osmolality indicates the presence of lipids or proteins that occupy space and reduce the total concentration but not the effective concentration of sodium, sodium not being soluble in fats.
  - This measurement error is possible in any sodium assay in which there is a dilution step prior to analysis such as in flame photometry. The problem is avoided with the use of direct ion specific electrode techniques.
  - Indirect assays, or any assay in which the serum is diluted prior to testing can deliver inaccurate results.
- A low serum osmolality confirms the presence of hyponatremia. The estimated and measured osmolalities should agree.
- Evaluation of the patient with hyponatremia begins with estimation of the volume status.
- Sodium can be lost via renal (diuretics, salt-wasting nephropathy, adrenal insufficiency) or nonrenal (diarrhea, diaphoresis, bleeding) routes.
- When free water is used to maintain hydration, hyponatremia results.
  - These patients are or have been hypovolemic.
- Urine sodium levels in diuretic cases reflect the time of the last diuretic dose.
- Hypokalemia is an important clue to diuretic use, not much else than diuretics can produce hyponatremia, hypoosmolality and hypokalemia.
- Urine testing for diuretics should be done if the patient denies their use.
- Treatment for hypovolemic hyponatremia is salt replacement usually with saline.
- Other causes of hypovolemic hyposmolarity will be easily spotted. Chronic interstitial nephritis, Bartter syndrome, polycystic kidney disease, obstruction, and Addison disease need to be considered.
- Hyperglycemia will result in translocation of free water to the intravascular space secondary to osmotic forces. The measured sodium concentration will be lower by 1.6 mEq/L for every 100 mg/dL the glucose has increased above normal.
- The anion gap should be performed on the nonadjusted data.

- These patients are frequently volume depleted because of the diuretic effect of hyperglycemia. Mannitol and glycine produce similar effects.

Normovolemic Patients

- Normal or low levels of uric acid and urea help to define normovolemia,
- Low urine sodium suggests sodium loss and in the euvolemic state repletion with free water.
- Hypothyroidism can present with low urine sodium.
- SIADH results in hyponatremia as the kidneys are unable to excrete free water properly.
  - ADH causes the collecting tubules to reabsorb water down the concentration gradient established by the loop of Henle resulting in hypoosmolality.
  - This is the most common causes of hypoosmolality.
  - Criteria to diagnose SIADH[100]
    - Low sodium and hypoosmolality without pseudohyponatremia
    - Inappropriately high urine osmolality (>100 mOsm)
    - Clinical euvolemia
    - High urine sodium concentration: more than 30 mEq/L
    - Normal thyroid, adrenal, and renal function
- Diagnosis
  - Confirm hypoosmolality and hyponatremia
  - Then test for urine osmolality, which will be high in SIADH (>100 mmol).
  - Other interesting confirmatory tests include:
    - The inability to excrete a free water load (80% of a 20 mL per kg over 4 hours)
    - Inability to dilute the urine to less than 100 mmol/kg
    - Elevated vasopressin levels
    - No correction of serum sodium after volume expansion, but improvement with fluid restriction.

Exercise-Induced Hyponatremia

- Experienced by long distance runners who overhydrate with hypotonic solutions during their run.
- This can be a fatal
- Euvolemic despite the long distance run, because of the aggressive fluid replacement.[101]
- Hyponatremia of any degree if associated with symptoms must be treated, the symptoms may be very subtle and noticed by family members who report on alterations in mood, attitude, and other changes from baseline that might go unnoticed by other observers.
- Headache and nausea, disorientation are common (nausea stimulates ADH release) and may progress to severe alteration in mental status and seizure. This "hyponatremic encephalopathy" reflects cerebral edema.
- Cerebral edema in severe cases can result in brainstem herniation
  - The brain can protect itself against hyposmolarity by making intracellular osmolytes via volume regulation.
- Severe symptoms do not usually occur at sodium levels greater than 125 mEq/L.
- Rapid development of hyponatremia is not as well tolerated as that attained over several days.
- Women young enough to be menstruating, particularly in the postoperative or postpartum period seem to be particularly susceptible to symptomatic hyponatremia and its complications.
- Treatment of severely symptomatic hyponatremia calls for infusion of 3% sodium chloride at a rate calculated to raise the sodium no more than 12 mE/L over 24 hours and no more than 18 mEq/L over 48 hours.
  - To accomplish this, the rate of 3% sodium chloride at 1 mL/kg of patient's weight per hour will raise the sodium 1 mEq/h; it will raise the sodium 0.5 mE/L per hour running at 0.5 mL/kg/h.
  - Loop diuretics should be started in patients at risk for CHF.
  - The object of the aggressive therapy is not only to relieve the severe symptoms but to prevent osmotic demyelination caused by too rapid correction of the low sodium.

- Current therapy calls for
  - Prompt bolus treatment of symptomatic hyponatremia with hypertonic saline.
  - After the initial treatment, overcorrection must be avoided.
  - Definitive treatment should be directed toward the nature of the underlying disorder.[102]
  - The mildly symptomatic may be treated with fluid restriction with the addition of loop diuretics and occasionally sodium chloride tablets.
  - The use of demeclocycline has fallen out of favor but works by inducing a counteractive DI.
  - Tolvaptan and conivaptan have shown promise as aquaphoretics in resolving hyposmolar states.
    - The cost of these medications remains concerning.
  - CHF, cirrhosis, and nephrosis have stages of pressure loss and free water retention in response to physiologically appropriate ADH release that leaves the patient euvolemic and hyponatremic.
    - These patients are, however, more frequently volume overloaded with ascites, edema, pleural effusions, and pulmonary edema.
    - Diagnosis is by history and physical, the urine sodium is usually low in spite of volume overload as the renal system is inadequately perfused.
    - ADH secretion, aldosterone activation, and the resultant water and sodium retention are high.
    - Therapy includes diuretic and underlying disease management.
    - These patients are sodium replete or overloaded in most cases.
- Psychogenic polydipsia (water intoxication) is a common problem with psychiatric patients and must be carefully separated from DI.
- Psychiatric patients frequently experience dry mouth as the result of their medications.
- The urine osmolality should be maximally dilute in this and in beer potomania. In beer potomania, the excretion of free water is limited by the body's inability to dilute urine because of lack of solute intake.
- Therapy is to remove offending agents and thiazides and to institute fluid restriction with a regular diet.
- Iatrogenic
  - Glycine solutions are used to irrigate the bladder in urologic procedures.
  - Occasionally they are absorbed into the bloodstream with severe hyponatremia resulting.
  - This usually resolves with discontinuation of the glycine irrigation.

Hypernatremia

- Hypernatremia is most often seen as the result of lost free water, it can also result from sodium overload usually resulting from pharmacologic misadventure.
  - Water is lost when insensible losses exceed water intake or when AVP (ADH) is underproduced.
- The most common clinical presentation is that of patients who have altered thirst sensation or those who depend on others for access to water.
- Diabetes insipidus (DI) is the absence of or the inability to respond to arginine vasopressin (AVP) (ADH) resulting in excretion of inappropriately dilute urine.
- Central DI is the result of surgery, trauma, or neoplasm.
  - A number of cases (50%) are idiopathic.
  - Familial cases are rare, autosomal dominant, and progress from partial to complete over time.
  - The typical patient is young, complains of nocturia, and prefers to drink cold water.
  - AVP testing will raise the urine osmolality 100 mmol above the level noted with water deprivation.
  - Complete DI patients cannot concentrate their urine above 200 mmol/kg with water restriction; partial DI patients can do better but cannot concentrate maximally.
  - Treatment is with nasally administered deamino-8-D-arginine vasopressin (desmopressin acetate; dDAVP). Clinically these patients do well without treatment

because the thirst mechanism is intact, stimulated by plasma osmolality, and so the sodium is near normal.

- The patients complain of is of polyuria or nocturia and polydipsia.
- Undiagnosed military personnel in training or without access to water in tactical situations are discovered as a result of volume depletion.
  - They are unfit for deployment.
- Nephrogenic DI is caused by lack of response to AVP in the collecting duct.
  - A genetic form in which cyclic adenosine monophosphate is not made in response to AVP has been found and is X linked. It is caused by mutations of the V2 receptor.
  - Other autosomal dominant forms have been found, all are rare.
- Acquired Nephrogenic DI is more common, but less severe than other forms of DI.
  - It is the result of chronic renal failure, hypercalcemia, lithium use, obstruction, and hypokalemia.
  - Lithium is a commonly used treatment for psychotic manic depressives, 20% to 30% of treated patients will develop severe side effects.
- Ethanol and phenytoin impair AVP release and induce an aquaphoresis.
- Lithium and demeclocycline induce AVP resistance.
- Pregnancy-induced DI is caused by the presence of placental vasopressinase.
  - This enzyme degrades AVP and oxytocin.
  - It appears in early pregnancy and increases in concentration until delivery, which cures the condition.
  - Treatment with dDAVP, which is resistant to vasopressinase may be useful.
- The typical hypernatremic patient is volume depleted.
  - The first step in the evaluation is to determine if thirst is intact.
    - If it is, was the patient capable of obtaining water?
    - If not then this is the likely explanation.
  - If thirst is not intact, was patient being given water appropriately?
    - If not, then water deprivation is once again the explanation.
    - If so, then evaluate the urine osmolality.
      - If the serum sodium is 147 mEq/L or greater then maximal stimulus to AVP release has been achieved, and the urine osmolality should be greater than 700 mmol/kg.
      - If not so, then some degree of DI is present.
      - If the urine osmolality is greater than 700, then the free water loss is not from the renal system.
- Urine osmolality may be (and usually is) between 300 and 699; in this not clearly diagnostic area the possibilities include psychogenic polydipsia, partial central or nephrogenic DI, and osmotic diuresis.
- Treatment of hypernatremia
  - Water deficits are corrected slowly to avoid sudden osmolar shifts that might induce cerebral edema. As in correction of hyponatremia, the hypernatremia should not be corrected faster than 10 mEq/L per day.
  - Free water needed is:

$$\text{Water needed} = (\text{Total Body Water}) \times [(\text{Measured Na/Desired Na}) - 1]$$

Hypokalemia

- Serious hypokalemia is almost always caused by potassium loss.
- This makes taking an accurate history important.
- Many causes are iatrogenic and easily corrected.
- The symptoms include diarrhea, vomiting, diuretic, and laxative abuse.
- The clinical findings focus on volume depletion.
  - If there is no volume loss, then suspect mineralocorticoid excess.
    - The presence of hypertension will help confirm this.
- Hypokalemia is frequently detected on routine testing; urine electrolytes must be checked to confirm renal losses.
- The danger of hypokalemia is cardiac dysrhythmia and muscle weakness, respiratory muscle paralysis is possible.

- Aggressive replacement is needed, when digitalis toxicity and metabolic acidosis are present, a shift of potassium back into the cells will occur in 1 or 2 hours; this mandates more aggressive potassium repletion.[103]
- Potassium shifts out of cells during metabolic acidosis and into the cells during metabolic alkalosis.

Hyperkalemia

- Hyperkalemia is a medical emergency.
- Diagnosis and treatment must be started immediately.
- If the patient is a dialysis patient plan to dialyze as soon as possible.
- Temporizing treatments include sodium polystyrene sulfonate (Kayexalate), IV NaHCO₃, β-agonists and IV CaCl₂ or calcium gluconate.
- Only dialysis and sodium polystyrene sulfonate (Kayexalate) remove the potassium, other measures only buy time.
- All potassium supplements should be stopped, most cases of hyperkalemia involve both reduced clearance of potassium coupled with increased intake.
- An electrocardiogram will help confirm hyperkalemia through the presence of tall peaked T waves, this is usually faster than a repeat potassium assay in the laboratory.
- Bedside electrolyte analyzers may be faster but are frequently the source of the suspect assay to begin with.
- Hemolysis will raise the serum potassium but cannot be discounted as an error if present. Intravascular hemolysis must be ruled out as a source; also a repeat normal potassium is adequate
- Elevated leukocyte and platelet counts can raise the potassium (this is a similar to hemolysis and usually not a clinical problem).
- Collection of the blood in a lithium (not potassium heparin) tube with gentle agitation of the collection tube will allow an accurate assay.
- Once hyperkalemia is confirmed, initiate therapy with dialysis, IV loop diuretics, sodium polystyrene ion exchange resin (sodium polystyrene sulfonate [Kayexalate]), and potassium restriction. ACEI and ARBs should be held if practical and renal insufficiency addressed.

Calcium Metabolism

- Skeleton houses 99% calcium as phosphate salt, hydroxyapatite [Ca10(PO4)6(OH)2].
- Approximately 500 mmol calcium is exchanged daily with extracellular fluid.
- Extracellular fluid calcium concentration is tightly regulated between 9 and 10.5 mg/dL (2.2–2.6 mmol/L) (40% bound to serum albumin; 15% is complexed to anions citrate, sulfate, phosphate; 45% as free ionized calcium—physiologically relevant, 4.5–5.6 mg/dL or 1.1–1.4 mmol/L).[104]
  - Calcium levels should be corrected for serum albumin: correction factor of 0.8 mg/dL decrease for every 1 g decrease in serum albumin.
  - Acidosis: decreased calcium binding to proteins; alkalosis increased calcium binding to proteins
- Approximately 25 mmol daily calcium intake, 10 mmol (40%) intestinal brush border absorption via TRPV6 channels, intracellular vitamin D-dependent calcium-binding protein, calbindin, and basolateral PCMA1 calcium pumps (duodenal active transport occurs with low calcium intake, passive paracellular diffusion in jejunum and ileum with high calcium intake).
- Urine and feces losses total 10 mmol/day; 1,25(OH)₂-VitD (25-hydroxyvitamin D; calcitriol) regulates calbindin absorption of calcium. Parathyroid hormone stimulates 1-α-hydroxylation of 25(OH) calcidiol to calcitriol in addition to increasing distal renal tubular calcium reabsorption.
- Calcitonin, produced by parafollicular cells of the thyroid in response to high serum calcium levels, stimulates bone to reabsorb calcium.

Calcium Disorders

- Hypercalcemia:
  - Clinical presentation: altered mentation, fatigue, muscle weakness, depression, dehydration

- Etiology:
  - Primary hyperparathyroidism (1° HPTH)
  - Adenoma (50% cases of hypercalcemia)
  - Carcinoma (<1%)
  - Hyperplasia (2.5% cases)
  - Clinical manifestations: increased calcium, decreased phosphate, increased phosphate excretion
- Malignancy-related humoral hypercalcemia of malignancy (HHM; 80% malignancy-related hypercalcemia [2° parathyroid hormone-related protein] frequently with advanced malignancy of squamous cell, breast, ovarian, renal cell, lymphomas [human T-cell lymphoma virus type 1 {HTLV-1}] and non-Hodgkin), lytic bone disease, ectopic $1,25(OH)_2$-VitD production.
- Inherited autosomal dominant disorders:
  - Multiple endocrine neoplasia (MEN) type I (gene defect in chromosome 11q13 called menin—characterized by pituitary pancreas parathyroid tumors)
  - MEN IIA (parathyroid hyperplasia, medullary thyroid carcinoma, pheochromocytoma—defective gene 10 encoding for tyr kinase)
  - Hyperparathyroidism (HPTH) jaw tumor syndrome (gene defect *HRPT2* tumor suppressor gene on chromosome 1q25–32 presents as hypercalcemia with parathyroid adenoma, fibroosseous jaw tumors), familial hypocalciuric hypocalcemia, neonatal severe
  - HPTH 4: granulomatous disorders (vitamin D production from nonrenal sites), sarcoidosis, macrophage 1_α-OH of $25(OH)D$
  - Others etiologies: leprosy, disseminated candidiasis, coccidiomycosis, acquired immunodeficiency syndrome (AIDS), *Pneumocystis*, pulmonary tuberculosus.
  - Medications: thiazides, lithium, vitamins D and A, estrogens, aminophylline
  - Immobilization (increase bone resorption during immobilization [parathyroid hormone and $1,25(OH)_2$-VitD levels normal] self-corrects with remobilization)
  - Milk: alkali (renal dysfunction with increased calcium and alkali intake)
  - Nonparathyroid endocrine disorders[4,105,106]
- Treatment:
  - Saline infusion to correct volume depletion and increase calciuria.
  - Loop diuretics (inhibit TAL calcium resorption) with saline diuresis only after volume repletion
  - Bisphosphonates 30 to 90 mg to decrease osteoclastic bone turnover, 4 to 8 units salmon calcitonin to inhibit osteoclastic bone turnover
  - Glucocorticoids
  - Calcimimetic agents to suppress parathyroid hormone (PTH) production for parathyroid hyperplasia and tumors, hemodialysis with low calcium bath in severe symptomatic refractory cases.

Hypocalcemia

- Acute signs and symptoms:
  - Positive Chvostek
  - Positive Trousseau sign
  - QT interval prolongation and dysrhythmias
  - Neuromuscular irritability with laryngeal or bronchospasm, tingling, numbness, muscle cramps, seizures, respiratory arrest
  - Chronic symptoms: brittle nails, dry skin, coarse hair, alopecia, loss or poor dentition
- Etiology:
  - Hypoparathyroid state (surgical, ablation, autoimmune, congenital)
  - Vitamin D deficiency or resistance
  - Increased calcium chelation (citrate, lactate) or protein binding (alkalemia), hypomagnesemia (PTH resistance)
  - Medications (bisphosphonates, cinacalcet, foscarnet, ketoconazole, cisplatinum via hypomagnesemia), phenytoin and phenobarbital (via vitamin D resistance) fluoride intoxication
  - Acute pancreatitis
  - Critical illness

- Treatment:
  - Acute symptomatic hypocalcemia: IV calcium gluconate 1 to 2 g in 50 mL of 5% dextrose in water over 20 minutes.
  - Chronic or nonacute hypocalcemia: 1.5 to 2 g elemental calcium supplementation (calcium carbonate or calcium citrate) in divided doses, correction of underlying cause including hypomagnesemia, vitamin D deficiency recommended.

Phosphate Metabolism

- Phosphate exists complexed in bone (hydroxyapatite) and intracellularly (phospholipids, phosphate esters, and inorganic phosphorus [Pi]; ratio 4:1 $H_2PO_4^2$:H_2PO_4, pH 7.4, normal levels 2.5–4.5 mg/dL).
- PTH stimulates phosphorous resorption from bone and gut, increases renal proximal tubular phosphaturia by effects on type 2 NaPi cotransporter.
- Vitamin D increases intestinal phosphorous reabsorption.
- Absorption can be blocked by increased doses of aluminum, calcium, and magnesium oral binders.
  - Hypophosphatemia
    - Clinical presentation:
      - Myopathy
      - Rhabdomyolysis
      - Encephalopathy
      - Respiratory and cardiac failure
      - Hematopoietic abnormalities including hemolysis granulocyte and platelet dysfunction
    - Etiology:
      - Poor intake
      - Anorexia
      - Malabsorption
      - Hungry bone syndrome
      - Refeeding
      - Excessive phosphate binder use
      - Vitamin D deficiency
      - Renal phosphate wasting (>5% fractional phosphate excretion or >100 mg/day in the face of hypophosphatemia)
      - Fanconi syndrome
      - HPTH (primary, secondary, tertiary)
      - Fibroblast growth factor 23 (FGF23), genetic abnormalities (X-linked hypophosphatemic rickets, FGF23 mutations, mutations of Na-H exchange regulatory factor, and type 2a NaPi transporter, G stimulatory protein-α subunit mutation).
    - Treatment:
      - Treat underlying etiology, phosphorus repletion.
      - Asymptomatic low phosphate
        - Serum phosphorous 1.5 to 2.0 mg/dL
          - Oral sodium phosphate (or potassium phosphate) supplementation 40 to 80 mmol/24 h
        - Serum phosphorous less than 1.5 mg/dL
          - Oral phosphate up to 100 mmol/24 h
      - Symptomatic low phosphate
        - IV phosphate 1.3 mg/dL or more, maximum 30 mmol/6 h
        - For phosphate IV less than 1.3 mg/dL, maximum 80 mmol/12 h

Hyperphosphatemia

- Clinical presentation:
  - Acute and marked increase in phosphate may lead to hypocalcemia and tetany
  - Chronic increased phosphate leads to vascular calcification, calcium-phospate deposition in skin with rash and pruritus, in joint leading to limited motion and pain, in tendons and ligaments with spontaneous rupture, in eyes presenting as band keratopathy or conjunctivitis; leads to increased PTH secretion.

- Etiology:
  - Rapid tissue or cell breakdown (rhabdomyolysis, tumor lysis syndrome)
  - Significant ingestion
  - Chronic kidney disease
  - Hypoparathyroidism
  - Vitamin D intoxication
  - Gene mutations (*FGF23*, *Klotho*, *GALNT3*).
- Treatment:
  - Acute phosphate elevation
    - IV saline if renal function intact
    - Consider hemodialysis (HD) if renal function compromised and associated hypocalcemia evident.
  - Chronic phosphate elevation: phosphate binders, dietary phosphate restriction.

Vitamin D

- Vitamin D, a steroid hormone, is mainly regulated by levels of calcium, phosphorus, PTH, and FGF23.
- PTH stimulated by low calcium and elevated phosphorous promotes renal phosphorous excretion and increased vitamin D synthesis.
- Vitamin D feeds back to suppress PTH production and secretion.
- Conversion in the liver of dietary ergocalciferol and pre-vitamin D precursor cholecalciferol from nonenzymatic conversion in the skin by sunlight to 25(OH) D provides substrate for 1α-hydroxylation to the active 1,25-dihydroxyvitamin D3 [1,25(OH)2 D3] in the kidney.
- FGF23 inhibits renal tubular 1α-hydroxylation (decreased mRNA expression) to decrease active 1,25(OH)2 D3 while increasing 24-hydroxylation to and 24,25(OH)2 D3 (inactive form) to counter vitamin D-mediated increased gut phosphorous reabsorption.
- Vitamin D receptors are present in various tissues, particularly in bone, gut, and parathyroid gland.
- Deficiency: decreased intake (elderly, children), decreased absorption (malabsorption syndromes, gastric bypass), decreased synthesis (advanced chronic kidney disease leads to low calcium level with secondary HPTH, decreased sunlight exposure, chronic hospitalization), increased conversion to inactive metabolites by drugs (anticonvulsants, rifampin, isoniazid, theophylline), increased losses via kidney of vitamin D and binding proteins.
- Resistance: genetic mutation of vitamin D receptor.
- Use of vitamin D and its analogs are useful in suppressing excess PTH production.
- Excess: zealous over repletion, peripheral conversion in granulomatous tissues associated with hypercalcemia.
- Treatment of low vitamin D levels:
  - Treat underlying cause if possible.
    - Oral vitamin D replacement with cholecalciferol or ergocalciferol.
    - For decreased levels of 25(OH)2 less than 20 ng/mL:
      - Oral ergocalciferol, 50,000 units once weekly for 6 to 8 weeks, then dosing daily 800 units. Total weekly or monthly to maintain vitamin D levels may also be tried.
      - Malabsorptive states may require 10,000 to 50,000 units daily.
      - Repeat levels at least after 3 months may suggest adequate repletion.
      - Hypercalciuria and hypercalcemia may result from excessive replacement.
      - Supplementary reading[104,107–110]

Renal Transplant

- Renal transplant is the best option for most patients with ESRD.
- The annual death rate is reduced by 50% after transplant.[111]
- Unfortunately, this benefit in not uniform for all transplant recipients.
- Patients who receive kidneys from live donors have improved survival over those who receive kidneys from deceased donors.
- Older recipients do not benefit as much as younger recipients. Additional factors such as deceased donor age, cause of death (eg, myocardial infarction, cerebrovascular accident),

length of time from removal to implantation, and human leukocyte antigen (HLA) match impact both graft and recipient survival.

- Absolute contradictions to transplantation:
  - Presence of anti-HLA antibodies to donor HLA antigens
  - Active infections
  - Malignant neoplasm
- Relative contraindications to transplantation:
  - Cardiovascular disease
  - Active hepatitis
  - Noncompliance
  - HIV
  - Advanced age
  - Glomerular diseases that may reoccur after transplantation
- Immunosuppression is required for all renal transplants except for identical twins.
- There is no universal immunosuppression protocol but can be divided into pretransplant, induction, maintenance, and rejection treatment.
  - Pretransplant immunosuppression is designed to remove or decrease identified immunologically active components.
  - Induction immunosuppression targets the initial immunological responses to foreign antigens.
  - Maintenance immunosuppression balances the need to maintain immunosuppression and limit the risk of opportunistic infections and drug toxicity.
  - Rejection immunosuppression must reverse T and/or B-cell mediated immune activation directed against the kidney.

Useful Formulae

- $AG = [Na - (Cl + HCO3)]$
- AG corrected for low albumin = $[Na - (Cl + CO_2)] - [4 - (\text{Measured Albumin})] \times 2.5$
- Clearance formula = $[\text{Urine Concentration/Serum Concentration}] \times (\text{Volume Urine/Minutes})$
  - The urine and serum concentrations are usually creatinine but may be urea or any solute of interest.
  - Fractional excretion formula is the clearance of the substance studied divided by the GFR or the commonly used clearance of creatinine
- $(\text{Urine Sodium/Serum Sodium}) \times \text{L}/1440 \text{ min}/(\text{Urine Creatinine/Serum Creatinine})/(\text{L}/1440 \text{ min})$
  - In this formula the denominators are identical and cancel out leaving:
    - (Urine Sodium/Serum Sodium)/(Urine Creatinine/Serum Creatinine), which is multiplied times 100 to make it a percentage.
    - FeNa is <1% in prerenal states with intact renal function, diuretics may make FeNa higher.
    - FeNa is >1% in ATN and in normal patients who are Na loaded.
    - FeUric acid is <10% in prerenal state and not affected by diuretics.
    - Fractional excretion of urea is <35% in prerenal states and not affected by diuretics.
- Cockcroft and Galt estimation of GFR[112]: $(140 - \text{Age})/\text{Serum Creatinine} \times (\text{kg}/72)$ ($\times 0.85$ for women)
- Osmolality + $[(2 \text{ Na}) + (\text{glucose}/18) + (\text{BUN}/2.8)]$
- Calcium Correction for Hypoalbuminemia = $0.8 \times (4 - \text{Measured Albumin}) + \text{Measured Calcium}$

Water Formulae

- Free Water Gain or Loss = $[0.6(\text{Weight in Kilograms})] - [0.6(\text{Weight in Kilograms}) \times \text{Osm}/290]$
- A formula to estimate the amount of free water needed is:

$$\text{Water Needed} = (\text{Total Body Water}) \times [(\text{Measured Na/Desired Na}) - 1]$$

- Electrolyte clearance (Ec)
  - Ec = $[(\text{UrNa} + \text{Ur K})/\text{SNa})] \times \text{Urine Volume}$

- Urine Volume = Ec + Water Clearance
- Osmolar and Free Water Clearance
  - The "clearance" of all osmotically active particles can be calculated in manner similar to the clearance of individual substances:
  - Cosm = Uosm × V/Posm
    - This is termed the osmolar clearance, and is the volume of plasma cleared of osmotically active particles per unit time.
    - Urine formation minus the osmolar clearance (Cosm), is the free water clearance, and can be viewed as the volume of pure water subtracted from (positive free water clearance) or added to (negative free water clearance) the plasma per unit time:
  - $CH_2O = V - Cosm$
- Transtubular potassium concentration gradient:
  - (Urine K/Serum K)/(Urine Osm/Serum Osm)
    - In hypokalemia
      - <2 = GI loss
      - >4 = renal loss, excess aldosterone
    - In hyperkalemia
      - <6 = renal loss, ineffective or absent aldosterone
      - >10 = nonrenal hyperkalemia

REFERENCES

1. Herrera-Gutierrez ME, Seller-Perez G, Maynar-Moliner J, et al: Variability in renal dysfunction defining criteria and detection methods in intensive care units: are the international consensus criteria used for diagnosing renal dysfunction? *Med Intensiva.* 2011

2. White SR: Amphetamine toxicity. *Semin Respir Crit Care Med.* 2002;23(1):27-36.

3. Lin PY, Lin CC, Liu HC, et al: Rasburicase improves hyperuricemia in patients with acute kidney injury secondary to rhabdomyolysis caused by ecstasy intoxication and exertional heat stroke. *Pediatr Crit Care Med.* 2011;12(6):e424-7.

4. Georges CG, Guthoff M, Wehrmann M, et al: Hypercalcaemic crisis and acute renal failure due to primary hyperparathyroidism. *Dtsch Med Wochenschr.* 2008;133(suppl 0):F3.

5. Ulett K, Wells B, Centor R: Hypercalcemia and acute renal failure in milk-alkali syndrome: a case report. *J Hosp Med.* 2010;5(2):E18-20.

6. Waked A, Geara A, El-Imad B: Hypercalcemia, metabolic alkalosis and renal failure secondary to calcium bicarbonate intake for osteoporosis prevention—"modern" milk alkali syndrome: a case report. *Cases J.* 2009;2:6188.

7. Uchiyama T, Inamori M, Iida H, et al: Renal dysfunction caused by oral sodium phosphate tablets for colonoscopy. *Digestion.* 2009;80(3):159.

8. Santos P, Branco A, Silva S, et al: Acute phosphate nephropathy after bowel cleansing: still a menace. *Nefrologia.* 2010;30(6):702-704.

9. Muslimani A, Chisti MM, Wills S, et al: How we treat tumor lysis syndrome. *Oncology (Williston Park).* 2011;25(4):369-375.

10. Nzerue CM: The tumor lysis syndrome. *N Engl J Med.* 2011;365(6):573; author reply 573-4.

11. Bagshaw SM, Langenberg C, Bellomo R: Urinary biochemistry and microscopy in septic acute renal failure: a systematic review. *Am J Kidney Dis.* 2006;48(5):695-705.

12. Graber M, Lane B, Lamia R, Pastoriza-Munoz E: Bubble cells: renal tubular cells in the urinary sediment with characteristics of viability. *J Am Soc Nephrol.* 1991;1(7):999-1004.

13. Levitov A, Mayo PH, Slonim AD: *Critical care ultrasonography.* New York: McGraw-Hill Medical; 2009.

14. Corwin HL, Bray RA, Haber MH: The detection and interpretation of urinary eosinophils. *Arch Pathol Lab Med.* 1989;113(11):1256-1258.

15. Goldsmith SR, Gilbertson DT, Mackedanz SA, Swan SK: Renal effects of conivaptan, furosemide, and the combination in patients with chronic heart failure. *J Card Fail.* 2011;17(12):982-989.

16. Radaelli G, Bodanese LC, Guaragna JC, et al: The use of inhibitors of angiotensin-converting enzyme and its relation to events in the postoperative period of CABG. *Rev Bras Cir Cardiovasc* 2011;26(3):373-379.

17. Vecchis RD, Di Biase G, Ariano C, et al: ACE-inhibitor therapy at relatively high doses and risk of renal worsening in chronic heart failure. *Arq Bras Cardiol.* 2011;97:507-516.

18. Ahn HS, Kim YS, Kim SG, et al: Cystatin C is a good predictor of hepatorenal syndrome and survival in patients with cirrhosis who have normal serum creatinine levels. *Hepatogastroenterology.* 2012;59:116:1168-1173.

19. Angeli P, Morando F, Cavallin M, Piano S: Hepatorenal syndrome. *Contrib Nephrol.* 2011;174:46-55.

20. Bittencourt PL, de Carvalho GC, de Andrade Regis C, et al: Causes of renal failure in patients with decompensated cirrhosis and its impact in hospital mortality. *Ann Hepatol.* 2012;11(1):90-95.

21. Dameron M: Hepatorenal syndrome: progressive renal failure in patients with cirrhosis. *JAAPA.* 2011;24(11):30-33.

22. Zheng YY, Xu XY: Progression on the use of vasoactive agents in the treatment of hepatorenal syndrome. *Zhonghua Gan Zang Bing Za Zhi.* 2011;19(9):718-720.

23. Narahara Y, Kanazawa H, Sakamoto C, et al: The efficacy and safety of terlipressin and albumin in patients with type 1 hepatorenal syndrome: a multicenter, open-label, explorative study. *J Gastroentero.* 2012;47(3)313-320.

24. Leung W, Wong F: Hepatorenal syndrome: do the vasoconstrictors work? *Gastroenterol Clin North Am.* 2011;40(3):581-598.

25. Ellison DH: The physiologic basis of diuretic synergism: its role in treating diuretic resistance. *Ann Intern Med.* 1991;114(10):886-894.

26. Yu H, Zhang D, Haller S, et al: Determinants of renal function in patients with renal artery stenosis. *Vasc Med.* 2011;16(5):331-338.

27. Dasari TW, Hanna EB, Exaire JE: Resolution of anuric acute kidney injury after left renal angioplasty and stenting for a totally occlusive in-stent restenosis of a solitary kidney. *Am J Med Sci.* 2011;341(2):163-165.

28. Chen T, Lv Y, Lin F, Zhu J: Acute kidney injury in adult idiopathic nephrotic syndrome. *Ren Fail.* 2011;33(2):144-149.

29. Rose BD, Black RM: *Manual of clinical problems in nephrology.* Boston: Little, Brown; 1988.

30. Fletcher A: Eosinophiluria and acute interstitial nephritis. *N Engl J Med.* 2008;358(16):1760-1761.

31. Nolan CR 3d, Anger MS, Kelleher SP: Eosinophiluria—a new method of detection and definition of the clinical spectrum. *N Engl J Med.* 1986;315(24):1516-1519.

32. Nolan CR 3d, Kelleher SP: Eosinophiluria. *Clin Lab Med.* 1988;8(3):555-565.

33. Essid A, Allani-Essid N, Rubinsztajn R, et al: A neonatal case of immunoallergic acute interstitial nephritis. *Arch Pediatr.* 2010;17(11):1559-1561.

34. Perazella MA, Markowitz GS: Drug-induced acute interstitial nephritis. *Nat Rev Nephrol.* 2010;6(8):461-470.

35. Jennette JC, Falk RJ: Diagnosis and management of glomerular diseases. *Med Clin North Am.* 1997;81(3):653-677.

36. Jennette JC, Falk RJ: Diagnosis and management of glomerulonephritis and vasculitis presenting as acute renal failure. *Med Clin North Am.* 1990;74(4):893-908.

37. Jennette JC, Falk RJ: Antineutrophil cytoplasmic autoantibodies and associated diseases: a review. *Am J Kidney Dis.* 1990;15(6):517-529.

38. Westberg NG, Michael AF: Immunohistopathology of diabetic glomerulosclerosis. *Diabetes.* 1972;21(3):163-174.

39. Alpers CE: Fibrillary glomerulonephritis and immunotactoid glomerulopathy: two entities, not one. *Am J Kidney Dis.* 1993;22(3):448-451.

40. Gibelin A, Maldini C, Mahr A: Epidemiology and etiology of Wegener granulomatosis, microscopic polyangiitis, Churg-Strauss syndrome and Goodpasture syndrome: vasculitides with frequent lung involvement. *Semin Respir Crit Care Med.* 2011;32(3):264-273.

41. Kunaparaju S, Okafor C, Cathro H, et al: Proteinuria in a patient with diabetes. *Kidney Int.* 2011;79(7):793-794.

42. Koyama A, Yamagata K, Makino H, et al: A nationwide survey of rapidly progressive glomerulonephritis in Japan: etiology, prognosis and treatment diversity. *Clin Exp Nephrol.* 2009;13(6):633-650.

43. Okuyama S, Wakui H, Maki N, et al: Successful treatment of post-MRSA infection glomerulonephritis with steroid therapy. *Clin Nephrol.* 2008;70(4):344-347.

44. Falk RJ, Jennette JC: Thoughts about the classification of small vessel vasculitis. *J Nephrol.* 2004;17(suppl 8):S3-9.

45. Jennette JC, Falk RJ: New insight into the pathogenesis of vasculitis associated with antineutrophil cytoplasmic autoantibodies. *Curr Opin Rheumatol.* 2008;20(1):55-60.

46. Sugino K, Kikuchi N, Muramatsu Y, et al: Churg-Strauss syndrome presenting with diffuse alveolar hemorrhage and rapidly progressive glomerulonephritis. *Intern Med.* 2009;48(20):1807-1811.

47. Falk RJ, Jennette JC: ANCA disease: where is this field heading? *J Am Soc Nephrol.* 2010; 21(5):745-752.

48. Ball GV: The history of ANCA-associated vasculitis. *Rheum Dis Clin North Am.* 2010;36(3):439-446.

49. Nadasdy T, Hebert LA: Infection-related glomerulonephritis: understanding mechanisms. *Semin Nephrol.* 2011;31(4):369-375.

50. Welch TR: An approach to the child with acute glomerulonephritis. *Int J Pediatr.* 2012;2012:Article 426192 DOI-10.1155/2012/426192

51. Uchida T, Oda T, Watanabe A, et al: Clinical and histologic resolution of poststreptococcal glomerulonephritis with large subendothelial deposits and kidney failure. *Am J Kidney Dis.* 2011;58(1):113-117.

52. Scolari F, Ravani P, Gaggi R, et al: The challenge of diagnosing atheroembolic renal disease: clinical features and prognostic factors. *Circulation.* 2007;116(3):298-304.

53. Pontier PJ, Patel TG: Racial differences in the prevalence and presentation of glomerular disease in adults. *Clin Nephrol.* 1994;42(2):79-84.

54. Freedman BI, Kopp JB, Langefeld CD, et al: The apolipoprotein L1 (APOL1) gene and nondiabetic nephropathy in African Americans. *J Am Soc Nephrol.* 2010;21(9):1422-1426.

55. Genovese G, Friedman DJ, Ross MD, et al: Association of trypanolytic ApoL1 variants with kidney disease in African Americans. *Science.* 2010;329(5993):841-845.

56. Meyrier A: Focal and segmental glomerulosclerosis: multiple pathways are involved. *Semin Nephrol.* 2011;31(4):326-332.

57. Reeves-Daniel AM, DePalma JA, Bleyer AJ, et al: The APOL1 gene and allograft survival after kidney transplantation. *Am J Transplant.* 2011;11(5):1025-1030.

58. Eirin A, Irazabal MV, Gertz MA, et al: Clinical features of patients with immunoglobulin light chain amyloidosis (AL) with vascular-limited deposition in the kidney. *Nephrol Dial Transplant.* 2012;27(3)1097-1101.

59. Zipfel PF, Wolf G, John U, et al: Novel developments in thrombotic microangiopathies: is there a common link between hemolytic uremic syndrome and thrombotic thrombocytic purpura? *Pediatr Nephrol.* 2011;26(11):1947-1956.

60. Chen J, Reheman A, Gushiken FC, et al: N-acetylcysteine reduces the size and activity of von Willebrand factor in human plasma and mice. *J Clin Invest.* 2011;121(2):593-603.

61. Artunc F, Amann K, Haap M: Hemolytic uremic syndrome following EHEC infection. *Dtsch Med Wochenschr.* 2011;136(38):1917.

62. Bitzan M, Schaefer F, Reymond D: Treatment of typical (enteropathic) hemolytic uremic syndrome. *Semin Thromb Hemost.* 2010;36(6):594-610.

63. Clark WF, Hildebrand A: Attending rounds: microangiopathic hemolytic anemia with renal insufficiency. *Clin J Am Soc Nephrol.* 2012;7(2):342-347.

64. Fremeaux-Bacchi V, Fakhouri F, Roumenina L, et al: Atypical hemolytic-uremic syndrome related to abnormalities within the complement system. *Rev Med Interne.* 2011; 32(4):232-240.

65. Loirat C, Fremeaux-Bacchi V: Atypical hemolytic uremic syndrome. *Orphanet J Rare Dis.* 2011;6:60.

66. Majdan M: Antiphospholipid syndrome and the kidney diseases. *Pol Merkur Lekarski.* 2010;28(167):341-344.

67. Ruiz-Irastorza G, Crowther M, Branch W, Khamashta MA: Antiphospholipid syndrome. *Lancet.* 2010;376(9751):1498-1509.

68. Sharma RK, Kaul A, Agrawal V, Jaisuresh K: Primary antiphospholipid syndrome presenting as thrombotic microangiopathy: Successful treatment with steroids, plasma exchange and anticoagulants. *Indian J Nephrol.* 2011;21(4):280-282.

MEDICAL SPECIALTIES

69. Roda-Safont A, Simeon-Aznar CP, Fonollosa-Pla V, et al: Clinical features and prognosis of patients with scleroderma renal crisis. *Med Clin (Barc).* 2011;137(10):431-434.

70. Hudson M, Baron M, Lo E, et al: An international, web-based, prospective cohort study to determine whether the use of ACE inhibitors prior to the onset of scleroderma renal crisis is associated with worse outcomes-methodology and preliminary results. *Int J Rheumatol.* 2010;2010:347402. Epub Sep 14, 2010.

71. Stojanovic V, Ihle S: Role of beta-hydroxybutyric acid in diabetic ketoacidosis: a review. *Can Vet J.* 2011;52(4):426-430.

72. Bayliss G: Dialysis in the poisoned patient. *Hemodial Int.* 2010;14(2):158-167.

73. Montjoy CA, Rahman A, Teba L: Ethylene glycol and methanol poisonings: case series and review. *W V Med J.* 2010;106(6):17-23.

74. Suchard JR, Grotsky TA: Fatal metformin overdose presenting with progressive hyperglycemia. *West J Emerg Med.* 2008;9(3):160-164.

75. Guven A, Cebeci N, Dursun A, et al: Methylmalonic acidemia mimicking diabetic ketoacidosis in an infant. *Pediatr Diabetes.* 2012;13(6):e22-25.

76. Seashore MR: The organic acidemias: an overview. In Pagon RA, Bird TD, Dolan CR, Stephens K, ed. *GeneReviews.* Seattle: University of Washington; 1993.

77. Hayward JN, Boshell BR: Paraldehyde intoxication with metabolic acidosis; report of two cases, experimental data and a critical review of the literature. *Am J Med.* 1957; 23(6):965-976.

78. Kraut JA, Xing SX: Approach to the evaluation of a patient with an increased serum osmolal gap and high-anion-gap metabolic acidosis. *Am J Kidney Dis.* 2011;58(3):480-484.

79. Platteborze PL, Rainey PM, Baird GS: Ketoacidosis with unexpected serum isopropyl alcohol. *Clin Chem.* 2011;57(10):1361-1364.

80. Cerda J, Tolwani AJ, Warnock DG: Critical care nephrology: management of acid-base disorders with CRRT. *Kidney Int.* 2012;82(1)9-18.

81. Burry LD, Tung DD, Hallett D, et al: Regional citrate anticoagulation for PrismaFlex continuous renal replacement therapy. *Ann Pharmacother.* 2009;43(9):1419-1425.

82. Chadha V, Garg U, Warady BA, Alon US: Citrate clearance in children receiving continuous venovenous renal replacement therapy. *Pediatr Nephrol.* 2002;17(10):819-824.

83. Henderson WR, Brubacher J: Methanol and ethylene glycol poisoning: a case study and review of current literature. *CJEM.* 2002;4(1):34-40.

84. Lundgaard P: Extreme metabolic acidosis after presumed intoxication with ethylene glycol. *Ugeskr Laeger.* 2009;171(22):1866-1867.

85. Peces R, Fernandez R, Peces C, et al: Effectiveness of pre-emptive hemodialysis with high-flux membranes for the treatment of life-threatening alcohol poisoning. *Nefrologia.* 2008;28(4):413-418.

86. Meier H, Gschwend S, Raimondi S, Giambarba C: Ethanol, sugar, acid and coma. *Praxis (Bern 1994).* 2011;100(13):797-799.

87. Mihai B, Lacatusu C, Graur M: Alcoholic ketoacidosis. *Rev Med Chir Soc Med Nat Iasi.* 2008;112(2):321-326.

88. Causso C, Arrieta F, Hernandez J, et al: Severe ketoacidosis secondary to starvation in a frutarian patient. *Nutr Hosp.* 2010;25(6):1049-1052.

89. Patel A, Felstead D, Doraiswami M, et al: Acute starvation in pregnancy: a cause of severe metabolic acidosis. *Int J Obstet Anesth.* 2011;20(3):253-256.

90. Lulsegged A, Saeed E, Langford E, et al: Starvation ketoacidosis in a patient with gastric banding. *Clin Med.* 2011;11(5):473-475.

91. Pearlman BL, Gambhir R: Salicylate intoxication: a clinical review. *Postgrad Med.* 2009; 121(4):162-168.

92. Khanna A, Kurtzman NA: Metabolic alkalosis. *J Nephrol.* 2006;19(suppl 9):S86-96.

93. Luke RG, Galla JH: It is chloride depletion alkalosis, not contraction alkalosis. *J Am Soc Nephrol.* 2012;23(2):204-207.

94. Wu MY, Hsu YH, Bai CH, et al: Regional citrate versus heparin anticoagulation for continuous renal replacement therapy: a meta-analysis of randomized controlled trials. *Am J Kidney Dis.* 201259(6):810-818.

95. Rossi E, Farnetti E, Debonneville A, et al: Liddle's syndrome caused by a novel missense mutation (P617L) of the epithelial sodium channel beta subunit. *J Hypertens.* 2008;26(5):921-927.

96. Vehaskari VM: Heritable forms of hypertension. *Pediatr Nephrol*. 2009;24(10):1929-1937.

97. Hebert SC, Gullans SR: "The molecular basis of inherited hypokalemic alkalosis: Bartter's and Gitelman's syndromes." *Am J Physiol*. 1996;271(5 Pt 2):F957-9.

98. Pollak MR, Delaney VB, Graham RM, Hebert SC: Gitelman's syndrome (Bartter's variant) maps to the thiazide-sensitive cotransporter gene locus on chromosome 16q13 in a large kindred. *J Am Soc Nephrol*. 1996;7(10):2244-2248.

99. Tolouian R, Alhamad T, Farazmand M, Mulla ZD: The correlation of hip fracture and hyponatremia in the elderly. *J Nephrol*. 2012;25(5)789-793.

100. Verbalis JG: Managing hyponatremia in patients with syndrome of inappropriate antidiuretic hormone secretion. *Endocrinol Nutr*. 2010;57(suppl 2):30-40.

101. Siegel AJ, Verbalis JG, Clement S, et al: Hyponatremia in marathon runners due to inappropriate arginine vasopressin secretion. *Am J Med*. 2007;120(5):461.e11-461.e17.

102. Overgaard-Steensen C: Initial approach to the hyponatremic patient. *Acta Anaesthesiol Scand*. 2011;55(2):139-148.

103. Halperin ML, Goldstein MB: *Fluid, electrolyte, and acid-base emergencies*. Philadelphia: Saunders; 1988:354.

104. Cooper MS, Gittoes NJ: Diagnosis and management of hypocalcaemia. *BMJ*. 2008; 336(7656):1298-1302.

105. Hutchison CA, Batuman V, Behrens J, et al: The pathogenesis and diagnosis of acute kidney injury in multiple myeloma. *Nat Rev Nephrol*. 2011;8(1):43-51.

106. Titan SM, Callas SH, Uip DE, et al: Acute renal failure and hypercalcemia in an athletic young man. *Clin Nephrol*. 2009;71(4):445-447.

107. Barbieri AM, Filopanti M, Bua G, Beck-Peccoz P: Two novel nonsense mutations in GALNT3 gene are responsible for familial tumoral calcinosis. *J Hum Genet*. 2007;52(5): 464-468.

108. Connor A: Novel therapeutic agents and strategies for the management of chronic kidney disease mineral and bone disorder. *Postgrad Med J*. 2009;85(1003):274-279.

109. Hruska KA, Mathew S, Lund R, et al: Hyperphosphatemia of chronic kidney disease. *Kidney Int*. 2008;74(2):148-157.

110. Hruska KA, Saab G, Mathew S, Lund R: Renal osteodystrophy, phosphate homeostasis, and vascular calcification. *Semin Dial*. 2007;20(4):309-315.

111. Wolfe RA, Ashby VB, Milford EL, et al: Comparison of mortality in all patients on dialysis, patients on dialysis awaiting transplantation, and recipients of a first cadaveric transplant. *N Engl J Med*. 1999;341(23):1725-1730.

112. Shoker A, Hossain MA, Koru-Sengul T, et al: Performance of creatinine clearance equations on the original Cockcroft-Gault population. *Clin Nephrol*. 2006;66(2):89-97.

CHAPTER 10

Neurology

Paul Marik

GATHERING DATA

Common Neurologic Signs and Symptoms

Syncope

Syncope is loss of consciousness caused by a reduced supply of blood to the cerebral hemispheres or brainstem. It can result from pancerebral hypoperfusion caused by vasovagal reflexes, orthostatic hypotension, or decreased cardiac output or from selective hypoperfusion of the brainstem resulting from vertebrobasilar ischemia. It is important to distinguish seizures from syncope because they have different causes, diagnostic approaches, and treatment.

The initial step in evaluating a patient who has suffered a lapse of consciousness is to determine whether the setting in which the event occurred, or associated symptoms or signs, suggests that it was a direct result of a disease requiring prompt attention, such as hypoglycemia, meningitis, head trauma, cardiac arrhythmia, or acute pulmonary embolism.

The onset of a syncopal episode is rapid, its duration brief, and recovery is spontaneous and complete. Other causes of transient loss of consciousness need to be distinguished from syncope; these include seizures, vertebrobasilar ischemia, hypoxemia, and hypoglycemia. The causes of syncope can be divided into three general categories: The clinical features, underlying pathophysiologic mechanisms, therapeutic interventions, and prognoses differ markedly among these three causes.

- Neurally mediated syncope (also called reflex syncope). Neurally mediated syncope comprises a heterogeneous group of functional disorders that are characterized by a transient change in the reflexes responsible for maintaining cardiovascular homeostasis. Episodic vasodilation and bradycardia occur in varying combinations, resulting in temporary failure of blood pressure control
- Orthostatic hypotension
- Cardiac syncope. Cardiac syncope may be due to arrhythmias or structural cardiac diseases that cause a decrease in cardiac output.

High-Risk Features Indicating Hospitalization or Intensive Evaluation

- Chest pain or evidence of coronary ischemia
- Features of heart failure
- Valvular disease
- History of arrhythmias
- Prolonged QT interval (>500 ms)
- Repetitive sinoatrial block or sinus pauses
- Persistent sinus bradycardia
- Atrial fibrillation
- Trifascicular block
- Family history of sudden death
- Preexcitation syndromes

Seizures

- A seizure is a transient disturbance of cerebral function caused by an abnormal neuronal discharge. Epilepsy is a group of disorders characterized by recurrent seizures.
- The presence or absence of prodromal symptoms, the patient's position when the episodes occur, and whether episodes are followed by periods of confusion are critical in evaluating episodic loss of consciousness.

TABLE 10-1. GLASGOW COMA SCALE

Score	1	2	3	4	5	6
Eye opening	None	To pain	To voice	Spontaneously		
Verbal response	None	Vocal but not verbal	Verbal but not conversational	Conversational but disoriented	Orientated	
Motor response	None	Extension	Flexion	Withdraws to pain	Localizes to pain	Obeys commands

- Confusion after the episode strongly suggests a seizure. Jerking body movements and urinary incontinence are not necessarily indicative of seizure, and can occur during vasovagal and other causes of syncope as well.
- Generalized tonic-clonic (grand mal, or major motor) seizures are characterized by loss of consciousness, accompanied initially by tonic stiffening, and subsequently by clonic (jerking) movements of the extremities. A period of confusion, disorientation, or agitation (postictal state) follows a generalized tonic-clonic seizure. The period of confusion is usually brief, lasting only minutes. Although such behavior is often strikingly evident to witnesses, it may not be recalled by the patient. Biting of the lateral aspect of the tongue is highly specific for grand mal seizure. Prolonged alteration of consciousness (prolonged postictal state) may follow status epilepticus.

Weakness and Paralysis

Weakness, paralysis and/or sensory loss are very common presenting features of neurologic diseases. Weakness is a reduction in the power that can be exerted by 1 or more muscles. Paralysis indicates weakness that is so severe that a muscle cannot be contracted at all, whereas paresis refers to weakness that is mild or moderate. The prefix "hemi-" refers to one-half of the body, "para-" to both legs, and "quadri-" to all 4 limbs. The distribution of weakness helps to indicate the site of the underlying lesion. The time of onset and the rapidity with which the symptoms developed must be determined as they play a critical role in both the diagnosis and therapeutic approach.

Confusion and Delirium

- *Confusion*, a mental and behavioral state of reduced comprehension, coherence, and capacity to reason, is one of the most common problems encountered in medicine, accounting for a large number of emergency department visits, hospital admissions, and inpatient consultations.
- *Delirium*, a term used to describe an acute fluctuating confusional state. The patient may be hyperactive or hypoactive. Delirium often goes unrecognized despite clear evidence that it is usually the cognitive manifestation of serious underlying medical or neurologic illness.

Headache and Facial Pain

- Headache results from disorders that affect pain-sensitive structures of the head and neck, such as meninges, blood vessels, nerves, and muscle.
- Headaches that are new in onset or different from previous headaches are those most likely to be caused by a serious illness, whereas headaches of long standing usually have a benign cause.
- Signs of meningeal irritation—such as neck stiffness on passive flexion in the anteroposterior direction or hip and knee flexion in response to passive neck flexion— must be sought in patients with acute headache; detecting these signs is critical in the rapid diagnosis of meningitis, and this directs the diagnostic evaluation toward urgent lumbar puncture and away from imaging procedures.
- Subarachnoid hemorrhage typically causes a "thunderclap headache" or "the worst headache of my life."
- High BP alone does not cause chronic headache.

Typical Causes of Headaches

Acute Onset

- *Common causes*
  - Subarachnoid hemorrhage
  - Other cerebrovascular diseases
  - Meningitis or encephalitis
  - Ocular disorders (glaucoma, acute iritis)
- *Less common causes*
  - Seizures
  - Lumbar puncture
  - Hypertensive encephalopathy
  - Coitus
- *Subacute onset*
  - Giant cell (temporal) arteritis
  - Intracranial mass (tumor, subdural hematoma, abscess)
  - Pseudotumor cerebri (benign intracranial hypertension)
  - Trigeminal neuralgia (tic douloureux)
  - Glossopharyngeal neuralgia
  - Postherpetic neuralgia
  - Hypertension (including pheochromocytoma and the use of monoamine oxidase inhibitors plus tyramine)
  - Atypical facial pain

Chronic

- Migraine
- Cluster headache
- Tension headache
- Cervical spine disease
- Sinusitis
- Dental disease

Coma

Coma refers to an altered level of consciousness in which the patient does not respond to external stimuli. Coma is produced by disorders that affect the cerebral hemispheres bilaterally or the brainstem reticular activating system. The possible causes of coma are limited: mass lesion, metabolic encephalopathy (hypoglycemia), infection of the brain (encephalitis) or its coverings (meningitis), and subarachnoid hemorrhage. When a patient presents in coma it is essential to obtain an accurate history from family members and friends as to the circumstances leading to the patient's present medical condition. The Glasgow Coma scale should be performed in all patients with an altered level of consciousness (see Table 10-1; http://www.mdcalc.com/glasgow-coma-scale-score).

Neurologic History and Review of Systems

A neurologic history should include the above symptoms as well as a review of systems that may alert the clinician to a systemic disease. A detailed cardiovascular history is particularly important as well as the use of medications, illicit drugs, and alcohol. In many instances, a detailed history cannot be obtained from the patient; in such circumstances family members or close friends should be contacted to obtain pertinent information.

Neurologic Examination

Despite recent advances in neuroscience and the continuing development of sensitive diagnostic procedures, the essential skill required for diagnosis of neurologic disorders remains the clinical neurologic examination. A screening neurologic examination should be performed in all medical patients (Table 10-2). In those presenting with neurologic symptoms, a more detailed examination should be performed. In those patients presenting with a stroke or cerebrovascular accident, the National Institutes of Health Stroke Scale

TABLE 10-2. OUTLINE OF THE SCREENING NEUROLOGIC EXAMINATION

Mental status Assessed while recording the history

Cranial nerves

I	Should be tested in all persons who experience spontaneous loss of smell, in patients suspected to have Parkinson disease, and in patients who have suffered head injury
II	Each eye: gross visual acuity, visual fields by confrontation, funduscopy
III, IV, VI	Horizontal and vertical eye movements
	Pupillary response to light
	Presence of nystagmus or other ocular oscillations
V	Pinprick and touch sensation on face, corneal reflex
VII	Close eyes, show teeth
VIII	Perception of whispered voice in each ear or rubbing of fingers; if hearing is impaired, look in external auditory canals and use tuning fork for lateralization and bone versus air sound conduction
IX, X	Palate lifts in midline, gag reflex present
XI	Shrug shoulders
XII	Protrude tongue

Motor Separate testing of each limb:

Presence of involuntary movements

Muscle mass (atrophy, hypertrophy) and look for fasciculations

Muscle tone in response to passive flexion and extension

Power of main muscle groups

Tendon reflexes

Plantar responses

Sensation

Pinprick and light touch on hands and feet

Double simultaneous stimuli on hands and feet

Joint position sense in hallux and index finger

Vibration sense at ankle and index finger

Coordination

Finger-to-nose and heel-to-shin testing

Performance of rapid alternating movements

Gait and balance Spontaneous gait should be observed; stance, base, cadence, arm swing, tandem gait should be noted

Postural stability should be assessed by the pull test

Romberg test Stand with eyes open and then closed

---

should be performed on admission and then daily until the neurologic signs have stabilized (http://learn.heart.org/ihtml/application/student/interface.heart2/nihss.html).

In patients with muscle weakness, the pattern of findings helps determine whether this is an upper or lower motor neuron lesion or caused by a myopathy (Table 10-3).

In patients with neurologic signs and symptoms, a more detailed examination needs to be performed. This nature of the examination depends to some degree on the presenting features but should include the following:

Level of Consciousness

Consciousness may be assessed as:

• Normal (patient awake and alert, attentive to surroundings and to the examiner)

• Depressed (patient sleepy, lethargic, stuporous—arousing only briefly in response to pain stimulation)

TABLE 10-3. SIGNS THAT DISTINGUISH THE ORIGIN OF WEAKNESS

Sign	Upper Motor Neuron	Lower Motor Neuron	Myopathic
Atrophy	None	Severe	Mild
Fasciculations	None	Common	None
Tone	Spastic	Decreased	Normal/decreased
Distribution of weakness	Pyramidal	Distal	Proximal
Distribution of weakness	Hyperactive	Hypoactive/absent	Normal/hypoactive
Babinski sign	Present	Absent	Absent

- Comatose—not arousable by pain stimulation
- Hyperalert (patient distractible, jittery, "jumpy")

    The patient's level of consciousness determines the extent to which many of the physical examination maneuvers can be performed.

Pupillary Reflexes

- A normal pupil will constrict:
  - In response to direct light
  - As a consensual response to light in the opposite eye
  - To accommodation (convergence to focus on a close object)
- A pupil that reacts to accommodation but not to light is an Argyll-Robertson pupil, signifying a lesion in the tectum of the midbrain.
- A Marcus-Gunn pupil is one with impaired constriction to direct light with preservation of the consensual response; in this case, an afferent light stimulus does not reach the lateral geniculate nucleus and a lesion should be sought in the optic tract, preoptic chiasm, optic nerve, or retina.

Constriction to Accommodation

- Consensual constriction (swinging flashlight test): After shining a flashlight into one eye to constrict the pupil, switch to the other eye and observe if that pupil constricts further (normal response) or dilates (abnormal response).

Nystagmus

Nystagmus is rhythmic oscillation of the eyes; it can be either conjugate or asymmetric. It can be a normal phenomenon (eg, at the extremes of lateral gaze) or may relate to weakness of an eye muscle or to lesions in the brainstem, cerebellum, or anywhere in the peripheral or central vestibular systems; each type has its characteristic pattern. Nystagmus is most easily observed—as are all disorders of smooth coordinated eye movements—while the patient is following the examiner's finger.

Doll's-Head (Oculocephalic) Maneuver

If the patient is unresponsive or otherwise unable to perform voluntary eye movements, the doll's-eye (doll's-head) maneuver (oculocephalic reflex) should be performed. The patient's head is held firmly and rotated from side to side, then up and down. If the brainstem is intact, the eyes will move conjugately away from the direction of turning (as if still looking at the examiner rather than fixed straight ahead).

Cognitive Functioning

Assessment of cognitive functioning aims not to determine "how smart the patient is," but how the patient's cognitive capacity has changed from a recent baseline. The examiner must have some way (recent work history, observations of family, other physicians, etc.) of assessing the patient's cognitive status before onset of the present illness. Assessment should include (at a minimum) informal evaluation of the following.

- Orientation is to person, place, and time.
- Fund of common knowledge: This is judged by the response to such questions as "Who is the president?" or "How many nickels are there in a dollar?"

- **Short-term memory:** Repeat the names of three common objects, then name them again after 5 minutes.
- **Long-term memory:** Recount verifiable events from the past.
- **Insight and judgment:** "Why have you come to see me?"
- **Concentration:** This can often be tested along with calculations (see below) or by instructing the patient (for example) to repeat a series of four to seven digits, arrange the letters in "world" in alphabetical order, or spell "world" backward.
- **Calculations:** The conventional test is serial sevens, but informal "real-life" problems may yield a more objective result.
  - **Serial sevens:** Count backward from 100, taking away 7 each time.
  - **Real-life problem:** for example, "If an apple costs 29 cents, how many can you buy for $1.50?" Then, "How much change do you have left over?"

Abstract Thought

Examples are proverb interpretation or "compare-and-contrast" tasks such as "How is an apple different from an orange?"

Verbal Fluency

This can be judged by listening to the patient talk or by asking such questions as "How many words can you say that start with the letter B?" (Time for 30 seconds.)

Function of Specific Hemispheres

Dominant Hemisphere

The most important function of the dominant hemisphere is language. Language skills include comprehension, repetition, naming, reading, and writing. Language mastery can be lost as a consequence of diffuse transient (eg, metabolic derangements) or degenerative (eg, dementia) diseases, but language impairment with otherwise normal cognitive function almost always suggests a focal lesion.

Aphasias or impairments of the expression or understanding of language are traditionally divided into categories depending on the pattern of the language deficit and the site of the damage (See Table 10-4). The three most frequently seen syndromes of clinical significance: Broca aphasia, Wernicke aphasia, and conduction aphasia. The three syndromes are tested as follows.

Nondominant Hemisphere

Tests for lesions of the nondominant hemisphere are chiefly concerned with the interpretation of incoming stimuli (other than language), visuospatial orientation, and perception of the contralateral body in space.

Defects of sensory interpretation can be evaluated in a number of ways, although all require reasonably intact primary sensation.

- **Graphesthesia:** Ask the patient to identify a letter or number written on the palm.
- **Object identification (stereognosis):** Have the patient name a common object placed in the hand (key, paper clip, coin, etc.).
- **Neglect:** Misperception of one side of space results in a number of abnormalities collectively called *neglect*. The patient may not heed information incoming from the side contralateral to the lesion (right brain affecting left side of body). Patients may deny that the left side of the body exists (even a dense hemiparesis may be cheerfully "overlooked"), fail to acknowledge as one's own the left arm held up in plain view by the examiner, or, most dramatically, fail to properly clothe or groom the left side of the body. Neglect may be tested as follows:
  - **Double simultaneous stimulation.** Touch the patient gently first on one hand and then the other while identifying the side. Then randomly vary the stimulus, asking the patient to say, with both eyes closed, "left," "right," or "both." If the patient correctly identifies each side in isolation but "extinguishes" the touch on the involved side when both are touched, neglect is present.
  - **Clock face exercise:** Draw (or have the patient draw) a large circle and ask the patient to write in the numbers of the hours of the day. Note if the patient writes all 12 numbers into the hemicircle opposite the neglected side.
  - **Reading and writing:** Ask the patient to read from a book or write on a sheet of paper. The patient may read only the right side of the page or squeeze the sentence into the

TABLE 10-4. COMMON APHASIA SYNDROMES

Fluency	Listen to spontaneous speech. Assess speech for fluency, errors of grammar or vocabulary, neologisms (meaningless words), or word substitutions (paraphasias). Determine whether the patient's speech makes sense in the current context. Alternatively, give the patient paper and pencil and say, "Write your name." "Write, 'The boy and the girl are happy about the dog.'" "Please write down your reason for being here."
Comprehension	Using only words (no gestures), instruct the patient to follow commands of increasing complexity: "Close your eyes." "Show me your left hand." "With your left hand, put a finger in your right ear." Alternatively, present a written command ("Go to the door, knock three times, and come back.") and assess whether the task is performed properly. If the patient does not comply, assess cooperation and physical capacity by repeating the commands with demonstration and miming.
Repetition	Ask the patient to repeat 3 common nouns ("bread, coffee, pencil") or "No ifs, ands, or buts."
Writing	With rare exceptions, every patient aphasic in speech is also aphasic in writing (agraphic). A patient who cannot speak but can write is mute, and the lesion is not in Broca area. Muteness occurs in a wide variety of disorders, including severe rigidity, vocal cord paralysis, bilateral corticobulbar lesions, and psychiatric disease.
Naming	Difficulty in naming familiar objects (anomia) may occur in expressive aphasia or other aphasic syndromes but by itself is not diagnostic of any specific entity. It is more likely a consequence of diffuse cerebral dysfunction of structural or metabolic origin. Ask patients to name, or mute patients to point to, a wristwatch, a typewriter keyboard, etc.

right half. Give the patient a sheet of lined notebook paper and say, "Cross out all the lines." Note whether lines on the left side of the page are ignored.

Diagnostic Tests

Laboratory

The patient's presenting symptoms determine which laboratory tests should be performed. In all patients presenting with an altered level of consciousness (altered mental status), metabolic and endocrine causes should be excluded; this includes

- Serum electrolytes including calcium, magnesium and phosphorus
- Glucose
- Liver function tests (including ammonia)
- Arterial blood gas (to exclude hypoxemia and hypercarbia)
- Thyroid function tests
- Serum cortisol
- Toxicology screen
- Serum vitamin B_{12}

Patients with non–central nervous system (CNS) infections may present with confusion; this warrants appropriate diagnostic testing including complete blood count, blood and urine cultures, chest x-ray, and so forth. In patients with unexplained altered mental status or those in whom there is a suspicion of a CNS infection, require a lumbar puncture (LP). It is important to exclude raised intracranial pressure (ICP) and mass lesion prior to performing a LP.

Lumbar Puncture

Indications

- Diagnosis of meningitis and other infective or inflammatory disorders
- Subarachnoid hemorrhage (with normal computed tomography [CT])
- Meningeal malignancies
- Paraneoplastic disorders
- Suspected abnormalities of ICP.
- Patients with suspected Guillain-Barre and chronic inflammatory demyelinating polyneuropathy
- Assessment of the response to therapy in meningitis and other infective or inflammatory disorders
- Administration of intrathecal medications or radiologic contrast media
- To reduce cerebrospinal fluid (CSF) pressure.

Contraindications

- Suspected intracranial mass lesion. In this situation, performing a LP can hasten incipient transtentorial herniation.
- Local infection overlying the site of puncture. Under this circumstance, cervical or cisternal puncture should be performed instead.
- Coagulopathy. The INR, partial thromboplastin time and platelet count must be checked prior to performing a LP. Patients with a coagulopathy can develop a spinal hematoma with consequent paralysis. The INR should be corrected in patients taking vitamin K antagonists. A platelet transfusion is indicated in patients with a platelet count below 20,000/mm^3. A LP appears to be safe in patients taking aspirin. However, adenosine diphosphate antagonists (clopidogrel [Plavix]) should ideally be stopped 7 days prior to performing a LP. In emergent situations a platelet transfusion should be considered.
- Suspected spinal cord mass lesion. Lumbar puncture in this case should be performed only in association with myelography, which is used to determine the presence and level of structural spinal pathology

Tests to Order on Spinal Fluid

- Glucose: CSF glucose concentration is usually more than 50% of serum concentration, but moderately reduced values are occasionally seen with herpes simplex virus (HSV), mumps, some enteroviruses, and lymphocytic choriomeningitis virus. Low levels are typical of bacterial meningitis.
- Protein: CSF protein concentration is typically less than 50 mg/dL.
- Cells: CSF is normally acellular. However, up to 5 white blood cells (WBCs) and 5 red blood cells (RBCs) are considered normal in adults when the CSF is sampled by LP. More than 3 polymorphonuclear leukocytes are abnormal in adults. An elevated CSF WBC concentration does not diagnose an infection, because increases in the CSF WBC concentration can occur in a variety of both infectious and noninfectious inflammatory states.
- Gram stain and culture: always preform.
- Bacterial antigens (meningococcal, streptococcal): perform in patients with suspected bacterial meningitis.
- Cytology: when suspecting malignancy.
- Immunoglobulins and oligoclonal bands: Immunoglobulins are almost totally excluded from the CSF in healthy individuals. The blood-to-CSF ratio of immunoglobulin G (IgG) is normally 500:1 or more. Elevations in oligoclonally expanded immunoglobulin concentrations in the CSF, termed *oligoclonal bands*, may occur in any disorder that disrupts the blood-brain barrier. Oligoclonal bands may also be caused by intrathecal production of IgG, and the presence of such bands is a diagnostic criterion for multiple sclerosis
- Polymerase chain reaction (PCR): With the advent of PCR technology, significant advances have been made in the ability to diagnose viral infections of the CNS. CSF PCR should be performed for HSV type 1 (HSV-1), HSV type 2 (HSV-2), and enteroviruses. PCR testing can also be requested for varicella-zoster virus and cytomegalovirus in the appropriate settings. PCR testing for other viruses will depend on the clinical situation, epidemiology, and availability.

Among patients with bacterial meningitis, the classic findings are (Table 10-5):

- CSF WBC count above 1000/μL, usually with a neutrophilic predominance
- CSF protein concentration above 250 mg/dL
- CSF glucose concentration below 45 mg/dL

TABLE 10-5. CEREBRAL SPINAL FLUID ANALYSIS IN CENTRAL NERVOUS SYSTEM INFECTIONS

	Glucose (mg/dL)				Protein (mg/dL)			Total WBC Count (cells/μL)		
	<10	10–45	>250	50–250		>1000	100–1000	5–100		
More Common	Bacterial meningitis	Bacterial meningitis	Bacterial meningitis	Viral meningitis Lyme disease Neurosyphillis		Bacterial meningitis	Bacterial or viral meningitis TB meningitis	Early bacterial meningitis Viral meningitis Neurosyphillis TB meningitis		
Less Common	TB meningitis Fungal meningitis	Neurosyphillis Some viral infections, such as mumps, LCMV	TB meningitis			Some cases of mumps and LCMV	Encephalitis	Encephalitis		

LCMV, lymphocytic choriomeningitis virus; TB, tuberculosus; WBC, white blood cell.

Among patients with viral meningitis, the typical findings include:

- The CSF WBC count is usually less than 250/μL, and almost always less than 2000/μL. The differential typically shows a predominance of lymphocytes, although early infection may reveal a predominance of neutrophils that, within the next 24 hours, generally shows a shift from neutrophils to lymphocytes.
- The CSF protein concentration is typically less than 150 mg/dL; it has been estimated that CSF protein concentrations greater than 220 mg/dL reduce the probability of viral infection to 1% or less.
- The CSF glucose concentration is usually more than 50% of serum concentration, but moderately reduced values are occasionally seen with HSV, mumps, some enteroviruses, and lymphocytic choriomeningitis virus.

Xanthochromia, a yellow or pink discoloration of the CSF, represents most often the presence of hemoglobin degradation products and indicates that blood has been in the CSF for at least 2 hours (eg, subarachnoid hemorrhage).

Radiography: CT and Magnetic Resonance Imaging (MRI)

The investigations that are performed in a particular case depend on the clinical context and the likely diagnosis.

Investigations are performed not only to suggest or confirm the diagnosis but also to exclude other diagnostic possibilities, aid prognostication, provide a guide to further management, and follow disease progression.

The results of investigations need to be interpreted in the context in which they were obtained.

Computed Tomography

CT scanning is a noninvasive computer-assisted radiologic means of examining anatomic structures. It permits the detection of structural intracranial abnormalities with precision and speed. It is thus of particular use in evaluating patients with progressive neurologic disorders or focal neurologic deficits in whom a structural lesion is suspected as well as patients with dementia or increased ICP. It is particularly important in the evaluation of patients with suspected stroke or with head injuries. Intravenous administration of an iodinated contrast agent improves the ability of CT scan to detect and define lesions, such as tumors and abscesses, associated with a disturbance of the blood-brain barrier.

Indications for Use

- Stroke: CT scan is particularly helpful in evaluating strokes because it can distinguish infarction from intracranial hemorrhage; it is particularly sensitive in detecting intracerebral hematomas, and the location of such lesions may provide a guide to their cause.
- Tumor: CT scans can indicate the site of a brain tumor, the extent of any surrounding edema, whether the lesion is cystic or solid, and whether it has displaced midline or other normal anatomic structures. It also demonstrates any hemorrhagic component.
- Trauma: CT scan is an important means of evaluating patients following head injury, in particular for detecting traumatic subarachnoid or intracerebral hemorrhage (ICH) and bony injuries. It also provides a more precise delineation of associated fractures than do plain x-rays.
- Dementia: In patients with dementia, CT scan may indicate the presence of a tumor or of hydrocephalus (enlarged ventricles), with or without accompanying cerebral atrophy. The occurrence of hydrocephalus without cerebral atrophy in demented patients suggests normal pressure or communicating hydrocephalus. Cerebral atrophy can occur in demented or normal elderly subjects.
- Subarachnoid hemorrhage: In patients with subarachnoid hemorrhage, the CT scan generally indicates the presence of blood in the subarachnoid space and may even suggest the source of the bleeding. CT angiography may demonstrate an underlying vascular malformation or aneurysm.

Magnetic Resonance Imaging

MRI is an imaging procedure that involves no radiation. The patient lies within a large magnet that aligns some of the protons in the body along the magnet's axis. The protons resonate when stimulated with radio-frequency energy, producing a tiny echo that is strong enough to be detected. The position and intensity of these radio-frequency emissions are recorded and mapped by a computer. The signal intensity depends on the concentration of mobile hydrogen nuclei (or nuclear-spin density) of the tissues. Spin-lattice (T1) and spin-spin (T2) relaxation times are mainly responsible for the relative differences in signal intensity of the various soft tissues; these parameters are sensitive to the state of water in biologic tissues. Pulse sequences with varying dependence on T1 and T2 selectively alter the contrast between soft tissues.

The soft-tissue contrast available with MRI makes it more sensitive than CT scanning in detecting certain structural lesions. MRI provides better contrast than does CT scan between the gray and white matter of the brain; it is superior for visualizing abnormalities in the posterior fossa and spinal cord and for detecting lesions associated with multiple sclerosis or those that cause seizures. Gadopentetate dimeglumine (gadolinium-diethylenetriamine pentaacetic acid [DPTA]) is stable, well-tolerated intravenously, and an effective enhancing MRI agent that is useful in identifying small tumors that, because of their similar relaxation times to normal cerebral tissue, may be missed on unenhanced MRI.

- Diffusion-weighted MRI: This technique, in which contrast within the image is based on the microscopic motion of water protons in tissue, provides information that is not available on standard MRI. It is particularly important in the assessment of stroke because it can discriminate cytotoxic edema (which occurs in strokes) from vasogenic edema (found with other types of cerebral lesion) and thus reveals cerebral ischemia early and with high specificity. Diffusion-weighted MRI permits reliable identification of acute cerebral ischemia during the first few hours after onset, before it is detectable on standard MRI.

- Perfusion-weighted MRI: Perfusion-weighted imaging measures relative blood flow through the brain by either an injected contrast medium (eg, gadolinium) or an endogenous technique (in which the patient's own blood provides the contrast). It allows cerebral blood-flow abnormalities to be recognized and can confirm the early reperfusion of tissues after treatment.

Indications for Use and Comparison with CT Scan

- Stroke: Within a few hours of vascular occlusion, it may be possible to detect and localize cerebral infarcts by MRI. These can be detected by T2-weighted imaging and fluid-attenuated inversion-recovery (FLAIR) sequences. CT scans, conversely, may be unrevealing for up to 48 hours. After that period, there is less advantage to MRI over CT scanning except for the former's ability to detect smaller lesions and its superior imaging of the posterior fossa. Nevertheless, CT scanning without contrast is usually the preferred initial study in patients with acute stroke, in order to determine whether hemorrhage has occurred. Intracranial hemorrhage is not easily detected by MRI within the first 36 hours, and CT scan is more reliable for this purpose. Hematomas of more than 2 to 3 days' duration, however, are better visualized by MRI.

- Tumor: Both CT scans and MRI are very useful in detecting brain tumors, but the absence of bone artifacts makes MRI superior for visualizing tumors at the vertex or in the posterior fossa and for detecting acoustic neuromas. Secondary effects of tumors, such as cerebral herniation, can be seen with either MRI or CT scan, but MRI provides more anatomic information.

- Trauma: In the acute phase following head injury, CT scan is preferable to MRI because it requires less time, is superior for detecting intracranial hemorrhage, and may reveal bony injuries.

- Dementia: In patients with dementia, either CT scan or MRI can help in demonstrating treatable structural causes, but MRI appears to be more sensitive in demonstrating abnormal white matter signal and associated atrophy.

- Multiple sclerosis: In patients with multiple sclerosis, it is often possible to detect lesions in the cerebral white matter or the cervical cord by MRI, even though such lesions may not be visualized on CT scans. The demyelinating lesions detected by MRI may have signal characteristics resembling those of ischemic changes, however, and clinical correlation is therefore always necessary. Gadolinium-enhanced MRI permits lesions of different ages to be distinguished. This ability facilitates the diagnosis of multiple sclerosis: the presence of lesions of different ages suggests a multiphasic disease, whereas lesions of similar age suggest a monophasic disorder, such as acute disseminated encephalomyelitis.

- Infections: MRI is very sensitive in detecting white-matter edema and probably permits earlier recognition of focal areas of cerebritis and abscess formation than is possible with CT scan.

Contraindications

Contraindications to MRI include the presence of intracranial clips, metallic foreign bodies in the eye or elsewhere, pacemakers, cochlear implants, and conditions requiring close monitoring of patients.

SPECIFIC NEUROLOGIC CONDITIONS

Coma

Coma is a sleeplike state in which the patient makes no purposeful response to the environment and from which he or she cannot be aroused. The eyes are closed and do not open spontaneously. The patient does not speak, and there is no purposeful movement of the face or limbs. Verbal stimulation produces no response. Painful stimulation may produce no response or nonpurposeful reflex movements mediated through spinal cord or brainstem pathways. Coma is produced by disorders that affect the cerebral hemispheres bilaterally or the brainstem reticular activating system. The most common causes of coma include: mass lesion, metabolic encephalopathy, infection of the brain (encephalitis) or its coverings (meningitis), subarachnoid hemorrhage, and drug overdose. Hypoglycemia must be excluded in all patients who present in coma. The management of coma depends on the specific causative factor. Endotracheal intubation must be considered to protect the airway and prevent aspiration pneumonitis and airway obstruction.

The most common causes of coma grouped by category are listed below:

Metabolic

- Hypoxia
- Hypercapnia
- Hypernatremia
- Hyponatremia
- Hypoglycemia
- Diabetic ketoacidosis
- Hyperglycemic nonketotic coma
- Hypercalcemia
- Hypocalcemia
- Hypothermia
- Wernicke encephalopathy
- Hepatic encephalopathy
- Uremia
- Addisonian crisis
- Myxedema coma

Infections

- Bacterial meningitis
- Viral encephalitis
- Postinfectious encephalomyelitis

Drugs

- Sedatives
- Barbiturates
- Opiates
- Anticholinergics
- Psychotropics
- Antidepressants
- Lithium
- Monoamine inhibitors

Illicit Drugs and Toxins

- Ethanol
- Methanol
- Ethylene glycol
- Carbon monoxide
- Amphetamines
- Phencyclidine
- Lead
- Thallium
- Mushrooms
- Cyanide

Central Nervous System Lesions

- Subarachnoid hemorrhage
- Intracerebral hemorrhage
- Brain stem hemorrhage
- Brain stem infarction
- Massive or bilateral supratentorial infarction
- Subdural hemorrhage
- Subdural empyema
- Head trauma with contusions
- Unilateral hemispheric mass (tumor, bleed) with herniation
- Hydrocephalus
- Cerebral abscess
- Cerebral vasculitis
- Acute disseminated encephalomyelitis
- Multiple sclerosis
- Brain stem tumor

Other

- Hypotension and/or shock
- Hypertensive encephalopathy
- Catatonia

Ischemic Strokes

- Stroke causes 9% of all deaths worldwide and is the second most common cause of death after ischemic heart disease. In over 75% of cases the stroke is ischemic in nature.
- Ischemic stokes may be conveniently classified as:
  - Large vessel atherosclerotic
  - Cardioembolic
  - Small artery (lacuna)
  - Stroke of other identified cause (eg vasculitis)
  - Stroke of undetermined cause.
- Unlike acute myocardial infarction, therapeutic interventions that attempt to limit infarct size have been of limited success. Apart from thrombolytic therapy in a highly select groups of patients (probably less than 5% of "stroke" patients) and aspirin, no therapeutic intervention has been demonstrated to impact the course of this illness.
- The most important aspects of care include determination of the underlying cause, anticoagulation when appropriate, assessment for the presence of and management of dysphagia and rehabilitation (speech therapy, physical therapy). In most cases, such treatment is best provided by specialized "low-technology" stroke units.
- At present, no intervention with putative neuroprotective actions has been established as effective in improving outcomes after stroke and therefore none currently can be recommended. Similarly, hemodilution, volume expansion, vasodilators, and induced hypertension cannot be recommended.
- For the overwhelming majority of patients suffering stroke, acute medical interventions in an intensive care unit (ICU) have not been established to improve outcome, and in fact, certain interventions may be harmful. Patients with an absent gag reflex on admission to hospital will almost always die from their stroke.
- The failure of specific intervention to improve the outcome of patients suffering a stroke should not imply that physicians should adopt a fatalistic approach when managing these patients. A number of well-conducted clinical trials have demonstrated that the mortality and functional recovery of patients following a stroke is significantly improved when these patients are cared for in a specialized stroke unit as compared to a general medical ward. These units provide specialized nursing care and a well-organized multidisciplinary rehabilitation program.
- Endotracheal intubation should be reserved for patients with reversible respiratory failure or comatose patients who are likely to have a good prognosis for a functional recovery.
- Patients who are likely to require a neurosurgical intervention including those with large middle cerebral artery (MCA) strokes at risk of "malignant cerebral edema" and cerebellar infarcts should be admitted to the ICU.

Workup on patients with stroke:

- Immediate CT scan to exclude hemorrhage or other intracranial lesions
- T2-weighted MRI, diffusion-weighted MRI and/or FLAIR sequences when clinically appropriate
- Echocardiogram to exclude cardiac emboli
- Bilateral carotid duplex studies
- Thrombophilia workup when clinically indicated/suspicion of clotting disorder
- Genetic testing when indicated (eg, cerebral autosomal dominant arteriopathy with subcortical infarcts and leukoencephalopathy [CADASIL])

Thrombolytic Therapy

- The National Institute of Neurological Disorders and Stroke (NINDS) rt-PA Stroke Trial demonstrated that recombinant tissue-type plasminogen activator (rtPA) given to patients within 3 hours of the onset of stroke resulted in an 11% to 13% absolute increase in the chance of minimum or no disability at 3 months.

- More recently the European Cooperative Acute Stroke Study III reported the results of a study in which alteplase (0.9 mg/kg) or placebo was administered between 3 and 4.5 hours after the onset of acute ischemic stroke. Patients with severe stroke were excluded from this trial. Although mortality did not differ between groups, more patients had a favorable outcome with alteplase than with placebo (52.4% vs 45.2%; odds ratio [OR] 1.34; 95% confidence interval [CI] 1.02 to 1.76; $P = 0.04$)

- This data demonstrates that the benefits of thrombolytic therapy decease with time while the risks (intracranial bleeding) increase with time; time is therefore of the essence. Thrombolytic therapy is best administered at regional centers that have experience with this therapy and where the timely evaluation and initiation of therapy can be instituted; selected patients may benefit when the window of treatment is extended up to 4.5 hours.

- The most recent guidelines from the Stroke Council of the American Heart Association (AHA) suggest the following inclusion and exclusion criteria for thrombolytic therapy:
  - Diagnosis of ischemic stroke causing measurable neurologic deficit.
  - The neurologic signs should not be clearing spontaneously.
  - The neurologic signs should not be minor or isolated.
  - Caution should be exercised in treating patients with major deficits.
  - The symptoms of stroke should not be suggestive of subarachnoid hemorrhage.
  - Onset of symptoms less than 3 hours before beginning treatment (this can now be extended up to 4.5 hours in selected patients).
  - No head trauma or stroke in previous 3 months.
  - No myocardial infarction in previous 3 months.
  - No gastrointestinal tract or urinary tract hemorrhage in previous 21 days.
  - No major surgery in previous 14 days.
  - No history of previous intracranial hemorrhage.
  - Blood pressure not elevated (systolic blood pressure [SBP] <185 mm Hg or diastolic blood pressure [DBP] <110 mm Hg)
  - Not taking an oral anticoagulant or, if anticoagulant being taken INR <1.5.
  - If receiving heparin in previous 48 hours, activated partial thromboplastin time must be normal.
  - Platelet count >100,000 per microliter.
  - No seizure.
  - CT does not show multilobar infarction (hypodensity > one-third of the cerebral hemisphere).
  - The patient or family members understand the potential risks and benefits from treatment.

- The role of intraarterial thrombolysis in patients with ischemic stroke is unclear. This treatment modality is, however, an option is selected patients who have had a major stroke of less than 4 hours duration caused by occlusion of the MCA and who are not otherwise candidates for intravenous (IV) rtPA (recent surgery, etc.). Treatment requires the patient to be at an experienced stroke center with immediate access to cerebral angiography and qualified interventionists.

Treatment of Acute Ischemic Stroke with IV rtPA

- Perform National Institutes of Health Stroke Scale assessment
- Infuse 0.9 mg/kg (maximum dose 90 mg) over 60 minutes with 10% of the dose given as a bolus over 1 minute.
- Admit the patient to an ICU or stroke unit for monitoring.
- Perform neurologic assessments every 15 minutes during the infusion and every 30 minutes thereafter for the next 6 hours, then hourly until 24 hours after treatment.
- If the patient develops severe headache, acute hypertension, nausea or vomiting, discontinue the infusion (if rtPA being administered) and obtain emergency CT scan.
- Measure BP every 15 minutes for the first 2 hours and subsequently every 30 minutes for the next 6 hours, then hourly until 24 hours after treatment.
- Increase the frequency of BP measurements if SBP is higher than 180 mm Hg or if DBP is higher than 105 mm Hg; administer antihypertensive medication to maintain BP below these levels (nicardipine or clevidipine preferred).

- Delay placement of nasogastric (NG) tubes and central venous, bladder, or intraarterial catheters.
- Obtain a follow-up CT scan at 24 hours before starting anticoagulants or antiplatelet drugs.

Antiplatelet Therapy and Anticoagulation

- The International Stroke Trial randomized (using a factorial design) more than 19,000 patients within 48 hours of an acute ischemic stroke to 14 days of treatment with placebo, heparin (5,000 or 12,500 units every 12 hours) or aspirin 300 mg daily. Aspirin resulted in a 1.1% absolute reduction in recurrent ischemic strokes at 14 days; both heparin regimens had no effect on outcome. Additional studies have demonstrated that heparin, low-molecular-weight heparin and heparinoids do not improve outcome following a stroke.
- The current AHA and American Stroke Association (ASA) guidelines do not recommend urgent anticoagulation for patients with moderate to severe strokes because of an increased risk of serious intracranial hemorrhage. Nor do they recommend anticoagulant therapy following rtPA. However, these guidelines recommend treatment with aspirin (initial dose of 325 mg) within 24 to 48 after stroke onset.

Anticoagulation in Cardioembolic Stroke

- Hemorrhage into the infarct occurs in approximately 30% of cases of all embolic infarcts; it may, however, require 3 or 4 days or longer to become apparent on the CT scan. However, MRI has demonstrated that by 3 weeks, hemorrhagic conversion occurs in up to 70% of patients. Hemorrhage ranges from the usual cortical petechiae to confluent hematomas. In nonanticoagulated patients, infarct volume seems to be the only independent predictor of hemorrhagic conversion.
- Chronic anticoagulant therapy has been demonstrated to reduce the risk of recurrent embolization in patients who have suffered an embolic stroke. Approximately 80% of patients who have suffered a cerebral embolic stroke will suffer a subsequent embolic stroke without anticoagulation.
- Because of the risk of infarct hemorrhage, it may be prudent to delay anticoagulation for 10 to 14 days, particularly in patients with large cerebral infarcts and hypertensive patients.
- The role of transesophageal echocardiography (TEE) is unclear. However, it may be prudent to perform TEE in patients at high risk of early recurrent embolization, and to commence anticoagulation earlier if clot is visualized within the cardiac cambers and CT scan does not show evidence of hemorrhagic transformation.

Decompressive Surgery

Hemispheric decompression in young patients with malignant MCA-territory infarction and space-occupying brain edema has been demonstrated to improve outcome. An individual patient meta-analysis demonstrated a marked improvement in neurologic recovery and survival with decompressive craniectomy. This combination occurs in approximately 1% to 10% of patients with supratentorial hemispheric infarcts and usually arises between 2 and 5 days after stroke.

Treatment of Hyperglycemia

Both animal and human data suggest that postinfarction hyperglycemia increases neuronal damage with an increase in infarct size. This data suggests that hyperglycemia should be treated, with careful monitoring of the serum glucose (hypoglycemia may extend infarct size). The optimal target blood glucose level in this group of patients has yet to be determined, however, a level between 110 and 150 mg/dL appears reasonable. Results of clinical trials in critically ill patients suggest improved outcome with early enteral nutrition. Prevention of hyperglycemia once feeding is initiated is important.

Treatment of Fever

Fever has been shown to worsen the prognosis in acute stroke. It is therefore important to treat fever (temperature >37.5°C [99.5°F]) in stroke patients with antipyretics. In patients who remain febrile after antipyretics, external cooling with cooling blankets and/or intravascular cooling should be instituted. The goal should be to keep patients normothermic. In animal models of focal cerebral ischemia, hypothermia significantly reduces infarct size and improves outcome; however, the role of induced hypothermia in patients with ischemic stroke has yet to be determined.

Treatment of Post-Stroke Hypertension

- The vast majority of patients with cerebral ischemia present with acutely elevated BP regardless of the subtype of infarct or preexisting hypertension. The BP elevation spontaneously decreases over time. The elevated BP is not a manifestation of a hypertensive emergency, but rather a protective physiologic response to maintain cerebral perfusion pressure to the vascular territory affected by ischemia.

- Lowering the BP in patients with ischemic strokes may reduce cerebral blood flow (CBF), which because of impaired autoregulation, may result in further ischemic injury. The common practice of "normalizing" the BP following a cerebrovascular accident is potentially dangerous.

- The Scandinavian Candesartan Acute Stroke Trial, which examined the use of the *angiotensin-receptor blocker, candesartan, for treatment of acute stroke,* randomized 2029 patients with acute stroke and a SBP of 140 mm Hg or higher to an escalating dose of candesartan or placebo. During 6 months' follow-up, the risk of the composite vascular end point did not differ between treatment groups. Analysis of functional outcome suggested a higher risk of poor outcome in the candesartan group (adjusted common OR 1.17; 95% CI, 1.00–1.38; $P = 0.048$). This study together with previous research in this area suggests that patients should not routinely be treated with antihypertensive agents following an ischemic stroke.

- ASA/AHA and the European Stroke Initiative do not recommend routine lowering of BP unless it is repeatedly exceeds 200 to 220 mm Hg SBP or 120 mm Hg DBP in the acute period. In these patients, the aim is to reduce the pressure by no more than 10% to 15% in the first 24 hours. While the drug of choice is unclear, a short-acting IV agent is currently recommended (ie, labetalol, nicardipine, or clevidipine).

- The ASA/AHA and European Stroke Initiative guidelines recommend the reduction of BP according to the eligibility thresholds for inclusion in the NINDS rtPA efficacy trial before thrombolytics are administered. Antihypertensive therapy is therefore required for SBP higher than 185 mm Hg or DBP higher than 110 mm Hg with a targeted SBP of 180 mm Hg and a DBP of 105 mm Hg.

Supportive Medical Therapy

- General measures are aimed at maintaining an adequate cerebral perfusion pressure and preventing complications.

- Maintain euvolemia; hypovolemia will compromise cardiac output and cerebral perfusion thereby extending the size of the infarct. Avoid hypotonic solutions, which will increase cerebral edema. Stroke patients may develop the "cerebral salt-wasting syndrome," which requires aggressive volume replacement.

- Bed rest with elevation of the head to 20 to 35 degrees.

- Laxatives

- Deep vein thrombosis prophylaxis (stockings, pneumatic boots) and low-molecular-weight heparin after 48 to 72 hours in nonambulating patients with no evidence of hemorrhagic transformation.

- Mild sedation and anxiolysis for agitated patients.

- Regular chest physiotherapy and physical therapy.

- Speech and swallowing assessment: The ability of the patient to swallow should be assessed as abnormalities of swallowing occur in up to 40% of patients. In patients with swallowing dysfunction, enteral feeding should be achieved using a small-bore feeding nasoenteric tube. In the majority of patients, swallowing function will recover in 7 to 10 days. Occasionally, prolonged supportive feeding may be required necessitating placement of a gastrostomy or gastrojejunostomy.

- Corticosteroids have no role in the management of cerebral edema and increased ICP after stroke.

- The frequency of seizures during the acute period after stroke is reported to be between 4% and 43%. Recurrent seizures occur in approximately 20% to 80% of cases. There are no data concerning the value of prophylactic administration of anticonvulsants after ischemic stroke. Until such data becomes available, stroke patients who are seizure-free should not receive anticonvulsant drugs.

Intracerebral Hemorrhages

• Approximately 15% of all strokes are hemorrhagic. The mortality rate in the first 30 days after ICH is 35% to 50% with more than half of the deaths occurring in the first 2 days. Clot volume is the most powerful predictor of outcome. Other important variables are baseline neurologic status and intraventricular hemorrhage volume.

• Although previously thought to be rare, recurrence or extension of ICH recently has been shown to be a relatively common occurrence affecting as many as one-third of patients in the early period after ICH. The principles of management of ICH are similar to those of acute ischemic stokes, with a few exceptions.

• A urine toxic screen should be obtained as part of the initial evaluation in ICH patients, particularly the young and the normotensive; substances implicated in the causation of ICH include cocaine, amphetamines, methylphenidate, pentazocine (Talwin)-tripelennamine (Pyribenzamine), phencyclidine and phenylpropanolamine.

• Two randomized trials showed no benefit on regional blood flow, neurologic improvement, mortality, and functional outcomes from the regular use of IV mannitol boluses.

• Those patients with ICH while receiving anticoagulant therapy should have emergent correction of the abnormal coagulation parameters to prevent further enlargement of the hematoma.

  • Vitamin K antagonists must be reversed with IV vitamin K, prothrombin concentrate, and fresh frozen plasma.

  • Patients' receiving aspirin and/or clopidogrel (Plavix) do not appear to benefit from platelet transfusion.

  • In patients with ICH and mechanical heart valves, temporary interruption of anticoagulation therapy seems safe in patients without previous evidence of systemic embolization. For most patients at risk of cardioembolic stroke, discontinuation of anticoagulation for 1 to 2 weeks should be sufficient to observe the evolution of a parenchymal hematoma.

• A phase II study demonstrated an improvement in neurologic outcome and mortality in patients with an ICH treated with activated recombinant factor VII (fVIIa). However, a large phase III trial (Recombinant Factor VII in Acute Intracerebral Hemorrhage Trial [FAST]) was unable to reproduce these findings.

Blood Pressure Control

• The acute hypertensive response in ICH is characterized by its high prevalence, self-limiting nature, and prognostic significance. The high BP might be secondary to uncontrolled chronic hypertension, with disruption of central autonomic pathways by ICH. High BP is associated with hematoma enlargement and poor outcome; however, an exact cause and effect relation is unproven.

• The current AHA Stroke Council guidelines recommend, "until ongoing clinical trials of blood pressure intervention for intracerebral hemorrhage are completed, physicians must manage blood pressure on the basis of the present incomplete evidence…" by http://www.acep.org/content.aspx?id=26716 maintaining SBP less than 180 mm Hg in the acute period with short half-life IV antihypertensive drugs. Great caution is advised about lowering BP too aggressively without concomitant management of cerebral perfusion pressure.

Surgical Interventions

• Routine surgical interventions include placing an ICP monitor in patients who have large hemorrhages or performing a ventriculostomy in patients who display evidence of obstructive hydrocephalus.

• Urgent surgical decompression is indicated in patients with cerebellar hematomas greater than 3 cm in diameter or with brain stem compression.

• Open craniotomy and decompression of cortical or lobar hemorrhages has been associated with a higher mortality over medical therapy. The AHA Stroke Council and European Stroke Organization guidelines do not recommend routine evacuation of supratentorial hemorrhage by standard craniotomy within 96 hours of ictus.

• Both guidelines recommend surgery for patients presenting with lobar hemorrhage within 1 cm of the surface, particularly for those with good neurologic status who are deteriorating clinically. The role of stereotactic approaches to clot evacuation has yet to be determined.

Profiles Predictive of Futility after Devastating Stroke

- Persistent coma after attempts to lower ICP
- Massive intraventricular hemorrhage with hydrocephalus
- Presence of delayed global edema on CT
- Lobar ICH
- Coma with extensor posturing and absent pontomesencephalic reflexes
- Coma with septum pellucidum shift more than 6 mm on CT
- Ganglionic ICH
- Coma with hydrocephalus and hematoma size more than 60 cc
- Pontine hemorrhage
- Coma with hyperthermia and tachycardia
- Coma with acute hydrocephalus and hemorrhage extension into thalamus
- Cerebellar hemorrhage
- Absent corneal reflexes
- Absent oculocephalic response with hydrocephalus
- Hemispheric ischemic infarction
- Clinical deterioration with coma and loss of pontomesencephalic reflexes
- Shift of pineal gland more than 4 mm on CT scan performed within 48 hours
- Cerebellar ischemic infarction
- Persistent coma after decompressive surgery

Subarachnoid Hemorrhage

- Subarachnoid hemorrhage (SAH) is a common and devastating condition. Patients who have suffered a SAH are best managed in an ICU or a specialized neurology/neurosurgical unit.
- Despite improved management, the outcome following SAH remains poor; with an overall mortality of approximately 25% and significant morbidity among the survivors. The most serious complications following the initial bleed are rebleeding and cerebral vasospasm; management of patients with SAH is therefore is largely directed to avoiding these complications.
- The risk of rebleeding (with conservative therapy) is highest in the first month, with a rate of between 20% and 30%. The mortality rate is approximately 70% for patients who rebleed.
- Angiographic vasospasm probably develops to some degree in most patients who suffer a SAH. However, clinically manifest vasospasm occurs in approximately 40% of patients; 15% to 20% of these patients will suffer a stroke or die despite aggressive management.

Diagnosis and Evaluation

Noncontrast CT scanning is the diagnostic test of choice following a suspected SAH. If the scan is performed within 24 hours of the event, clot can be demonstrated in the subarachnoid space in approximately 90% of patients. The diagnostic sensitivity of the CT scan declines after the first day. A diagnostic LP should be performed in a patient with a suspected SAH if the initial CT scan is negative. A normal CT scan and a normal spinal fluid examination excludes a SAH and predicts a favorable prognosis in the setting of the sudden onset of a severe headache.

Clinical Classification

The Hunt and Hess Classification system is the most commonly used grading system to assess the severity of a SAH. The Hunt and Hess grade has important therapeutic and prognostic implications:

- I = asymptomatic or slight headache
- II = moderate to severe headache, nuchal rigidity, no neurologic deficit other than cranial nerve palsy
- III = drowsiness, confusion, or mild focal deficit
- IV = stupor, moderate to severe hemiparesis
- V = deep coma, decerebrate rigidity

Cerebral Angiography

Selective catheter angiography is currently the standard for diagnosing cerebral aneurysms as the cause of SAH. Approximately 20% to 25% of cerebral angiograms performed for SAH will not indicate a source of bleeding. It is generally recommended to repeat the angiogram in 2 weeks, because vascular spasm may have obscured the aneurysm. However, only a very small percentage of repeat angiograms will demonstrate an aneurysm. The risk of rebleeding in patients with normal angiograms is low; less than 4% are reported to rebleed when followed for up to 10 years. CT angiography has improved to the point where some centers use it as the primary test to identify an aneurysm.

Initial Management: General Measures and Measures to Prevent Rebleeding

- Bed rest with elevation of the head to 20 to 35 degrees.
- Mild sedation and anxiolysis for grade I and II patients.
- Pain management with morphine sulphate or codeine. Meperidine should be avoided as it can precipitate seizures.
- Maintain euvolemia. Careful fluid management is required to avoid hypovolemia; this may reduce the risk of delayed cerebral ischemia. Despite being widely advocated, data supporting the use of hypervolemia are scant.
- Laxatives.
- Deep vein thrombosis prophylaxis (stockings, pneumatic boots).
- Nimodipine 60 mg every 4 to 6 hours.
- Ventriculostomy for acute obstructive hydrocephalus; consider in all patients with Hunt and Hess grades IV and V.
- The routine use of anticonvulsants has been associated with cognitive impairment in patients with SAH and heralded the growing acceptance of reduced use of anticonvulsants. Anticonvulsants (preferably levetiracetam [Keppra]) should be considered in patients with MCA aneurysms.
- Corticosteroids have no proven benefit in SAH.

Antihypertensive Agents

The role of antihypertensive agents in preventing rebleeding is controversial. Rebleeding may be related to variations or changes in BP rather than the absolute BP. However, it is generally advised that the SBP be kept below 150 mm Hg. Mild sedation and control of pain may adequately control an elevated BP. If antihypertensive agents are used, these should be used with extreme caution. Intravenous agents that can be closely titrated are preferred; an excessive reduction of BP may cause cerebral ischemia. Nicardipine, clevidipine, and labetalol are preferred agents.

Antifibrinolytic Therapy

The role of antifibrinolytic agent in preventing rebleeding is unclear. While antifibrinolytic agents reduce the rate of bleeding, the benefits are offset by a higher incidence of cerebral infarction. In a prospective, randomized trial of the antifibrinolytic drug, tranexamic acid, early rebleeding rates and adverse outcomes were reduced when the drug was administered immediately after the diagnosis of SAH and stopped when the aneurysm was secure.

Surgical and Endovascular Methods of Treatment

In 1991, Guglielmi et al described the technique of occluding aneurysms by an endovascular approach with electrolytically detachable platinum coils (Guglielmi detachable coils). Guglielmi detachable coils are introduced directly into the aneurysm through a microcatheter and detached from a stainless steel microguidewire by an electric current. The aneurysm is packed with several coils. The coils induce thrombosis, thereby excluding the aneurysm from the circulation. The International Subarachnoid Aneurysm Trial compared neurosurgical clipping versus endovascular coiling in 2143 patients with ruptured aneurysms. In this study, which enrolled patients with ruptured intracranial aneurysms suitable for both treatments, endovascular coiling was more likely to result in independent survival at 1 year than neurosurgical clipping; the survival benefit continued for at least 7 years.

Management of Cerebral Vasospasm

After aneurysmal SAH, angiographic vasospasm is seen in 30% to 70% of patients, with a typical onset 3 to 5 days after the hemorrhage, maximal narrowing at 5 to 14 days, with a gradual resolution over 2 to 4 weeks. Cerebral vasospasm is associated with reduced

CBF. The changes in CBF are coupled to changes in oxygen delivery so that cerebral hypoperfusion leads to inadequate oxygen delivery. In approximately one-half of cases, vasospasm is manifested by the occurrence of a delayed neurologic ischemic deficit, which may resolve or progress to cerebral infarction. In contemporary series, 15% to 20% of such patients suffer stroke or die of vasospasm despite maximal therapy. Monitoring for vasospasm with transcranial Doppler technology, in addition to clinical observation in the ICU, has been controversial. The literature is inconclusive regarding its sensitivity and specificity.

The goal for the management of cerebral vasospasm is to reduce the threat of ischemic neuronal damage by controlling ICP, decreasing the metabolic rate of oxygen use, and improving CBF. Cerebral autoregulation is disturbed in patients after SAH, with cerebral perfusion being directly dependent on cerebral perfusion pressure. Vasoactive agents are used to increase the cerebral perfusion pressure. Norepinephrine or phenylephrine may achieve this goal. The SBP should be kept between 160 and 200 mmHg (120–150 mm Hg for unclipped aneurysms) and titrated to the patients' neurologic state. The patient should be closely monitored, and serial transcranial Doppler imaging performed to monitor the progress of the patient's condition. It is important to ensure that patients are adequately hydrated (euvolemic); hypovolemia must be avoided. Angioplasty of the implicated vessel, high-dose IV nicardipine, and intraarterial papaverine should be attempted in patients with refractory vasospasm.

Subdural Hematoma

The collection of fresh blood under the dura mater is referred to as an *acute subdural hematoma*. Data from the traumatic Coma Data Bank indicates the 21% of all severely injured patients have subdural hematomas. Subdural hematoma is usually caused by injury to an artery or vein within or over the brain surface. The clinical presentation includes a wide spectrum of neurologic findings secondary to either mass effect or direct brain injury. On CT scan the lesion is seen as a hyperdense extraaxial collection that is crescent shaped. Patients presenting with acute neurologic deficits and a CT scan demonstrating an acute subdural hematoma should undergo emergent surgery. Surgical intervention may not be required for patients with small lesions less than 3-mm thick on CT scan or those who present neurologically after a significant delay.

Epidural Hematoma

Like subdural hematoma, epidural hematomas are most commonly associated with head trauma, especially in association with skull fractures. They are rarely seen in adults older than the age of 60 years, because after this age the dura adheres tightly to the inner table of the calvarium. The most common locations are temporal and frontal. When identified, the most common source is the middle meningeal artery. The primary therapy for an acute epidural hematoma is surgery, usually urgently. Mannitol, furosemide, and hyperventilation are used when patients deteriorate clinically from an awake state to one of decreased arousal or agitation.

Seizures

Seizures are a common neurologic problem. Seizures may be the patient's primary presenting medical condition or the patient may develop seizures as a complication of an underlying neurologic disease or a complication of a coexisting medical or surgical condition. Seizures may occur in association with drug and substance toxicity or alcohol withdrawal. Epilepsy is defined as a condition of recurrent unprovoked seizures.

International Classification of Seizures

- Generalized seizures (bilaterally symmetrical and without local onset)
  - Tonic, clonic, or tonic-clonic (grand mal)
  - Absence (petit mal)
    - With loss of consciousness only
    - Complex—with brief tonic, clonic, or automatic movements
  - Lennox-Gastaut syndrome
  - Juvenile myoclonic epilepsy

- Infantile spasms (West syndrome)
- Atonic (astatic, akinetic) seizures (sometimes with myoclonic jerks)
- Partial, or focal, seizures (seizures beginning locally)
  - Simple (without loss of consciousness or alteration in psychic function)
    - Motor-frontal lobe origin (tonic, clonic, tonic-clonic; jacksonian; benign childhood epilepsy; epilepsia partialis continua)
    - Somatosensory or special sensory (visual, auditory, olfactory, gustatory, vertiginous)
    - Autonomic
    - Pure psychic
  - Complex (with impaired consciousness)
  - Beginning as simple partial seizures and progressing to impairment of consciousness
  - With impairment of consciousness at onset
- Special epileptic syndromes
  - Myoclonus and myoclonic seizures
  - Reflex epilepsy
  - Acquired aphasia with convulsive disorder
  - Febrile and other seizures of infancy and childhood
  - Hysterical seizures

Seizures from Primary Neurologic Diseases

- Hemorrhagic stroke
- Large cortical infarct
- Intracranial tumor
- Traumatic head injury

Seizures Occurring as a Complication of Acute Illness

- Cerebral hypoxia and ischemia
- Eclampsia
- Posterior reversible encephalopathy syndrome
- Drug and substance abuse and withdrawal
  - Alcohol
  - Barbiturates
  - Benzodiazepines
  - Opioids
  - Cocaine
  - Amphetamines
- Metabolic
  - Hypoglycemia
  - hypocalcemia
  - Hypophosphatemia
  - Hyponatremia
  - Renal failure
- Antibiotics
  - Carbapenems, especially imipenem
  - Penicillins
  - Cephalosporins
  - Aztreonam
  - Fluoroquinolones
  - Metronidazole
- Drug related
  - Tricyclic antidepressants
  - Chlorpromazine
  - Tacrolimus
  - Cyclosporine
  - Theophylline

Management

Many seizures manifest as single, self-limited episodes. The first step is to terminate the ictal activity followed by an evaluation as to the cause of the seizure. In patients with known epilepsy, noncompliance with mediation and/or the use of alcohol and recreational drugs are common precipitating causes. Neuroimaging (CT scan) is always required in patients with new onset seizures and those who develop seizures in hospital to exclude a structural lesion even in the context of an identifiable metabolic or drug etiology. This is particularly important in patients with alcohol withdrawal seizure who may have an underlying subdural hematoma. An urgent electroencephalogram (EEG) is required in patients who do not fully regain conscious (see status epilepticus) and in those patients whose level of consciousness is difficult to assess (due to sedation, underlying disease, etc.).

Seizure Therapy

- Acute termination of ictal activity
  - Lorazepam 0.05 to 0.1 mg/kg or midazolam 0.05 to 0.2 mg/kg
- Treatment of underlying cause
  - Meningitis
  - Encephalitis
  - SAH
  - Drug induced: stop drug, consider hemodialysis if recurrent (theophylline)
  - Lorazepam for drug withdrawal
  - Alcohol withdrawal: lorazepam
  - INH: IV pyridoxine
  - Serotonin inhibitors (see serotonin syndrome)
  - Cocaine: benzodiazepine
- Prophylaxis if risk persists (consult neurology for input)
  - Phenytoin
  - Levetiracetam
  - Gabapentin
  - Lamotrigine
  - Topiramate

Levetiracetam (Keppra) has distinct advantages over the other IV and oral anticonvulsants in the acutely ill patient as it has few drug interactions and is usually well tolerated.

Status Epilepticus

- Status epilepticus is usually defined as continuous seizure activity lasting 30 minutes or as 2 or more discrete seizures between which consciousness is not fully regained. Lowenstein, D. H., Bleck, T. and Macdonald, R. L. (1999), It's Time to Revise the Definition of Status Epilepticus. Epilepsia, 40:120-122, have proposed that status epilepticus be defined as a continuous, generalized, convulsive seizure lasting longer than 5 minutes or 2 or more seizures during which the patient does not return to baseline consciousness
- Because only a small fraction of seizures go on to become status epilepticus, the probability that a given seizure will proceed to status is small at the start of the seizure and increases as the seizure duration increases. If a seizure lasts longer than 5 minutes, clinical experience suggests that the likelihood of spontaneous termination decreases.
- Status epilepticus is a major medical emergency associated with significant morbidity and a mortality of up to 76% in elderly patients with refractory status epileptics. This clinical entity requires prompt management. The complications of status epilepticus include:
  - Cardiac dysrhythmias
  - Derangements of metabolic and autonomic function
  - Neurogenic pulmonary edema
  - Hyperthermia
  - Rhabdomyolysis
  - Pulmonary aspiration
  - Permanent neurologic damage

- Refractory status epilepticus is usually defined as seizures lasting longer than 2 hours, or seizures recurring at a rate of two or more episodes per hour without recovery to baseline between seizures, despite treatment with conventional antiepileptic drugs. However, from a clinical perspective it is preferable to consider refractory status epilepticus as any patient who has failed first-line therapy.

- Status epilepticus may be classified by the presence of motor convulsions (convulsive status epilepticus) or their absence (nonconvulsive status epilepticus). They may be further divided into status epilepticus that affects the whole brain (generalized status epilepticus) or only part of the brain (partial status epilepticus). Status epilepticus appears to be more frequent among males, African Americans, and the aged.

Etiology of Status Epilepticus

In many patients with a preexistent seizure disorder, no obvious precipitating factor can be determined. A decrease in serum levels of antiepileptic drugs because of poor compliance with medications or to because of increased clearance associated with concurrent illness has been implicated in some patients. Adult patients with a new diagnosis of epilepsy may first present in status epilepticus.

Common Causes of Status Epilepticus

- Antiepileptic drug noncompliance
- Alcohol
- Cerebrovascular accidents
- Drug toxicity
  - Cephalosporins
  - Carbapenems
  - Penicillins
  - Ciprofloxacin
  - Tacrolimus
  - Cyclosporine
  - Theophylline
  - Cocaine
- Central nervous system infections
  - Meningitis
  - Encephalitis
- Central nervous system tumors (primary or secondary)
- Metabolic disturbances (ie, electrolyte abnormalities, uremia)
- Head trauma
- Cerebral anoxia and hypoxia
- Hypoglycemia or hyperglycemia

Management Principles of Status Epilepticus

- Status epilepticus is a medical emergency that requires rapid and aggressive treatment to prevent neurologic damage and systemic complications. The longer status epilepticus remains untreated, the greater the neurologic damage. In addition, the longer an episode of status epilepticus continues, the more refractory to treatment it becomes and the greater is the likelihood of chronic epilepsy.

- The management of status epilepticus involves the rapid termination of seizure activity, airway protection, measures to prevent aspiration, management of potential precipitating causes, treatment of complications, prevention of recurrent seizures and the treatment of any underlying conditions.

- Despite the periods of apnea and cyanosis that occur during the tonic or clonic phases of their seizure, most patients in status epilepticus breathe sufficiently as long as the airway remains clear. An oral airway may be required once the seizure has terminated to prevent airway obstruction.

- Once the seizures are controlled and if the patient is oxygenating and ventilating adequately, endotracheal intubation may not be required for "airway protection" even if the patient remains comatose. However, in this situation, precautions should be taken to avoid aspiration and a NG tube should be placed to ensure that the stomach is empty.

- Endotracheal intubation will be required in patients who continue to seizure despite first-line therapy (see below).
- Hypoglycemia must be excluded rapidly and corrective measures instituted if serum levels of glucose are low. If prompt measurement of blood glucose levels is not possible, the patient should receive 100 mg of IV thiamine followed by a 50-mL bolus of 50% dextrose.
- Blood pressure, electrocardiogram, and temperature should be monitored. If the patient develops significant hyperthermia (>40°C [104°F]), then passive cooling is required.
- Blood specimens should be obtained for the determination of serum chemistries.
- Continuous motor seizures may lead to muscle breakdown with the release of myoglobin into the circulation. Maintenance of adequate hydration is necessary to prevent myoglobin-induced renal failure. Forced saline diuresis should be considered in presence of myoglobinuria or significantly elevated serum creatine kinase levels (>5,000 U/l).
- Brain imaging with CT and/or MRI, as well as a LP, will be required in patients presenting with a previously undiagnosed seizure disorder once the seizure activity has been controlled. It is important to emphasize that the first priority is to control the seizures. Imaging studies should only be performed once the seizure activity has been controlled. Endotracheal intubation and neuromuscular paralysis for the sole purpose of imaging the patient may increase morbidity and is strongly discouraged.
- Continuous EEG monitoring is required in patients who do not recover consciousness once the convulsive seizure has aborted
- Once status epilepticus is controlled, attention turns to preventing its recurrence. The best regimen for an individual patient will depend on the cause of the patient's seizure and any previous history of antiepileptic drug therapy. A patient who develops status epilepticus in the course of ethanol withdrawal may not need antiepileptic drug therapy once the withdrawal has run its course. In contrast, patients with new, ongoing epileptogenic stimuli (eg, encephalitis) may require high dosages of antiepileptic drugs to control their seizures.

Pharmacotherapy for Status Epilepticus

- The goal of pharmacologic therapy is to achieve rapid and safe termination of the seizure and prevention of its recurrence without adverse effects on the cardiovascular and respiratory systems or altering the level of consciousness. Diazepam, lorazepam, midazolam, phenytoin, fosphenytoin, and phenobarbital have all been used as first-line therapy for the termination of status epilepticus.
- The results of the Veterans Administration Cooperative Trial in 1998 demonstrated that lorazepam 0.1 mg/kg was the best first-line therapy for status epilepticus.
- Many authorities recommend phenytoin 20 mg/kg (or fosphenytoin) following the administration of lorazepam. Although there is no data that demonstrates that phenytoin increases the response rate following the use of lorazepam, this agent may prevent recurrent seizures and is recommended in patients without a rapidly reversible process (eg, the effect of subtherapeutic antiepileptic-drug concentrations).

Management of Refractory Status Epilepticus

- A variety of agents have been recommended for the treatment of refractory status epilepticus including, midazolam, propofol, high-dose thiopentone or pentobarbital, IV levetiracetam, IV valproate, topiramate, tiagabine, ketamine, isoflurane, and IV lidocaine.
- Currently a continuous IV infusion of midazolam or propofol together with continuous EEG monitoring is the preferred mode of treatment.
  - Midazolam is given as a loading dose of 0.2 mg/kg, followed by an infusion of 0.1 to 2.0 mg/kg/h titrated to produce seizure suppression by continuous EEG monitoring.
  - Propofol is given as a loading dose of 3 to 5 mg/kg, followed by an infusion of 30 to 100 µg/kg/min titrated to EEG seizure suppression. After 12 hours of seizure suppression, the dose is gradually titrated by 50% over the next 12 hours, and then titrated to off over the subsequent 12 hours.
- Recently IV valproic acid and IV levetiracetam (Keppra) have become available and may have particular usefulness in status epilepticus both as second-line agents and as "add-ons" to another second-line agent (midazolam or propofol).

Acute Bacterial Meningitis

- Bacterial meningitis is an acute purulent infection within the subarachnoid space. It is associated with a CNS inflammatory reaction that may result in decreased consciousness, seizures, increased ICP, and stroke. The meninges, the subarachnoid space, and the brain parenchyma are all frequently involved in the inflammatory reaction (meningoencephalitis).
- The organisms most often responsible for community-acquired bacterial meningitis are
  - *Streptococcus pneumoniae*, 50%
  - *Neisseria meningitidis*, 25%
  - Group B streptococci, 15%
  - *Listeria monocytogenes*, 10%
  - *Haemophilus influenzae* type b, less than 10%
- The classic clinical triad of meningitis is fever, headache, and nuchal rigidity. A decreased level of consciousness occurs in more than 75% of patients and can vary from lethargy to coma.
- Fever and either headache, stiff neck, or an altered level of consciousness will be present in nearly every patient with bacterial meningitis. Nausea, vomiting, and photophobia are also common complaints.
- Seizures occur as part of the initial presentation of bacterial meningitis or during the course of the illness in 20% to 40% of patients.
  - The presence of petechial or purpuric skin lesions can provide an important clue to the diagnosis of meningococcal infection. In some patients the disease is fulminant, progressing to death within hours of symptom onset.
  - Otitis, mastoiditis, and sinusitis are predisposing and associated conditions for meningitis because of *Streptococcus* sp., gram-negative anaerobes, *Staphylococcus aureus*, *Haemophilus* sp., and Enterobacteriaceae.
  - *L. monocytogenes* is an increasingly important cause of meningitis in pregnant women, individuals older than 60 years, and immunocompromised individuals of all ages. Infection is acquired by ingesting foods contaminated by *Listeria*.
  - *S. aureus* and coagulase-negative staphylococci are important causes of meningitis that occurs following invasive neurosurgical procedures.
- When bacterial meningitis is suspected, blood cultures should be immediately obtained and empirical antimicrobial and adjunctive dexamethasone therapy initiated without delay.
- The diagnosis of bacterial meningitis is made by examination of the CSF (see the section "Lumbar Puncture" and Table 10-5).
- The need to obtain neuroimaging studies (CT or MRI) prior to LP requires clinical judgment. In an immunocompetent patient with no known history of recent head trauma, a normal level of consciousness, and no evidence of papilledema or focal neurologic deficits, it is considered safe to perform LP without prior neuroimaging studies.
- If LP is delayed to obtain neuroimaging studies, empirical antibiotic therapy should be initiated after blood cultures are obtained.
- Bacterial meningitis is a medical emergency. The goal is to begin antibiotic therapy within 60 minutes of a patient's arrival in the emergency room. Empirical antimicrobial therapy is initiated in patients with suspected bacterial meningitis before the results of CSF Gram stain and culture are known (Table 10-6).
- The role of adjunctive treatment with dexamethasone in adults is controversial. A prospective European trial of adjunctive therapy for acute bacterial meningitis in 301 adults found that dexamethasone reduced the number of unfavorable outcomes (15% vs 25%; $P = 0.03$) including death (7% vs 15%, $P = 0.04$). The benefits were most striking in patients with pneumococcal meningitis. Dexamethasone (10 mg IV) was administered 15 to 20 minutes before the first dose of an antimicrobial agent, and the same dose was repeated every 6 hours for 4 days.

Acute Viral Meningitis

- Immunocompetent adult patients with viral meningitis usually present with headache, fever, and signs of meningeal irritation coupled with an inflammatory CSF profile (see Table 10-5).

TABLE 10-6. EMPIRIC THERAPY OF BACTERIAL MENINGITIS

Age 3 mo–18 y	Third-generation cephalosporin plus vancomycin
Age 18–50 y	Third-generation cephalosporin plus vancomycin
Age >50 y	Third-generation cephalosporin plus vancomycin plus ampicillin
Immunocompromised state	Vancomycin plus ampicillin and ceftazidime
Basilar skull fracture	Third-generation cephalosporin plus vancomycin
Head trauma, neurosurgery	Vancomycin plus ceftazidime
CSF shunt	Vancomycin plus ceftazidime

- Patients often have mild lethargy or drowsiness; however, profound alterations in consciousness, such as stupor, coma, or marked confusion do not occur in viral meningitis and suggest the presence of encephalitis or other alternative diagnoses. Similarly, seizures or focal neurologic signs or symptoms or neuroimaging abnormalities indicative of brain parenchymal involvement are not typical of viral meningitis and suggest the presence of encephalitis or another CNS infectious or inflammatory process.
- The most important causes are enteroviruses (including echoviruses and coxsackieviruses in addition to numbered enteroviruses), HSV-2, human immunodeficiency virus (HIV), and arboviruses.
- CSF cultures are positive in 30% to 70% of patients, the frequency of isolation depending on the specific viral agent. Approximately two-thirds of culture-negative cases of "aseptic" meningitis have a specific viral etiology identified by CSF PCR testing.
- Treatment of almost all cases of viral meningitis is primarily symptomatic and includes use of analgesics, antipyretics, and antiemetics. Fluid and electrolyte status should be monitored. Patients with suspected bacterial meningitis should receive appropriate empirical therapy pending culture results Tables 10-7 and 10-8).

Viral Encephalitis

- In contrast to viral meningitis, where the infectious process and associated inflammatory response are limited largely to the meninges, in encephalitis, the brain parenchyma is also involved. Many patients with encephalitis also have evidence of associated meningitis (meningoencephalitis) and, in some cases, involvement of the spinal cord or nerve roots (encephalomyelitis, encephalomyeloradiculitis).
- In addition to the acute febrile illness with evidence of meningeal involvement characteristic of meningitis, the patient with encephalitis commonly has an altered level of consciousness (confusion, behavioral abnormalities), or a depressed level of consciousness ranging from mild lethargy to coma, and evidence of either focal or diffuse neurologic signs and symptoms.
- Focal or generalized seizures occur in many patients with encephalitis.
- Virtually every possible type of focal neurologic disturbance has been reported in viral encephalitis.
- Despite comprehensive diagnostic efforts, the majority of cases of acute encephalitis of suspected viral etiology remain of unknown cause.
- Hundreds of viruses are capable of causing encephalitis, although only a limited subset is responsible for most cases in which a specific cause is identified.
- The most commonly identified viruses causing sporadic cases of acute encephalitis in immunocompetent adults are herpesviruses (HSV, varicella-zoster virus, Epstein-Barr virus).
- Epidemics of encephalitis are caused by arboviruses, which belong to several different viral taxonomic groups including Alphaviruses (eg, eastern equine encephalitis virus, western equine encephalitis virus), Flaviviruses (eg, West Nile virus, St. Louis encephalitis

**TABLE 10-7. SPECIFIC ANTIMICROBIAL THERAPY FOR ACUTE
MENINGITIS**

Microorganism		Standard Therapy	Alternative Therapy
Haemophilus influenzae	β-lactamase negative	Ampicillin	Third-generation cephalosporin
	β-lactamase positive	Third-generation cephalosporin	cefepime
Neisseria meningitidis		Penicillin G or third-generation cephalosporin	
Streptococcus pneumoniae	Penicillin MIC <0.1 ug/mL	Penicillin G or ampicillin	Third-generation cephalosporin
	Penicillin MIC 0.1–1 ug/mL	Third-generation cephalosporin	Vancomycin, meropenem
	Penicillin MIC ≥2.0 ug/mL	Vancomycin plus third-generation cephalosporin	Meropenem
Enterobacteriaceae		Third-generation cephalosporin	Meropenem, fluoroquinolone, cefepime
Pseudomonas aeruginosa		Ceftazidime or cefepime	Meropenem, fluoroquinolone, piperacillin
Listeria monocytogenes		Ampicillin	
Streptococcus agalactiae		Ampicillin	Third-generation cephalosporin, vancomycin
Staphylococcus aureus	Methicillin-sensitive	Nafcillin or oxacillin plus third-generation cephalosporin	Vancomycin
	Methicillin-resistant	Vancomycin plus third-generation cephalosporin	Linezolid, tigecycline
Staphylococcus epidermidis		Vancomycin	Linezolid, tigecycline

MIC, minimum inhibitory concentration.

virus, Japanese encephalitis virus, Powassan virus), and Bunyaviruses (eg, California encephalitis virus serogroup, LaCrosse virus).

- CSF examination should be performed in all patients with suspected viral encephalitis unless contraindicated by the presence of severely increased ICP (see Table 10-5). The characteristic CSF profile is indistinguishable from that of viral meningitis and typically consists of a lymphocytic pleocytosis, a mildly elevated protein concentration, and a normal glucose concentration. A CSF pleocytosis (>5 cells/L) occurs in more than 95% of immunocompetent patients with documented viral encephalitis.
- Approximately 20% of patients with encephalitis will have a significant number of RBCs (>500/L) in the CSF in a nontraumatic tap. The pathologic correlate of this finding may be a hemorrhagic encephalitis of the type seen with HSV.

TABLE 10-8. VIRUSES CAUSING ACUTE MENINGITIS AND ENCEPHALITIS IN NORTH AMERICA

	Common	Less Common
Acute Meningitis	Enterovirus (coxsackie, echovirus and human enteroviruses 68–71)	VZV
	HSV-2	EBV
	Arbovirus HIV	Lymphocytic choriomeningitis virus
Acute Encephalitis	HSV-1	Rabies
	VZV	EEEV
	EBV	Western equine encephalitis virus
	Arbovirus	Powassan virus
	LaCrosse virus	Enteroviruses
	West Nile Virus	Colorado tick fever
	St. Louis encephalitis virus	Mumps

EBV, Epstein-Barr virus; EEEV, eastern equine encephalitis virus; HIV, human immunodeficiency virus; HSV, herpes simplex virus; VZV, varicella-zoster virus.

- CSF PCR has become the primary diagnostic test for CNS infections caused by HSV, cytomegalovirus, Epstein-Barr virus, human herpesvirus type 6, and enteroviruses.
- Patients with suspected encephalitis almost invariably undergo neuroimaging studies and often EEG. These tests help identify or exclude alternative diagnoses and assist in the differentiation between a focal, as opposed to a diffuse, encephalitic process. Focal findings in a patient with encephalitis should always raise the possibility of HSV encephalitis.
- Specific antiviral therapy should be initiated when appropriate. Acyclovir is of benefit in the treatment of HSV and should be started empirically in patients with suspected viral encephalitis, especially if focal features are present, while awaiting viral diagnostic studies. Adults should receive a dose of 10 mg/kg of acyclovir intravenously every 8 hours for 14 to 21 days.

Guillain-Barré Syndrome

- Guillain-Barré syndrome (GBS) is an acute, frequently severe, and fulminant polyradiculoneuropathy that is autoimmune in nature.
- Approximately 70% of cases of GBS occur 1 to 3 weeks after an acute infectious process, usually respiratory or gastrointestinal.
- GBS manifests as a rapidly evolving areflexic motor paralysis with or without sensory disturbance. The usual pattern is an ascending paralysis that may be first noticed as rubbery legs. Weakness typically evolves over hours to a few days and is frequently accompanied by tingling dysesthesias in the extremities. The legs are usually more affected than the arms, and facial diparesis is present in 50% of affected individuals.
- The lower cranial nerves are also frequently involved, causing bulbar weakness with difficulty handling secretions and maintaining an airway; the diagnosis in these patients may initially be mistaken for brainstem ischemia.
- Pain in the neck, shoulder, back, or diffusely over the spine is also common in the early stages of GBS, occurring in 50% of patients. Most patients require hospitalization, and in different series up to 30% require ventilatory assistance at some time during the illness.
- The need for mechanical ventilation is associated with more severe weakness on admission, a rapid tempo of progression, and the presence of facial and/or bulbar weakness during the first week of symptoms.

- Once clinical worsening stops and the patient reaches a plateau (almost always within 4 weeks of onset), further progression is unlikely.

- Autonomic involvement is common and may occur even in patients whose GBS is otherwise mild. The usual manifestations are loss of vasomotor control with wide fluctuation in BP, postural hypotension, and cardiac dysrhythmias.

- CSF findings are distinctive, consisting of an elevated CSF protein level (100–1000 mg/dL) without accompanying pleocytosis. The CSF is often normal when symptoms have been present for 48 hours; by the end of the first week, the level of protein is usually elevated. Similarly electrodiagnostic tests may be normal initially but progress to that typical of a demyelinating pattern.

- In the vast majority of patients with GBS, treatment should be initiated as soon after diagnosis as possible. Either high-dose IV immune globulin (IVIg) or plasmapheresis can be initiated, as they are equally effective for typical GBS. A combination of the 2 therapies is not significantly better than either alone. IVIg is often the initial therapy chosen because of its ease of administration and good safety record.

- Glucocorticoids have not been found to be effective in GBS.

- Patients require close monitoring of respiratory reserve; clinically and by measurement of forced vital capacity and negative inspiratory force. The following parameters warn of impending respiratory arrest and are an indication for intubation:
  - Forced vital capacity less than 20 mL/kg
  - Maximum inspiratory pressure less than 30 cm/H_2O
  - Maximum expiratory pressure less than 40 cm/H_2O

- The following factors were identified as predictors of respiratory failure:
  - Time of onset to admission less than 7 days
  - Inability to cough
  - Inability to stand
  - Inability to lift the elbows
  - Inability to lift the head
  - Liver enzyme increases

Delirium

- Delirium is defined in the American Psychiatric Association's *Diagnostic and Statistical Manual of Mental Disorders, 4th edition* (*DSM-IV*) as a disturbance of *consciousness and cognition* that develops over a short period of time (hours to days) and *fluctuates* over time.

- Delirium is a common problem in hospitalized patients, particularly the elderly. Delirium is particularly common in ICU patients and following major surgery.

- Delirium is an independent predictor of the length of hospital stay as well as hospital and 6-month mortality rates. In addition, delirium may be a predictor of long-term cognitive impairment.

- Delirium can be categorized into subtypes according to psychomotor behavior, and the high prevalence of hypoactive delirium probably contributes to clinician's lack of recognition of delirium. Hypoactive delirium is characterized by decreased responsiveness, withdrawal and apathy, whereas hyperactive delirium is characterized by agitation, restlessness, and emotional lability.

- Sleep deprivation, sepsis, hypoxemia, use of physical restraints, fluid and electrolyte imbalances, and metabolic and endocrine derangements have been implicated in the causation of delirium. The use of meperidine and benzodiazepines has been independently associated with the development of delirium in ICU and postoperative patients.

- Postoperative delirium is associated with a poor long-term functional outcome. Some patients may progress into a long-term confusional state.

Management of Delirium

Although no placebo-controlled clinical trials have been conducted to evaluate its efficacy, haloperidol is recommended as the drug of choice for the treatment of delirium by the American Psychiatric Association. Haloperidol blocks D_2-dopamine receptors, resulting in amelioration of hallucinations, delusions, and unstructured thought patterns. Patients are typically treated with 2 mg IV followed by repeated doses (doubling the previous dose) every 15 to 20 minutes while agitation persists. Once agitation subsides, scheduled doses (every 4–6 hours) may be continued for a few days, followed by tapered doses for several days. The most important side effects of haloperidol are dystonia, extrapyramidal effects, laryngeal spasm, and QTc prolongation. A baseline and daily 12-lead electrocardiogram is recommended to follow the QTc interval; magnesium deficiency should be aggressively treated, and other drugs that prolong the QTc interval used with caution.

Olanzapine, quetiapine, and dexmedetomidine have also been successfully used to manage delirium.

Neuroleptic Malignant Syndrome

- Neuroleptic malignant syndrome (NMS) is a life-threatening neurologic emergency associated with the use of neuroleptic agents and characterized by a distinctive clinical syndrome of mental status change, rigidity, fever, and dysautonomia.
- Muscular rigidity is generalized and is often extreme.
- Temperatures higher than 38°C (100.4°F) are typical, but even higher temperatures, greater than 40°C (104°F), are common.
- Autonomic instability typically takes the form of tachycardia, labile or high BP and tachypnea.
- NMS is most often seen with the "typical" high-potency neuroleptic agents (eg, haloperidol, fluphenazine). However, every class of neuroleptic drug has been implicated, including the low-potency (eg, chlorpromazine) and the newer "atypical" antipsychotic drugs (eg, clozapine, risperidone, olanzapine), as well as antiemetic drugs (eg, metoclopramide, promethazine).
- Antiparkinson medication withdrawal: NMS is also seen in patients treated for parkinsonism in the setting of withdrawal of L-dopa or dopamine-agonist therapy, as well as with dose reductions and a switch from 1 agent to another.
- Because of the class of agents with which NMS is associated, dopamine receptor blockade is central to most theories of its pathogenesis. Central dopamine receptor blockade in the hypothalamus may cause hyperthermia and other signs of dysautonomia.
- Removal of the causative agent is the single most important treatment in NMS. Other potential contributing psychotropic agents (lithium, anticholinergic therapy, serotonergic agents) should also be stopped if possible. When the precipitant is discontinuation of dopaminergic therapy, it should be reinstituted.
- The need for aggressive and supportive care in NMS is essential and uncontroversial.
- Recommendations for specific medical treatments in NMS are based on case reports and clinical experience, and their use is, therefore, controversial.
  - Dantrolene is a direct-acting skeletal muscle relaxant and is effective in treating malignant hyperthermia. Doses of 0.25 mg/kg to 2 mg/kg are given intravenously every 6 to 12 hours.
  - Bromocriptine, a dopamine agonist, is prescribed to restore lost dopaminergic tone. It is well tolerated in psychotic patients. Doses of 2.5 mg (through NG tube) every 6 to 8 hours are titrated up to a maximum dose of 40 mg/day. It is recommended that this be continued for 10 days after NMS is controlled and then tapered slowly.

Serotonin Syndrome

- Serotonin syndrome is characterized by the triad of neuromuscular hyperactivity, autonomic hyperactivity, and change in mental status. It is not an idiosyncratic drug reaction but is a predictable response to serotonin excess in the CNS.
- Hyperthermia develops in approximately half of cases and results from increased muscle activity because of agitation and tremor. A core temperature as high as 40°C (104°F) is common in moderate to severe cases. Tachycardia, hypertension, mydriasis, hyperactive bowel sounds, myoclonus, and ocular clonus are common; however, not all of these symptoms are present in every patient.
- It can occur from an overdose, drug interaction, or adverse drug effect involving serotonergic agents.
- Most severe cases result from a drug combination especially the combination of selective serotonin reuptake inhibitors (SSRIs) and monoamine oxidase inhibitors (MAOIs).
- It occurs in approximately 15% of patients with SSRI overdose.

- Serotonin syndrome may result from a large number of drugs and drug combinations including:
  - SSRIs
  - MAOIs
  - Phenelzine, moclobemide, tranylcypromine, clorgyline, isocarboxazid
  - Linezolid (an MAOI)
  - Meperidine, fentanyl, tramadol
  - Ondansetron, granisetron, metoclopramide

Treatment

- Most important step is the removal of the offending drug.
- Mild cases (eg, tremors and hyperreflexia) are managed with supportive care and treatment with benzodiazepines. Control of agitation with benzodiazepine is an essential step in the management.
- 5-HT$_{2A}$ antagonists (cyproheptadine and chlorpromazine) have been used in moderate to severe cases. There are however no randomized clinical trials demonstrating the effectiveness of these agents.
  - Cyproheptadine is only available in oral form; the initial dose is 12 mg followed by 2 mg every 2 hours until symptoms improve, and patients may require up to 12 to 32 mg of the drug in a 24-hour period
  - Chlorpromazine is the only 5-HT$_{2A}$ antagonist available in the parenteral form; 50 to 100 mg of intramuscular chlorpromazine may be administered.

CHAPTER 11

Oncology

Shrirang Ajvalia, Shilpa Amara, and Anthony D. Slonim

DATA GATHERING

Patients are generally hospitalized for conditions that require acute care. On occasion, a cancer diagnosis may be made during an index hospitalization. Given that cancer patients often present with vague or nonspecific symptoms, it is important that physicians consider an underlying cancer diagnosis when gathering patient data and performing diagnostic testing. Alternatively, cancer patients may require hospitalization because of complications arising from multimodal therapy, including surgical care, radiation, and chemotherapy. These treatments, while potentially lifesaving, have a profound affect on the body, and often complicate a patient's recovery.

Epidemiology of Cancer

Cancer is a disease that can affect many organs and systems. Epidemiologic data may provide clinicians with an understanding of commonly encountered malignancies, as well as resultant prognoses and mortality rates.

- Incidence and mortality rates (National Cancer Institute—Surveillance Epidemiology and End Results [SEER], http://seer.cancer.gov/statfacts/, accessed July 11, 2012)
  - Prostate cancer:
    - Estimated incidence: 241,740 men in 2012
    - Estimated mortality: 28,170 men in 2012
  - Breast cancer:
    - Estimated incidence: 226,870 women in 2012
    - Estimated mortality: 39,510 women in 2012
  - Lung cancer:
    - Estimated incidence: 226,160 men and women in 2012
    - Estimated mortality: 160,340 men and women in 2012
  - Colorectal cancer:
    - Estimated incidence: 143,460 men and women in 2012
    - Estimated mortality: 51,690 men and women in 2012

History

The history is an important component of gathering data from the patient and family. Although no single symptom or complaint may lead directly to a cancer diagnosis, a thorough patient history, in combination with specific diagnostic testing, helps the physician formulate a differential diagnosis that may include cancer.

- Chief complaints
  - Specific patient complaints that may trigger an investigation for an oncologic diagnosis (Table 11-1)
- Past medical history—components of the medical history that may predispose patients to various cancer types
  - Radiation exposure
    - Leukemia is the most common radiation-induced cancer.
    - Other strongly linked cancers include lung cancer, skin cancer, thyroid cancer, multiple myeloma, breast cancer, stomach cancer.
    - Breast cancer risk increased with less than 0.5 Gy.
    - Risk of head and neck tumors increased with less than 1 Gy.
    - Ultraviolet radiation from sun is linked to carcinoma and melanoma.
  - Precancerous syndromes place patients at higher risk for certain malignancies:
    - Neurofibromatosis and other phacomatoses can lead to nervous system cancer.

TABLE 11-1. A LISTING OF SPECIFIC COMPLAINTS AND ASSOCIATED POTENTIAL MALIGNANCIES

Complaint	Potential Malignancy
Back pain	Adrenal cancer
Anal bleeding	Anal cancer
Difficulty urinating	Bladder cancer
Joint pain	Bone cancer/myeloma
Severe headaches	Brain tumors
Breast lumps/swelling	Breast cancer
Abnormal vaginal bleeding	Cervical/endometrial cancer
Constipation	Colorectal cancer
Difficulty swallowing	Esophageal cancer
Jaundice	Gallbladder/liver cancer
Abdominal pain	Gastrointestinal cancer
Hematuria	Kidney cancer
Easy bleeding/bruising	Leukemia/myelodysplastic syndrome
Difficulty breathing	Lung cancer
Chest pain	Lymphoma
Frequent urination	Ovarian cancer
Erectile dysfunction	Prostate cancer
Abnormal lumps/growths	Sarcoma
Redness/rough skin/growths	Skin cancer
Testicular pain/swelling	Testicular cancer
Hemoptysis	Throat/lung cancer
Difficulty swallowing/lumps in neck	Thyroid cancer
Bleeding in mouth	Tongue cancer

- Xeroderma pigmentosum can lead to skin cancer.
- Ataxia-telangiectasia can lead to lymphoma.
- Bloom syndrome can lead to leukemia.
- Fanconi anemia can lead to leukemia.
- Certain infectious agents may predispose patients to cancer
  - Hepatitis B virus can predispose to hepatocellular carcinoma.
  - Human papilloma virus can predispose to cervical or oral cancer.
  - Herpes simplex virus can predispose to cervical cancer.
  - Epstein-Barr virus can predispose to lymphoma or nasopharyngeal cancer.
  - *Schistosoma haematobium* can predispose to bladder cancer.
  - *Helicobacter pylori* can predispose to gastric cancer.
- Signs and symptoms: When attempting to identify a specific type of cancer, the clinician may ask the patient about signs and symptoms that, when taken together, may be indicative of a specific malignancy (Table 11-2)

TABLE 11-2. A LIST OF MALIGNANCIES AND ASSOCIATED SIGNS AND SYMPTOMS

Malignancy	Associated Signs and Symptoms
Adrenal cancer	· Muscle weakness/numbness · Abdominal/lower back pain · Insomnia · Weight fluctuations (rapid gain or loss) · Deepening of voice/increased hair growth in women
Anal cancer	· Anal bleeding · Anal growths · Anal pain/itching
Bladder cancer	· Back/pelvic pain · Dysuria · Hematuria
Bone cancer—Chondrosarcoma (in cartilage)	· Headaches · Pain and swelling in cancerous region · Diplopia
Bone cancer—Ewing sarcoma (in tissue surrounding bone)	· Fever · Weight loss · Abnormal joint growth/swelling · Joint pain
Brain tumor—Astrocytoma	· Seizures · Unbearable headaches · Numbness/loss of sensation in arms and legs · Personality changes · Memory problems · Diplopia · Difficulty thinking clearly · Difficulty speaking
Brain tumor—Brain cancer	· Fainting · Loss of total muscle control · Vision disturbances · Stiffening and spasms of arms/legs · Personality changes
Brain tumor—Glioblastoma (fast-growing)	· Memory lapses · Difficulty speaking · Diplopia · Headaches · Seizures
Breast cancer—Common	· Breast lumps · Nipple discharge · Breast pain · Nipple inversion

(continued on next page)

TABLE 11-2. A LIST OF MALIGNANCIES AND ASSOCIATED SIGNS AND SYMPTOMS *(Continued)*

Malignancy	Associated Signs and Symptoms
Breast cancer—Inflammatory	· Red/swollen breast · Pits/dimples in skin · Orangelike skin (peau de orange)
Breast cancer—Lymphedema (post-breast cancer therapy)	· Swelling/fluid buildup in arms and hands · Difficulty moving hands and fingers · Heavy feeling in arms
Cervical cancer	· Abnormal vaginal bleeding (eg, midmenstrual cycle, postcoital, postmenopausal)
Colon and rectal cancer	· Fatigue · Weakness · Shortness of breath · Diarrhea · Constipation · Abdominal pain · Weight loss
Endometrial (uterine) cancer	· Abnormal vaginal bleeding (eg, midmenstrual cycle, postcoital, postmenopausal)
Esophageal cancer	· Dysphagia · Hoarse voice · Fluctuating weight · Chest/throat pain
Gallbladder cancer	· Nausea/vomiting · Abdominal pain · Jaundice · Anorexia · Fluctuating weight
Kidney cancer	· Pink or red urine (because of hematuria) · Growth or lump in lower back · Abnormal weight loss/gain · Pain in abdomen or side of back
Laryngeal cancer	· Difficulty breathing · Ear and sinus pain · Hoarse voice · Dysphagia
Leukemia—Acute lymphoblastic leukemia	· Weakness/fatigue · Vulnerability to sickness · Vulnerability to bleeding
Leukemia—Acute myeloid leukemia	· Weakness/fatigue · Vulnerability to sickness · Vulnerability to bleeding

TABLE 11-2. A LIST OF MALIGNANCIES AND ASSOCIATED SIGNS AND SYMPTOMS *(Continued)*

Malignancy	Associated Signs and Symptoms
Leukemia—Chronic lymphoblastic leukemia	• Weakness/tenderness • Vulnerability to bleeding • Swollen lymph nodes in neck • Fevers • Night sweats • Fluctuating weight
Leukemia—Chronic myeloid leukemia	• Weakness/fatigue • Profuse sweating • Fevers • Vulnerability to bleeding
Liver cancer	• Lump in abdomen • Pain in upper abdominal region • Jaundice • Swelling of arms/legs
Lung cancer	• Coughing • Chest pain • Wheezing • Shortness of breath • Drooped eyelid • Weakness in arms
Lymphoma—Diffuse large B-cell	• Profuse night sweating • Fever • Weight loss
Lymphoma—Follicular	• Cough • Weakness/fatigue • Difficulty breathing • Chest pain • Intestinal obstruction
Lymphoma—Hodgkin disease	• Cough • Difficulty breathing • Chest pain
Multiple myeloma	• Nausea/vomiting • Vulnerability to sickness • Fluctuating weight • Bone pain/weakness • Blurry vision
Myelodysplastic syndrome	• Often asymptomatic • Dizziness • Difficulty with recall • Vulnerability to bleeding • Difficulty breathing

MEDICAL SPECIALTIES

(continued on next page)

TABLE 11-2. A LIST OF MALIGNANCIES AND ASSOCIATED SIGNS AND SYMPTOMS *(Continued)*

Malignancy	Associated Signs and Symptoms
Ovarian cancer	Stomach swelling/bloating "Full" feeling/bloating Frequent urination
Pancreatic cancer	Jaundice Diarrhea Stomach pain Weight loss
Prostate cancer	Urinary frequency Erectile dysfunction Blood in urine/semen Leg swelling
Sarcoma	Gradually forming lump from soft tissues
Skin cancer—Actinic keratosis	Swollen/red skin Crusty/scaly skin Skin that sticks up like a fingernail
Skin cancer—Melanoma	ABCD criteria of mole: asymmetry, border irregularity, color variegation, diameter >6 mm (http://www.ncbi. nlm.nih.gov/pubmed/15585738, accessed July 5, 2012)
Stomach cancer	Abdominal pain Dysphagia Nausea/vomiting Shortness of breath (caused by anemia) Weight loss
Testicular cancer	Lump on testicles Testicular pain Heavy feeling near pelvis, anus, or scrotum
Throat cancer	Mouth bleeding Hoarse voice Difficulty swallowing Otalgia Hemoptysis Lump in neck region
Thyroid cancer	Nodule on thyroid gland Difficulty breathing Difficulty speaking Dysphagia Hemoptysis
Tongue cancer	Bleeding from tongue Abnormal lump on tongue Mouth or tongue pain

- Past surgical history—Surgery is a primary treatment modality for malignancies; a surgical history can help to identify potential areas for recurrence
  - Past surgeries for breast or colon cancer recurrence increase likelihood of metastasis.
- Family history
  - Lung, colon, and breast cancer have a strong genetic component
  - Skin cancer rarely appears on inherited dark-pigmented skin
  - Familial dysplastic nevi may place patients at risk for melanoma
  - Inherited precancerous syndromes
    - Neurofibromatosis and other phacomatoses places patient at risk for nervous system cancer.
    - Ataxia telangiectasia places patient at risk for lymphoma.
    - Bloom syndrome places patient at risk for leukemia.
    - Fanconi anemia places patient at risk for leukemia.
    - Multiple endocrine neoplasia (MEN) syndromes (http://www.endocrineweb.com/conditions/endocrine-disorders/men-syndromes-multiple-endocrine-neoplasia, accessed July 5 2012):
      - Multiple endocrine neoplasia type 1 (MEN-1) places patient at risk for parathyroid tumors, pancreatic tumors, and pituitary tumors.
      - MEN-2a places patient at risk for medullary thyroid cancers, pheochromocytoma, and parathyroid tumors.
      - MEN-2b places patient at risk for medullary thyroid cancers, pheochromocytoma, and neuromas.
- Social history
  - Diet
    - Increased consumption of fruits and vegetables reduces the risk of oral, esophageal, stomach, and lung cancer because carotenoids and vitamin E reduce cancer risk.
    - Increased consumption of fast food and saturated fats increases the risk of colon and other cancers.
    - High-fat, low-fiber diets are linked to breast cancer.
  - Smoking
    - Increases susceptibility to carcinoma.
    - Associated with 20-fold increase in lung cancer risk
    - Associated with pharyngeal, esophageal, laryngeal, bladder, and pancreatic cancer.
    - Increases risk for intestinal polyps, which may lead to colorectal cancer.
    - Second-hand smoke increases lung cancer risk by 30%.
  - Alcohol
    - Linked to liver, rectal, and breast cancer
    - When combined with tobacco use, 35-fold increased risk for oral cancer
  - Occupational hazards (Table 11-3)
- Gynecologic history
  - Increased estrogen exposure linked to breast and uterine cancer
    - Women who begin menstruating prior to the age of 12 years
    - Women who undergo menopause after the age of 50 years
  - Potential pregnancy-related malignancies
    - Cervical cancer: Pap smear recommended to check for dysplastic lesions, squamous cells, atypical glandular cells.
    - Breast cancer: Biopsy recommended as needed.
    - Melanoma: Review tanning safety with patient.
    - Thyroid and colorectal cancer: Diagnostic testing recommended as needed.
  - Oral contraceptive risks (National Cancer Institute: http://www.cancer.gov/cancertopics/factsheet/Risk/oral-contraceptives, accessed July 5, 2012)
    - Increased risk of breast cancer
    - Decreased risk of ovarian cancer (by 10%–20%)
    - Decreased risk of endometrial cancer
    - Increased risk of cervical cancer

TABLE 11-3. OCCUPATIONAL HAZARDS AND ASSOCIATED
               MALIGNANCIES

Exposure	Cancer Site
4-Amino biphenyl	Bladder
Arsenic	Lung, skin
Benzene	Leukemia
Benzidine	Bladder
β-Naphthylamine	Bladder
Bischloromethylether	Lung
Chromium	Lung
Coal	Lung, skin
Mineral oil	Skin
Mustard gas	Pharynx, lung
Nickel compounds	Lung, nasal sinus
Radon	Lung
Soot, tars, oils	Lung, skin
Strong inorganic acid mist	Lung
Tac containing asbestiform fibers	Lung
Vinyl chloride	Liver
Wood dusts (furniture)	Nasal sinuses

- Medication history: Certain medications (including various chemotherapeutic agents) are associated with cancer development, so physicians should always obtain a thorough medication history when evaluating patients (Table 11-4).

Review of Systems

A comprehensive review of systems can provide a systematic approach for uncovering clues to an underlying cancer diagnosis (Table 11-5).

TABLE 11-4. MEDICAL AGENTS ASSOCIATED WITH SPECIFIC
               MALIGNANCIES

Drug	Associated Malignancy
Chlorambucil	Leukemia
Chlornaphazine	Bladder cancer
Combined chemotherapy for lymphoma using MOPP (mustargen, vincristine, procarbazine, prednisone)	Leukemia
Cyclophosphamide	Leukemia, bladder cancer
Cyclosporine	Lymphoma
Estrogen (steroid)	Liver tumors

TABLE 11-4. MEDICAL AGENTS ASSOCIATED WITH SPECIFIC
MALIGNANCIES *(Continued)*

Drug	Associated Malignancy
Estrogens (conjugated)	Endometrial cancer
Estrogen (synthetic; eg, diethylstilbestrol)	Vagina, cervical cancer
Melphalan	Leukemia
Methoxsalen	Skin cancer
Busulfan	Leukemia
Phenacetin	Renal, pelvis cancer
Tamoxifen	Uterine cancer
Thiotepa	Leukemia
Treosulfan	Leukemia

TABLE 11-5. A REVIEW OF SYMPTOMS AND THEIR POTENTIAL FOR
UNDERLYING MALIGNANCY

Site or System	Symptoms
Cardiovascular	• Shortness of breath • Difficulty breathing • Difficulty laying down (pain/breathing issues) • Chest pain • Tachycardia • Swollen arms or legs
Constitutional	• Weight gain/loss • Fever • Fatigue
Ear, nose, and throat	• Sore throat • Mouth sores • Unbearable headaches • Hemoptysis • Wheezing • Ringing in the ear • Masses
Endocrine and Hematologic	• Easy bleeding/bruising • Night sweats • Intolerance to cold/heat • Frequent fevers
Eyes	• Dryness • Vision changes/diplopia

(continued on next page)

MEDICAL SPECIALTIES

TABLE 11-5. A REVIEW OF SYMPTOMS AND THEIR POTENTIAL FOR UNDERLYING MALIGNANCY *(Continued)*

Site or System	Symptoms
Gastrointestinal	· Diarrhea · Blood in stool · Nausea/vomiting · Constipation · Bleeding in anus · Abdominal pain
Gynecologic	· Abnormal breast lumps · Nipple discharge · Vaginal discharge
Musculoskeletal	· Joint/muscle pain · Muscle weakness · Swollen lymph nodes · Paralysis · Numbness
Neurologic	· Seizures · Dizziness · Frequent headaches · Numbness/weakness
Skin	· Pruritus · Rash · Redness/discoloration · Roughness · Raised skin · Lumps/moles/cysts
Urologic	· Frequent urination · Hematuria · Dysuria

Physical Examination

The physical examination is an important component of establishing a malignant diagnosis. While the physical examination may be completely normal in a patient with cancer, potential cancer-related findings are outlined in Table 11-6. Importantly, these findings are not specific to cancer, and must be considered in conjunction with the entire clinical picture (http://meded.ucsd.edu/clinicalmed/ros.htm, accessed July 5, 2012).

Diagnostic Testing

Although clinical findings are important, diagnostic testing must be conducted to establish a definitive cancer diagnosis. Specific screening and diagnostic guidelines for breast, colorectal, lung, and prostate cancer are outlined below.

Breast Cancer

- Preventive guidelines and screening
  - Clinical breast examination

TABLE 11-6. PHYSICAL EXAMINATION FINDINGS ASSOCIATED WITH SPECIFIC SITES OF MALIGNANCY

Site	Physical Findings
Head and neck	• Inflamed/firm/tender lymph nodes upon palpation (differentiate from infectious disease)
Mouth/throat	• Mouth sores/ulcers (differentiate from viral/fungal causes) • Tracheal deviation
Thyroid	• Thyroid nodules • Thyromegaly
Ears	• Growths or abnormalities in canal • Abnormalities in hearing quality/tone (may be caused by growths or obstructions)
Eyes	• Diplopia/blurred vision • Discharge from eye • Eye pain
Voice	• Cough • Hoarseness • Hemoptysis
Pulmonary	• Wheezing (differentiate from asthma) • Bronchial breath sounds • Chest tenderness • Tachypnea • Dullness from effusions • Stridor—upper airway obstruction
Cardiovascular	• Chest pain • Tachycardia • Muffled heart tones • Cardiomegaly
Gastrointestinal	• Nausea • Vomiting • Dysphagia • Jaundice • Black, tarry stools • Constipation • Abdominal tenderness • Abdominal masses • Hepatomegaly • Splenomegaly • Dullness to percussion • Fluid accumulation
Genitourinary	• Scrotal tenderness • Hematuria • Masses

(continued on next page)

MEDICAL SPECIALTIES

TABLE 11-6. PHYSICAL EXAMINATION FINDINGS ASSOCIATED WITH SPECIFIC SITES OF MALIGNANCY *(Continued)*

Site	Physical Findings
Rectal	• Fissures • Bleeding • Rectal masses • Prostate masses/swelling
Hematologic	• Abnormal bruising/bleeding (easily occurring) • New lumps or growths
Gynecologic	• Vaginal discharge • Breast changes[a]
Neurologic	• Numbness in extremities • Weakness • Dizziness • Growths
Musculoskeletal/ Integumentary	• Joint pain/swelling/redness • Muscle aches • Back pain • Skin changes • Rashes • Bruising

[a]Physical breast examination findings described in next section.

- Every 3 years for women age 20 to 40 years, and yearly for women age 40 years and older (http://www.cancer.org/Healthy/FindCancerEarly/CancerScreeningGuidelines/american-cancer-society-guidelines-for-the-early-detection-of-cancer, accessed July 12, 2012)
- Mammography
  - Only method of breast imaging that consistently has been found to decrease breast cancer-related mortality (http://www.uptodate.com/contents/breast-imaging-mammography-and-ultrasonography?source=see_link, accessed July 5 2012)
  - Yearly screening for women age 40 years and older according to American Cancer Society guidelines (http://www.cancer.org/Healthy/FindCancerEarly/CancerScreeningGuidelines/american-cancer-society-guidelines-for-the-early-detection-of-cancer, accessed July 12, 2012)
- Biennial screening for women aged 50 to 74 years according to U.S. Preventive Services Task Force (USPSTF) guidelines (http://www.uspreventiveservicestaskforce.org/uspstf/uspsbrca.htm#summary, accessed July 5 2012)
  - Sensitivity based on:
    - Lesion size
    - Lesion conspicuity
    - Breast tissue density
    - Age of patient
    - Image quality
    - Hormone status of tumor
  - Sensitivity and specificity are approximately 79% and 90%, respectively (http://webcache.googleusercontent.com/search?q=cache:soODFpbDBOcJ:www.cancer.gov/cancertopics/pdq/screening/breast/healthprofessional/page4+&cd=1&hl=en&ct=clnk&gl=us, accessed July 12, 2012)
    - Both values are lower in younger women with dense breast tissue.[1]
    - High density is associated with 10% to 29% reduction in sensitivity.[2]

- Mammogram abnormalities include masses, calcifications, asymmetry, and architectural distortion (http://www.uptodate.com/contents/breast-imaging-mammography-and-ultrasonography?source=see_link, accessed July 5 2012)
  - Most specific mammographic feature of malignancy is a spiculated soft tissue mass; nearly 90% of these lesions represent invasive cancer.
  - Clustered microcalcifications seen in approximately 60% of cancers detected mammographically.
  - Linear branching microcalcifications have higher predictive value for malignancy than granular calcifications.
- Breast Imaging Reporting and Data System (BIRADS) mammography findings:[3]
  - Category 0: Need additional imaging evaluation and/or prior mammograms for comparison
  - Category 1: Negative
  - Category 2: Benign findings
  - Category 3: Probably benign finding—short-interval follow-up suggested
  - Category 4: Suspicious abnormality—biopsy should be considered
  - Category 5: Highly suggestive of malignancy—appropriate action should be taken
  - Category 6: Known biopsy—proven malignancy and appropriate action should be taken
- Ultrasound
  - Much research including that done by the European Group for Breast Cancer has found little evidence to support the use of ultrasound for screening. Mammography is most efficient.[4]
- Magnetic resonance imaging (MRI)[3]
  - Not for routine use in average-risk women
  - Used as an adjunct to mammography for high-risk women
    - BRCA 1 or 2 mutation
    - First-degree relative with BRCA 1 or 2 mutation and are untested
    - Based on family history, 20% to 25% or greater lifetime risk of breast cancer
    - Received radiation to chest between the ages of 10 and 30 years
    - Carry or have a first-degree relative who carries a genetic mutation in the *TP53* or *PTEN* genes
  - When combined with conventional testing, 86% to 100% sensitivity[5]
  - When combined with conventional testing, 77% to 96% specificity[5]
- Diagnostic
- Diagnostic mammography[3]
- Used to evaluate patients with positive clinical findings
  - Includes additional views (eg, spot compression, magnification) not present in screening mammogram
- Breast ultrasonography[3]
  - Does not detect most microcalcifications
  - Recommended for:
    - Women younger than 30 years of age presenting with dominant mass or asymmetric thickening and nodularity
    - Women 30 years of age and older with a dominant mass and diagnostic mammogram assessed as Breast Imaging Reporting and Data System (BIRADS) categories 1 through 3
    - Adjunct to diagnostic mammography for women 30 years and older with asymmetric thickening and nodularity
    - Adjunct to diagnostic mammography in women with skin changes, nipple discharge
  - Results classified according to BIRADS categories
- Diagnostic Breast MRI[3]
  - Recommended for patients with skin changes consistent with serious breast disease, when biopsy is benign and lesion is classified as BIRADS categories 1 through 3
- Biopsy
  - If diagnostic mammogram and/or ultrasound is suggestive of malignancy
    - Fine-needle aspiration biopsy

- Core needle biopsy
- Excisional biopsy
- A study comparing accuracy of diagnostic tests found the following results:[6]
  - Mammography: 67.8% sensitivity; 75% specificity
  - Ultrasound: 83% sensitivity; 34% specificity
  - MRI: 94.4% sensitivity; 26% specificity
- Colon and Rectal Cancer
  - Preventative guidelines and screening (http://www.uspreventiveservicestaskforce.org/uspstf08/colocancer/colors.htm, accessed July 12, 2012)
    - The USPSTF recommends screening for colorectal cancer using fecal occult blood testing, sigmoidoscopy, or colonoscopy, beginning at age 50 years and continuing until age 75 years.
    - Fecal occult blood test
      - Detects hidden blood in stool samples
      - Should be performed annually
      - Guaiac smear versus immunochemical tests: Guaiac smear reacts to peroxidase activity of heme, but may yield false positives (low specificity) because of other peroxidase activity. Immunochemical tests detect hemoglobin.
      - Guaiac smear sensitivity: 50% to 60% for one-time use; up to 90% when used annually over many years (http://www.worldgastroenterology.org/assets/downloads/en/pdf/guidelines/06_colorectal_cancer_screening.pdf, accessed July 12, 2012)
    - Sigmoidoscopy
      - Flexible sigmoidoscope used to view interior walls of rectum and part of colon
      - Polyp removal and tissue sampling possible
      - Should be performed every 5 years
      - 35% to 70% sensitivity; 98% to 100% specificity (http://www.worldgastroenterology.org/assets/downloads/en/pdf/guidelines/06_colorectal_cancer_screening.pdf, accessed July 12, 2012)
    - Colonoscopy
      - Flexible colonoscope used to view interior walls of rectum and entire colon
      - Allows detection and removal of polyps and biopsy of cancer throughout colon
      - Should be performed every 10 years
      - Over 95% sensitivity and specificity for large polyps (http://www.worldgastroenterology.org/assets/downloads/en/pdf/guidelines/06_colorectal_cancer_screening.pdf, accessed July 12, 2012)
  - Diagnostic
    - Colonoscopy[7]
      - Reference standard technique
      - Can detect cancer, premalignant adenomas, other symptomatic colonic diseases
      - Facilitates biopsy of suspected lesions
      - Highest sensitivity and specificity
    - Flexible sigmoidoscopy followed by barium enema[7]
      - Facilitates biopsy of suspected lesions
      - Combination comparable in sensitivity to colonoscopy
    - CT colonography[7]
      - Cross-sectional images of abdomen and pelvis obtained following insufflation of large bowel
      - Subsequent colonoscopy may be obtained at later date for biopsies
      - Sensitivity approaches that of colonoscopy for detection of larger polyps (>1 cm)
      - Meta-analysis found:[8]
        - 88% sensitivity for polyps larger than 10 mm, 84% for polyps 6 to 9 mm, 65% for polyps 5 mm or smaller
        - 95% specificity for polyps larger than 10 mm

- Biopsy
- Check carcinoembryonic antigen levels
  - Check for elevation
  - Nonsmoker range: less than 2.5 micrograms/L
  - Smoker range: less than 5.0 micrograms/L
- Lung Cancer
  - Preventive guidelines and screening
    - American College of Chest Physicians recommends against serial chest radiographs and sputum cytologic evaluation for lung cancer screening[9]
      - Sensitivity and specificity of chest x-ray are 26% and 93%, respectively (http://www.uspreventiveservicestaskforce.org/3rduspstf/lungcancer/lungcanrs.htm, accessed July 13, 2012)
    - Helical low-dose computed tomography (CT) screening (http://www.medscape.org/viewarticle/753395, accessed July 13, 2012)
      - Data indicates that screening heavy smokers with low-dose CT scans is associated with a 20% reduction in lung cancer-specific mortality
      - Recommended for select, high-risk patients only
        - Those aged 55 to 74 years with at least a 30-pack-year history and smoking cessation for less than 15 years
        - Those aged 50 years or older with a 20 or more pack-year history of smoking and 1 additional risk factor
      - Patients with no lung nodule on baseline low-dose CT scan should have annual low-dose CT screening for 3 years and until age 74 years
      - Patients with a solid or part-solid lung nodule on baseline low-dose CT scan should have low-dose CT screening frequency based on the size of the nodule
      - Nodules that increase in size or become solid during follow-up should be excised
      - Sensitivity 4 times greater than chest x-ray; decreased specificity versus chest x-ray but false-positives (5%–41%) generally resolved with high-resolution CT (http://www.uspreventiveservicestaskforce.org/3rduspstf/lungcancer/lungcanrs.htm, accessed July 13, 2012)
  - Diagnostic[10]
    - Preferred diagnostic technique depends on cancer type, tumor size and location, and patient's clinical status
    - For patients suspected of having small-cell lung cancer, diagnosis should be confirmed by one of the following:
      - Sputum cytology
      - Thoracentesis
      - Fine-needle aspiration
      - Bronchoscopy including transbronchial needle aspiration
      - Endobronchial ultrasound-needle aspiration
      - Esophageal ultrasound
    - For patients suspected of having accessible pleural effusion, thoracentesis recommended (followed by thoracoscopy if fluid cytology is negative)
    - For patients suspected of having solitary extrathoracic metastasis, tissue confirmation with fine-needle aspiration or biopsy recommended
    - For patients with multiple suspected metastases who cannot undergo biopsy of a metastatic site, one of the following is recommended:
      - Sputum cytology
      - Bronchoscopy
      - Transthoracic needle aspiration
    - For patients suspected of having extensive infiltration of mediastinum, one of the following is recommended:
      - Bronchoscopy with transbronchial needle aspiration
      - Endobronchial ultrasound needle aspiration
      - Esophageal ultrasound needle aspiration
      - Transthoracic needle aspiration

- Mediastinoscopy
- Sensitivities and specificities:
  - Sputum cytology: 66% sensitivity (but varies by cancer location); 99% specificity
  - Flexible bronchoscopy: 88% sensitivity for central, endobronchial lesions and 34% to 63% sensitivity for peripheral lesions; endobronchial ultrasound may increase diagnostic yield for peripheral lesions
  - Transthoracic needle aspiration: 90% sensitivity (reduced for lesions <2 cm); 97% specificity
  - Diagnostic accuracy in distinguishing between small-cell and nonsmall-cell lung cancer for various diagnostic modalities: 98%
- Prostate cancer
  - Preventive guidelines and screening
    - USPSTF recommends against routine screening for prostate cancer in men older than 75 years of age and states that the evidence is insufficient to recommend for or against screening for men younger than 75 because screening often results in overdiagnoses and overtreatment of prostatic tumors that will not progress to cause illness or death (http://www.uspreventiveservicestaskforce.org/uspstf/uspsprca.htm, accessed July 13, 2012)
    - American Cancer Society recommends that men make an informed decision with their health care provider regarding screening; (http://www.cancer.org/Cancer/ProstateCancer/MoreInformation/ProstateCancerEarlyDetection/prostate-cancer-early-detection-acs-recommendations, accessed July 13, 2012) discussion should occur:
      - At age 50 years for men at average risk who are expected to live for at least 10 years
      - At age 45 years for men at high risk (eg, African Americans, those with a first-degree relative who was diagnosed with prostate cancer before the age of 65 years)
      - At age 40 years for men at higher risk (eg, those with more than 1 first-degree relative who was diagnosed with prostate cancer before the age of 65 years)
      - Those who opt to be screened should use prostate-specific antigen (PSA) test and/or digital rectal examination (DRE)
    - PSA test
      - Measures blood levels of PSA (protein produced by prostate)
      - PSA less than 2.5 ng/mL: Retest every 2 years
      - PSA more than 2.5 ng/mL: Retest annually
      - Test is not cancer-specific, and may indicate infection, inflammation, or enlargement
      - Traditionally, a value higher than 4 ng/mL is considered abnormal, corresponding to a sensitivity of 67.5% to 80% and specificity of 60% to 70% (http://emedicine.medscape.com/article/457394-overview#aw2aab6b8, accessed July 13, 2012)
      - Sensitivity may be improved by lowering cutoff value
      - Specificity may be improved by using age-adjusted values
    - Digital Rectal Examination (DRE)
      - Finger examination done to detect abnormalities in texture, size, and shape
      - 59% sensitivity; 94% specificity (http://www.uptodate.com/contents/screening-for-prostate-cancer, accessed July 13, 2012)
  - Diagnostic[11]
    - Prostate biopsy
    - Note: May detect clinically insignificant cancers that are unlikely to cause symptoms or affect life expectancy
  - Imaging recommendations are based on treatment intent, which is determined by staging (Table 11-7)
  - Pelvic CT or MRI
    - Recommended for men with high-risk localized or locally advanced prostate cancer who are being considered for radical treatment
  - Isotope bone scans
    - Performed when hormonal therapy is being deferred through watchful waiting in asymptomatic men at high-risk of developing bone complications

TABLE 11-7. CLINICAL STAGING FOR PROSTATE CANCER

	PSA		Gleason Score		Clinical Stage
Low risk	<10 ng/mL	and	<6	and	T1-T2a
Intermediate risk	10–20 ng/mL	or	7	or	T2b-T2c
High risk	>20 ng/mL	or	8–10	or	T3-T4[a]

[a]Clinical stage T3-T4 represents locally advanced disease.

Differential Diagnoses

It is also important that physicians consider other conditions that may be confused with malignancies. Specific symptoms and tests that may be used to obtain a differential diagnosis are described in Table 11-8. (http://www.uptodate.com/index, accessed July 5, 2012)

Staging

Once cancer is diagnosed, staging can help determine prognosis and appropriate treatment (Tables 11-9 and 11-10).

TABLE 11-8. DIFFERENTIAL DIAGNOSES

Condition	Differentiating Signs and Symptoms	Differentiating Tests
Breast Cancer Differential		
Fibrocystic changes	• Unlike breast cancer, fibrocystic changes are typically symmetrical and are related to breast pain	• Ultrasound scan can differentiate cysts from solid lesions
Fibroadenoma	• Worsens during periods of elevated estrogen levels (such as pregnancy) • Decreases in size during menopause • Physical examination shows well-demarcated and mobile mass • Fibroadenoma has a defined oval curvature, while breast carcinomas have no well-defined margins	• Excisional biopsy shows that fibroadenomas are well defined and have a shiny, bulging surface
Colorectal Cancer Differential		
Irritable bowel syndrome (IBS)	• Recurrent abdominal pain or discomfort • Abdominal pain with defecation • Change in frequency of stools • Change in appearance of stools	• There is no specific diagnostic test for IBS • Check for differentiating symptoms • Patients >50 years of age have higher risk of cancer
Crohn disease	• Watery diarrhea • Target age is 20–40 years (younger than the typical cancer patient)	• Colonoscopy will show mucosal inflammation, and discrete deep superficial ulcers appearing like a cobblestone walkway

MEDICAL SPECIALTIES

(continued on next page)

TABLE 11-8. DIFFERENTIAL DIAGNOSES *(Continued)*

Condition	Differentiating Signs and Symptoms	Differentiating Tests
Lung Cancer Differential		
Carcinoid tumor	• Causes cough, dyspnea, wheezing (unilateral), or pneumonia	• CT chest: 80% of carcinoid tumors appear as an endobronchial nodule • Bronchoscopy shows raised, pink, vascular, lobulated lesions
Metastatic cancer	• May include pain, weight loss, malaise, cough, dyspnea, clubbing, or focal wheezing. • Physical examination findings depend on the origin of the primary tumor	• CT chest shows one or multiple nodules of variable sizes from ill-defined to well-defined masses • Sputum cytology reveals malignant cells. • PET-FDG scan shows increased uptake in both primary and distant sites • Renal cell carcinoma has a lower probability of FDG uptake • Bronchoscopy has high yield of endobronchial lesions • Needle aspiration (TTNA) reveals malignant cells in lesions based on size, location, and risks
Prostate Cancer Differential		
Benign prostatic hyperplasia	• BPH prostate has a rubbery feeling with no palpable nodules • Hard nodules are indicative of malignancy	• A positive prostate biopsy is the best test to perform to differentiate between BPH and prostate cancer
Chronic prostatitis	• This illness manifests itself over more than a 3-month period • Symptoms include increased urinary frequency, dysuria, male dyspareunia, and hematospermia	• Microscopic examination of a biopsy may show presence of leukocytes suggestive of inflammation • Serum PSA is usually elevated in chronic prostatitis • Course of antibiotics will resolve chronic prostatitis

BPH, benign prostatic hyperplasia; CT, computed tomography; IBS, irritable bowel syndrome; PET-FDG, positron emission tomography with ^{18}F-labeled fluorodeoxyglucose; PSA, prostate-specific antigen; TTNA, transthoracic needle aspiration.

TABLE 11-9. GENERAL TNM STAGING

T	**Tx**: Tumor cannot be evaluated
	T0: No evidence of a primary tumor
	Tis: Carcinoma in situ (preinvasive cancer)
	T1, T2, T3, T4: Size or extent of primary tumor
N	**Nx**: Lymph nodes cannot be evaluated
	N0: Tumor cells absent from regional lymph nodes
	N1, N2, N3: Involvement of regional lymph nodes (number of lymph nodes and/or extent of spread)
M	**Mx**: Distant metastasis cannot be evaluated
	M0: No distant metastasis
	M1: Metastasis to distant organs (beyond regional lymph nodes)

TABLE 11-10. CANCER SPECIFIC STAGING

Breast Cancer Staging		
Stage	**Survival (%)**	**Characteristics**
I	90	Tumor <2 cm
IIA	80	Tumor >2 cm
IIB	65	Tumor >5 cm
IIIA	50	Internal mammary
IIIC	40	Infraclavicular
IV	15	Distant metastases

Colorectal Cancer Staging			
TNM	**Criteria**	**Treatment**	**Survival (%)**
I	Into submucosa	Surgery	94–97
IIA	Into serosa	Surgery, preoperative XRT	83
IIB	Into peritoneum	Surgery; preoperative XRT	74
IIC	Direct invasion	Surgery; preoperative XRT	56
IIIA	<6 LNs	Surgery + chemotherapy	86
IIIB	Varying degrees of LNs	Surgery + chemotherapy	51–77
IIIC	Varying degrees of LNs	Surgery + chemotherapy	15–47
IV	Distant metastases	Chemotherapy	5

(continued on next page)

MEDICAL SPECIALTIES

TABLE 11-10. CANCER SPECIFIC STAGING *(Continued)*

Breast Cancer Staging			
Stage	**Survival (%)**	**Characteristics**	
Lung Cancer Staging			
Stage	**Definition**	**Treatment**	**Survival (%)**
I	Isolated lesion	Surgery + chemotherapy	>60
II	Hilar node spread	Surgery + radiation + chemotherapy	50
III A	Mediastinal spread but resectable	Surgical resection + chemoradiation	25–30
IIIB	Unresectable	Chemoradiation + biologic + surgery	10–20
IV	Metastatic	Chemotherapy + palliative radiation	1
Prostate Cancer Staging			
Stage	**Tumor**	**Treatment**	
I	T1a	• Active surveillance, radiation • Radical prostatectomy	
II	T1/T2	• Active surveillance, radiation • Radical prostatectomy	
III	T3	Radiation	
IV	T4	• Radiation • Androgen deprivation • Chemotherapy	

LN, lymph node; XRT, x-ray therapy.

SPECIFIC CONDITIONS ASSOCIATED WITH MALIGNANCY

Certain malignancy-related complications require emergency treatment in the intensive care unit. Appropriate acute management can improve short-term outcomes by facilitating definitive treatment of the underlying malignancy or the institution of appropriate palliative measures. Three such malignancy-related complications include febrile neutropenia, spinal cord compression, and tumor lysis syndrome.

Febrile Neutropenia

Febrile neutropenia is defined as:

- **Fever:** Temperature 38.3°C (100°F) or higher or 38°C (100.4°F) if taken 1 h or more apart
- **Neutropenia:** absolute neutrophil count less than 500 cells/mm^3

Presentation

- Chief complaint: fever—potential manifestation of a serious infection in an immunocompromised patient
- Signs and symptoms:
  - Tachycardia
    - Treat immediately; may be sign of sepsis or shock
  - Hypotension:
    - Treat immediately; may be sign of shock and increased risk of mortality

- Pneumonia
  - Cough
  - Shortness of breath
- Gastrointestinal tract infections
  - Abdominal pain
  - Nausea and vomiting
  - Diarrhea
- Urinary tract infection
  - Dysuria
- Mucositis or oral ulcers

Risk Factors

- Patient-related risk factors
  - Female (odds ratios of 2.00 and 1.32) (http://bestpractice.bmj.com/best-practice/monograph/950.html, accessed July 5, 2012)
  - Age older than 65 years
- Past medical history
  - Recent chemotherapy (particularly full-dose chemotherapy)
  - Patients with:
    - Breast cancer
    - Non-Hodgkin lymphoma
    - Hematologic malignancy (fivefold increased risk)
  - Past episodes of neutropenia
  - Absolute neutrophil count nadir less than 500 PMN/μL after first cycle of chemotherapy
  - Concurrent radiotherapy
- Medications
  - Patients who have taken prior antibiotic regimens have an increased risk for fungal infections
- Predisposing factors
  - Skin breakdown
  - Gastrointestinal mucositis
  - Obstructions
  - Immune defects
  - Pretreatment anemia (hemoglobin 12.0 g/L)
  - Low baseline albumin (<35 g/L [3.5 g/dL])
  - Zubrod score Eastern Cooperative Oncology Group (ECOG) ≥1

Classification

- Low risk for serious infection:
  - Age younger than 60 years
  - Temperature lower than 39°C (102.2°F)
  - No tachypnea
  - No dehydration
  - Solid tumor
  - No history of fungal infection
- High risk for serious infection:
  - Profound neutropenia of long duration (>10 days)
  - History of splenectomy
  - Additional perturbations in host defenses
  - Hypogammaglobulinemia
  - Infant acute lymphoblastic leukemia
  - Acute myeloid leukemia induction therapy
  - Concern for sepsis

Diagnosis[14]

- History and physical examination (repeat daily in high-risk patients)

TABLE 11-11. FEBRILE NEUTROPENIA ACTION[12]

Type	Name	Notes
Empiric regimen		Include antipseudomonal activity
PO antibiotics	Cipro + amoxicillin-clavulanate	May be used in low risk
IV antibiotics	Mono: ceftazidime, cefepime, imipenem, or meropenem 2 drug: aminoglycoside + antipseudomonal β-lactam PCN-allergy: levofloxacin + aztreonam or aminoglycoside	Monotherapy or 2-drug regimens may be used[5]
	Vancomycin	Add in select cases (eg, severe mucositis, hypotension, MRSA colonization, indwelling catheter); discontinue when cultures negative over 48 h

IV, intravenous; MRSA, methicillin-resistant *Staphylococcus aureus*; PCN, penicillin; PO, oral.

- Hematologic
  - Complete blood count with differential
    - High white blood cell (WBC) count signifies infection
    - Low WBC count usually after chemotherapy
  - Platelets
  - Coagulation studies (may be considered in high-risk patients only)
- Microbiologic
  - Nose and throat (when symptoms are present)
  - Urine
  - Blood
- Radiologic
  - Chest (for high-risk patients and symptomatic low-risk patients)
  - Sinus (may be considered in high-risk patients only)
  - CT and MRI (when symptoms are present)
- Prevention: levofloxacin (500 mg daily) to reduce risk of bacterial infections and febrile episodes

Action[14]

- Low-risk patients: Broad-spectrum antibiotic therapy with a single parenteral agent (eg, ceftazidime, cefepime, imipenem, meropenem) or possible oral therapy (ciprofloxacin and amoxicillin-clavulanate)
- High-risk patients: Broad-spectrum antibiotic therapy with a single parenteral agent (eg, ceftazidime, cefepime, imipenem, meropenem) or a combination regimen
- Additions and modifications likely in patients with persistent fever or prolonged neutropenia
  - For progressive disease, add vancomycin.
  - For neutropenic fever lasting longer than 5 days, use antifungal therapy.
  - Specific antibiotic regimens are outlined in the Table 11-11.

Spinal Cord Compression[15]

Malignant spinal cord compression occurs in approximately 5% of terminal cancer patients within the last 2 years of life, and most cases are epidural in origin (because of thecal sac impingement by spinal epidural masses or locally advanced cancer). Prompt treatment usually palliates pain and prevents paralysis.

Presentation
- Chief complaint: Local or radicular pain
- Signs and symptoms:
  - Back pain (first symptom in 95% of cases)
  - Sensory abnormalities (40%–90% of afflicted patients)
  - Bowel and bladder dysfunction (50% of afflicted patients)
  - Focal weakness (75% of afflicted patients) progresses to ataxia and paralysis if left untreated

Risk Factors
- Past medical history
  - Patients with:
    - Lung cancer (15%–20% of all cases)
    - Breast cancer (15%–20% of all cases)
    - Prostate cancer (15%–20% of all cases)
    - Multiple myeloma (5%–10% of all cases)
    - Non-Hodgkin lymphoma (5%–10% of all cases)
    - Renal cell carcinoma (5%–10% of all cases)
  - Incontinence
  - Disc herniation
  - Osteoporosis
  - Hyperreflexia
  - Paralysis
- Medications
  - Intravenous (IV) drug use (eg epidural)

Diagnosis
- Physical examination: Evaluate patient for stiffness, hypotension, tachycardia, back and chest pain, abdominal tightness, pain and weakness of extremities
- Radiology:
  - MRI
    - Gold standard (93% sensitivity; 97% specificity)
    - T1- and T2-weighted imaging in axial, sagittal, and coronal planes
    - Gadolinium-enhancement improves identification of leptomeningeal and intramedullary metastases but are unnecessary for evaluation of epidural spinal cord compression
  - CT with myelography (>95% sensitivity and specificity)
  - Bone scintigraphy with plain radiography (98% sensitivity; poor specificity)
  - Noncontrast spinal CT
- Laboratory test results:
  - Complete blood count with differential: raised WBC count
  - Blood or cerebrospinal fluid cultures: raised in epidural abscess
  - Tumor biopsy: to diagnose malignant tissues

Action
- Treatment goals: maintenance of neurologic function, control of local tumor growth, spine stabilization, pain control
- *Do not* wait for neurologic signs and disorders before giving treatment; rapid treatment initiation improves short-term prognosis
- Corticosteroids mitigate vasogenic edema
  - High-dose dexamethasone (96 mg IV bolus, then 24 mg by mouth every 6 hours for 3 days, then 10-day taper) for patients with abnormal neurologic examination
  - Moderate-dose dexamethasone (10 mg IV bolus, then 4 mg 4 times daily with 2-week taper) for all other patients
- Radiotherapy of sensitive tumors
  - 50% of survivors ambulatory at 1 year after radiation

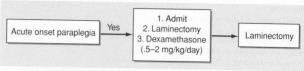

Figure 11-1 Acute onset paraplegia action.[13]

- Indications for radiation alone:
  - Prior radical spinal decompression
  - No spinal compression or instability
  - Subclinical cord compression
  - Poor surgical candidate
- Surgical decompression followed by postoperative radiation
  - Indications:
    - Spinal instability
    - Previous radiation therapy to area
    - Disease progression despite radiation
    - Radioresistant tumor
    - Unknown primary tumor
    - Paraplegia less than 48 hours
    - Single area of cord compression
- Figures 11-1 and 11-2 depict appropriate action for patients with acute onset paraplegia and no acute onset paraplegia.

Tumor Lysis Syndrome[15]

Acute tumor lysis syndrome is a potentially life-threatening emergency characterized by metabolic derangements resulting from the death of malignant cells and release of intracellular contents.

Presentation

- Chief complaint: weakness
- Signs and symptoms:
  - Nausea and vomiting
  - Diarrhea
  - Muscle weakness/cramps
  - Hyperkalemia (6–72 hours after initiation of cytotoxic chemotherapy; exacerbated by acute kidney injury)

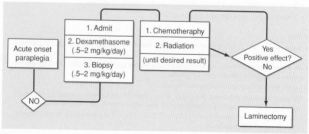

Figure 11-2 New acute onset paraplegia.[13]

- Hyperphosphatemia (24–48 hours after chemotherapy)
- Hypocalcemia
- Hyperuricemia

Risk Factors

- Past medical history
  - Primarily associated with hematological malignancies with high proliferative rate and tumor burden (eg, high-grade non-Hodgkin lymphoma, acute lymphoblastic leukemia)
  - Also associated with low- and intermediate-grade hematologic malignancies (eg, multiple myeloma, acute myeloid leukemia, chronic lymphocytic leukemia)
  - Uncommon in solid tumors *except* those with high proliferative rates and rapid response to cytotoxic chemotherapy (eg, testicular cancer, small-cell lung cancer, neuroblastoma, breast cancer)
  - Preexisting renal dysfunction
  - Elevated serum lactate dehydrogenase
  - Dehydration
  - Severe hypocalcaemia
  - Chemotherapy: systemic, intrathecal, glucocorticoids, biologic agents, ionizing radiation
- Family history
  - Cardiac arrhythmia
    - Indicative of hyperkalemia or hypocalcaemia
  - Seizures
    - Severe hypocalcaemia or hypophosphatemia
- Medications
  - Calcium supplements
  - Aminoglycoside antibiotics and nonsteroidal antiinflammatory drugs
    - Cause or worsen existing renal impairment
    - Increase the risk of tumor lysis syndrome

Diagnosis

- Physical examination: Check for tumors and tumor size, arrhythmias, tachycardia
- Laboratory test results:
  - Serum uric acid level higher than 476 mmol/L (8 mg/dL)
  - Serum calcium level lower than 1.75 mmol/L (7 mg/dL)
  - WBC count higher than 25,000/μL (increased risk)
  - Serum creatinine level higher than 1.5 times upper normal limit
- Radiology:
  - Electrocardiogram:
    - Arrhythmia with hyperkalemia
    - Hypophosphatemia
    - Hypocalcaemia
- Prevention:
  - High-risk patients: rasburicase 0.15 mg/kg or 6 mg fixed-dose
  - Intermediate-risk patients: allopurinol 300 mg daily or 200 to 400 mg/m^2
  - Low-risk patients: watch and wait

Action

- Volume loading with fluid at twice maintenance rate to increase glomerular filtration rate, urine flow, and uric acid, and calcium phosphate solubility
- Hyperkalemia
  - Enteral sodium polystyrene (ion exchange resin)
  - For symptomatic patients: Rapid treatment with insulin and dextrose or sodium bicarbonate to shift potassium intracellularly and calcium gluconate to stabilize cardiac cell membranes

TABLE 11-12. POSTTREATMENT SYMPTOMATIC MANAGEMENT[a]

Symptom	Drug	Dose and Route	Side Effects
Nausea and vomiting	1. 5-HT$_3$ antagonists 2. Aprepitant 3. Dexamethasone 4. Dronabinol 5. Metoclopramide 6. Promethazine	1. PO, IV 2. PO 3. PO, IV 4. PO 5. PO, IV 6. PO, IV	Constipation, headache
Electrolyte abnormalities	Supplemental electrolytes or diuretics (low-high)	IV	Muscle spasms, weakness, twitching
Depression	1. SSRIs (citalopram) 2. SNRIs (venlafaxine)	1. PO 2. PO	Upset stomach, fatigue, insomnia, weight change
Mucositis	1. Morphine PCA 2. Mouthwash (chlorhexidine)	1. IV 2. PO	Headache
Acral erythema	1. Corticosteroids 2. Pyridoxine	IV	

IV, intravenous; PCA, patient-controlled analgesia; PO, oral; SNRI, selective noradrenergic reuptake inhibitor; SSRI, selective serotonin reuptake inhibitor.
[a]Treatments include chemotherapy, radiation, and surgery.

- Hyperphosphatemia
  - Phosphate removal from fluids
  - Volume loading
  - Phosphate binders
  - Renal replacement therapy (for severe cases)
- Hypocalcemia—treat only if symptomatic
- Hyperuricemia
  - Recombinant urate oxidase (rasburicase) 0.2 mg/kg IV daily for 5 days
    - Contraindicated in patients with glucose-6-phosphate dehydrogenase deficiency because it may cause hemolytic anemia or methemoglobinemia
- Significant acute kidney injury—renal replacement therapy

Table 11-12 is a quick reference guide for other commonly occurring posttreatment symptoms.

REFERENCES

1. Carney PA, Miglioretti DL, Yankaskas BC, et al. Individual and combined effects of age, breast density, and hormone replacement therapy use on the accuracy of screening mammography. *Ann Intern Med.* 2003;138(3):168-75.
2. Rosenberg RD, Hunt WC, Williamson MR, et al. Effects of age, breast density, ethnicity, and estrogen replacement therapy on screening mammographic sensitivity and cancer stage at diagnosis: review of 183,134 screening mammograms in Albuquerque, New Mexico. *Radiology.* 1998;209(2):511-18.
3. Bevers TB, Anderson BO, Bonaccio E, et al. Breast cancer screening and diagnosis. *J Natl Compr Canc Netw.* 2009;7:1060-96.
4. Teh W, Wilson AR: The role of ultrasound in breast cancer screening. A consensus statement by the European Group for Breast Cancer Screening. *Eur J Cancer.* 1998;34(4):449-50.

5. Lord SJ, Lei W, Craft P, et al. A systematic review of the effectiveness of magnetic resonance imaging (MRI) as an addition to mammography and ultrasound in screening young women at high risk of breast cancer. *Eur J Cancer*. 2007;43(13):1905-17.

6. Berg WA, Gutierrez L, NessAiver MS, et al. Diagnostic accuracy of mammography, clinical examination, US, and MR imaging in preoperative assessment of breast cancer. *Radiology*. 2004;233(3):830-49.

7. National Institute for Health and Clinical Excellence (NICE). *Colorectal cancer. The diagnosis and management of colorectal cancer.* London (UK): National Institute for Health and Clinical Excellence (NICE); 2011 Nov. 42 p. (Clinical guideline; no. 131). This is the citation requested by the governmental agency.

8. Sosna J, Morrin MM, Kruskal JB, et al. CT colonography of colorectal polyps: a metaanalysis. *AJR Am J Roentgenol*. 2003;181(6):1593-98.

9. Bach PB, Silvestri GA, Hanger M, Jett JR, American College of Chest Physicians. Screening for lung cancer: ACCP evidence-based clinical practice guidelines (2nd ed.). *Chest*. 2007;132(3 suppl):69S-77S.

10. Rivera MP, Mehta AC. Diagnosis and management of lung cancer: ACCP guidelines (2nd ed.). *Chest*. 2007;132(3):S131-48.

11. National Collaborating Centre for Cancer. *Prostate Cancer: Diagnosis and Treatment.* NICE clinical guideline no. 58. London: National Institute for Health and Clinical Excellence (NICE); 2008:146.

12. Sabatine, MS. *Pocket Medicine.* Philadelphia: Wolters Kluwer Health/Lippincott Williams and Wilkins; 2011.

13. Lowry AW, Kushal YB, Nag PK. *Texas Children's Hospital Handbook of Pediatrics and Neonatology.* New York: McGraw-Hill; 2011.

14. Pizzo PA. Fever in immunocompromised patients. *N Engl J Med*. 1999;341(12):893-900.

15. McCurdy MT, Shanholtz CB. Oncologic emergencies. *Crit Care Med*. 2012;40(7):2212-22.

CHAPTER 12

Pulmonology

Himanshu Desai, Michael Hooper, and Jeffrey Schnader

GATHERING DATA

Common Respiratory Signs and Symptoms

Dyspnea

Defined as "subjective experience of breathing discomfort that consists of qualitatively distinct sensations that vary in intensity. The experience derives from interactions among multiple physiological, psychological, social, and environmental factors and may induce secondary physiological and behavioral responses."

Causes of Dyspnea

- *Acute:* pneumothorax, pneumonia, pulmonary embolism (PE), asthma exacerbation, myocardial infarction
- *Subacute:* pleural effusion, pulmonary hypertension (HTN), congestive heart failure (CHF) exacerbation
- *Chronic:* interstitial lung diseases such as interstitial pulmonary fibrosis (IPF), chronic obstructive pulmonary disease (COPD), chronic pulmonary thromboembolic disease
- Orthopnea (dyspnea in supine position): CHF, obesity
- Platypnea (dyspnea in upright position): hepatopulmonary syndrome, left atrial myxoma

Cough

Causes of Cough

- *Acute (<3 weeks):* respiratory tract infection, aspiration, inhalation, or smoke injury
- *Subacute (3–8 weeks):* tracheobronchitis, pertussis
- *Chronic (>8 weeks):* interstitial lung diseases, CHF, tuberculosis and other chronic infections. *Consider cough-variant asthma, gastroesophageal reflux, nasopharyngeal drainage, and angiotensin-converting enzyme inhibitors in patients with normal chest x-ray.*

Pleuritic Chest Pain

Sharp and/or stabbing, increased by deep inspiration and cough

Causes of pleuritic chest pain: pleurisy, pleural effusion, pneumonia, PE with pulmonary infarct

Hemoptysis

- Important to distinguish from epistaxis and hematemesis

Causes of hemoptysis: bronchitis, pneumonia, pulmonary edema, coagulopathies, PE, bronchiectasis, lung cancer, tuberculosis, atrioventricular malformation, aspergilloma, pulmonary alveolar hemorrhage (Wegener granulomatosis, microscopic polyangiitis, Goodpasture disease, systemic lupus erythematosus, etc.)

Fever

Pulmonary causes of fever include bacterial and viral pneumonia, lung cancer, tuberculosis, and PE

Respiratory System History and Review of Systems

Smoking

Most important risk factor for COPD and lung cancer (adenocarcinoma) although 10% to 15% of patients with COPD are nonsmokers. Always calculate pack years (packs per day per years of smoking). Lung cancer risks return to baseline after 20 years of smoking cessation.

Allergies

Asthma is frequently associated with atopic symptoms. Allergic rhinitis, eczema, and hay fever are more common in patients with asthma.

Occupation and Environment

Exposures to asbestos (pleural effusion, asbestosis, and mesothelioma), silica (silicosis), and beryllium are associated with various pulmonary conditions. Passive smoking is also important.

Immunization

Flu shot annually. Pneumococcal polysaccharide vaccine is recommended for COPD patients 65 years and older and for COPD patients younger than age 65 with a forced expiratory volume at 1 second (FEV_1) less than 40% predicted.

Family History

Important for cystic fibrosis, α_1-antitrypsin deficiency. Asthma is also commonly seen in family members.

Immunosuppression

Pneumocystis, tuberculosis, fungal infections are more common in immunocompromised (human immunodeficiency virus [HIV], chemotherapy, transplant, steroids).

Sleep Apnea

Assess for daytime sleepiness with Epworth Sleepiness Score: http://www.stanford.edu/~dement/epworth.html

Medications

Check for pulmonary toxicity: http://pneumotox.com/indexf.php?fich=drugs&lg=en&nf=

Important Physical Examination Findings

- Barrel-shaped chest: COPD, obstructive lung disease
- Cyanosis: chronic hypoxia
- Clubbing: IPF, lung cancer, bronchiectasis
- Pursed-lip breathing: COPD
- Pulsus paradoxus: severe asthma exacerbation
- Dull percussion: pleural effusion, collapse or atelectasis of lung, consolidation
- Hyperresonant percussion: pneumothorax
- Prolonged expiration: COPD, asthma
- Bronchial breath sounds: major airways, consolidation, partial collapse
- "Velcro" rales: pulmonary fibrosis
- Inspiratory rales: pulmonary edema
- Rhonchi and wheezes: COPD, asthma exacerbation
- Egophony and increased vocal resonance: consolidation, partial collapse

Diagnostic Tests

Laboratory

- Blood gas analysis: hypoxia, CO_2 retention, alveolar-arterial (A-a) gradient. Helps identifying cause for respiratory failure.
- D-dimer: High sensitivity and low specificity for diagnosis of PE. Should be reserved for patients with low pretest probability for PE and no other significant comorbidities.

Radiology

- Review basic concepts of chest radiology here: http://chestradiology.net/
- Chest x-ray: Helps in the diagnosis of COPD (hyperinflation, flattened diaphragm, emphysematous bullae), asthma exacerbation (hyperinflation), pneumonia (consolidation with air bronchogram), atelectasis and collapse (consolidation with shift of mediastinum to same side), bronchiectasis, pulmonary fibrosis, pleural effusion, pneumothorax, pulmonary edema (cardiogenic and noncardiogenic), lung nodule and mass
- Computed tomography (CT) scan: Especially helpful with interstitial lung diseases, lung nodules. CT pulmonary angiogram (CTPA) is useful for the diagnosis of PE

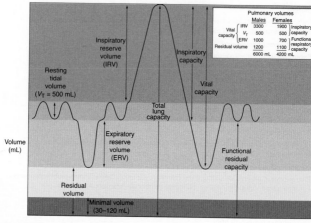

Figure 12-1 Lung volumes and capacities.

- Ventilation-perfusion (VQ) scan: Helps with the diagnosis of PE when CTPA is contraindicated and in patients without underlying lung parenchymal abnormalities.
- Positron emission tomography (PET) scan: Helps differentiating malignant (hypermetabolic) and nonmalignant nodule of more than 1-cm size. Not reliable for very small nodules.
- Gallium scan: Helps detecting alveolitis (active inflammation), especially useful for amiodarone toxicity.

Special Tests

- Pulmonary Function Tests (Figures 12-1 and 12-2)
- For American Thoracic Society and European Respiratory Society (ATS/ERS) guidelines: http://www.thoracic.org/statements/resources/pfet/pft5.pdf
- Cardiopulmonary exercise tests: Useful in patients with unexplained dyspnea. Helps differentiating respiratory, cardiac, or vascular causes for limitation of exercise capacity.
- For ATS and American College of Chest Physicians (ACCP) guidelines: http://www.thoracic.org/statements/resources/pfet/cardioexercise.pdf
- Right heart catheterization: help in the diagnosis of pulmonary hypertension and to evaluate response to vasodilator therapy. Also helps identifying left heart failure as a cause of pulmonary HTN (elevated pulmonary capillary wedge pressure).

Bronchoscopy

Diagnostic

- Infection (with bronchoalveolar lavage)
- Malignancy (endobronchial biopsy, transbronchial needle aspiration from lymph nodes)
- Interstitial lung disease (ie, sarcoidosis with transbronchial lung biopsy)
- For British Thoracic Society guidelines: http://thorax.bmj.com/content/56/suppl_1/i1.full.pdf

Therapeutic

- Removal of foreign body or mucus plug
- Difficult intubation
- Stent for tracheal or bronchial narrowing or compression
- Bronchial thermoplasty for severe anemia

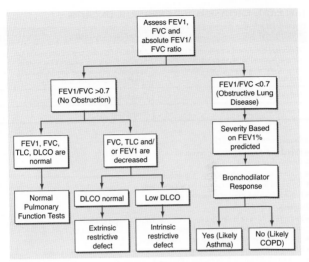

Figure 12-2   Interpretation of pulmonary function tests. COPD, chronic obstructive pulmonary disease; DLCO$_2$, diffusing capacity of lungs for carbon dioxide; FEV$_1$, forced expiratory volume at 1 second; FVC, forced vital capacity; TLC, total lung capacity.

MEDICAL SPECIALTIES

- Palliative laser or phototherapy for endobronchial malignancies
- For ATS/ERS guidelines: http://www.ers-education.org/pages/default.aspx?id=2451

SPECIFIC CONDITIONS

Chronic Obstructive Pulmonary Disease

Definition

COPD is a preventable and treatable disease with some significant extrapulmonary effects that may contribute to the severity in individual patients. Its pulmonary component is characterized by airflow limitation that is not fully reversible. The airflow limitation is usually progressive and associated with an abnormal inflammatory response of the lungs to noxious particles or gases.

Epidemiology

- Third most common killer in United States
- Only leading cause of death increasing in prevalence
- 10% prevalence in persons 55 to 85 years of age
- Rare in persons younger than 40 years of age
- Mortality of hospitalized is 5% to 14%
- Occurs in men more than women

Risk Factors

- Smoking, passive smoking: 80% to 90% of those with COPD are smokers. 15% of smokers develop clinically significant COPD.
- Ambient air pollution
- Occupational dust and chemicals
- Childhood infections (severe respiratory, viral)
- α$_1$-antitrypsin deficiency (<1%)

TABLE 12-1. EMPHYSEMA AND CHRONIC BRONCHITIS

Emphysema	Chronic Bronchitis
Abnormal permanent enlargement of the air spaces distal to the terminal bronchioles accompanied by destruction of their walls and without obvious fibrosis.	Presence of chronic productive cough for 3 months in each of 2 successive years in a patient in whom other causes of chronic cough have been excluded.
Pathological diagnosis	Clinical diagnosis
"Pink Puffer"	"Blue Blotter"

Clinical Features (Table 12-1)

- Exertional dyspnea, chronic cough
- Weight loss, fatigue
- Tachypnea, accessory respiratory muscle use
- Barrel-shaped chest, decreased breath sounds
- Pursed-lip exhalation, prolonged expiration

Diagnosis

- PFTs: FEV_1/forced vital capacity (FVC) less than 0.7, hyperinflation (increased total lung capacity), air trapping (increased residual volume), decreased $DLCO_2$
- Chest x-ray: Hyperinflation, flattened diaphragm
- CT scan: Shows early emphysematous changes, more sensitive than chest x-ray
- Arterial blood gas analysis (ABG): Hypoxia, hypercarbia

Treatment (Figure 12-3)

Read more guidelines at: http://www.goldcopd.org/guidelines-global-strategy-for-diagnosis-management.html and http://www.annals.org/content/155/3/179.full

COPD Exacerbation

Defined as an acute change in dyspnea, cough and/or sputum sufficient enough to warrant therapy change.

- Increase dose and/or frequency of short-acting bronchodilator therapy
- Supplemental oxygen, if needed

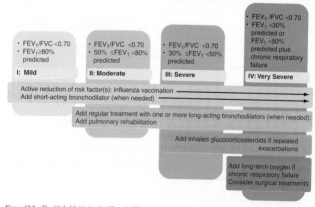

Figure 12-3 The Global Initiative for Chronic Obstructive Lung Disease (GOLD) guidelines for therapy at each stage of chronic obstructive pulmonary disease. FEV_1, forced expiratory volume at 1 second; FVC, forced vital capacity.

- Systemic glucocorticosteroid
- Antibiotics
- Noninvasive mechanical ventilation is preferred over invasive mechanical ventilation.

Prevention of Exacerbation

- Long-acting bronchodilators
- Inhaled corticosteroids
- Phosphodiesterase inhibitors: roflumilast
- Immunizations: influenza vaccine, pneumococcal vaccine
- Macrolides

Lung Volume Reduction Surgery (LVRS)

- Patients with predominantly **upper-lobe emphysema** who had **low exercise capacity** who underwent LVRS had **significant improvements in survival** and functional outcomes as compared with medical therapy.
- Patients with **$FEV_1/DLCO_2$ 20% or less** of predicted AND **homogeneous (diffuse) distribution of emphysema** are **at high risk for death** after surgery and are unlikely to benefit from LVRS.

Asthma

Definition

Asthma is a chronic inflammatory disease characterized by variable airflow obstruction and bronchial hyperresponsiveness. Airflow obstruction is reversible, either spontaneously or with treatment.

Epidemiology

- 300 million asthmatics worldwide
- Estimated prevalence of asthma in United States is 29.8 million
- 500,000 hospitalizations each year
- Ninth leading cause of hospitalization nationally
- Worldwide costs of asthma are greater than acquired immunodeficiency syndrome and tuberculosis combined
- Asthma accounts for 1 in every 250 deaths worldwide

Pathophysiology (Figure 12-4)

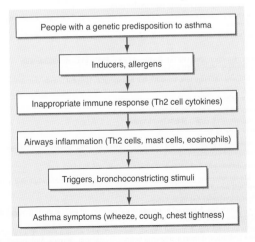

Figure 12-4 Th2, T-helper cell 2.

TABLE 12-2. ASTHMA SEVERITY CLASSIFICATION

		Persistent		
	Intermittent	Mild	Moderate	Severe
Symptoms	<2 days per week	>2 days per week, but not daily	Daily	Throughout the day
Nighttime awakenings	<2 times per month	3–4 times per month	>1 times per week, but not every night	>7 times per week
Short-acting β_2 agonist use	<2 days per week	> 2 days per week, but not daily	Daily	Several times per day
Interference with normal activity	None	Minor limitation	Some limitation	Extremely limited
Lung functions	FEV_1 >80% FEV_1/FVC normal	FEV_1 >80% FEV_1/FVC normal	FEV_1 60%–80% FEV_1/FVC reduced by 5%	FEV_1 <60% FEV_1/FVC reduced by >5%
Exacerbations requiring systemic steroids	0–1 per year	≥2 per year		

FEV_1, forced expiratory volume at 1 second; FVC, forced vital capacity.

Clinical Features (Table 12-2)

- Characteristic symptoms: wheezing, dyspnea, and coughing, which are variable.
- Chest tightness, thick mucus expectoration
- Worsening of symptoms on exposure to allergens
- Characteristic physical examination findings: inspiratory and expiratory rhonchi, hyperinflation
- Physical examination may be normal with stable asthma without exacerbation

Diagnosis

- Pulmonary function tests (PFTs): Reduced FEV1, FEV_1/FVC. Reversible with bronchodilators. Normal $DLCO_2$.
- Methacholine challenge test: sensitive but not specific. Helpful to rule out asthma as a cause of patient's symptoms
- Chest x-ray: Hyperinflation
- Skin allergy tests: To identify allergens, triggers
- Immunoglobulin E (IgE): Might be elevated

Treatment (Figure 12-5)

For evidence-based guidelines: visit http://www.ginasthma.org/guidelines-gina-report-global-strategy-for-asthma.html

Acute Severe Asthma and Asthma Exacerbation

- May be life-threatening. Patients have worsening shortness of breath, wheezing, unable to complete full sentences.
- Severely reduced peak expiratory flow.
- Hypoxia, hypocarbia. A normal or rising partial pressure of carbon dioxide suggests impending respiratory failure.
- Treatment includes supplemental oxygen, nebulized and inhaled short-acting β-agonists, nebulized and inhaled short-acting anticholinergic, systemic steroids. Aminophylline

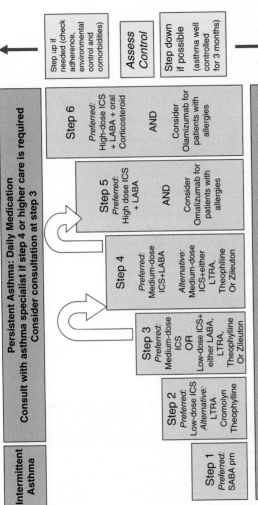

Figure 12-5 Stepwise approach for the treatment of asthma. ICS, inhaled corticosteroid; LABA, long-acting β-agonist; LTRA, leukotriene receptor agonist; prn, as needed; SABA, short-acting β-agonist.

infusion and magnesium sulfate could also be tried in severe cases. Patients with acute respiratory failure require mechanical ventilation.

Allergic Bronchopulmonary Aspergillosis

- Poorly controlled asthma.
- Elevated IgE. Skin test to *Aspergillus fumigatus* is positive.
- Fleeting infiltrates and centrilobular bronchiectasis on imaging.
- Treatment includes systemic steroids and itraconazole.

Pneumonia

Definition

- Community-acquired pneumonia (CAP) is defined as an acute infection of the lung parenchyma accompanied by symptoms of acute illness acquired outside of hospitals or extended-care facilities.
- Ventilator-associated pneumonia (VAP) is defined as a pneumonia that develops after 48 hours of mechanical ventilation.
- Health care-associated pneumonia (HCAP) is defined as an outpatient onset pneumonia with likely multidrug-resistant (MDR) pathogens because of various risk factors.

Epidemiology

- CAP results in more than 600,000 hospitalizations, 64 million days of restricted activity, and 45,000 deaths annually.
- The overall yearly cost associated with CAP is estimated at $9 to $10 billion.
- The incidence rates are highest at the extremes of age
- VAP is the commonest nosocomial infection in the intensive care unit (ICU) and an important cause of morbidity.
- VAP complicates the hospital course of approximately 20% of patients receiving mechanical ventilation or about 5 episodes per 1000 ventilator days.
- VAP increases the number of days requiring mechanical ventilation as well as ICU and hospital length of stay

Pathophysiology (Tables 12-3, 12-4, 12-5 and 12-6)

Clinical Features

- Common clinical features of CAP include cough, fever, sputum production, and pleuritic chest pain.
- Patients may have gastrointestinal symptoms such as nausea, vomiting, and/or diarrhea. Other symptoms may include fatigue, headache, myalgias, and arthralgias.
- Various prediction scores including the Pneumonia Severity Index and CURB-65 criteria (confusion, urea >19 mg/dL, respiratory rate >30 breaths/min, low blood pressure [systolic <90 mm Hg or diastolic <60 mm Hg], and age >65 years) have been shown to reliably predict mortality in patients with CAP.

TABLE 12-3. PATHOGENS IN COMMUNITY-ACQUIRED PNEUMONIA BY LEVEL OF CARE (IN ORDER OF FREQUENCY)

Outpatients	Inpatients (non-ICU)	Inpatients (ICU)
Streptococcus pneumoniae	S. pneumoniae	S. pneumoniae
Mycoplasma pneumoniae	M. pneumoniae	Legionella spp.
Haemophilus influenzae	C. pneumoniae	H. influenzae
Chlamydia pneumoniae	H. influenzae	Gram-negative bacilli
Respiratory viruses	Legionella spp. Respiratory viruses	Staphylococcus aureus

ICU, intensive care unit.

TABLE 12-4. COMMUNITY-ACQUIRED PNEUMONIA PATHOGENS ASSOCIATED WITH UNDERLYING COMORBID CONDITIONS

· *Streptococcus pneumoniae*
  Dementia
  Congestive heart failure
  Chronic obstructive pulmonary disease
  Cerebrovascular disease
  Institutional crowding
  Seizures

· Penicillin-resistant and drug-resistant *S. pneumoniae*
  Age >65 years
  Alcoholism
  Immunomodulating illness or therapy (including steroids)
  Previous β-lactam therapy within 3 months
  Multiple medical comorbidities
  Exposure to a child in day care center

· Gram-negative bacilli
  Residence in long-term care facility
  Underlying cardiopulmonary disease
  Recent antibiotic therapy
  Multiple medical comorbidities

· *Pseudomonas aeruginosa*
  Broad-spectrum antibiotics for >7 days in past month
  Structural lung disease (bronchiectasis)
  Corticosteroid therapy
  Malnutrition
  Undiagnosed HIV infection
  Neutropenia

· *Legionella* spp.
  AIDS
  Hematologic malignancy
  End-stage renal disease

AIDS, acquired immunodeficiency syndrome; HIV, human immunodeficiency virus.

MEDICAL SPECIALTIES

- The clinical manifestations are generally the same in VAP as in all other forms of pneumonia: fever, leukocytosis, increase in respiratory secretions, and pulmonary consolidation on physical examination, along with a new or changing radiographic infiltrate.

Diagnosis

- Chest x-ray shows consolidation, lobar and patchy infiltrates
- Blood cultures: To identify pathogen causing pneumonia
- Urinary antigen tests for *Legionella pneumophila* and *Streptococcus pneumoniae*
- Expectorated sputum for culture
- Intubated patients require endotracheal aspirate (fresh) or mini-bronchoalveolar lavage and blind bronchoalveolar lavage
- Nasopharyngeal swab for influenza during seasonal influenza (rapid antigen test and viral polymerase chain reaction

TABLE 12-5. PATHOGENS IN VENTILATOR-ASSOCIATED PNEUMONIA

Common Pathogens	Less Common Pathogens
Pseudomonas aeruginosa	*Escherichia coli*
MRSA	*Enterobacter* spp.
Klebsiella pneumoniae	*Citrobacter* spp.
Acinetobacter spp.	*Serratia* spp.
Stenotrophomonas maltophilia	*Legionella* spp.
Streptococcus pneumoniae (early VAP)	
Haemophilus Influenzae (early VAP)	

MRSA, methicillin-resistant *Staphylococcus aureus*; VAP, ventilator-associated pneumonia.

Treatment
- For ATS and Infectious Diseases Society of America (IDSA) guidelines on CAP, visit http://www-archive.thoracic.org/sections/publications/statements/pages/mtpi/idsaats-cap.html
- For ATS/IDSA guidelines on VAP, HCAP, and hospital-acquired pneumonia (HAP), visit http://www-archive.thoracic.org/sections/publications/statements/pages/mtpi/guide1–29.html
- See Figures 12-6 and 12-7.

Empiric Therapy for Early Onset Hospital- and Ventilator-Acquired Pneumonia
See Table 12-7.

Empiric Therapy for Late-Onset Hospital-, Ventilator-, and Health Care-Acquired Pneumonia
See Table 12-8.

Pleural Effusion

Definition
Presence of excess quantity of fluid in pleural space is called *pleural effusion*. Pleural fluid accumulates when pleural fluid formation exceeds pleural fluid absorption.

TABLE 12-6. RISK FACTORS FOR INFECTION BY MULTIDRUG-RESISTANT ORGANISMS

Intubation for longer than 7 days
Previous broad-spectrum antibiotics
Hemodialysis
Hospitalization for 2 days or more in the last 90 days
Prior admission to the ICU
Nursing home residence
Immunosuppression
Chronic wound care

ICU, intensive care unit.

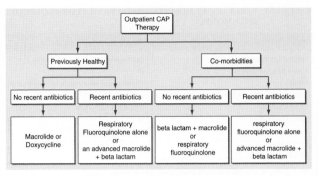

Figure 12-6 American Thoracic Society and Infectious Diseases Society of America guidelines for outpatient community-acquired pneumonia treatment. CAP, community-acquired pneumonia.

Epidemiology and Pathophysiology

Mechanisms underlying development of pleural effusion include:

- Change in transpleural pressure balance (transudate): CHF
- Increase in capillary permeability (exudate): pneumonia
- Impairment in lymphatic drainage (exudate): malignancy
- Movement of fluid from extravascular spaces (transudate or exudate): peritoneal dialysis, chylothorax

Exudative pleural effusions meet at least one of the following criteria, whereas transudative pleural effusions meet none:

- The ratio of pleural fluid protein to serum protein is greater than 0.5
- The ratio of pleural fluid lactate dehydrogenase (LDH) to serum LDH is greater than 0.6
- Pleural fluid LDH is more than two-thirds of normal upper limit for serum

Serum-pleural fluid protein gradient greater than 3.1 and/or serum-pleural fluid albumin gradient greater than 1.2 favor transudative pleural effusion.

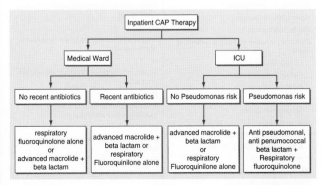

Figure 12-7 American Thoracic Society and Infectious Diseases Society of America guidelines for inpatient community-acquired pneumonia treatment. ICU, intensive care unit.

TABLE 12-7.   EARLY ONSET HOSPITAL- AND VENTILATOR-ACQUIRED
              PNEUMONIA[a]

Potential Pathogen	Recommended Antibiotic
Streptococcus pneumoniae	Ceftriaxone
Haemophilus influenzae	or
MSSA	Ciprofloxacin, levofloxacin or moxifloxacin
Antibiotic-sensitive enteric gram-negative bacilli:	or
Escherichia coli	Ampicillin/sulbactam
Klebsiella pneumoniae	or
Enterobacter spp.	Ertapenem
Proteus spp.	
Serratia marcescens	

MDR, multidrug resistant; MSSA, methicillin-sensitive *Staphylococcus aureus*.
[a]No risk factors for MDR pathogens, any disease severity.

Transudative Pleural Effusion

Imbalance in hydrostatic and oncotic pressures, normal pleura, limited differential, cause apparent from clinical presentation.

Causes

CHF, hepatic hydrothorax, hypoalbuminemia, trapped lung, nephrotic syndrome, atelectasis, peritoneal dialysis, constrictive pericarditis, urinothorax, duropleural fistula, ventriculopleural shunt

TABLE 12-8.   LATE-ONSET HOSPITAL-, VENTILATOR-, AND HEALTH
              CARE-ACQUIRED PNEUMONIA[a]

Potential Pathogen	Combination Antibiotic Therapy
Streptococcus pneumoniae	Antipseudomonal cephalosporin (cefepime, ceftazidime)
Haemophilus influenzae	
Staphylococcus aureus	or
Antibiotic-sensitive enteric gram-negative bacilli:	Antipseudomonal carbapenem (imipenem or meropenem)
Escherichia coli	or
Klebsiella pneumoniae	β-Lactam/β-lactamase inhibitor (piperacillin-tazobactam)
Enterobacter spp.	
Proteus spp.	plus
Serratia marcescens	Antipseudomonal fluoroquinolone (ciprofloxacin or levofloxacin)
MDR pathogens:	or
Pseudomonas aeruginosa	Aminoglycoside (amikacin, gentamicin, or tobramycin)
K. pneumoniae (ESBL positive)	
Acinetobacter spp.	plus
MRSA	Linezolid or vancomycin
Legionella pneumophila	

ESBL, extended-spectrum β-lactamase; MDR, multidrug resistant; MRSA, methicillin-resistant *S. aureus*.
[a]Risk factors for MDR pathogens, any disease severity.

Exudative Pleural Effusion

Caused by infection, malignancy, inflammation or impaired lymphatic drainage; broad differential

Exudative Effusions with LDH Level Greater Than 1000 U/liter

Empyema, complicated parapneumonic effusion, cholesterol effusion, rheumatoid pleurisy, primary pleural lymphoma

Exudative Effusions with Pleural Fluid Neutrophilia

Parapneumonic, early tuberculosis, trauma, inflammation (lupus)

Exudative Effusions with Lymphocyte-Predominant Pleural Fluid

Acute lung rejection, chronic rheumatoid pleurisy, chylothorax, lymphoma, post-coronary artery bypass graft (2–12 months), sarcoidosis, tuberculous pleural effusion, uremic pleural effusion, yellow nail syndrome

Exudative Effusions with Pleural Fluid Eosinophilia

Pneumothorax (within hours), hemothorax (delayed: 10–14 days), benign asbestos related pleural effusion, pulmonary infarction, parasitic disease, fungal disease, drug-induced, lymphoma, and carcinoma

Clinical Features

- Shortness of breath on exertion
- Symptoms of underlying condition causing pleural effusion
- Dull percussion, absent breath sounds on physical examination

Diagnosis

- Chest x-ray: "meniscus" sign, mediastinal shift.
- Ultrasound can detect small amounts of pleural fluid, helps with thoracentesis, identifies loculated effusion.
- CT scan more sensitive to detect minimal amount, loculations, other pleural pathologies
- Thoracentesis to identify cause etiology of pleural effusion. Pleural fluid diagnostic studies: pH, LDH, protein, albumin, cell count and differential, glucose, cytology, gram stain and culture, acid-fast bacillus, adenosine deaminase, amylase, triglycerides, cholesterol.
- Simultaneous serum LDH, protein, and albumin.
- Video-assisted thoracic surgery, pleural biopsy: May be required for undiagnosed cases.

Treatment

- Treat underlying condition.
- Therapeutic thoracentesis for symptomatic pleural effusion.
- See Figures 12-8 and 12-9.

Deep Venous Thrombosis-Pulmonary Embolism

Epidemiology

- Deep vein thrombosis (DVT) and PE account for 100,000 to 300,000 deaths per year in United States.
- Venous thromboembolism (VTE) can cause death from PE or, among survivors, chronic thromboembolic pulmonary HTN and postphlebitic syndrome.
- Ninety to ninety-five percent of pulmonary emboli originate in the deep venous system of the lower extremities. Other rare locations include:
  - Uterine and prostatic veins
  - Upper extremities
  - Renal veins
  - Right side of the heart

Risk Factors

- CHF
- Venous stasis
- Prior DVT
- Age older than 70 years
- Prolonged bed rest
- Surgery requiring more than 30 minutes general anesthesia

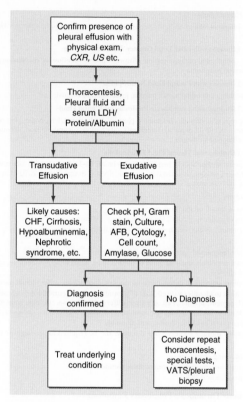

Figure 12-8   Diagnostic approach for pleural effusion. AFB, acid-fast bacillus; CHF, congestive heart failure; CXR, chest x-ray; US, ultrasound; VATS, video-assisted thoracic surgery.

- Orthopedic surgery
- Malignancy
- Obesity
- Estrogen; oral contraceptives
- Pregnancy
- Lower extremity injury
- Coagulopathy

Pathophysiology

- Virchow triad—Factors predisposing venous thrombosis are:
  - Local trauma to the vessel wall
  - Hypercoagulability (factor V Leiden mutation, protein C deficiency, protein S deficiency, antithrombin deficiency, prothrombin gene mutation *A20210*, anticardiolipin antibodies, lupus anticoagulant, hyperhomocystinemia)
  - Stasis of blood flow

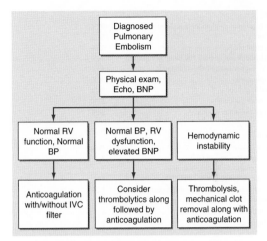

Figure 12-9 Algorithm for management of pulmonary embolism. BNP, B-type natriuretic peptide; BP, blood pressure; Echo, echocardiogram; IVC, inferior vena cava; RV, respiratory volume.

- When venous emboli become dislodged from their site of origin, they embolize to the pulmonary arterial circulation or, paradoxically to the arterial circulation through a patent foramen ovale. PE can cause:
  - Increased pulmonary vascular resistance
  - Impaired gas exchange
  - Alveolar hyperventilation
  - Increased airway resistance
  - Decreased pulmonary compliance
  - Right ventricular dysfunction

Clinical Features

- Symptoms of DVT include lower extremity swelling, redness, or pain
- Classic triad of hemoptysis, dyspnea, and pleuritic chest pain is not commonly present.
- Dyspnea is the most frequent symptom of PE.
- Tachypnea is the most frequent physical finding.
- Dyspnea, syncope, hypotension, or cyanosis suggest a massive PE.
- Symptoms:
  - Dyspnea   84%
  - Chest pain, pleuritic   74%
  - Anxiety   59%
  - Cough   53%
  - Hemoptysis   30%
  - Sweating   27%
  - Chest pain, nonpleuritic   14%
  - Syncope   13%

- Signs:
  - Tachypnea more than 20 breaths per minute   92%
  - Rales   58%
  - Accentuated S_2 53%
  - Tachycardia more than 100 beats per minute   44%
  - Fever higher than 37.8°C (100.04°F)   43%
  - Diaphoresis   36%
  - S_3 or S_4 gallop   34%
  - Thrombophlebitis   32%
  - Lower extremity edema   24%

Diagnosis

• Clinical feature	Points
• Clinical symptoms of DVT	3
• Other diagnosis less likely than PE	3
• Heart rate greater than 100 beats per minute	1.5
• Immobilization or surgery within past 4 weeks	1.5
• Previous DVT or PE	1.5
• Hemoptysis	1
• Malignancy	1

Pretest probability: More than 6 points indicates high risk (78.4%); 2 to 6 points indicates moderate risk (27.8%); fewer than 2 points indicates low risk (3.4%).

- Imaging Studies
  - Chest x-ray: nonspecific and low sensitivity. May see "Hampton's hump" (wedge-shaped density) or "Westermark sign" (focal oligemia).
  - Ventilation-perfusion scans: Noninvasive; helpful in pregnant patients and in patients with contraindication to intravenous (IV) contrast. Useful if normal (or near normal) with low pretest probability or high probability. Otherwise, scan should be followed by a confirmatory test.
  - Spiral chest CT: Modality of choice; rapid, sensitive; identifies other pathologies. Needs IV contrast.
  - Pulmonary angiography: Considered gold standard; useful when spiral CT is nondiagnostic and high pretest probability.
  - Echocardiography should be done in all patients with PE for risk stratification; can identify high-risk patients (with respiratory volume dysfunction).
  - Venous ultrasonography: Approximately one-third of patients with PE have no evidence of DVT. If DVT is present with clinical suspicion of PE, further workup of PE may not be required. However, workup for PE should continue in high pretest probability with negative ultrasound.
- Laboratory analysis
  - Complete blood count, erythrocyte sedimentation rate, hemoglobin and hematocrit generally not useful.
  - D-dimer very sensitive but nonspecific with false positives; has high negative predictive value. Can be helpful if negative in patients with low pretest probability.
  - ABG: Hypoxia, high A-a gradient; might be normal.
- Electrocardiogram: Tachycardia or nonspecific ST-T-wave changes. $S_1Q_3T_3$ is present only in 20% of cases.

Treatment

For ACCP evidence-based guidelines, please visit http://chestjournal.chestpubs.org/content/141/2_suppl/7S.full?etoc

- Goals of therapy include preventing death from a current embolic event, reducing the likelihood of recurrent embolic events, and minimizing the long-term morbidity of the event.
- Start treatment with unfractionated heparin or low-molecular-weight heparin as soon as possible, if not contraindicated. Could start treatment while undergoing workup in

high-risk patients. Start oral anticoagulation as soon as possible. Continue unfractionated heparin or low-molecular-weight heparin for at least 5 days and therapeutic INR for 24 hours.

- Thrombolytics and mechanical clot removal in patients with massive PE and hemodynamic instability.
- Duration of anticoagulation depends on risk of recurrent VTE (3 months for provoked DVT and PE, longer for unprovoked PE without risk factors, prolonged for patients with risk factors for recurrent VTE).
- Consider insufficient ventilatory drive filter when anticoagulation is contraindicated with DVT or in patients with massive or submassive PE and large DVT in addition to anticoagulation.

Lung Cancer

Definition

Uncontrolled growth of malignant cells in one or both lungs and tracheobronchial tree

Epidemiology

- Leading cause of cancer-related death in men and women in North America and Europe.
- Five-year survival rate is approximately 16%.
- Rare before age 40 years.
- Tobacco consumption is the primary cause of lung cancer. However, it can affect nonsmokers and passive smokers.
- Only 10% to 15% of active smokers develop lung cancer and 10% to 15% of lung cancers occur in never smokers.
- Risk factors
  - Smoking (80%–90%)
  - Exposure to asbestos, arsenic, bischloromethyl ether, hexavalent chromium, mustard gas, nickel, and polycyclic aromatic hydrocarbons
  - Ionizing radiation
  - Passive smoking
  - Genetic and inherited factors
  - Hormonal factors and oncogenic viruses

Pathophysiology

- Small cell lung cancer: 18%, almost 100% of patients are smokers; centrally located
- Non-small cell lung cancer:
  - Squamous cell cancer: 29%, 95% of patients are smokers; centrally located
  - Adenocarcinoma: 32%, 50% of patients never smokers; peripherally located
  - Large cell carcinoma: 9%, 90% of patients smokers; peripherally located
- Unclassified or undifferentiated: 12%

Clinical Features

- Common symptoms:
  - Cough
  - Dyspnea
  - Hemoptysis
  - Recurrent infections
  - Chest pain
- Symptoms and signs caused by regional metastases:
  - Esophageal compression: dysphagia
  - Laryngeal nerve paralysis: hoarseness
  - Symptomatic nerve paralysis: Horner syndrome
  - Cervical and thoracic nerve invasion: Pancoast syndrome
  - Lymphatic obstruction: pleural effusion
  - Vascular obstruction: superior vena cava syndrome
  - Pericardial and cardiac extension: pericardial effusion, tamponade

TABLE 12-9. STAGING AND TREATMENT FOR NON-SMALL CELL LUNG CANCER

Stage	Description	Treatment Options
Stage I a/b	Tumor of any size is found only in the lung	Surgery
Stage II a/b	Tumor has spread to lymph nodes associated with the lung	Surgery + chemotherapy
Stage III a	Tumor has spread to the lymph nodes in the tracheal area, including chest wall and diaphragm	Chemotherapy followed by radiation or surgery
Stage III b	Tumor has spread to the lymph nodes on the opposite lung or in the neck	Combination of chemotherapy and radiation
Stage IV	Tumor has spread beyond the chest	Chemotherapy and/or palliative (maintenance) care

Diagnosis

- Chest x-ray and CT scan: Lung nodule or mass, mediastinal or hilar lymphadenopathy, pleural or pericardial effusion
- Bronchoscopy and transthoracic needle biopsy to confirm diagnosis
- Bone scan and PET scan for staging
- Mediastinoscopy and endobronchial ultrasound for lymph node staging

Treatment (Table 12-9)

Staging and Treatment for Small Cell Lung Cancer

Limited Disease

- Defined as tumor involvement of 1 lung, the mediastinum and ipsilateral and/or contralateral supraclavicular lymph nodes or disease that can be encompassed in a single radiotherapy port.
- Approximately 25% of cases; treated with chemotherapy plus radiotherapy.

Extensive Disease

- Defined as tumor that has spread beyond 1 lung, mediastinum, and supraclavicular lymph nodes. Common distant sites of metastases are the adrenals, bone, liver, bone marrow, and brain.
- Approximately 75% of cases; treated with chemotherapy alone.

Solitary Pulmonary Nodule

Definition

A solitary pulmonary nodule (SPN), or "coin lesion," is an approximately round lesion that is less than 3 cm in diameter and that is completely surrounded by pulmonary parenchyma, without other abnormalities.

Epidemiology

- Lesions larger than 3 cm are called *masses* and are often malignant.
- An SPN is noted on 0.09% to 0.20% of all chest radiographs. An estimated 150,000 such nodules are identified each year.
- The incidence of cancer in patients with SPNs ranges from 10% to 70%.
- Infectious granulomas cause approximately 80% of the benign lesions, and hamartomas approximately 10%.

Causes of SPN

- Malignant:
  - Bronchogenic carcinoma

- Metastatic lesions
- Pulmonary carcinoid
- Benign:
  - Infectious granuloma (histoplasmosis, tuberculosis, coccidioidomycosis, etc.)
  - Other bacterial and parasitic infections (bacterial abscesses, echinococcus cyst, *Pneumocystis carinii*, aspergilloma, etc.)
  - Benign neoplasms (hamartoma, lipoma, fibroma)
  - Atrioventricular malformation
  - Bronchogenic cyst
  - Wegener granulomatosis
  - Rheumatoid nodule
  - Round atelectasis
  - Hematoma
  - Pseudotumor
  - Pulmonary infarct

Clinical Features
- Helps differentiating between malignant and benign lesions.
- Age, smoking, and another malignancy favor malignant etiology.
- Signs and symptoms suggestive of infection, history of granulomatous disease favor benign etiology.

Diagnosis

Diagnosis can be confirmed with biopsy (bronchoscopy, transthoracic needle aspiration, surgical resection).

- Chest x-ray and CT scan:
  - Try to obtain old films for comparison. More than 2 years of stability on chest x-ray or CT scan favors benign etiology.
  - Lesions larger than 3 cm are particularly likely to be malignant.
  - "Corona radiata" sign (very fine linear strands extending 4 to 5 mm outward from the nodule) and speculated appearance favor malignancy whereas smooth border favors benign etiology.
  - Diffuse homogeneous, central, lamellated (concentric) or "popcorn" calcification favor benign lesion.
  - Malignant lesions tend to have a doubling time between 20 and 400 days whereas benign lesions generally have a doubling time of less than 20 days (infectious causes) or more than 450 days (old granulomatous lesions).
- PET scan:
  - More accurate than CT scan in differentiating benign from malignant lesions as small as 1 cm. PET has sensitivity of 96% and specificity of 79%.
  - False negative with slow growing tumors, small lesions and hyperglycemia.
  - False positive with inflammatory conditions and granulomatous diseases.

Workup and Follow-Up (Figure 12-10)

Fleischner Society guidelines for radiological follow-up of SPN:
- For nodules 4 mm or smaller, serial CT scans are not required if the patient is low risk. Patients who are high risk should have a CT scan performed at 12 months with no further follow-up if the nodule is unchanged.
- For nodules 4 to 6 mm, a CT scan should be performed at 12 months if the patient is low risk, with no further follow-up if the nodule is unchanged. Patients who are high risk should have a CT scan performed at 6 to 12 months and at 18 to 24 months if the nodule is unchanged.
- For nodules 6 to 8 mm, a CT scan should be performed at 6 to 12 months and at 18 to 24 months if the nodule is unchanged and the patient is low risk. Patients who are high risk should have a CT scan performed at 3 to 6 months, 9 to 12 months, and 24 months if the nodule remains unchanged.
- For nodules greater than 8 mm, a CT scan should be performed at 3, 9, and 24 months if the nodule remains unchanged, regardless of whether the patient is low or high risk.

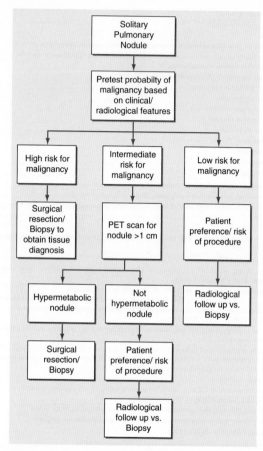

Figure 12-10 Workup and follow-up. PET, positron emission tomography.

Bronchiectasis

Definition

Abnormal, permanent focal or diffuse dilation of airways that could be cylindrical or tubular, varicose, or cystic.

Epidemiology

• Prevalence increases with age, except for patients with cystic fibrosis.
• More common in women than in men.
• Tuberculosis in developing countries is a common cause.
• Approximately 110,000 individuals in the United States have bronchiectasis.

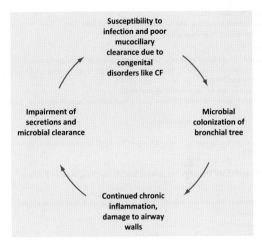

Figure 12-11   Vicious cycle hypothesis. CF, cystic fibrosis.

Pathophysiology
- Vicious cycle hypothesis (Figure 12-11)
- Etiologies
  - Airway obstruction: foreign body aspiration
  - Defective host defenses: hypogammaglobulinemia, common variable immunodeficiency
  - Cystic fibrosis
  - α_1-antitrypsin deficiency
  - Young syndrome
  - Rheumatic and systemic diseases: rheumatoid arthritis, Sjögren syndrome
  - Dyskinetic cilia: Kartagener syndrome
  - Pulmonary infections: tuberculosis, *Mycobacterium avium* complex
  - Allergic bronchopulmonary aspergillosis
  - Cigarette smoking

Clinical Features
- Most common clinical presentation is a persistent productive cough.
- Other symptoms include shortness of breath, fatigue, hemoptysis.
- Clubbing of fingers.
- Crackles and wheezing on physical examination.
- Acute exacerbations of bronchiectasis are characterized by changes in the nature of sputum production with increased volume and purulence, worsening shortness of breath or fatigue.

Diagnosis
- Chest x-ray: thick, dilated airways ("tram tracks"), mucus plugging
- High-resolution computed tomography (HRCT) of the chest is very sensitive and specific: airway dilation (detected as parallel "tram tracks" or as the "signet-ring sign"), lack of bronchial tapering, bronchial wall thickening in dilated airways, inspissated secretions (eg, the "tree-in-bud" pattern), or cysts emanating from the bronchial wall.
- Complete blood count and differential
- Workup for rheumatoid arthritis, other systemic diseases
- Sweat chloride test, genetic testing for cystic fibrosis, α_1-antitrypsin level

- Immunoglobulin levels
- Sputum culture including acid-fast bacillus, fungal cultures
- PFTs: May show airway obstruction

Treatment

- Prolonged (10–14 days) antibiotic therapy with exacerbation of antibiotics.
- Chronic suppressive antibiotic therapy for patients with frequent exacerbations and significant symptoms.
- Prolonged therapy for mycobacterial infections.
- Pulmonary hygiene: bronchodilators, chest physiotherapy, mucolytic agents, hypertonic saline
- Treatment of underlying conditions
- Pulmonary rehabilitation
- Surgical resection in case of very symptomatic localized bronchiectasis or intractable hemoptysis.

Acute Respiratory Distress Syndrome and Acute Respiratory Failure

Definition

Acute respiratory distress syndrome (ARDS) is a clinical syndrome characterized by:

- Acute onset
- Bilateral infiltrates
- No evidence of elevated left atrial pressure
- A ratio of arterial oxygen tension to fraction of inspired oxygen (PaO_2/FiO_2) of less than 200.

A PaO_2/FiO_2 between 200 and 300 identifies patients with acute lung injury (ALI). ALI is a less severe disorder but has the potential to evolve into ARDS.

Epidemiology

- The annual incidences of ALI and ARDS are estimated to be up to 80:100,000 and 60:100,000, respectively.
- Approximately 10% of all ICU admissions suffer from acute respiratory failure, with approximately 20% of these patients meeting criteria for ALI or ARDS.
- The incidence increases with advancing age.

Etiology

- Direct lung injury:
  - Pneumonia
  - Aspiration
  - Pulmonary contusion
  - Near drowning
  - Inhalation injury
- Indirect lung injury:
  - Sepsis **(most common cause)**
  - Severe trauma
  - Multiple bone fractures
  - Flail chest
  - Head trauma
  - Burns
  - Transfusion-related ALI
  - Drug overdose
  - Pancreatitis
  - Cardiopulmonary bypass
  - Lung and hematopoietic stem cell transplant

Pathophysiology

- Exudative phase: Initial 7 days. Accumulation of protein-rich fluid in alveoli and interstitial spaces; release of cytokines, pulmonary vascular injury.

- Proliferative phase: 1 to 3 weeks. Initiation of lung repair, organization of alveolar exudates, and a shift from a neutrophil- to a lymphocyte-predominant pulmonary infiltrate. Proliferation of type II pneumocytes along alveolar basement membranes that differentiate in to type I pneumocytes.
- Fibrotic phase: 3 weeks onward. Extensive alveolar duct and interstitial fibrosis. Acinar architecture is markedly disrupted, leading to emphysema-like changes with large bullae. Intimal fibroproliferation in the pulmonary microcirculation can lead to pulmonary HTN.

Clinical Features

- Initial symptoms are caused by underlying condition.
- Respiratory symptoms start in 48 to 72 hours after inciting event.
- Hypoxia, dyspnea, tachypnea, cough, chest pain may be present.
- Most of the patients require mechanical ventilation.
- Prolonged course with slow recovery.
- Complete recovery may require many months after initial symptoms.

Diagnosis

- ABG: hypoxia, PaO_2/FiO_2 less than 200. The saturation of peripheral oxygen (SpO_2) to FiO_2 less than 235 is correlated with PaO_2/FiO_2 of less than 200.
- Chest x-ray: bilateral infiltrates, no cardiomegaly
- CT chest: patchy infiltrates in dependent areas of lungs, sparing of some areas of lungs.
- Echocardiogram and B-type natriuretic peptide: to rule out cardiac causes of pulmonary edema

Treatment

- Management of underlying condition (ie, sepsis, pneumonia, pancreatitis)
- Nutrition support, DVT prophylaxis, stress ulcer prophylaxis.
- Precautions to avoid aspiration, ventilator associated pneumonia, catheter-related infections.
- Sedation holiday, early physical therapy, protocols for weaning from ventilators.
- Avoid fluid overload.
- Mechanical ventilation (also see the section "Mechanical Ventilation"):
  - Low tidal volume (6–8 mi/kg of ideal body weight).
  - Set initial respiratory rate to achieve baseline minute ventilation.
  - Adjust FiO_2 and positive end-expiratory pressure (PEEP) to achieve oxygenation goal.
  - Adjust respiratory rate, tidal volume, PEEP to achieve pH and plateau pressure goals.
  - Oxygenation goal: PaO_2 55 to 80 mm Hg; SpO_2 88% to 95%
  - Plateau pressure goal less than 30 cm of H_2O
  - pH goal: 7.3 to 7.45. Allow permissive hypercapnia.
- For ARDSnet protocol, please visit http://www.ardsnet.org/system/files/Ventilator%20 Protocol%20Card.pdf
- Use of glucocorticoids is controversial in the treatment of ARDS
- Can try other modes of ventilator: airway pressure release ventilation, high frequency oscillator ventilation, extracorporeal membrane oxygenation in severe cases not responding to traditional modes of mechanical ventilation.

Prognosis

- Overall mortality 26% to 44%
- Mortality is higher with advanced age, chronic liver disease, cirrhosis, chronic alcohol abuse, chronic immunosuppression, sepsis, chronic renal disease, any nonpulmonary organ failure, and increased Acute Physiology and Chronic Health Evaluation (APACHE) III scores.
- PaO_2/FiO_2 ratio is not helpful in predicting mortality.

Interstitial Lung Disease

Classification and Etiology

The interstitial lung diseases (ILDs) also called *diffuse parenchymal lung diseases,* are a heterogeneous group of disorders that are classified together because of similar clinical, radiographic, physiologic, or pathologic manifestations. ILDs are classified into 4 major categories:

MEDICAL SPECIALTIES

- Idiopathic interstitial pneumonia:
  - Usual interstitial pneumonia (UIP) or IPF: most common cause
  - Desquamative interstitial pneumonia
  - Nonspecific interstitial pneumonia
  - Acute interstitial pneumonia
  - Respiratory bronchiolitis interstitial lung disease
  - Cryptogenic organizing pneumonia
  - Lymphoid interstitial pneumonia
- ILD of known etiology:
  - Collagen vascular diseases (systemic sclerosis, rheumatoid arthritis, polymyositis, dermatomyositis, ankylosing spondylitis, etc.)
  - Drug-induced ILDs (methotrexate, amiodarone, nitrofurantoin, etc.)
  - Environmental causes (asbestosis, silicosis, berylliosis, coal worker's pneumoconiosis)
- Granulomatous ILDs:
  - Sarcoidosis
  - Bronchocentric granulomatosis
  - Granulomatous vasculitides
  - Lymphomatoid granulomatosis
- Other forms of ILDs
  - Lymphangioleiomyomatosis (LAM)
  - Pulmonary Langerhans cell histiocytosis (PLCH) and histiocytosis X
  - Eosinophilic pneumonia

History and Clinical Features

- Subacute to chronic presentation except for ILDs caused by allergy (drugs, fungi, helminths), acute interstitial pneumonia, eosinophilic pneumonia, and hypersensitivity pneumonitis where it can be acute.
- Most patients with sarcoidosis, ILD associated with connective tissue disease (CTD), LAM, PLCH present between the ages of 20 and 40 years. Most patients with IPF are older than 60 years of age.
- LAM is exclusively seen in postmenopausal women.
- PLCH, respiratory bronchiolitis and desquamative interstitial pneumonia, Goodpasture syndrome, respiratory bronchiolitis, and pulmonary alveolar proteinosis are more common in smokers.
- Occupational and environmental exposure helps identifying etiology of ILDs.
- Typical symptoms include progressive dyspnea on exertion and nonproductive cough.
- Hemoptysis may be seen with diffuse alveolar hemorrhage syndromes, lymphangioleiomyomatosis.
- Wheezing and chest pain are uncommon but may be present in some patients.
- Symptoms of CTDs and other underlying causes may be present.
- Clubbing present in patients with IPF, asbestosis.
- Cyanosis might be present in patients with advanced disease.
- "Velcro rales" are present in most cases: mainly at bases.
- Scattered late inspiratory high-pitched rhonchi (inspiratory squeaks) are heard in patients with bronchiolitis.
- The cardiac examination may show findings of pulmonary HTN and cor pulmonale in later stages.

Diagnosis

- Chest x-ray: May show reticulonodular pattern, honeycombing. Nonspecific, not very useful in diagnosis.
- HRCT:
  - Useful in early detection and confirmation of suspected ILD.
  - In appropriate clinical settings, HRCT may preclude the need for lung biopsy in IPF, sarcoidosis, hypersensitivity pneumonitis, asbestosis, lymphangitic carcinoma, and PLCH.
  - When a lung biopsy is required, HRCT scanning is useful for determining the most appropriate area from which biopsy samples should be taken.

- PFTs: restrictive defect with reduced $DLCO_2$. Prognostic value in patients with IPF, nonspecific interstitial pneumonia.
- ABG: May show hypoxia and respiratory alkalosis.
- Bronchoscopy and bronchoalveolar lavage: Cellular analysis of bronchoalveolar lavage fluid may be useful in some cases of sarcoidosis, hypersensitivity pneumonitis, diffuse alveolar hemorrhage syndrome, cancer, pulmonary alveolar proteinosis.
- Lung biopsy: Helpful in confirming the diagnosis and assessing disease activity. Biopsy should be obtained before the initiation of treatment. Fiberoptic bronchoscopy with multiple transbronchial lung biopsies is often the initial procedure of choice, especially when sarcoidosis, lymphangitic carcinomatosis, eosinophilic pneumonia, Goodpasture syndrome, or infection is suspected. If a specific diagnosis is not made by transbronchial biopsy, surgical lung biopsy by video-assisted thoracic surgery or open thoracotomy is indicated.

Treatment

- Treatment of underlying condition (ie, collagen vascular disease) if possible.
- Removal of offending agent (drugs, environmental factors, allergens, etc.) when known.
- Supplemental oxygen for hypoxia.
- Pulmonary rehabilitation.
- Glucocorticoid therapy is recommended for symptomatic ILD patients with eosinophilic pneumonias, cryptogenic organizing pneumonia, CTD, sarcoidosis, hypersensitivity pneumonitis, acute inorganic dust exposures, acute radiation pneumonitis, diffuse alveolar hemorrhage, and drug-induced ILD.
- Glucocorticoids have not been shown to be beneficial in patients with UIP (IPF).
- Other immunosuppressive agents (methotrexate, azathioprine, cyclophosphamide) can be tried in patients not responding to glucocorticoids.
- Patients with UIP (IPF) have poor prognosis and generally do not respond to pharmacotherapy.
- Lung transplant can be considered in severe cases with failed pharmacotherapy.

Pulmonary Hypertension

Definition

Pulmonary HTN is defined as a mean pulmonary artery pressure greater than 25 mmHg at rest on right heart catheterization.

Etiology and Classification

- World Health Organization classification of pulmonary HTN.

Pulmonary Arterial HTN (PAH)

- Idiopathic PAH
- Heritable
- Drug- and toxin-induced
- Associated with CTDs, HIV infection, portal HTN, congenital heart diseases, schistosomiasis, chronic hemolytic anemia
- Persistent pulmonary HTN of the newborn
- Pulmonary venoocclusive disease and/or pulmonary capillary hemangiomatosis

Pulmonary HTN Owing to Left Heart Disease

- Systolic dysfunction
- Diastolic dysfunction
- Valvular disease

Pulmonary HTN Owing to Lung Diseases and/or Hypoxia

- COPD
- Interstitial lung disease
- Other pulmonary diseases with mixed restrictive and obstructive pattern
- Sleep-disordered breathing
- Alveolar hypoventilation disorders
- Chronic exposure to high altitude
- Developmental abnormalities

MEDICAL SPECIALTIES

Chronic Thromboembolic Pulmonary HTN

Pulmonary HTN with Unclear Multifactorial Mechanisms

- Hematologic disorders: myeloproliferative disorders, splenectomy
- Systemic disorders: sarcoidosis, pulmonary Langerhans cell histiocytosis (lymphangioleiomyomatosis, neurofibromatosis, vasculitis)
- Metabolic disorders: glycogen storage disease, Gaucher disease, thyroid disorders
- Others: tumoral obstruction, fibrosing mediastinitis, chronic renal failure on dialysis

Clinical Features

- Initial symptoms include exertional dyspnea, lethargy, and fatigue. With progression of disease exertional chest pain (ie, angina), exertional syncope, and peripheral edema may develop because of worsening right ventricular function.
- Passive hepatic congestion may cause anorexia and abdominal pain in the right upper quadrant. Less common symptoms of pulmonary HTN include cough, hemoptysis, and hoarseness because of compression of the left recurrent laryngeal nerve by a dilated main pulmonary artery.
- Symptoms of underlying causes (CTDs, left heart failure, lung diseases) may be present.
- Loud P_2 and wide split of second heart sound might be present on physical examination.
- Systolic murmur of TR and diastolic murmur of PR are also present on auscultation.
- Elevated jugular venous pressure, a right ventricular third heart sound, and a prominent V wave in the jugular venous pulse might be present.
- Hepatomegaly, a pulsatile liver, peripheral edema, ascites, and pleural effusion may exist.

Diagnosis

- Chest x-ray: Enlargement of the central pulmonary arteries with attenuation of the peripheral vessels, right ventricular enlargement and right atrial dilatation may be seen.
- Echocardiogram: Useful screening test. Can assess pulmonary artery systolic pressure from TR jet. Also helpful in assessing right and left ventricular function, valvular heart diseases, pericardial effusion, intracardiac shunts.
- Electrocardiogram might show right ventricular hypertrophy or strain, right axis deviation, incomplete or complete right bundle branch block, or increased P wave amplitude in lead II (P pulmonale) because of right atrial enlargement.
- Right heart catheterization required to confirm the diagnosis and to determine the severity of the hemodynamic derangements. It is helpful in assessing vasodilator response.
- CT scan chest to evaluate pulmonary parenchymal abnormalities associated with underlying cause of pulmonary HTN (CTDs, ILDs, sarcoidosis, etc.)
- PFTs to assess severity of underlying pulmonary disease.
- VQ scan to rule out chronic thromboembolic disease causing pulmonary HTN.
- Workup for CTD: erythrocyte sedimentation rate, rheumatoid arthritis, antinuclear antibody, and so forth.
- HIV test
- Six-minute walk test: prognostic value and also to assess response to therapy.
- ABG: hypoxia.

Treatment

- Treatment of underlying cause.
- All patients with pulmonary HTN should be treated with:
  - Diuretics
  - Supplemental oxygen
  - Anticoagulation
  - Digoxin
  - Exercise
- Pulmonary vasodilator therapy is indicated for patients with World Health Organization group 1 and group 4 pulmonary HTN.
  - Calcium channel blockers: Long-acting nifedipine, diltiazem, or amlodipine. Can be used in patients with significant response to vasodilator on right heart catheterization.
  - Prostanoids:
    - Epoprostenol: IV. Can be used in severe cases; mortality benefit.

- Treprostinil: IV or subcutaneous.
- Iloprost: Inhaled.
- Endothelin receptor antagonist:
  - Bosentan
  - Ambrisentan
  - Sitaxsentan
- Phosphodiesterase-5 inhibitors:
  - Sildenafil
  - Tadalafil
  - Vardenafil
- Atrial septostomy: May be considered in patients with refractory severe PAH and right heart failure, despite aggressive advanced therapy and maximal diuretic therapy.
- Lung transplant: Considered in patients with idiopathic pulmonary arterial HTN.

Noninvasive Positive Pressure Ventilation

Definition

- Application of external device that performs work to support or assist ventilator function through the upper airway through a noninvasive airway (eg, sealed facemask). The inspiratory and expiratory pressure support are considered and ordered separately in noninvasive positive pressure ventilation. The operator assigns inspiratory and expiratory pressures and FiO_2. This form of ventilatory support is used in acute settings, but variations are also used in obstructive sleep apnea and some types of chronic hypercarbic respiratory failure. When inspiratory and expiratory pressures are equivalent, the term *continuous positive airway pressure* is commonly used.

Epidemiology

This form of ventilatory support has become increasingly common, but is still used in a small fraction (~3%–5%) of critically ill patients because of limited indications.

Pathophysiology

- Noninvasive positive pressure ventilation (NIPPV) is primarily used to support ventilation and maintain an open upper airway. Improvements in oxygenation are also common, however.
- NIPPV maintains constant positive pressure that stents open upper airway tissue to prevent collapse as seen in obstructive sleep apnea. The positive expiratory pressure is equivalent to PEEP used in mechanical ventilation and can aid in recruitment of atelectatic alveoli. Positive inspiratory pressure decreases the work of breathing in patients with hypercarbic respiratory failure.

Clinical Features

- The indication for NIPPV in the acute setting is an awake patient with hypercarbic respiratory failure in a patient suffering from cardiogenic pulmonary edema or COPD exacerbation. These ailments are generally quick to respond to therapy and thus lead to a short duration of illness.
- Use of NIPPV in other disease processes is not supported by published data, but may be reasonable if the disease process is expected to reverse quickly and the patient has the ability to protect his or her airway. Use may also be considered in patients who are not candidates for endotracheal intubation.
- Chronic use may be considered in patients with obstructive sleep apnea, obesity-hypoventilation syndrome, neuromuscular weakness, or other documented chronic hypercarbic respiratory failure.

Mechanical Ventilation

Definition

- Application of external device that performs work to support or assist ventilator function. This may be performed through an invasive airway (eg endotracheal tube) or a noninvasive airway (eg sealed facemask), although typically an invasive airway is implied. All forms of modern mechanical ventilation apply positive pressure to the airway to support the work of breathing.

- Variations in the methods for delivery of positive pressure are common. The various "modes" are determined by the parameters that must be set by an operator. The main parameters may include tidal volume, peak inspiratory pressure, PEEP, respiratory rate, pressure support, FiO_2, flow rate, inspiratory time, and expiratory time. Whether these parameters are fixed or variable is determined on the mode of ventilation one chooses.

Epidemiology

- Approximately one-half of ICU patients are supported by mechanical ventilation at the time of admission. Approximately 3% of all hospitalized patients require mechanical ventilation at some point during their stay.

- Among ICU patients, mechanically ventilated patients suffer a 100% increased unadjusted mortality rate versus nonmechanically ventilated patients. The risk is equivalent if adjusted for severity of illness.

Pathophysiology

- Mechanical ventilation is an intervention used to support ventilation, and/or support oxygenation. This is usually performed in conjunction with an artificial airway (eg endotracheal tube).

- Mechanical ventilation is continued so long as the patient is unable to maintain or protect his or her innate airway, sustain the work of breathing necessary to eliminate adequate CO_2, or efficiently exchange O_2 at a FiO_2 that is easily reproduced without mechanical ventilation. Data support the regular (daily) assessment of these criteria by use of spontaneous breathing trials when the patient is not sedated.

Clinical Features

- Patterns of use of mechanical ventilation to support ventilation and oxygenation are variable.

- Management of hypoxic respiratory failure: Mechanical ventilation is often a successful strategy for the management of hypoxic respiratory failure related to poor diffusion of gas through the alveolar-capillary membrane or VQ mismatch. Hypoxemia caused by true right-to-left shunt is not typically improved by mechanical ventilation.

  - Acute increases in PaO_2 (and SpO_2) in the pulmonary venous circulation is determined by 2 primary variables:

    - FiO_2: Increasing FiO_2 improves the diffusion of O_2 from alveolar spaces into the pulmonary capillaries with increases in hemoglobin saturation and dissolved O_2 in the blood.

    - Mean airway pressure: Manipulation of ventilator modes and settings that increase the mean airway pressure (over the respiratory cycle) also increase diffusion of O_2 from alveolar spaces into the pulmonary capillaries.

  - Alveolar recruitment (opening of atelectatic alveoli) will also typically improve hypoxemia by providing increased diffusion capacity. Alveolar recruitment is largely determined by the PEEP. Mean airway pressure and peak pressures may also play a role.

- Management of hypercarbic respiratory failure: The pH of the blood is determined by dissolved acids, including CO_2. Inadequate minute ventilation will lead to a falling pH by failing to exhale CO_2 in equilibrium with production (primary respiratory acidosis). In the setting of a metabolic production of copious amount of organic acids, the failure of minute ventilation to increase proportionally will also lead to a falling pH (secondary respiratory acidosis). If a patient is unable to reverse or stabilize a respiratory acidosis then mechanical ventilation is a necessary supportive measure.

  - Increases in respiratory rate or tidal volume will increase minute ventilation and improve elimination of CO_2.

- Airway protection: Aspiration of gastric contents, secretions, or foreign objects may lead to pneumonia, pneumonitis, airway obstruction, and/or death. In patients who lack cough, gag, or normal pharyngeal muscle activity, the use of an artificial airway (usually paired with mechanical ventilation) should be considered.

CHAPTER 13

Rheumatology

Joan K. Kowalec and Robert G. Lahita

Rheumatology encompasses a wide variety of musculoskeletal conditions and systematic diseases including arthritis. A careful history and physical examination will allow a diagnosis in the majority of cases. Laboratory testing and imaging play a supporting role in most cases.

CLINICAL APPROACH TO THE PATIENT WITH RHEUMATIC DISEASE

History

A history of present illness that includes complaint of stiffness, arthralgia, back pain, myalgia, or paresthesias suggests the possibility of rheumatologic disease.

Stiffness

• Widespread, to suggest inflammatory polyarthritis.
• Localized to joint (gelling of osteoarthritis).
• To proximal muscles (polymyalgia rheumatica).
• To areas around joints (nonarticular rheumatism).

Arthralgia

• Without swelling of joint(s): Consider osteoarthritis, overuse, systemic rheumatic disease (systemic lupus erythematosus, scleroderma), medical illness hypothyroidism, infection, renal failure, etc.).
• With swelling of joint(s): Consider noninflammatory causes such as osteoarthritis, trauma and osteonecrosis and inflammatory causes including rheumatoid arthritis, crystal-induced arthritis, seronegative spondyloarthropathy, arthritis with connective tissue disease (may also be noninflammatory).
• With constitutional symptoms: infection or malignancy.

Back Pain

• With overuse or trauma, with or without neurologic deficit, aggravated with activity: mechanical back pain (degenerative, disc herniation, fracture).
• With prolonged morning stiffness, improvement with activity: inflammatory back pain (seronegative spondyloarthropathy).
• With constitutional symptoms: infection, malignancy.

Myalgia

• Localized: strain, localized myofascial syndrome, trauma, polymyalgia rheumatica.
• Widespread: systemic rheumatic disease (systemic lupus erythematosus, inflammatory myopathy), drug-induced (statins, biologics, etc.) medical illness (endocrine/metabolic, malignancy, infection).

Paresthesias

• Localized: Entrapment neuropathy (carpal tunnel syndrome, tarsal tunnel syndrome, etc.), radiculopathy.
• Diffuse without constitutional symptoms, peripheral neuropathy; with constitutional symptoms, systemic rheumatic disease or vasculitis syndrome.

Past Medical History

Additional past medical history can reveal conditions presaging certain rheumatic disease: Consider psoriasis (psoriatic arthritis), inflammatory bowel disease (arthritis of inflammatory bowel disease), uveitis (seronegative spondyloarthropathy), chronic systemic corticosteroid therapy such as for asthma or organ transplant (a vascular necrosis), hepatitis C (cryoglobulinemia), recurrent deep vein thrombosis, or miscarriage (antiphospholipid syndrome).

Medications

Consider hydralazine and drug-induced lupus, oral contraceptives and erythema nodosum, statins and myopathy, allopurinol and hypersensitivity syndrome, colchicine and neuromyopathy, chronic systemic corticosteroid therapy, and avascular necrosis among others.

Family History

Certain rheumatic diseases that are likely to have occurred in relatives of the patient with rheumatic disease include rheumatoid arthritis, systemic lupus erythematosus, psoriasis and psoriatic arthritis, and ankylosing spondylitis.

Social History

- Occupation or recreational activity predisposing to osteoarthritis, internal derangement of the knee, lumbar disc herniation, entrapment neuropathy.
- Recreational drug use: marijuana (myopathy), cocaine (vasculopathy), septic arthritis.
- Sexual exposure: disseminated gonococcal infection and gonococcal septic arthritis, reactive arthropathy, arthritis with hepatitis B antigenemia, vasculitis with hepatitis B infection.

Review of Systems

Review of systems is helpful for missed clues. Did you forget abdominal pain (mesenteric vasculitis), oral ulcers (Behçet disease), dry eyes and mouth (sicca syndrome, Sjögren's syndrome)?

Physical Examination

- The complete general examination is always necessary to reveal manifestations of systemic rheumatic disease and extraarticular manifestations of joint disease.
- The musculoskeletal examination.
  - Examination of both involved and uninvolved joints to determine:
    - Articular (diffuse tenderness, pain on active and passive motion in all directions, usually swelling) versus periarticular disease (focal tenderness, pain on motion in less than all planes, swelling not common).
    - Presence of joint swelling
    - Range of motion (Table 13-1). Be mindful that full painless range of motion of a painful joint can mean referred pain such as hip disease for knee pain, cholecystitis for shoulder pain, abdominal aortic aneurysm for low back pain.
    - Contracture or deformity
    - Stability
  - Muscle examination to determine:
    - Tenderness
    - Atrophy
    - Strength
      - 5:5 normal
      - 4:5 active motion
      - 3:5 active motion possible against gravity
      - 2:5 active motion possible gravity eliminated
      - 1:5 trace of contraction
      - 0:5 no muscle contraction

Laboratory Testing

General Laboratory Tests

The serum chemistry including uric-acid level, complete blood count and urinalysis will not be diagnostic but may suggest organ system involvement in systemic rheumatic disease and will be a necessary consideration in arriving at a safe therapeutic approach.

Acute Phase Reactants

The erythrocyte sedimentation rate (ESR) is a nonspecific marker of inflammatory process. While the markedly elevated ESR is commonly associated with giant cell (temporal)

**TABLE 13-1. RANGE OF MOTION FOR UPPER AND LOWER
          EXTREMITY JOINTS**

Upper Extremities	Lower Extremities
Distal Interphalangeal: • Flexion 75° • Extension 0°	Metatarsalphalyngeal: • Flexion 30° • Extension 80°
Proximal Interphalangeal: • Flexion 110° • Extension 0°	Subtalar: • Inversion 30° • Eversion 20°
Metacarpophalangeal: • Flexion 80° • Extension 25°	Ankle: • Flexion 45° • Extension 20°
Wrist: • Flexion 80° • Extension 60° • Ulnar deviation 60° • Radial deviation 25°	Knee: • Flexion 130° • Extension 0°
Elbow: • Flexion 150° • Extension 0–5°	Hip: • Flexion 120° • Extension 15° • Abduction 45° • Rotation 45°
Shoulder: • Flexion 180° • Abduction 90° • Rotation 90°	Spine: • Cervical forward flexion 40° • Lateral bending 30° • Extension 30° • Lateral rotation 60°
	Lumbar: • Forward flexion 90° • Lateral bending 30° • Extension 30°

arthritis, rheumatologic disease is not the most common association. Infection (33%), malignancy (17%), and renal disease (17%) have been demonstrated to exceed rheumatic disease (14%).[1] The C-reactive protein (CRP) also serves as a nonspecific marker for inflammatory activity, which rises and falls quicker than the ESR. Both the ESR and CRP are best used to monitor activity of an inflammatory disease and assess response to a therapeutic approach; which works best in a given clinical situation will need to be determined.

Specific Rheumatologic Tests

• Autoantibodies
  • Rheumatoid factor (RF) and anticyclic citrullinated peptide (anti-CCP): RF, an antibody against the Fc portion of immunoglobulin G (IgG) antibodies is positive in at least 60% of patients with rheumatoid arthritis, but it is also detected in 4% of the normal population and 25% of older individuals as well as in patients with a variety of illnesses including other rheumatic disease, mixed cryoglobulinemia, chronic liver disease, and subacute bacterial endocarditis. The anti-CCP is an enzyme-linked immunosorbent assay (ELISA) that demonstrates presence of antibodies to CCPs; it is more specific than RF for rheumatoid arthritis (95% vs 85%) with similar sensitivity (67% vs 69%).[2]
  • Antinuclear antibodies (ANA): The test demonstrates antibodies directed against the cell nucleus, and the presence of ANA is most commonly associated with systemic

TABLE 13-2. ASSOCIATION OF SPECIFIC DISEASES WITH
              ANTINUCLEAR ANTIBODIES

ANAs/Disease Association

1. Anti-dsDNA/SLE

2. Antihistone /SLE, drug-induced lupus

3. Anti-Smith/SLE (most specific)

4. Anti-RNP/SLE, mixed connective tissue disease, myositis

5. Anti-SSA/Sjögren syndrome, SLE

6. Anti-SSB/Sjögren syndrome

7. Anti-Scl-70 (antitopoisomerase)/diffuse systemic sclerosis

8. Anticentromere/limited systemic sclerosis

9. Anti-Jo-1/polymyositis/dermatomyositis, antisynthetase disorder

ANA, antinuclear antibody; SLE, systemic lupus erythematosus.

lupus erythematosus; however, they are detected in many other systemic rheumatic and autoimmune disorders as well as in the normal population with up to 30% of the latter demonstrating levels of 1:40 and 13% at 1:80 (Table 13-2).[3]

- Antineutrophil cytoplasmic antibodies (ANCAs): Testing for ANCA aids in the diagnosis of Wegener granulomatosis and microscopic poly arthritis. The c-ANCA correlates with antibodies to proteinase-3, the p-ANCA with antibodies to myeloperoxidase. A positive ANCA test is significant only if the screening test is associated with specific antibodies to proteinase-3 and myeloperoxidase (Table 13-3).

Churg-Strauss Syndrome

- Antiphospholipid antibodies are antibodies detected against phospholipids, and their presence is associated with the antiphospholipid syndrome (arterial and venous clotting events, miscarriage, thrombocytopenia) but also and in greater proportion in other specialty patients as well as in up to 5% of the general population:[4]
  - Rheumatology – antiphospholipid syndrome, systemic lupus erythematosus, rheumatoid arthritis, Sjögren syndrome, Behçet disease
  - Hematology and Oncology – arterial and venous thrombosis, thrombocytopenia, Coombs-positive hemolytic anemia, malignancy
  - Cardiology – Libman-Sacks endocarditis, coronary thrombosis
  - Pulmonary – pulmonary embolus, pulmonary hypertension
  - Neurology – cerebral thrombosis, transient ischemic attack, chorea, transverse myelopathy, migraine
  - Dermatology – livedo reticularis, digital gangrene
  - Infectious Disease – acquired immunodeficiency syndrome, mononucleosis
- Serum complement levels
  The most commonly measured are CH50, which demonstrates function of the classical pathway, and individual components C3 and C4; the most common abnormality is

TABLE 13-3. ANTINEUTROPHIL CYTOPLASMIC ANTIBODIES: TESTING
              AND CORRELATION WITH SPECIFIC ANTIBODIES

ANCA Disease	Positivity (%)	PR3 (%)	MPO (%)
Wegener Granulomatosis	90 (c)	85	10
Limited Wegener Granulomatosis	50 (c)	Mostly	
Microscopic Polyangiitis	75 (c,p)	10	70
Churg-Strauss Syndrome	50 (p)	More often	

ANCA, antineutrophil cytoplasmic antibodies; MPO, myeloperoxidase; PR3, proteinase 3; c, cytoplasmic; p, peripheral.

hypercomplementia as an acute phase reactant, while depressed levels are seen in disease states associated with immune complex deposition.

- Synovial fluid analysis

  Examination of the synovial fluid includes the only two diagnostic tests in rheumatology, the identification of crystals including monosodium urate (gout) and calcium pyrophosphate dehydrate (pseudogout) and the finding of organisms (bacterial septic arthritis); in addition, synovial fluid may be classified as follows:

  - Normal: yellow, clear, high viscosity, nucleated cells less than 200 with less than 25% neutrophils
  - Group 1 (noninflammatory): yellow, clear, high viscosity, nucleated cells less than 2000 with less than 25% neutrophils; consider osteoarthritis, traumatic arthritis
  - Group 2 (inflammatory): yellow, slightly turbid-turbid, 2000 to 50,000 (but may be higher), nucleated cells with more than 50% neutrophils: consider rheumatoid arthritis, crystal-induced arthritis, reactive arthropathy
  - Group 3 (infectious inflammatory): yellow indicates purulent, more than 50,000 nucleated cells with more than 90% neutrophils

Note: The arthritis of systemic lupus erythematosus may be noninflammatory and when mildly inflammatory associated with a predominantly mononuclear differential.

Imaging

- Plain radiology: Plain films are more important for the diagnosis of bony conditions (fracture, tumor, osteonecrosis) than for articular conditions except for ankylosing spondylitis for which the presence of bilateral sacroiliitis is a necessary criterion; they are more helpful in following the progression of joint disease.
- Magnetic resonance imaging (MRI) is the study of choice for imaging soft tissue structures of joints and the diagnosis of early osteonecrosis and valuable for investigating disorders affecting the axial skeleton; cost is an issue, and the test has been precluded by the presence of pacemakers.
- Computed tomography (CT) is useful for evaluating the bony architecture of the spine especially mechanical disorders such as spinal stenosis, spondylolisthesis, trauma.
- Ultrasound is valuable for assessing fluid collections including popliteal cysts and ganglion cysts and guiding their aspiration.
- Scintigraphy can be used to assess extent of musculoskeletal disease such as Paget disease of bone and osteonecrosis and may be used to qualify persistent arthralgia with a normal joint examination.

Electrodiagnostic Testing

- Electromyography may demonstrate characteristic findings in inflammatory myopathy (polymyositis, dermatomyositis) and exclude neuropathy as cause for muscle weakness.
- Nerve conduction testing is appropriate for assessing peripheral neuropathies; diagnostic findings are seen with entrapment neuropathy (carpal tunnel syndrome, tarsal tunnel syndrome), Guillain-Barre syndrome, Eton-Lambert syndrome, myasthenia gravis.

ASPECTS OF DIFFERENTIAL DIAGNOSIS IN RHEUMATOLOGY

Number of Joints Involved

- Acute or chronic
- Inflammatory or noninflammatory
- Monoarticular acute noninflammatory: trauma, internal derangement of knee, sickle cell arthropathy.
- Acute inflammatory: septic arthritis, crystal-induced arthritis, viral arthritis, reactive arthritis, lyme disease.
- Chronic noninflammatory: osteoarthritis, osteonecrosis, pigmented villonodular synovitis, Charcot arthropathy.
- Chronic inflammatory: tuberculous arthritis, fungal arthritis, psoriatic arthritis, lyme disease, pseudogout.

Oligoarticular and Polyarticular

- Acute inflammatory: sickle cell crisis
- Acute inflammatory: viral arthritis, septic arthritis, acute rheumatic fever, reactive arthritis.

- Chronic noninflammatory: osteoarthritis, hemochromatosis, hypertrophic osteoarthropathy.
- Chronic inflammatory: rheumatoid arthritis, psoriatic arthritis, crystal-induced arthritis with connective tissue disease (may be noninflammatory)

Joint Distribution: Symmetry and Location

Symmetry

- Symmetric noninflammatory: osteoarthritis
- Symmetric inflammatory: rheumatoid arthritis, psoriatic arthritis, viral arthritis, arthritis of connective disease.
- Asymmetric noninflammatory: osteoarthritis, osteonecrosis, traumatic arthritis, internal derangement of knee.
- Asymmetric inflammatory: septic arthritis, crystal-blood arthritis, psoriatic arthritis.

Location

Upper Extremity

- Distal interphalangeal joint: osteoarthritis, psoriatic arthritis
- Proximal interphalangeal joint: osteoarthritis, rheumatoid arthritis, psoriatic arthritis, gout, arthritis of connective tissue disease, arthritis of inflammatory bowel disease
- Metacarpophalangeal joint: rheumatoid arthritis, psoriatic arthritis, hemochromatosis, gout, viral arthritis, arthritis of connective tissue disease, arthritis of inflammatory bowel disease
- First carpometacarpal joint: osteoarthritis
- Wrist: rheumatoid arthritis, psoriatic arthritis, crystal-induced arthritis, viral arthritis, arthritis of connective tissue disease, arthritis of inflammatory bowel disease, de Quervain tenosynovitis
- Elbow: rheumatoid arthritis, gout, medial and lateral epicondylitis, triceps tendonitis, olecranon bursitis
- Shoulder: glenohumeral or acromioclavicular arthritis, osteonecrosis, subacromial bursitis, rotator cuff or bicipital tendonitis, referred (cervical radiculopathy), brachial plexopathy, thoracic outlet (impingement), polymyalgia rheumatica

Lower Extremity

- Hip: osteoarthritis, rheumatoid arthritis, arthritis of inflammatory bowel disease, ankylosing spondylitis, trochanteric bursitis, ischiogluteal bursitis, iliopsoas bursitis, polymyalgia rheumatica
- Knee: osteoarthritis, rheumatoid arthritis, crystal-induced arthritis, reactive arthritis, arthritis of inflammatory bowel disease, osteonecrosis, anserine bursitis, pre and infrapatellar bursitis, internal derangement
- Ankle: gout, rheumatoid arthritis, Achilles tendonitis, retrocalcaneal bursitis, plantar fasciitis
- Metatarsophalangeal joint: osteoarthritis, (great toe), gout, rheumatoid arthritis, psoriatic arthritis, reactive arthritis, viral arthritis, arthritis of connective tissue disease, arthritis of inflammatory bowel disease
- Proximal interphalangeal joint: rheumatoid arthritis, crystal-induced arthritis, reactive arthritis, arthritis of inflammatory bowel disease, arthritis of connective tissue disease
- Distal interphalangeal joint: osteoarthritis, psoriatic arthritis.
Note: Realize that any joint may become infected.

Arthritis with Eye Involvement

- Conjunctivitis: reactive arthritis
- Uveitis: ankylosing spondylitis and other seronegative spondyloarthropathy, Lyme and Behçet disease
- Scleritis and episcleritis: rheumatoid arthritis, Wegener granulomatosis, relapsing polychondritis
- Corneal ulceration: rheumatoid arthritis, vasculitis
- Keratoconjunctivitis sicca (dry eye): rheumatoid arthritis and other connective tissue disease, primary Sjögren syndrome

Arthritis and Dermatology

- Gottron papules, heliotrope, shawl or V-neck signs: dermatomyositis
- Psoriasis: arthritis, reactive arthritis
- Erythema nodosum: Behçet disease, arthritis with inflammatory bowel disease
- Pyoderma gangrenosum: rheumatoid arthritis, Behçet disease, arthritis with inflammatory bowel disease
- Palpable purpura: leukocytoclastic vasculitis associated with rheumatoid arthritis, systemic lupus erythematosus, Sjögren syndrome
- Erythema chronica migrans: Lyme disease
- Nodular lesions: rheumatoid arthritis (rheumatoid nodule), gout (tophus), rheumatic fever associated nodules, Achilles tendonitis (cholesterol nodules), necrotizing arthritis

Arthritis and Pulmonary Disease

- Bibasilar interstitial lung disease: rheumatoid arthritis, diffuse systemic sclerosis, polymyositis.
- Upper lobe pulmonary fibrosis: ankylosing spondylitis.
- Cavitary lung disease: Wegener granulomatosis.
- Alveolar hemorrhage: microscopic polyangiitis, system lupus erythematosus.

Arthritis and Abdominal Pain and Diarrhea

- Arthritis with inflammatory bowel disease
- Reactive arthritis
- Whipple disease
- Celiac disease

Arthritis with Renal Disease

- Systemic lupus erythematosus
- Diffuse systemic sclerosis
- Polyarteritis nodosa
- Wegener granulomatosis

Arthritis and Hematologic Disease

- Sickle cell disease: severe arthralgia with crisis, bone infarcts, avascular necrosis, sickle cell arthropathy
- Hemophilia: destructive arthropathy
- Hemochromatosis: osteoarthritis involving unusual joints including Metacarpophalangeal joints, shoulders, elbows, ankles

Arthritis and Infection

- Bacterial septic arthritis: acute monoarticular arthritis
- Parvovirus B19 and rubella: symmetrical polyarthritis
- Human immunodeficiency virus infection: acute mils arthritis with initial viremia, persistent oligoarthritis or polyarthritis with acquired immunodeficiency syndrome (AIDS)
- Hepatitis A, B: small joint arthritis subsiding with the onset of jaundice
- Lyme disease: arthralgia early, episodic oligoarthritis late
- Tuberculosis: spondylitis (Pott disease), monoarticular arthritis of weightbearing joints, osteomyelitis, reactive arthritis (Poncet disease)
- Subacute bacterial endocarditis: positive rheumatoid factor, immune complex mediated arthralgia and arthritis
- Multisystem disease: Think vasculitis
- Second and third decades of life: aortic arch arteritis (Takayasu disease)
- Fifth decade of life: Wegener granulomatosis, polyarteritis nodosa, allergic granulomatous arteritis
- Sixth decade of life: essential cryoglobulinemia, isolated central nervous system vasculitis.

- Seventh and eight decade of life: giant cell (temporal) arteritis
- Any age: hypersensitivity vasculitis and serum sickness vasculitis with connective tissue disease, infection, and malignancy-associated vasculitis

SPECIFIC RHEUMATOLOGIC DISEASES

Ankylosing Spondyloarthropathy

- Ankylosing spondylitis (AS) is primarily an inflammatory arthritis of the back.
  - Sacroiliac and apophyseal joints of the spine affected
  - Occurs in men more than women in a 9:1 ratio
  - Age of onset: late teens.
  - AS begins gradually with pain and stiffness in the low back.
  - Nocturnal back pain is the most characteristic feature
  - Deformities result as AS progresses to involve the whole spine and includes:
    - Flattening of the lumbar lordosis, kyphosis of the thoracic spine
    - Hyperextension of the cervical spine
    - These result in flexion contractures of the hips and knees with significant morbidity and disability.
- Peripheral arthritis is not common, but when it develops early in the disease course is a predictor of progression.
- The presentation of arthritis in the lower extremities is asymmetric.
- The "axial" joints include the shoulders and hips and are more common than involvement of the distal joints.
- Enthesitis is inflammation of tendons and their insertions.
- In AS, the Achilles tendon and the insertion of the tendon or plantar fascia, into the calcaneus can be affected.
- It is inflammatory in nature and aggravated by rest and improves with activity.
- Extraarticular features include:
  - Iritis
  - Anterior uveitis
  - Dilatation of the aortic root and conduction defects
  - Fibrosis of the upper lobes of the lungs
  - Cauda equina syndrome from multiple thecal diverticulum or dilated lumbar sacs
  - Amyloidosis late in the course of disease

Radiographic Findings

- Sacroiliac joints show erosions with subsequent ankylosis
- In the spine, the thoracolumbar junction is an early site of involvement, and subsequent progression affects the whole spine.
- An early radiologic sign is squaring of the vertebra, followed by the development of syndesmophytes (the result of ossification of the outer layer of the nucleus fibrosus of the intervertebral disc).
- In the late stages of the disease, total ankylosis of the spine occurs with ossification of the longitudinal ligaments.

Etiology

- The cause of ankylosing spondylitis is unknown.
- Genetic, environmental, and immunological factors play a role in its pathogenesis.
- There have been multiple studies of human leukocyte antigen (HLA)-B27 in ankylosing spondylitis, showing increased frequencies in patients with ankylosing spondylitis in most populations studied.
- In individuals who clearly have "bamboo spine," HLA-B27 is irrelevant.

Clinical Diagnosis

There are new criteria for the diagnosis of axial spondyloarthropathy. Entry criteria that need to be satisfied:

- Back pain for at least 3 months.
- Age of onset before 45 years.

Once entry criteria are satisfied, a second group of criteria become relevant:

- Sacroiliitis on imaging studies (with one or more of the features given in the list below).
- HLA-B27 positive (with two or more of the features listed below).
- The Assessment of Spondyloarthritis International Society list of classification criteria include:
  - Inflammatory back pain
  - Arthritis—diagnosed by a clinician
  - Enthesitis—diagnosed by a clinician
  - Uveitis—past or present anterior uveitis, diagnosed by an ophthalmologist
  - Dactylitis—diagnosed by a clinician
  - Psoriasis—diagnosed by a clinician
  - Inflammatory bowel disease
  - Good response to nonsteroidal antiinflammatory drugs (NSAIDs)
  - Family history of spondyloarthropathy
  - HLA-B27 positive
  - Elevated CRP

The sensitivity and specificity of this set of criteria are 84% and 83%, respectively.

Treatment

- NSAIDs are the first line of therapy.
- Exercise programs are particularly important for these patients to maintain functional spinal outcomes.
- Disease-modifying medications like sulfasalazine have been used with benefits.
- Intraarticular corticosteroid injections may be of benefit for individual peripheral joints
- Anti-tumor necrosis factor (TNF) agents are useful in treating severe ankylosing spondylitis.

Reactive Arthritis

- Begins after an infection of the genitourinary or gastrointestinal tract
- Manifests at least one other extraarticular feature.
- Majority of patients are males who carry the HLA-B27 antigen
- The old term "Reiter's syndrome" refers to the clinical triad of nongonococcal urethritis, conjunctivitis, and arthritis first described by Reiter in 1916.
- Reactive arthritis were documented following infections with *Shigella*, *Salmonella*, *Campylobacter*, and *Yersinia*.
- Reactive arthritis is asymmetric.
- Distal interphalangeal joint involvement and the sacroiliitis is often asymmetric.
- Skin lesions seen are sometimes difficult to distinguish from pustular psoriasis, both clinically and pathologically; both lesions affect the palms and soles and have similar pathological features.
- Dactylitis is a feature of reactive arthritis.

Radiography

- Spinal changes and peripheral joint changes.
  - Spine:
    - Asymmetric sacroiliitis and paramarginal syndesmophytes are seen, in contrast to the symmetric sacroiliitis and marginal syndesmophytes, which typify ankylosing spondylitis.
  - Peripheral Joints:
    - Erosive changes in distal interphalangeal joints, which in extreme cases lead to "pencil-in-cup" changes.
    - There may also be periosteal reaction.
    - These changes are similar to those seen in psoriatic arthritis.
    - Like patients with ankylosing spondylitis, patients with reactive arthritis manifest enthesitis, particularly around the ankle joints.
    - Reactive arthritis erosions at the Achilles tendon insertion may be noted.

Other Findings

- Pathology of the eye:
  - Conjunctivitis in 30% to 60% of the patients.

- Conjunctivitis appears to be more common among patients with sexually acquired and post-*Shigella* reactive arthritis than in patients with other prior infections.
- Urethritis is a sterile urethritis
  - In many cases *Chlamydia trachomatis* and *Ureaplasma urealyticum* have been isolated.
- Circinate balanitis is a painless erythematous lesion of the glans penis seen in 25% of patients.
- Oral ulcers are superficial and painless.
- Skin manifestations
  - Keratodermia blenorrhagica
    - A hyperkeratotic lesion that progresses to macules, papules, and nodules.
    - Found on the palms and soles
    - Bacteria have seldom been isolated from the joints of patient with this condition, so it is called *reactive arthritis*.

Diagnosis

- Presence of a typical arthritis, affecting the lower limbs and asymmetrical.
- Evidence of a preceding infection with either diarrhea or urethritis is important.
- The presence of conjunctivitis and urethritis are also helpful in making the diagnosis.

Treatment

- NSAIDs
- Severe cases, sulfasalazine
- Methotrexate or azathioprine (Imuran) may be used in those patients with refractive disease
- Use of antibiotics is not appropriate.
- Reactive arthritis is self-limited and can last 3 to 12 months.

Psoriatic Arthritis

- An inflammatory arthritis associated with psoriasis
- One-third of patients with psoriasis can develop an inflammatory form of arthritis
- Actual disease prevalence is unknown
- Skin manifestations precede the joint features in 80% of patients.
- Etiology: Unknown but, genetic, immunologic, and environmental factors are considered important.

Presentation

Several patterns of presentation of psoriatic arthritis:

- Distal interphalangeal joints are involved.
- An oligoarticular pattern, affecting four or fewer joints.
- Polyarticular disease, affecting five or more joints often in an asymmetric distribution.
- Arthritis mutilans, a destructive form of arthritis.
- A spondyloarthropathy involving the sacroiliac joints and the joints of the spine.

Clinical Features

- Psoriatic arthritis is asymmetrical.
- Can be distinguished from rheumatoid arthritis by the absence of rheumatoid factor, the presence of distal joint disease, and the spondyloarthropathy.
- A feature of psoriatic arthritis is the presence of skin and nail lesions.
  - The majority of patients present with their skin lesions prior to the joint manifestations.
  - They may be hidden and the patient carefully examined to achieve the correct diagnosis.
  - Nail lesions; include pits and onycholysis, in more than 80% of the patients.
  - Dactylitis or sausage digit occurs in 35% of patients.
  - Iritis occurs in patients with psoriatic arthritis as it does in the other spondyloarthropathies.
  - Urethritis can also be found.
- Patients with psoriatic arthritis have an erosive arthritis.
  - Unlike rheumatoid arthritis there is no juxtaarticular osteopenia
  - Classically, there is the presence of pencil-in-cup changes, ankylosis, and periosteal reaction.
  - Erosive disease in the distal interphalangeal joints is typical for psoriatic arthritis.

- RF is negative.
- It is more difficult to make the diagnosis of psoriatic arthritis in a patient not known to have psoriasis.
- Clinical and radiographic features, including the pattern of the arthritis, the distribution, the joints involved, and the presence of a spondyloarthropathy, may facilitate the diagnosis. It is therefore crucial to perform a careful history and physical examination.

Treatment

- One must treat the skin and joint aspects of the disease simultaneously.
- Use NSAIDs for joint disease.
- Topical therapies for the skin.
- Disease-modifying drugs like the anti-TNF agents are appropriate for early use.
- Use of drugs like methotrexate, retinoic acid derivatives, psoralen with ultraviolet A light treatment and cyclosporine are also appropriate in conjunction with the anti-TNF agents.
- Infliximab is effective in controlling severe psoriasis.
- Etanercept is approved by the U.S. Food and Drug Administration for use in psoriatic arthritis.
- There is no role for antimalarial agents in the treatment of psoriatic arthritis.

Arthritis of Inflammatory Bowel Disease

- The arthritis that complicates inflammatory bowel disease, including Crohn disease and ulcerative colitis occurs in up to 20% of patients.
- Some patients actually present with the inflammatory arthritis before the diagnosis of inflammatory bowel disease is recognized.
- May begin at any age, most often in young males and females in an equal distribution.
- The arthritis is migratory or additive, is commonly asymmetric, and affects primarily the lower extremity joints.
  - It may be indistinguishable from rheumatoid arthritis in those with ulcerative colitis.
  - Deformities are rare.
  - The activity of the arthritis parallels the activity of the bowel inflammation.
  - There can also be granulomas of bones and joints and periostitis.
  - Spondyloarthropathy of inflammatory bowel disease is very similar to that of idiopathic AS.
    - It occurs more commonly in men than women and is not affected by the bowel inflammation.
- Skin lesions are more likely to be erythema nodosum in Crohn disease and pyoderma gangrenosum in ulcerative colitis.
- An extraarticular manifestation includes clubbing, which may occur in patients with either Crohn disease or ulcerative colitis and may be associated with the presence of erythema nodosum, granulomatous vasculitis, amyloidosis, osteoporosis, and osteomalacia.
- Both genetic and environmental factors lead to inflammatory bowel disease and spondyloarthropathy.
- The peripheral arthropathy of inflammatory bowel disease usually does not lead to deformity or damage.
- The axial disease often follows the course of ankylosing spondylitis with fusion of the spine and sacroiliac joints with associated deformity and disability.

Treatment

- Treatment of the inflammatory arthritis includes the treatment of the underlying bowel disease.
- Sulfasalazine (Salazopyrin) controls the arthritis.
- Azathioprine and methotrexate are used to treat inflammatory arthritis and may be effective in the enteropathic arthropathy as well.
- Anti-TNF agents in the treatment of inflammatory bowel disease is currently the treatment of choice. The antirheumatic use of such agents is historically derived from their use in treating inflammatory bowel disease.

Infectious Arthropathies

- The bone, joints, bursae, muscle, or tendon sheaths can be infected.
- Osteomyelitis, infectious arthritis, and bursitis are by far the most common musculoskeletal infections.

- Microorganisms including bacteria, viruses, fungi, and parasites may infect joints and other musculoskeletal tissues.
- *Staphylococcal aureus* is the most common cause of all types of musculoskeletal infection.

Acute Bacterial Arthritis

- Acute bacterial arthritis (septic arthritis) remains a medical emergency and the cause of significant morbidity and mortality.
- Bacteria commonly infect the synovium through hematogenous spread from a distant site or occasionally directly from penetrating trauma, iatrogenic joint needling, or an adjacent osteomyelitis focus.
- Age (>80 years), serious chronic illness such as diabetes mellitus, cancer and chronic renal failure, rheumatoid arthritis, the presence of a prosthetic joint, intravenous drug use, skin infection, and an immunosuppressed state predispose patients to septic arthritis.
- Males and females are equally affected.
- Polyarticular septic arthritis occurs in 15% of cases of septic arthritis.
- Polymicrobial infections occasionally occur with penetrating trauma and in patients with joint prostheses.
- While *S. aureus* is the most common cause of septic arthritis, it generally occurs in joints that were abnormal because of arthritis, trauma, prosthesis, and/or surgery prior to infection
- *Neisseria gonorrhoeae* is more likely to infect previously intact joints and otherwise healthy individuals.
- *S. aureus* causes the majority of joint infections in the elderly and in patients with rheumatoid arthritis.

Clinical Manifestations

- In approximately 70% to 80% of patients the clinical picture of septic arthritis is that of an acutely painful monoarthritis: a red, hot, swollen joint, mainly the knee.
- Associated systemic symptoms of chills and fever, and a high peripheral white cell count.
- Lack of fever and high peripheral white cell count and other atypical presentations are common and depend on the age and demographics of the patient population, the infecting organism, associated systemic illnesses, and coincident treatment such as the use of NSAIDs or inadequate doses of antibiotics.

Diagnostic Testing

- The definitive diagnostic test for infectious arthritis is synovial fluid aspiration for Gram stain and culture.
- Synovial fluid leukocytosis can be helpful.
  - Counts of more than 50,000 white blood cells (WBCs)/mm^3 suggest an infectious process.
  - "Pseudoseptic" fluids may occasionally be seen with crystal synovitis, rheumatoid arthritis, and spondyloarthropathies.
  - Approximately 10% of patients with proven intraarticular infections may have an initial synovial fluid WBC count of less than 25,000/mm^3.
  - The percentage of neutrophils is usually greater than 90% and often greater than 95%.
  - Synovial fluid lactic acid, produced by bacteria and synovial cells, is elevated in septic arthritis but also in other inflammatory arthropathies.
  - A normal synovial fluid lactic acid level virtually excludes septic arthritis.
  - In nongonococcal septic arthritis, organisms can be seen on Gram stain in 50% to 70% of cases
  - Gram-positive organisms are more frequently visualized than gram negative.
  - Synovial fluid cultures generally yield positive results in more than 70% of patients as do blood cultures in 50% of cases.
  - MRI has become the standard when making the diagnosis of osteomyelitis.

Treatment

- The initial antibiotic regimen will depend on the clinical setting.
- Coverage for *S. aureus* using β-lactamase-resistant penicillin or cefazolin, or vancomycin for suspected *methicillin-resistant S. aureus* is generally indicated until definitive bacteriologic identification is made.
- More than 25% of *S. aureus* joint infections are methicillin resistant.

- If a gram-negative organism is suspected, then a third-generation cephalosporin should be used.
- In clinically accessible joints, such as the knee, daily aspiration is preferable to open surgical drainage because of faster recovery of joint mobility.
- Arthrotomy with surgical drainage is generally indicated in infections of the hip, especially in children, or other joints that are difficult to monitor because of poor accessibility and for patients who exhibit an inadequate response to antibiotics and repeated joint aspiration within about 7 days.
- A clinical response to therapy should be seen within 2 to 3 days.
- Within 5 to 7 days, synovial fluid WBC should have decreased by 50%, with negative culture.
- Usually 4 weeks or longer is recommended for therapy; intravenously for 2 weeks followed by a course of high-dose oral antibiotics.

Disseminated Gonococcus Infection

- Occurs in approximately 1% of the 1 to 3 million cases of gonococcus infections in the United States annually.
- *N. gonorrhoeae* is a common cause of infectious arthritis, has a characteristic clinical picture, and responds well to antibiotic therapy.
- Patients with inherited deficiency of the complement components of the membrane attack complex (C5-C9) are susceptible to Neisserial infections including disseminated disease.
- Women are affected approximately 3 to 4 times more commonly than men.
- Asymptomatic rather than symptomatic urogenital or other mucosal infection precedes dissemination.
- In women, dissemination tends to occur at the time of menses, during pregnancy or immediately postpartum.
- Clinically 65% to 70% of patients with disseminated gonococcus infection have a syndrome characterized by fever, migratory polyarthralgia, tenosynovitis of the wrists, hands, ankles, or feet, and dermatitis with scattered, usually painless, pustular, vesicopustular, or hemorrhagic macular lesions.
- Septic monoarthritis occurs in 30% to 40% of patients, involving knees, wrists, and ankles most commonly.
- With gonococcal arthritis, the synovial fluid is often in the inflammatory range, with WBC counts less than 50,000, rather than frankly purulent. An asymmetric oligoarthritis can occur in approximately 10% of patients.

Treatment

- Penicillin-resistant strains of *N. gonorrhoeae* are common.
- A third-generation cephalosporin given parenterally, such as ceftriaxone or cefotaxime, is indicated.
- Spectinomycin may be used in penicillin-allergic patients.
- The duration of therapy is empiric, but generally 7 days are recommended for the bacteremia phase and 7 to 14 days for patients with septic arthritis.
- These latter patients often require daily joint aspiration and monitoring similar to nongonococcal septic arthritis.
- Concurrent treatment for chlamydial infection with oral doxycycline for 7 days is also recommended.

Prosthetic Joint Infections

- The overall infection rate in total joint replacement is approximately 1%, slightly higher for the knee than for the hip.
- Bacteria can adhere to the inert solid surface of the prosthetic joint, elaborate polysaccharides to cover the joint, and coalesce to form a protective biofilm.
  - This accounts for persistent infection despite antibiotic therapy and normal humoral and cellular immunity.
- Bacterial seeding of the prosthesis during hematogenous spread is one reason for late-onset infection of prosthesis.
- The most common organisms are *S. aureus* (45%), streptococci (25%), gram-negative bacilli (15%), coagulase-negative staphylococci (10%), and anaerobes (5%).

- Most of the time, surgical removal of the prosthetic joint is required for a cure.
- Debridement of the joint, a prolonged course of parenteral antibiotic therapy (6–8 weeks), and subsequent reimplantation of a new prosthesis employing antibiotic-impregnated cement is appropriate therapy.
- The reinfection rate may be very high (up to 30%) and arthrodesis may be necessary in those patients who are unable to have reimplantation because of mechanical factors in the joint.
- Initial parenteral antibiotic therapy followed by long-term oral suppressive antibiotic therapy with a cephalosporin or fluoroquinolone may be needed for those unable or unwilling to undergo prosthesis removal.

Septic Arthritis with Other Conditions

- Drug abuse
  - Intravenous drug abusers have many risk factors for septic arthritis or osteomyelitis.
    - These may include the development of soft tissue infections and transient bacteremias, and the presence of serious comorbid conditions such as hepatitis, bacterial endocarditis, and human immunodeficiency virus (HIV) infection.
  - Septic arthritis and osteomyelitis in this population may occur at unusual sites with atypical organisms.
  - The fibrocartilaginous joints (sternoclavicular, costochondral, symphysis pubis) and axial skeleton (vertebral osteomyelitis, sacroiliitis) are much more commonly affected than in other patient populations.
  - After *S. aureus*, gram-negative infections (*Pseudomonas aeruginosa*, *Enterobacter* spp., *Serratia marcescens*) are the next most common, and may be indolent.
  - Systemic candidiasis with costochondral or sternoclavicular joint infection has been described in addicts using contaminated brown heroin.
- Rheumatoid Arthritis
  - Patients with longstanding erosive, seropositive rheumatoid arthritis on corticosteroid therapy are particularly prone to polyarticular septic arthritis and account for a disproportionately high percentage of cases because of ulcerated rheumatoid nodules, and wound infections.
- Sjögren syndrome
  - Patients with lupus or Sjögren syndrome who are on chronic immunosuppressive therapy are also prone to septic arthritis.
  - Particular attention must be paid to patients receiving cytokine inhibitors such as anti-TNF, anti-interleukin 6 (IL-6) or anti-BLyS therapy, because these agents are associated with severe infections involving encapsulated bacteria. Any one of those agents with an infection can prove fatal if not recognized in time.
- Immunodeficiency
  - Congenital humoral immunodeficiency is occasionally associated with infectious arthritis involving unusual organisms.
  - Hypogammaglobulinemia predisposes patients to acute septic arthritis caused by *Mycoplasma* and *Ureaplasma*.
  - Deficiency of the late complement components (C5-C9) can result in joint infections with *Neisseria* species.
  - Patients with acquired cellular immunodeficiency either related to infection (AIDS) or immunosuppressant drugs, may get acute septic arthritis or chronic tuberculous or fungal arthritis.
  - Both gout and pseudo-gout can cause a pseudoseptic arthritis with fever, leukocytosis, and synovial fluid WBC count greater than 50,000/mm^3.
  - Patients in renal failure are also prone to severe joint infections.

Lyme Disease

- Lyme disease is the most common vector-borne (*Ixodes* tick) infection in the United States.
- 15,000 new cases reported yearly.
- Originally identified in Connecticut, found along the eastern seaboard and in parts of Wisconsin and Minnesota.
- Lyme disease is caused by infection with the spirochete *Borrelia burgdorferi*.

Clinical Manifestations

- The clinical picture can be classified as:
  - Early (localized or disseminated) and late.
  - Early disease occurs most frequently from spring through early fall when nymphal and adult ticks are abundant and feeding.
  - Early localized disease is characterized by an expanding, often asymptomatic, erythematous rash—erythema migrans—starting at the site of the tick bite.
- The rash often accompanied by fever (usually less than 38.9°C [102°F]) and a viral-like syndrome characterized by arthralgia, myalgia, and the occasional sore throat.
- The rash is present in 80% to 90% of patients.
- Early disseminated disease, related to hematogenous spread of *Borrelia*, is characterized predominately by involvement of any of three organ systems—skin, nervous system, heart—and includes disseminated erythema migrans lesions, facial palsy, meningitis, or radiculoneuropathy, and rarely heart block of any degree.
- Facial palsy may be isolated or accompanied by subtle or flagrant meningitis and be bilateral.
- If untreated, more than 50% of patients develop late features: mainly arthritis or neurologic involvement (peripheral neuropathy, encephalopathy).
- Coinfection with *Babesia microti*, an intraerythrocytic microorganism, or with the agent of human granulocytic ehrlichiosis (HGE), a rickettsia-like organism, may occur with Lyme disease because all 3 microorganisms use the *Ixodes* tick as vector.
- However, in areas highly endemic for Lyme disease, *B. burgdorferi* is found 3 to 5 times more commonly in ticks than the ehrlichiosis agent, reflecting the relative frequencies of the clinical illnesses.
- *Babesia* parasitemia may be silent but can be fatal in splenectomized individuals.
- HGE often presents with an acute illness with high fever, arthralgia, and myalgia.
- Leucopenia, thrombocytopenia, and high transaminases, which are not features of Lyme disease, occur quite commonly with HGE.
- HGE may be particularly severe and even fatal in the elderly but is responsive to doxycycline therapy.
- In early Lyme disease, arthralgia and myalgia are common.
- More than 50% of patients with untreated or incompletely treated Lyme disease develop arthritis.
- Initially, this is an intermittent migratory asymmetric mono- or oligoarthritis, appearing within weeks to months after infection.
- Recurrent joint inflammation may continue over many months, eventually becoming persistent in 10% of patients, with large effusions in one or both knee joints.
- The differential diagnosis includes juvenile rheumatoid arthritis (children and adolescents), spondyloarthropathy such as Reiter syndrome, other causes of bacterial arthritis, and crystal arthritis.
- The synovial fluid is inflammatory and tests for Lyme disease are positive.
- Arthritis that persists after antibiotic treatment may be related to slow resolution of the inflammatory response.

Diagnostic Testing

- Testing for the disease involves an ELISA followed, in equivocal and positive cases, by a more specific Western blot test.
- All patients with Lyme arthritis are IgG Western blot positive, making it an excellent diagnostic test for patients in a Lyme endemic area who present with an oligoarthritis or monoarthritis.
- However, antibodies to *B. burgdorferi*, once present, may persist in serum for many years, reducing the value of serological tests alone in distinguishing active from past infection.

Treatment

- Early Lyme disease (erythema migrans) is generally treated with 2 to 4 weeks of doxycycline 100 mg twice daily or amoxicillin 500 mg 3 times daily (in children).
- Doxycycline is also active against HGE.
- Patients with early disseminated or late disease are usually treated with oral or parenteral antibiotics depending on the severity of illness and the organ system involved.

- In general, neurologic involvement is treated with intravenous ceftriaxone, 2 g daily for 3 to 4 weeks.
- Isolated facial palsy may be treated with oral antibiotics.
- Carditis may be treated with intravenous antibiotics, initially followed by oral antibiotics when the heart block reverses.
- Lyme arthritis may be treated with oral antibiotics for 28 days, followed, if there is no response, by another course of antibiotics, oral or intravenous.
- There is no scientific evidence that more prolonged courses of antibiotics alter the course of Lyme disease infection.

Acute Bacterial Infections of Other Musculoskeletal Structures

Osteomyelitis

- Osteomyelitis is an infection in bone characterized by progressive inflammatory destruction and relative resistance to medical treatment.
- Bacteria gain access to bone either through hematogenous seeding, contiguous spread of infection, or direct trauma (compound fractures).
- Otherwise healthy children are more frequently affected than adults with osteomyelitis after bacteremia, and it most commonly involves the metaphysis of the femur, tibia, and humerus.
- In adults, especially intravenous drug abusers and the elderly, hematogenous infection may involve the axial skeleton: vertebrae, sacrum and sacroiliac joints, symphysis pubis, clavicle, and sternoclavicular joints.
- Diabetic patients with peripheral vascular insufficiency or foot ulcers and often both are especially susceptible to osteomyelitis of the bones of the feet.
- Prosthetic joint infections as described above involve bone and joints.
- Needle biopsy or open surgical biopsy is generally required to identify the appropriate organism for treatment.
- The predominate organism is *S. aureus*, but the clinical situation often dictates other likely organisms, such as Pseudomonas in intravenous drug abusers, streptococci or anaerobic bacteria in the diabetic foot, Salmonella or Streptococcus pneumoniae in sickle cell disease, opportunistic infections and *Mycobacterium tuberculosis* in immunocompromised patients.

Diagnostic Testing

- Imaging both helps to anatomically localize the infection and to aid in diagnosis.
- Plain radiographs may be normal
- Technetium bone scanning is sensitive for an inflammatory process but is not specific
- CT scanning can identify the extent of bone edema, inflammation, and destruction or presence of necrotic bone.
- MRI is the best modality to diagnose osteomyelitis of all bones.

Treatment

- Acute osteomyelitis may be cured with parenteral antibiotics alone.
- The principles of therapy are to employ the appropriate parenteral antibiotics in adults for 4–6 weeks.
- For S. aureus infections, there is some evidence that a higher cure rate is obtained when rifampin is added to standard antistaphylococcal regimens.
- Children may be treated with a shorter course of parenteral antibiotics followed by several weeks of oral therapy.
- Chronic osteomyelitis, by definition, is refractory to medical treatment and usually requires surgical debridement and removal of necrotic bone, in addition to appropriate antibiotic therapy.
- Therapy with fluoroquinolones, with or without rifampin, given for some months, has been used to suppress the symptoms and signs of chronic refractory osteomyelitis, as in the diabetic foot.

Septic Bursitis and Tenosynovitis

- Septic bursitis usually post traumatic is a common clinical problem.
- Diabetes, alcoholism, and systemic corticosteroid therapy are risk factors.

- Involvement of the olecranon and prepatellar bursae account for the majority of the cases.
- A cellulitis is common and must be distinguished from septic arthritis of the elbow or knee.
- The clue is that passive extension of the infected joint is full and pain free.
- Bursal fluid WBC counts are elevated, although lower on average than synovial fluid counts in septic arthritis, and the bursal fluid is not usually purulent.
- S. aureus is the most common cause of septic bursitis with streptococci second in frequency and together they account for over 90% of cases.

Treatment

- Uncomplicated olecranon bursitis, with little overlying cellulitis, in an otherwise healthy individual may be treated with a course of oral antibiotics (eg, dicloxacillin or cephalexin) and close follow up, including repeat bursal aspirations.
- Treatment should continue until the bursal fluid is sterile, usually 7 to 10 days.
- Older and immunocompromised patients, patients with accompanying cellulitis or systemic symptoms, and those with prepatellar septic bursitis are best treated initially with parenteral antibiotics; the duration of therapy should be about 2 weeks.
- Occasionally septic bursitis may require surgical drainage.
- Acute digital flexor tenosynovitis is a true emergency since delay in treatment will result in tendon necrosis.
- Patients almost always have a history of a cut or puncture wound on the palmar side of a finger or a chronic hand condition with skin ulceration, such as scleroderma.
- S. aureus and Streptococcus pyogenes are the most likely causes.
- Pyomyositis, an acute bacterial infection of muscle, is usually caused by S. aureus.
- Patients present with fever, constitutional symptoms, and localized muscle pain. The muscle is tender and indurated, not fluctuant.
- Blood cultures are rarely positive but cultures of the muscle aspirate usually reveal the infecting organism.
- The creatine phosphokinase levels may be normal or slightly elevated and local asymmetric muscle pain, not weakness, is the main clinical feature.

Osteoarticular Tuberculosis

- With HIV, the incidence of tuberculosis (TB) and the frequency of extrapulmonary TB have risen dramatically.
- Skeletal TB occurs in approximately 1% to 3% of cases.
- Osseous infection with M. tuberculosis typically occurs during hematogenous spread, either with primary infection or after many years with late reactivation.
- Spinal osteomyelitis with seeding to the vertebral bodies is the most common skeletal manifestation of TB.
- Joint involvement occurs secondary to hematogenous spread or from a contiguous focus of tuberculous osteomyelitis.
- Pulmonary involvement is found in only 30% of patients with skeletal TB, the tuberculin skin test is positive in almost all immunocompetent patients.
- Treatment of osteoarticular TB is by combination chemotherapy, usually for 12–18 months.
- Spine involvement accounts for 50% of all osteoarticular TB.
- It commonly begins in the anterior portion of a vertebral body in the thoracic or lumbar spine.
- The inflammation and caseation necrosis lead to destruction of the vertebral end plates, contiguous disc involvement with narrowing, and vertebral collapse.
- Infection often extends to one or two adjoining discs and vertebrae eventually leading to kyphosis.
- Soft tissue extension with abscess formation may occur resulting in pressure on neurologic structures and, if left untreated, cord compression with paraplegia can be the outcome.
- Tuberculous sacroiliitis can also occur.
  - The cardinal symptom is the subacute onset of back pain, gradually increasing over weeks to months.
  - Constitutional symptoms of fever and weight loss are present in less than half the patients, although the ESR is usually elevated.

- MRI defines the vertebral, disc, and soft tissue involvement of TB.
- The diagnosis is best made by bone biopsy for histology and culture.
- Patients can have tuberculosis of a single joint.
- This usually presents with an indolent monoarthritis of a weight-bearing joint, occasionally with mild constitutional features.
- Radiographic changes may show mild joint space and marginal erosions but often only paraarticular osteopenia.
- Adjacent osteomyelitis may be present.
- While the synovial fluid is inflammatory and TB cultures may be positive, the diagnosis is best made by synovial biopsy where histology shows a granulomatous synovitis and acid fast stains and culture are more likely to be positive.
- Prosthetic joint infections with M. tuberculosis can occur.
- Tuberculous osteomyelitis generally involves the long bones in adults and may be multifocal, especially in immunocompromised patients.
- Poncet's disease is a "reactive" polyarthritis, mainly in the hands and feet, in the setting of active TB which resolves with antituberculous therapy.
- Articular infections with atypical mycobacteria, especially M. marinum, M. kansasii, M avium intracellulare, may occur with a predominance of arthritis and tendinitis in the hands and wrists.
- Definitive diagnosis is often delayed and treatment usually requires combination chemotherapy and surgical debridement.

Fungal Arthritis

- Fungal musculoskeletal infections, especially osteomyelitis and arthritis, often create diagnostic difficulties because of a lack of clinical suspicion.
- Candidal organisms can cause arthritis by a number of mechanisms and in a number of settings including hematogenous spread in intravenous drug abusers or in seriously ill, immunosuppressed, hospitalized patients with indwelling vascular lines, direct intraarticular inoculation, and infection of prosthetic joints.
- Acute monoarthritis, especially of the knee, can be seen with Candida whereas most other fungal infections cause an indolent chronic monoarthritis.
- Treatment with ketoconazole or fluconazole is effective for Candida albicans. other fungi including coccidioidomycosis, sporotrichosis, blastomycosis, cryptococcosis, and histoplasmosis may cause arthritis.

Viral Arthritis

- Arthralgia commonly accompanies many viral infections, but actual arthritis is a well-recognized feature of only a few viral illnesses.
- The arthritis often occurs during the viral prodrome, at the time of the rash.
- Viral arthritis is generally characterized by the sudden onset of symmetrical small and medium joint pain and stiffness with or without joint swelling, lymphocytic/monocytic joint fluids, and a self-limited, nondestructive course.

Parvovirus B19

- Parvovirus, a single-stranded DNA virus, is the cause of erythema infectiosum (fifth disease) in children and a rheumatoidlike polyarthritis in adults.
- Clinically it presents with acute and occasionally persistent joint pain, morning stiffness, and occasional swelling most often involving the hands, wrists, and knees. Symptoms usually resolve within 1 to 2 weeks in most patients, but in some 10% it persists for weeks to many months, waxing and waning and mimicking seronegative rheumatoid arthritis.

Rubella Virus

- Rubella virus infection is commonly associated with arthralgia and arthritis, especially in adult women.
- Joint symptoms usually begin within one week of the German measles rash as an abrupt symmetrical polyarthralgia or polyarthritis syndrome with stiffness involving the hands, wrists, knees, and ankles.
- Periarthritis, tenosynovitis, and carpal tunnel syndrome may be seen.
- These symptoms resolve within a few weeks.
- Chronic and recurrent arthritis may occur for months to years in some patients.

Alphaviruses (Arboviruses)

- The alphaviruses are mosquito-borne viruses that can cause epidemics of febrile polyarthritis in Africa, Asia, Australia, and New Zealand (Ross River virus), Northern Europe, and South America.
- Patients typically develop fever, arthritis, and a morbilliform rash.
- The onset of the arthritis may be abrupt (chikungunya, o'nyong-nyong) or gradual.
- Typically, the hands, feet, and medium size joints of the upper and lower extremities are involved. The acute disease usually resolves within 10 days but it may recur or persist for months.

Hepatitis Viruses

- Arthralgia occasionally occurs with hepatitis A infection but arthritis is very rare.
- In about 30% of acutely infected patients, hepatitis B causes a serumlike illness in the preicteric phase of hepatitis, characterized by urticaria and arthritis. It is sudden in onset, symmetric, and additive.
- Pain, stiffness, and swelling of the hands and knees are common.
- Symptoms usually last from 1–3 weeks, occasionally persisting after the onset of jaundice.
- Soluble antigen-antibody complexes of HbsAg and HbsAb can be detected in both serum and synovial fluid.
- Patients with chronic HBV infection, including those who develop a polyarteritis nodosa like syndrome, may have recurrent arthralgia or arthritis.
- Hepatitis C infection is common and often asymptomatic.
- Hepatitis C arthritis is unusual except in those patients who develop circulating immune complex disease where the triad of arthritis, vasculitic purpura, and cryoglobulinemia are common.

Retroviruses

- Human T lymphotrophic virus type I (HTLV-1)
  - HTLV-1 is endemic in Japan and has also been associated with acute and chronic oligoarthritis accompanied by a nodular skin rash.
  - Direct infection is likely since these patients have antibodies to HTLV; type C viral particles are seen in the skin lesions and the synovium has atypical synovial cells with lobulated nuclei.
- Human Immunodeficiency Virus (HIV)
  - Rheumatic features accompanying HIV and AIDS are very varied.
  - Nonspecific joint and muscle pains are common in AIDS patients, as part of acute HIV, or a superimposed infectious process.
  - There are three arthritic syndromes associated with HIV:
    - A severe, intermittent, and short-lived (hours) oligoarticular joint pain syndrome
    - A lower extremity oligoarthritis
    - An arthrocutaneous syndrome with enthesopathy.
  - Treatment with NSAIDs is appropriate for the idiopathic arthralgias and arthritis of AIDS

Other Viral Illnesses

- Mumps virus infection causes a migratory polyarthritis affecting large joints beginning 1–3 weeks after infection and subsiding after 2 weeks without joint damage.
- Enterovirus (coxsackie and echovirus) infections are common but are uncommonly associated with arthritis.
- A self-limited polyarthritis involving large and small joints is seen at the peak of the viral clinical illness.
- Varicella-zoster infection, both chickenpox and zoster, may rarely be associated with an inflammatory arthritis.
- An acute monoarthritis has been described with chickenpox and virus has been isolated from the joint.
- Patients with zoster may have severe nerve root pain mimicking joint disease. Epstein-Barr virus infection (infectious mononucleosis) frequently causes arthralgia but rarely arthritis.
- A patient has been described with an acute polyarthritis associated with hantavirus infection (hemorrhagic fever with renal syndrome).

- Diagnosis in most cases of viral arthritis is made by the typical clinical picture, serological testing for viral antibodies when needed, and synovial fluid analysis to rule out other causes of inflammatory arthritis

Crystal-Induced Arthropathies

- The crystal-induced arthropathies are a collection of clinical syndromes characterized by the deposition of crystals in articular and periarticular tissues.
- The inflammatory response in and around affected joints is dependent upon the complex interplay of a host of issues including local tissue damage, associated diseases, genetic factors, lifestyle, and provocative stimuli.
- The main species of crystals found in synovial fluids of arthritis patients include monosodium urate (MSU), calcium pyrophosphate, and apatite crystals.
- These may also be found in bursal fluid and soft tissues. Less commonly noted species include calcium oxalate, amyloid, aluminum, cystine, xanthine, hypoxanthine, and cholesterol and liquid lipid crystals.
- Proteins such as cryoglobulins can crystallize in blood vessels and tissues.
- Not all crystals can be identified using compensated polarizing microscopy.
- Monosodium urate crystals are strongly birefringent and are seen as yellow when the crystal in question is parallel to the axis of slow vibration on the first order color compensator (negatively birefringent).
- In contrast, calcium pyrophosphate crystals are positively birefringent and hence yellow in appearance when perpendicular to the compensator.
- Furthermore, such crystals are only weakly birefringent.
- Liquid lipid crystals may display intense birefringence in the pattern of a Maltese cross.
- Calcium hydroxyapatite crystals do not manifest birefringence under polarized light.
- Crystals are capable of stimulating the release of inflammatory mediators from cells such as phagocytes and synoviocytes via nonspecific activation of signal transduction pathways.
- Among the soluble mediators can be found arachidonic acid metabolites, interleukins (IL-1, IL-6, IL-8), and (TNF-α).

Gout

- Gout represents a diverse group of diseases that can be characterized by arthritis, tophi, kidney stones, and nephropathy.
- Gout is a metabolic disorder due to a defect in the handling of uric acid.
- Predictive factors for gout include increasing uric acid levels, alcohol consumption, diuretics, and body mass index.
- Epidemiological studies associate hyperuricemia with renal impairment, lipoprotein abnormalities, increasing body mass, and excessive alcohol intake.
- The prevalence of gout in the United States is estimated at 8.4 per 1000 persons (all ages).
- Only 10% of patients with hyperuricemic gout are overproducers of uric acid.
- In general, this clinical state can be seen in the setting of increased nucleic acid turnover such as in myeloproliferative disease and psoriasis.
- Overproduction is seen in the situation of inherited disorders of purine nucleotide synthesis such as in HGPRT (hypoxanthine-guanine phosphoribosyltransferase) deficiency or in PRPP (5-phosphoribosyl-1-pyrophosphate) synthetase superactivity.
- The vast majority of patients have disease characterized by uric acid under excretion.
- Under excretion can be distinguished from overproduction by measuring the 24-hour urine uric acid secretion.
- On a normal diet, excess excretion is defined as 800 mg or more.
- Any disease that predisposes to renal insufficiency may contribute to gout.
- Diabetes mellitus and hypertension can be associated with decreased uric acid excretion.
- Organic acids can compete for renal tubular secretion as can be seen in ethanol intoxication with lactic acidosis or starvation diet with ketosis.
- Pharmaceutical agents, which can impair renal tubular handling of uric acid, include diuretics, cyclosporine, and low dose salicylates.
- Cyclosporine is an especially noteworthy cause of gout when used in patients who have had organ transplants ("transplantation gout").

- A combination of overproduction and under excretion of uric acid likely accounts for many cases of gout.
  - An example involves alcohol consumption.
    - In this situation, both mechanisms of disease physiology are in play because alcohol intake accelerates urate production through accelerated ATP breakdown while alcohol induced lactic acidemia blocks uric acid excretion.
    - Beer is particularly injurious to gouty physiology owing to the presence of guanosine, which is an intermediary in the nucleic acid catabolism pathway.
- Over a period of years, untreated hyperuricemia leads to an increase in the total body burden of uric acid.
- Collections of noninflammatory crystalline material, called tophi, can be found in soft tissues.
- Shedding of microtophi and intraarticular precipitation of crystals are two mechanisms whereby an acute attack of inflammation is initiated.
- Metabolism of purine nucleotides provides the substrate for the chemical reactions that ultimately produce uric acid.
  - The sources of purine nucleotides can be exogenous (dietary) or endogenous (de novo synthesis).
  - Oxidative catabolism of degradation products derived from these purine nucleotides results in the generation of uric acid catalytic pathways involve the enzyme xanthine oxidase, whereby xanthine is ultimately converted to uric acid.
  - Therefore xanthine oxidase inhibitors, such as allopurinol, exert a profound antihyperuricemic effect.
  - On the other hand, enzymatic deficiencies, such as in Lesch-Nyhan syndrome (HGPRT deficiency), can result in enhanced purine de novo synthesis with ultimate overproduction of uric acid.
  - Excessive enzymatic activity, such as with PRPP synthetase superactivity, augments PRPP availability and thereby drives uric acid production. These two enzymes (HGPRT and PRPP synthetase) are X-linked.
- Hyperuricemia is a risk factor for gout.
- Men have higher serum levels of uric acid.
- The relative protected status enjoyed by women may reflect the uricosuric effect of estrogen.
- After menopause, this gender discrepancy in the serum uric acid level regresses.
- The determination of serum uric acid level is predictive of gout.
- The incidence of gouty arthritis exceeds 5% when the uric acid level is above 9 mg/dL.
- At a serum level of 13 mg/dL, the annual incidence of renal stone formation is 50%.
- Serial monitoring of the serum uric acid is particularly helpful for assessing the effectiveness of antihyperuricemic therapy.

Clinical Presentation

- The classic presentation of clinical gout is that of acute, intermittent attacks of intense joint inflammation.
- Factors include trauma, surgery, alcohol, and certain drugs (diuretics, low dose aspirin). Initial twinges of discomfort rapidly develop into warmth, redness, and swelling. Intensity peaks within 12 hours and the time to resolution may be as long as 2 weeks in untreated cases.
- Attacks most frequently involve the metatarsophalangeal joint (podagra) but polyarticular presentations as well as involvement of other joints are not uncommon
- Systemic symptoms of an attack include fever and chills.
- Subcutaneous tophi, a sign of an increased total body burden of urate, take many years to develop.
- They may be seen over extensor surfaces including the digits and olecranon bursae, but also on the helix of the ears and the Achilles tendon.
- Renal stones occur in up to 25% of patients with gout.

Treatment

- Acute management of gout is rapid relief of pain and inflammation, whereas long term management seeks to reduce the frequency and severity of attacks as well as to reduce the risk for joint damage and kidney stones, and, where necessary, resolve tophi.

- Treatment for the acute attack largely relies upon judicious use of NSAIDs, colchicine, and corticosteroids.
- Indomethacin has been employed to ameliorate an acute gout attack.
- Other NSAIDs may be equally effective, especially when higher dosing is employed during the first 24–48 hours of an attack.
- The use of colchicine to treat acute gouty arthritis is limited by toxicity especially if there concomitant renal disease.
- Care with regard to colchicine dosing is especially important for individuals with renal or hepatic impairment or for those on concomitant P-450 inhibitors.
- The major route of elimination of colchicine is renal.
  - Therefore dosages should be halved in individuals with reduced creatinine clearance.
  - Owing to the enterohepatic circulation of colchicine, patients with liver disease are also at increased risk for toxicity.
  - Common manifestations of acute colchicine toxicity include abdominal cramps and diarrhea.
  - Other less common toxicities include marrow suppression and neuromyopathy with vacuolar changes in muscle.
  - The effectiveness of colchicine exceeds 90% when given within the first 24 hours of an attack.
- Corticosteroids have efficacy when provided orally, parenterally, or intraarticularly.
- The case for intervention with corticosteroid therapy is particularly compelling when colchicine and NSAIDs are relatively contra-indicated, such as in the situation of renal insufficiency or in patients with attacks of gout in the postsurgical period.
- Weight loss, avoidance of alcohol-containing products, and a low purine diet can be helpful.
- Blood pressure management should be carefully reviewed, especially the necessity for diuretics.
- In certain instances, prophylaxis with daily use of colchicine (up to 1.2 mg daily), NSAIDs, or combinations of the two are effective.
- In the case of either sustained hyperuricemia, chronic tophaceous gout, destructive arthropathy, or nephrolithiasis, uric acid lowering therapy is indicated.
- The mainstay of drug therapy centers on uricosurics and xanthine oxidase inhibitors and more recently a monoclonal antibody.
- Uricosuric agents include probenecid and sulfinpyrazone.
  - Uricosurics increase urinary urate excretion until a lower serum uric acid level results.
  - Their side effects include rash and gastrointestinal disturbance but in general are relatively safe.
  - The potential risk of uricosuric intervention also includes the formation of uric acid crystals in the urinary collection system. a high alkaline urine helps reduce this risk.
  - The uricosuric effect of probenecid declines with the glomerular filtration rate (GFR) and therefore will be of little use when the GFR drops below 50 cc/min.
- Salicylates also reduce the uricosuric effect of probenecid.
- Probenecid enhances the excretion of allopurinol and should be used carefully when giving that drug.
- Allopurinol is a hypoxanthine analogue that inhibits xanthine oxidase.
  - Side effects of allopurinol therapy include rash, nausea, diarrhea, and headache.
  - An allopurinol hypersensitivity syndrome is manifested as an exfoliative dermatitis that may be fatal.
  - An individual at increased risk for such reaction includes those with renal insufficiency and those on diuretic therapy.
  - Rare adverse experiences with allopurinol include marrow suppression and hepatitis.
  - Most patients can be controlled with a daily dose of 300 mg or less.
  - However, because patients may experience increased gouty attacks with dropping uric acid levels, it is best to institute uric acid lowering therapy gradually, eg, allopurinol 100 mg/day, increasing by 100 mg/day each month until the desired serum uric acid level is achieved.
  - Furthermore, colchicine prophylaxis is best used during the initial during the initial phases of uric acid lowering therapy to reduce the likelihood of a gouty arthritis flare.

- There are a new series of agents directed at prophylaxis of acute gouty arthritis.
- One of these is febuxostat which is used at 40 or 80 mg per day and is useful for patients with decreased renal function.
- No matter which uric acid lowering therapy is used, none should be initiated during an acute attack because such attack may worsen in terms of severity or duration.

Pseudogout

- Calcium pyrophosphate dehydrate (CPPD) crystal deposition may include the inflammatory syndrome termed pseudogout.
- When calcium-containing crystals are present in cartilage this is termed chondrocalcinosis.
- CPPD deposition is associated with aging and degenerative arthritides and suspected to be associated with various endocrinopathies, like hyperparathyroidism.
- Metabolic syndromes such hemochromatosis have been associated with pseudogout, and this disorder in particular may be of significance in the differential diagnosis of the younger patient (under age 55) presenting with chondrocalcinosis.
- Overproduction of inorganic pyrophosphate, a component of CPPD, is associated with crystal formation.
- Shedding of preformed articular crystalline deposits and the intracellular dissolution of calcium- containing crystals, with subsequent release of calcium, play a role in the initiation and maintenance of the inflammatory process.
- Under compensated polarizing microscopy, CPPD crystals are typically rhomboid or rectangularly shaped and demonstrate weakly positive birefringence.
- Crystals may be intracellular.
- Synovial fluid cell counts are predominately polymorphonuclear and may range upward of 80,000/mm^3.
- The radiographic finding of chondrocalcinosis is most commonly seen in the menisci and hyaline cartilage of the knees, the intervertebral disks, and the fibrocartilage of the wrists and symphysis pubis.
- Osteoarthritic change of the knees is also frequently seen radiographically.
- As compared to control subjects without CPPD, significant associations have been found between CPPD deposition and trapezioscaphoid arthropathy as well as 1st carpometacarpal arthropathy.
- Other areas of association include disease of the various bones of the wrist.
- Acute pseudogout may be indistinguishable in clinical appearance from gout except for a predilection for larger joint involvement.
- Abrupt onset of self-limited attacks may individually last for up to two weeks.
- Rarely, a mix of MSU and CPPD crystals may be seen within the same synovial fluid specimen.
- Similarly, the possibility of coexistent joint infection dictates that appropriate microbiological studies be performed upon new, atypical, or persistent cases of pseudogout arthritis.
- Major illness, surgery, joint lavage, and trauma are all precipitating factors.
- Monoarticular and polyarticular presentations are possible.
- A small percentage of patients follow a pseudo-rheumatoid pattern with stiffness, fatigue, and persistent, symmetric, synovial inflammation.
- Systemic features of acute and chronic pyrophosphate arthropathy may include fever, elevated acute phase reactants, and leukocytosis thereby mimicking a septic process.
- NSAIDs are the mainstay of management for CPPD related diseases.
- Colchicine may reduce the severity or frequency of attacks and hence may be of benefit both for the acute presentation as well as for prevention of episodic disease.

Apatite Arthropathy

- Hydroxyapatite is an example of a basic calcium phosphate crystal and crystals may deposit in cartilage and periarticular structures and may be asymptomatic.
- The most commonly recognized site of clinical involvement is in tendons near the shoulder joints.
- Besides this type of acute periarthritis, basic calcium phosphate crystals can be associated with frozen shoulder, acute articular inflammation, large joint destructive arthropathy (eg, Milwaukee shoulder), and calcinosis cutis.

- The end result of an acute calcific periarthritis of the shoulder may be a frozen shoulder.
- Basic calcium phosphate crystals are also associated with OA, especially in the small joints of the hands.
- These crystals do not demonstrate birefringence but they may be seen on light microscopy alone when aggregated together to form coinlike clumps.
- The pathophysiology of these crystals is poorly understood and mixtures of different types of crystals are frequently reported in the same tissue.
- Management of these syndromes traditionally relies upon NSAIDs but colchicine and corticosteroids (especially as intraarticular injection) have been employed.
- Care must be exercised if intraarticular injection is contemplated owing to the possibility of dislodging crystals and increasing the risk for future attacks.
- Improvement in calcific periarthritis has been reported following EDTA treatment.
- Milwaukee shoulder is a (commonly the shoulder or the knee) destructive arthropathy, which is associated with basic calcium phosphate crystals.
  - The Milwaukee shoulder (also termed "apatite-associated destructive arthritis" and "cuff tear arthropathy") is predominately a disease in older women or in patients with glenohumeral instability and can be characterized by limited flexibility, pain, and swelling.
  - A large, bloody, effusion may be present.
  - Management may be difficult.
  - Analgesics, antiinflammatory agents, and nerve blocks have been employed.

Cholesterol and Liquid Lipid Crystals

- Cholesterol crystals are commonly observed in chronic olecranon bursitis.
- Bone and joint trauma, especially fracture, may also result in the finding of cholesterol crystals in synovial fluid.
- The microscopic appearance of birefringent liquid lipid spherules seen in joint fluid aspirates has been likened to that of a "Maltese Cross."
- When cholesterol crystals are implicated in the pathogenesis of monoarticular synovitis, neutrophils are the predominant cell type on synovial fluid analysis.
- Cholesterol crystals take on greater clinical significance in the cholesterol crystal embolization syndrome.
- This syndrome may be precipitated by endovascular instrumentation and by anticoagulation.
- It may be characterized by calf pain, blue toes, leg ulcers, gastrointestinal bleeding, renal impairment, and eosinophilia.
- Because of these manifestations, cholesterol emboli syndrome has been termed pseudovasculitis.

Cryoglobulin Crystals

- Immunoglobulins may crystallize.
- Temperature dependent, reversible crystallization is a characteristic of cryoglobulins.
- These crystals are found in serum, and rarely, in synovial fluid.
- They may be comprised of monoclonal or mixed cryoglobulins and may be seen in autoimmune, neoplastic, and chronic infectious (such as hepatitis C) disorders.
- Monoclonal cryoglobulins tend to be associated with lymphoproliferative disorders or multiple myeloma.
- Mixed cryoglobulins are associated with connective tissue diseases, viral hepatitis, infective endocarditis, and chronic parasitic syndromes.
- Mixed cryoglobulins often contain IgM molecules with rheumatoid factor activity.
- Cryoglobulins may cause some symptoms by virtue of hyperviscosity.
- Cryoglobulinemia must be considered in the differential diagnosis of Raynaud phenomenon.
- Other features may include arthritis, glomerulonephritis, palpable purpura, livido reticularis, and ischemic acral ulcers.
- Resolution of the inciting chronic infection may lead to resolution of cryoglobulin generation.

Oxalate Gout

- Inborn errors of glyoxylate metabolism may lead to hyperoxaluria.
- These rare syndromes present with nephrolithiasis, renal failure, and systemic oxalosis.
- Systemic oxalosis may be characterized by bone pain, compression fracture, arthritis, and vascular calcification or insufficiency.
- They stain with Alizarin red S and hence may be confused with apatite crystals.

REFERENCES

1. Coblyn JS, Weinblatt J, Helfgott S, Bermas B. *Brigham and Women's Experts' Approach to Rheumatology*. Sudbury, MA: Jones & Bartlett Learning; 2011.

2. Nishmura K, Sugiyama D, Kogata Y, et al. Meta-analysis: diagnostic accuracy of anti-cyclic citrullinated peptide and rheumatoid factor for rheumatoid arthritis. *Ann Intern Med.* 2007;146(11):797-808.

3. Tan EM, Feltkamp TE, Smolen JS. Range of antinuclear antibodies in "healthy" individuals. *Arthritis Rheum.* 1997;40(9):1601-11.

4. Vlachoyiannopoulos PG, Samarkos M, Sikara M, Tsiligros P. Antiphospholipid antibodies: laboratory and pathogenetic aspects. *Crit Rev Clin Lab Sci.* 2007;44(3): 271-338.

MEDICAL SPECIALTIES

Section 3: Special Populations

CHAPTER 14

Obstetrics

Allison R. Durica, Amanda B. Murchison, and Patrice M. Weiss

GENERAL PRINCIPLES IN THE MANAGEMENT OF PREGNANT PATIENTS

- All pregnant patients should have an obstetric (OB) provider involved in their care during an acute hospitalization.
- Otherwise routine illnesses in nonpregnant women may lead to serious complications during pregnancy (eg, respiratory illness, influenza, and pyelonephritis may result in acute respiratory distress syndrome).
- Most medical therapy and intervention is reasonable during pregnancy if indicated for the health of the mother. OB providers should be consulted for guidance if needed.
- Patients who are at a viable gestational age (24 weeks or greater) should be cared for on an OB unit if possible during acute hospitalizations.
- Patients who are at a viable gestational age (24 weeks or greater) should have daily fetal monitoring. This may be continuous or intermittent, and should be determined and interpreted by an OB provider.
- If a pregnant patient is experiencing an acute illness requiring hospitalization, and her OB provider is not an obstetrician, consult to an OB service should be considered based on severity of her illness.
- Patients with severe disease or illness, such as preeclampsia, *h*emolysis, *e*levated *l*iver function, and *l*ow *p*latelets (HELLP) syndrome, acute fatty liver, heart disease, uncontrolled hypertension (HTN), respiratory failure, and so forth, should have a high-risk (maternal fetal medicine) physician involved for consultation. Transfer to a center where this service is available should be considered in such cases.

Normal Physiologic Changes in Pregnancy (Table 14-1)

SPECIFIC CONDITIONS OF IMPORTANCE TO THE INTERNIST

Neurology and Pregnancy

Seizures and Epilepsy

- Most pregnant women (>90%) with epilepsy experience favorable outcomes.
- Epilepsy is not a contraindication to pregnancy.

Preconception Counseling

- Use of some antiepileptic drugs (AEDs) may increase risk of failure of hormonal contraceptives.
- Possible fetal risks associated with medications should be reviewed.
- Consideration should be given for withdrawal of AEDs if indicated at least 6 months prior to conception.
- If continued AED therapy is necessary, monotherapy at the lowest doses to control symptoms is encouraged.
- Advise 4 mg folic acid supplementation daily, 3 months prior to conception.
- Continue the AED that best controls the patient's seizures. Avoid valproate and phenytoin if possible.

Management during Pregnancy

- Do not discontinue current AED therapy. Fetal effects are early in gestation (usually prior to the recognition of pregnancy) and abrupt changes may precipitate seizures.
- Consider consultation with a genetic counselor or high-risk obstetrician for further discussion regarding possible fetal effects of exposure.

TABLE 14-1. NORMAL PHYSIOLOGIC CHANGES IN PREGNANCY

Hematologic Changes

	Increased	· Blood volume · Increase in plasma and erythrocytes · Water and sodium retention · Red blood cell mass

	Decreased	· Systemic vascular resistance
		· Whole blood viscosity
		· Systemic blood pressure
		· Hemoglobin and hematocrit
		  · Caused by great plasma augmentation
		  · Hemoglobin <11.0 g/dL at term abnormal
		· Platelets—slight decrease

Immunologic Changes

	Increased	· C-reactive protein · Erythrocyte sedimentation rate · Complement C3 and C4
	Decreased	· Humoral immunity · Cellular immunity · T-helper cells · PMNL chemotaxis

Metabolism

	Water	· Increased water retention caused by decreased osmolality · Increased volume approximately 6.5 L
	Carbohydrates	· Mild fasting hypoglycemia · Postprandial hyperglycemia · Postprandial hyperinsulinemia · "Accelerated starvation" · Switch in glucose fuels to lipids

	Fat	· Free fatty acids
		  · Triglycerides
		  · Cholesterol
		· Fat
		  · Lipids
		  · Lipoproteins
		  · Apo lipoproteins
		  · LDL
		  · VLDL
		  · HDL
		  · Total cholesterol

(continued on next page)

TABLE 14-1.   NORMAL PHYSIOLOGIC CHANGES IN PREGNANCY *(Continued)*

Cardiovascular System (changes begin as early as 8 weeks of gestation)

	Increased	· Blood volume
		· Basal metabolic rate
		· Cardiac output at rest
		· Heart rate
		· Vascular tone
		· Because of increased prostaglandins
		· Renin and angiotensin II
	Decreased	· Mean arterial pressure
		· Venous return from lower body
		· Uterine blood flow (supine position)
		· Systemic vascular resistance
		· Pulmonary vascular resistance
		· Serum colloid osmotic pressure
		· COP-PCWP gradient

Respiratory System

	Physical Changes	· Diaphragm rises 4 cm
		· Subcostal angle widens approximately 2 cm
		· Thoracic circumference increases 6 cm
	Increased	· Tidal volume
		· Resting minute ventilation
		· Airway conductance
	Decreased	· Functional residual capacity
		· Residual volume
		· Peak expiratory flow rates
		· Total pulmonary resistance
		· Expiratory reserve volume
	Unchanged	· Respiratory rate
		· Lung compliance
		· Forced or timed vital capacity
		· Closing volume

Urinary System

	Increased	· Kidney size
		· Glomerular filtration rate
		· Renal plasma flow
		· Creatinine clearance
		· Ureteral dilation (right greater than left)
	Decreased	· Serum creatinine

TABLE 14-1. NORMAL PHYSIOLOGIC CHANGES IN
PREGNANCY (Continued)

Gastrointestinal System

	Increased	• Pyrosis (heartburn)
		• Epulis (gum swelling)
		• Hemorrhoids
		• Gastric emptying time in labor
		• Total alkaline phosphatase activity
		• Total albumin
	Decreased	• AST
		• ALT
		• GGT
		• Bilirubin levels
		• Serum albumin concentration
		• Gallbladder contractility
	Unchanged	• Gastric emptying time (each trimester)
		• Liver size

Endocrine System

	Increased	• Pituitary gland size (135%)
		• Maternal plasma prolactin levels
		• Thyroid gland size
		• Thyroxine-binding globulin
		• Total serum thyroxine
		• Free serum T_4
		• Total T_3
		• Serum cortisol concentration
		• Deoxycortisone
		• Aldosterone secretion
		• Androstenedione
		• Testosterone
	Decreased	• Thyrotropin
		• TSH
	Unchanged	• Incidence of pituitary prolactinomas
		• Thyroid-releasing hormone
		• Adrenal cortisol secretion

ALT, alanine aminotransferase; AST, aspartate aminotransferase; COP-PCWP, colloid oncotic pressure-pulmonary capillary wedge pressure; GGT, γ-glutamyltransferase; HDL, high-density lipoprotein; LDL, low-density lipoprotein; PMNL, polymorphonuclear neutrophilic leukocyte; T_3, triiodothyronine; T_4, thyroxine; TSH, thyroid-stimulating hormone; VLDL, very-low-density lipoprotein.

- AED metabolism, clearance, and absorption may be altered in pregnancy.
- Plasma AED levels (total and free) should be monitored monthly to guide needed adjustments to dosing.
- Generalized seizure activity after 20 weeks should be evaluated as an exacerbation of underlying epilepsy versus eclampsia (proteinuria, HTN, laboratory evaluation).

Postpartum Management

- If AED doses are adjusted during pregnancy, prepregnancy doses are anticipated during first few weeks postpartum. Postpartum levels to guide dose adjustment are recommended.
- Counsel the patient regarding importance of adequate rest, hydration, and medication compliance.
- Use of AEDs is not an absolute contraindication to breast feeding.

New-Onset Seizures during Pregnancy

- Evaluation and management is similar to the nonpregnant patient.
- In patients greater than 20 weeks estimated gestational age, evaluate for a diagnosis of eclampsia.
- Electroencephalogram and neuroimaging should be done as indicated for evaluation.
- AED treatment, if needed, should be started. Lowest dose needed to control symptoms is recommended.

Headache

Although most headaches affecting women of childbearing age are migraine or tension, new-onset and severe headaches during pregnancy should be evaluated for the possibility of more dangerous conditions (Table 14-2).

- Even in patients who report a history of headaches, pain that is more severe or different in character indicates need for further evaluation.
- In patients at more than 20 weeks of gestation with complaints of a diffuse headache associated with hypertension (HTN), vision changes, epigastric pain, or proteinuria, should be evaluated for severe preeclampsia.
- Severe headache (especially associated with focal neurologic signs) should be evaluated by neuroimaging.
- If indicated, lumbar puncture is not contraindicated by pregnancy.

Migraine Headache

- Most women with migraine headaches experience some improvement during pregnancy, and only 5% report worsening of symptoms.
- Postpartum recurrence is common. Women who experience menstrual migraines are more likely to have a postpartum recurrence. This may be linked to the fluctuation in estrogen levels.
- Various treatments are reasonable in pregnancy including: avoidance of triggers and medication (acute and prophylactic).
- Use of ergotamine is contraindicated during pregnancy, but may be used postpartum.
- Use of nonsteroidal antiinflammatory drugs should be limited, and used for less than 48 hours if necessary.
- Chronic use of opiates is discouraged because of potential for maternal addiction and neonatal withdrawal.

TABLE 14-2. HEADACHE TREATMENT OPTIONS DURING PREGNANCY

Acute Therapy	Prophylaxis
· Acetaminophen (do not exceed 4 g/day) · Hydration · Acetaminophen with codeine · Fioricet · Short term narcotics (IV or PO) · Antiemetics (PO or IV) · Metoclopramide · Sumatriptan (for moderate to severe symptoms)	· Beta-blockers (metoprolol or propranolol preferred) · Calcium channel blockers (avoid hypotension) · Antidepressants (SSRI, tricyclic) · Behavioral interventions (relaxation, biofeedback, massage)

IV, intravenous; PO, oral; SSRI, selective serotonin reuptake inhibitor.

- Prophylaxis is reasonable if indicated. Beta-blockers (avoid atenolol because of greater risk for fetal growth restriction) and calcium channel blockers (avoid hypotension) are common therapies, and safe during pregnancy.

Tension Headache

- These headaches tend to wax and wane, and unlike migraine headaches, are less likely to involve gastrointestinal symptoms, or light, smell, and sound hypersensitivity.
- Tension headaches are not hormonally mediated, and are unlikely to improve during pregnancy.
- Treatment is similar to migraine headache, but may also benefit from biobehavioral interventions (relaxation and biofeedback).

Preeclampsia

- A diagnosis should be considered in all women at more than 20 weeks of gestation with a headache.
- Headache associated with a diagnosis of preeclampsia is most often diffuse, and severity may vary.
- Scotomata or other vision changes may also be evident.
- Evaluation for HTN, proteinuria, and characteristic laboratory abnormalities is indicated.
- If preeclampsia is diagnosed, the presence of headache indicates severe disease.

New-Onset Headache during Pregnancy

- New headaches during pregnancy are not common.
- Rule out a diagnosis of preeclampsia if patient is at more than 20 weeks of gestation.
- In absence of a prior headache history, or report of severe or uncharacteristic headache pain, further evaluation is indicated.
- Focal neurologic signs further indicate need for evaluation.
- Neuroimaging is appropriate during pregnancy as indicated by clinical presentation. Angiogram may also be done safely if indicated.
- If indicated, lumbar puncture is not contraindicated by pregnancy.

Note: Avoid long-term narcotic use, which may lead to maternal dependence and neonatal withdrawal. Ergotamine is contraindicated during pregnancy. Avoid use of nonsteroidal antiinflammatory drugs during pregnancy.

Diagnostic Imaging during Pregnancy (Table 14-3)

- Human studies regarding safe levels of ionizing radiation exposure during pregnancy are limited. Recommendations are based on historic high-level exposures (eg, Hiroshima) and animal studies.

TABLE 14-3. DIAGNOSTIC IMAGING STUDIES

Imaging Study	Fetal Exposure (mrad)
Chest x-ray	<1
Abdominal x-ray	200–300
Dental x-ray	0.01
IV pyelogram	400–900
Chest CT	30
Abdominal CT	250
Cerebral angiography	<10
Helical chest CT	37
VQ, ^{99}Tc	50
Head imaging/pelvic shielding	Negligible

IV, intravenous; CT, computed tomography; ^{99}Tc, technetium 99; V/Q, ventilation-perfusion scan.

- Effects are related to type of exposure, duration, dose, and gestational age.
- Most diagnostic imaging procedures result in low level exposure to the fetus.
- No increased risk for fetal anomalies, growth delay, pregnancy loss, or IQ deficit is expected with radiation doses less than 5 rads.
- Radiation effects within the first 14 days after conception results in an unaffected embryo or loss: "all or none" effect.
- Possible effects of ionizing radiation beyond 14 days gestation may include: malformations, growth restriction, microcephaly (most common). Threshold for possible effects at less than 16 weeks of gestation is 10 to 20 rads. Threshold is greater after 16 weeks of gestation.
- Contrast materials may be used when necessary for diagnosis. Gadolinium and iodine 131 should be avoided.
- Magnetic resonance imaging use has been discouraged during the first trimester (National Radiologic Protection Board); however, use is not contraindicated if the benefit exceeds the possible risk.
- Coordination of care with radiology is recommended to time use of contrast agents, limit number of images or time of exposure, and increase hydration, in efforts to decrease radiation exposure to fetus.

Gastrointestinal Illness during Pregnancy (Table 14-4)

- Fifty to ninety percent of all pregnancies are complicated by some degree of nausea (with or without emesis).
- Symptoms peak by 9 weeks of gestation, and abate in most cases by 18 weeks.
- Up to 20% of pregnant patients may have persistent symptoms until the third trimester.
- Symptoms may occur at any time of the day or night.
- Dehydration must be recognized and corrected in pregnant patients experiencing severe or chronic nausea and emesis.

Hyperemesis Gravidarum

- Persistent, severe nausea and emesis, 5% or greater weight loss from prepregnancy weight, and ketonuria.
- Usually improves as gestation progresses. Resolves after delivery.
- Etiology is uncertain.
- May be associated with the increased levels of β-human chorionic gonadotropin complicating gestational trophoblastic disease and multiple gestation.
- Ultrasound to should be done to assess pregnancy viability.
- Altered gastric motility in cases of diabetic gastroparesis may exacerbate this condition.
- Electrolyte abnormalities (hypokalemia) should be corrected.
- Liver enzymes may be mildly elevated and will correct with resolution of emesis.
- Thyroid-stimulating hormone may be suppressed. Treatment for hyperthyroidism should not be started without associated free thyroxine (T_4), antithyroid antibodies, goiter, or other evidence of primary thyroid disorder.

TABLE 14-4. TREATMENT OF NAUSEA AND EMESIS DURING PREGNANCY

Encourage oral intake as tolerated, with attention to hydration
Antiemetic therapy: promethazine (Phenergan) oral, rectal, IM
ondansetron (Zofran) oral, IV
metoclopramide (Reglan) oral, IV
Vitamin B_6 10–25 mg + doxylamine 12.5 mg
H_2 blocker (eg, famotidine [Pepcid])

H_2, histamine 2; IM, intramuscular; IV, intravenous.

Persistent, Severe Nausea and Emesis during Pregnancy

- Provide medical therapy similar to treatment for nausea and emesis during pregnancy.
- Evaluate for ketonuria: rehydrate (may need to provide substrate) until urine ketones cleared.
- Evaluate for, and correct, electrolyte abnormalities.
- Resistant nausea and vomiting may necessitate steroid therapy, partial parenteral nutrition, nasogastric tube, or outpatient intravenous (IV) hydration.

Endocrine Diseases in Pregnancy

Diabetes

Preexisting Diabetes

- Maintain normal glycated hemoglobin in patient's planning pregnancy to minimize fetal and pregnancy risks.
- Obtain baseline maternal studies in early pregnancy: maternal electrocardiogram and echocardiogram, ophthalmologic examination, 24-hour urine protein, serum creatinine.
- Thyroid function tests (TFTs) are recommended if not previously evaluated in insulin-dependent diabetes mellitus patient.
- Blood sugar should be monitored fasting and 2 hours postprandial. Premeal values may be indicated in cases of carbohydrate counting.
- Blood sugar targets: less than 90 to 95 mg/dL fasting, less than 120 mg/dL 2 hours postprandial.
- Preferred medications for blood sugar control: Glyburide or insulin.
- Patients maintained on an insulin pump should continue with pregnancy blood sugar targets observed.

Gestational Diabetes

- Diagnosis confirmed by 2 or more abnormal values on a 100 g glucose tolerance test.
  - Fasting: 95 mg/dL
  - 1 hour: 180 mg/dL
  - 2 hour: 155 mg/dL
  - 3 hour: 140 mg/dL
- Blood sugar should be monitored fasting and 2 hours postprandial.
- Blood sugar targets: less than 90 to 95 mg/dL fasting, less than 120 mg/dL 2 hours postprandial.
- Medical therapy for blood sugar control: Glyburide or insulin.
- Gestational diabetes increases lifetime risk of type II diabetes. A 75-g glucose tolerance test is recommended 6 to 8 weeks postpartum. Routine screening with the patient's primary care provider is recommended thereafter.

Thyroid Disease in Pregnancy (Table 14-5)

Hypothyroidism

- Some symptoms may mimic those of normal pregnancy: fatigue, constipation, muscle cramps, dry skin, and cold intolerance.
- Treatment: levothyroxine

TABLE 14-5. THYROID FUNCTION TESTS IN PREGNANCY

	TSH	Free T$_4$	Total T$_4$	Total T$_3$
Hypothyroid	Increased	Decreased	Decreased	Decreased
Hyperthyroid	Decreased	Increased	Increased	Increased
Normal	No change	No change	Increased	Increased

T$_3$, triiodothyronine; T$_4$, thyroxine; TSH, thyroid-stimulating hormone.

- Evaluate TFTs each trimester in stable patients; evaluate TFTs within 4 to 6 weeks of any change in dose.
- Goal: Normalize thyroid-stimulating hormone

Hyperthyroidism

- Symptoms: tachycardia, heat intolerance, weight loss, palpitations, HTN, sweating, insomnia, goiter.
- Graves disease is most common cause.
- Thyroid-stimulating antibody titers may be evaluated if diagnosis of Graves is uncertain. Serial titers do not change OB management, or fetal surveillance.
- Suboptimal treatment may increase risk for pregnancy loss and fetal growth delay.
- Transient subclinical hyperthyroidism related to elevated human chorionic gonadotropin levels in early pregnancy does not require treatment. Reevaluate TFTs in the second trimester to ensure resolution.
- Treatment: thioamide at lowest dose to maintain free T_4 at upper limits of normal.
- Beta-blocker may be used to control maternal tachycardia if needed. Beta-blocker should be weaned when symptoms are controlled by thioamide dose.
- Radioiodine ablation is absolutely contraindicated during pregnancy.
- Thyroidectomy is reasonable during pregnancy if the patient cannot tolerate medical management.

Thioamide Therapy

Preconception

- Methimazole (MMI) most often used in nonpregnant adults.
- Consider conversion to propylthiouracil (PTU) if planning pregnancy.
- Both medications cross the placenta.
- Reports of aplasia cutis, tracheoesophageal fistulas, and choanal atresia in newborns of mothers treated with MMI.

Pregnancy

- Consider conversion to PTU at least during the first trimester.
- Treatment beyond the first trimester may be by PTU or MMI.
- Evaluate monthly TFTs. Adjust treatment to maintain free T_4 at the upper limits of normal.
- Serial antithyroid antibody titers are not necessary.
- Reports of hepatotoxicity related to PTU have been reported. Liver function test evaluation should be done after initiation of this medication.

Postpartum

- Graves hyperthyroidism may worsen postpartum, and patients in remission may experience relapse.
- Pediatrics should be notified of the maternal diagnosis to ensure appropriate newborn evaluation.

Thyroid Storm: Signs and Symptoms

- Metabolic: Fever, flushed skin, excessive perspiration
- Central nervous system: Irritability, tremor, mental status changes (psychosis, delirium)
- Cardiovascular: Tachycardia, congestive heart failure, arrhythmia
- Gastrointestinal: Nausea and emesis, diarrhea, jaundice (elevated liver function test results)

Management of Thyroid Storm

General Measures

- Admit to intensive care unit
  - OB consult
  - Cardiac monitoring
  - Cooling measures
  - Laboratory evaluation

- Oxygen as needed
- Nasogastric tube if needed

Pharmacologic Therapy
- Propranolol to control tachycardia
  - 20 to 80 mg orally every 4 to 6 hours or
  - 1 to 10 mg IV every 4 hours
- Oral PTU (by nasogastric tube if necessary)
  - 300 to 600 mg load; 150 to 200 mg every 4 to 6 hours
- Iodide 1 to 2 hours after starting PTU
  - Oral Lugol iodine solution (8 drops every 6 hours) or
  - IV sodium iodide (500–1000 mg every 8 hours) or
  - Oral lithium carbonate (300 mg every 6 hours)
- Adrenal glucocorticoids
  - Dexamethasone (2 mg IV every 6 hours × 4 doses) or
  - Hydrocortisone (100 mg IV every 8 hours) or
  - Prednisone (60 mg orally daily)

Infectious Diseases and Pregnancy

Vaccination
- Increased morbidity and mortality in pregnant patients with certain infections (eg, influenza).
- Efficacy and safety of inactive, killed, or recombinant vaccines has been shown.
- Live vaccines should not be given during pregnancy.
- All pregnant patients should receive the influenza vaccine, and hepatitis B vaccine (if nonimmune).
- At-risk pregnant patients should receive the pneumococcal and hepatitis A vaccines.
- Tetanus-diphtheria-pertussis vaccination should be encouraged for postpartum patients to provide protection to the infant.

Influenza
- All pregnant patients should be vaccinated against seasonal influenza and H_1N_1.
- The vaccine is safe and effective in all trimesters of pregnancy.
- Pregnant patients with fever and flulike symptoms should be treated empirically.
- Initiation of treatment is best if within 48 hours of symptom onset. Do *not* wait for influenza test results if performed.
- Treatment: oseltamivir (Tamiflu) 75 mg orally, twice daily for 5 days.
- Observation for symptoms of developing pneumonia is necessary.
- Oxygen should be used to maintain saturation at more than 95%.
- Superimposed bacterial respiratory infection should be treated if present (more common in smokers and asthma).
- Encourage smoking cessation.
- Treat asthma exacerbations as indicated.
- Intubation for respiratory support should be employed as necessary.

Asthma in Pregnancy (Table 14-6)

- One-third of patients improve, one-third of patients worsen, and one-third of patients remain unchanged.
- Patients should be instructed on daily peak flow monitoring, and baseline values should be recorded by provider.
- Environmental triggers should be reviewed and eliminated.
- Smoking cessation should be encouraged if indicated.
- In cases of acute exacerbation, partial pressure of carbon dioxide higher than 35 mm Hg or partial pressure of oxygen lower than 70 mm Hg indicates respiratory distress given the baseline changes in pregnancy.

TABLE 14-6. STEP THERAPY FOR CHRONIC ASTHMA DURING
            PREGNANCY

Mild Intermittent	Short-Acting Beta-Agonist PRN
Mild persistent	Inhaled glucocorticoid Short-acting β-agonist PRN
Moderate persistent	Inhaled glucocorticoid Long-acting β-agonist Short-acting β-agonist PRN
Severe persistent	Inhaled glucocorticoid Long-acting β-agonist Leukotriene receptor antagonist (or oral prednisone if needed) Short-acting β-agonist PRN

PRN, as needed.

Cardiovascular Disease in Pregnancy

Hypertensive Disease in Pregnancy

Chronic Hypertension

- Elevated blood pressure recognized prior to pregnancy or before 20 weeks of gestation.
- Hypertension defined as systolic blood pressure higher than 140 mm Hg or diastolic blood pressure higher than 90 mm Hg.
- Persistent HTN after postpartum recovery.

Mild Preeclampsia

- Usually diagnosed at more than 20 weeks of gestation.
- Blood pressure 140 mm Hg systolic or higher, or 90 mm Hg diastolic or higher *and*
- Proteinuria defined as 300 mg or greater on 24-hour collection.

Severe Preeclampsia

One or more of the following criteria:

- Blood pressure 160 mm Hg systolic or higher, or 110 mm Hg diastolic or higher on more than 1 occasion 6 hours apart at rest.
- Proteinuria 5 g or greater on 24-hour collection.
- Mild preeclampsia with at least one of the following:
  - Oliguria defined as less than 500 mL in 24 hours
  - Vision changes (scotomata)
  - Persistent epigastric pain or right upper quadrant pain
  - Elevated aspartate aminotransferase or alanine aminotransferase
  - Fetal growth restriction
  - Persistent diffuse headache
  - New-onset thrombocytopenia

Eclampsia

- The presence of generalized seizure in the presence of preeclampsia.
- Transient loss of vision or mental status changes may also be seen.
- Preeclampsia and eclampsia may be noted antepartum, peripartum, or postpartum (usually <2–4 weeks post delivery).
- Treatment for eclamptic seizure: magnesium sulfate IV bolus 6 g, then 2 g/h.
  - Chronic antihypertensive therapy (starting dose) in pregnancy:
    - Labetalol 100 mg twice daily
    - Methyldopa 250 mg twice daily

- Nifedipine 10 mg twice daily

  Note: Use of angiotensin-converting enzyme inhibitors and angiotensin receptor blockers is contraindicated. Avoid use of diuretics for chronic treatment during pregnancy.

- Acute antihypertensive therapy in pregnancy:
  - Labetalol 10 to 40 mg IV every 10 to 15 minutes
  - Hydralazine 5 to 10 mg IV every 20 minutes
  - Nifedipine 10 to 20 mg orally every 20 to 30 minutes (maximum dose 50 mg)

Opiate Addiction in Pregnancy

- There is a growing addiction to prescription opiates in reproductive-age women.
- May affect women of all socioeconomic, racial, and age groups.
- Patients with addiction issues may use more than one substance.
- Screen all pregnant patients by asking them about drug use.
- Testing may include urine, hair, blood, saliva, or sweat.
- Urine testing is most widely used.
- Inquire about drugs used, amounts, and routes.
- Test for sexually transmitted diseases, human immunodeficiency virus, and hepatitis; especially if IV drug use or prostitution is reported.
- Illicit drug use may increase risk for pregnancy complications including HTN, vaginal bleeding, poor fetal growth, and fetal distress.
- Detoxification from opiates is *not* recommended during pregnancy. Risks for fetal loss and distress have been suggested.
- Maintenance on methadone or buprenorphine is recommended. These medications require a special U.S. Drug Enforcement Administration license for prescription, unless being given to an established patient hospitalized for other pregnancy reasons.
- Methadone and buprenorphine are not associated with fetal anomalies, and may improve fetal growth because of consistent dosing.
- Neonatal withdrawal is expected with prenatal methadone and buprenorphine therapy and with illicit opiate use as well. This often occurs within 2 to 4 days of delivery.
- Consensus on breastfeeding on methadone or buprenorphine is not clear, and should be discussed with pediatrics.

CHAPTER 15

Gynecology

Amanda B. Murchison, Allison R. Durica, and Patrice M. Weiss

WELLNESS AND IMMUNIZATIONS FOR THE FEMALE PATIENT

- Adolescent: Age 13 to 18 years
  - History screening
    - Dietary assessment
    - Physical activity and exercise
    - Tobacco, alcohol, or drug use
    - Sexual practices
    - Depression
  - Laboratory testing and cancer prevention and screening
    - Chlamydia and gonorrhea testing if sexually active
  - Counseling
    - Contraceptive counseling if sexually active
    - Prevention of sexually transmitted infections (STIs)
    - Folic acid supplementation 0.4 mg daily
    - Dental hygiene
    - Safety belt and helmet use
  - Immunizations
    - Tetanus-diphtheria-pertussis booster (once between ages 11 and 16 years)
    - Hepatitis B series if not completed
    - Human papillomavirus (HPV) series if not completed
    - Meningococcal vaccine prior to starting high school
    - Consider offering influenza vaccine yearly
  - Leading causes of death
    - Accidents
    - Malignant neoplasms
    - Homicide
    - Suicide
- Adult: Age 19 to 39 years
  - History screening
    - Dietary assessment
    - Physical activity and exercise
    - Tobacco, alcohol, or drug use
    - Sexual practices
    - Depression
  - Laboratory testing and cancer prevention and screening
    - Cervical cytology screening to start at age 21 years (see Papanicolaou Test Screening and Management)
    - Chlamydia screening if 25 years or younger and sexually active
    - Offer complete STI screening (chlamydia, gonorrhea, *Trichomonas*, human immunodeficiency virus, syphilis, hepatitis B)
    - Monthly self breast examinations
  - Counseling
    - Contraceptive options
    - Preconception counseling (consider referral to obstetrics and gynecology if planning pregnancy)
    - Prevention of STIs

- Folic acid supplementation 0.4 mg daily
- Dental hygiene
- Safety belts and helmets
- Immunizations
  - HPV if patient is 26 years of age or younger and not yet vaccinated
  - Tetanus-diphtheria-pertussis booster every 10 years
  - Offer influenza vaccine yearly
- Leading causes of death
  - Malignant neoplasms
  - Accidents
  - Heart disease
  - Suicide
- Adult: Age 40 to 64 years
  - History screening
    - Dietary assessment
    - Physical activity and exercise
    - Tobacco, alcohol, or drug use
    - Sexual practices
    - Urinary and fecal incontinence
    - Depression
  - Laboratory testing and cancer screening
    - Cervical cytology screening (see Papanicolaou Test Screening and Management)
    - Monthly self breast examinations
    - Mammography yearly
    - Lipid profile: every 5 years starting at age 45
    - Thyroid-stimulating hormone (TSH): every 5 years starting at age 50 years
    - Colorectal cancer screening starting at age 50 years
    - Bone density screening if risk factors exist
  - Counseling
    - Contraceptive counseling until menopause
    - Folic acid supplementation 0.4 mg daily until menopause
    - Calcium supplementation
    - Menopausal management (see Menopause)
  - Immunizations
    - Offer Influenza Vaccine Yearly
    - Tetanus-diphtheria-pertussis booster every 10 years
    - Shingles vaccine at age 60 years
  - Leading causes of death
    - Malignant neoplasms
    - Heart disease
    - Cerebrovascular disease
    - Chronic lower respiratory diseases
- Adult: Age 65 years and older
  - History screening
    - Dietary assessment
    - Physical activity and exercise
    - Tobacco, alcohol, or drug use
    - Sexual practices
    - Urinary and fecal incontinence
    - Depression
  - Laboratory testing and cancer screening
    - Cervical cytology screening if appropriate (see Papanicolaou Test Screening and Management)
    - Monthly self breast examinations
    - Mammography yearly
    - Urinalysis

- Lipid profile: every 5 years starting at age 45 years
- TSH: every 5 years starting at age 50 years
- Colorectal cancer screening starting at age 50 years
- Bone density screening age 65 years
- Counseling
  - Sexual function
  - Calcium supplementation
  - Menopausal management (see Menopause)
- Immunizations
  - Influenza vaccine yearly
  - Tetanus-diphtheria-pertussis booster every 10 years
  - Pneumococcal vaccine (once)
  - Shingles vaccine if older than 60 years and not vaccinated
- Leading causes of death
  - Heart disease
  - Malignant neoplasms
  - Cerebrovascular disease
  - Chronic lower respiratory diseases

PAPANICOLAOU TEST SCREENING AND MANAGEMENT (TABLE 15-1)

- Screening guidelines (As recommended in ACOG practice Bulletin 131)
  - Begin screening at age 21
  - Ages 21-29
    - Screen every 3 years using cervical cytology (pap smear)
  - Ages 30 and over
    - Preferred Screening: Screen every 5 years using cervical cytology plus Human Papilloma Virus (HPV) testing for high risk types
    - Acceptable Screening: Screen every 3 years using cervical cytology
  - Women with history of Cervical Intraepithelial Neoplasia (CIN) 2 or higher should receive routine screening for at least 20 years
  - May stop screening at age 65 if last 3 paps normal and no history of CIN 2 or higher in the previous 20 years
    - Reassess annually for new risk factors (such as new sexual partner) and reinitiate screening if indicated
    - May stop screening if hysterectomy has been done for benign indications and no prior history of high grade cervical dysplasia (CIN 2 or higher)
- Human Papilloma Virus
  - DNA virus
    - Low-oncogenic
    - High-oncogenic types 16 and 18 responsible for 70% cervical cancer in the United States
  - Usually transient
    - In 8 months, 50% cleared
    - In 2 years, 90% cleared
  - Infects immature basal cells at cervical squamocolumnar junction
- Cervical cytology
  - Negative for intraepithelial lesion

TABLE 15-1. NATURAL HISTORY OF DYSPLASIA

PAP	Regress	Persist	Progress
LSIL	60%	30%	10% to HSIL
HSIL	30%	60%	10% to carcinoma

HSIL, high-grade squamous intraepithelial lesion; LSIL, low-grade squamous intraepithelial lesion; PAP, Papanicolaou.

- Atypical squamous cells of undetermined significance
- Atypical squamous cells, high-grade
- Low-grade squamous intraepithelial lesion
- High-grade squamous intraepithelial lesion
- Atypical glandular cells
- Management of abnormal Papanicolaou tests (Figure 15-1)
- Cervical cancer prevention
  - HPV vaccine
    - Quadrivalent recombinant vaccine (Gardasil) approved by the U.S. Food and Drug Administration (FDA) in 2006
    - Protects against HPV types 6, 11, 16, 18
    - Noninfectious, DNA-free virus-like particles
    - Produces high level of serum antibodies
    - Three injections (0, 2, 6 months)
    - Approved for ages 9 through 26 years

CONTRACEPTION (TABLE 15-2)

- Review of hormonal agents
  - Estrogens
    - Suppresses release of follicle-stimulating hormone (FSH)
    - Accelerates ovum transport
  - Progestins
    - Suppresses release of luteinizing hormone (LH)
    - Increases cervical mucus
    - Prevents capacitation of sperm
    - Thins lining of uterus

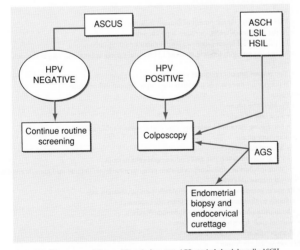

Figure 15-1 Management of abnormal Papanicolaou tests. AGS, atypical glandular cells; ASCH, high-grade atypical squamous cells; ASCUS, atypical squamous cells of undetermined significance; HPV, human papillomavirus; HSIL, high-grade squamous intraepithelial lesion; LSIL, low-grade squamous intraepithelial lesion; Pap, Papanicolaou test.

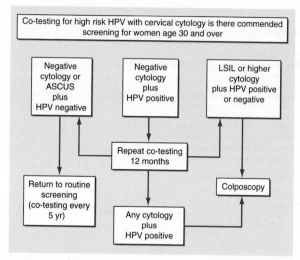

Co-testing for high risk HPV with cervical cytology is there commended screening for women age 30 and over

Negative cytology or ASCUS plus HPV negative

Negative cytology plus HPV positive

LSIL or higher cytology plus HPV positive or negative

Repeat co-testing 12 months

Return to routine screening (co-testing every 5 yr)

Any cytology plus HPV positive

Colposcopy

MENSTRUAL CYCLE

- Hypothalamic-pituitary-ovarian axis (Figure 15-2)
  - Hypothalamus releases gonadotropin-releasing hormone in a pulsatile fashion.
  - Pituitary releases FSH and LH.
- Ovary
  - FSH stimulates development of ovarian follicles.
  - As the follicles develop, estrogen is produced.
  - Increasing FSH levels cause negative feedback to the pituitary.
  - Increasing estrogen levels lead to the LH surge resulting in ovulation (approximately day 14).
  - The corpus luteum produces progesterone.
  - If pregnancy does not occur, then the corpus luteum will involute.
- Uterus
  - Proliferative phase
    - First half of cycle.
    - Increasing estradiol levels stimulate endometrial proliferation.
  - Secretory phase
    - Second half of cycle.
    - Progesterone levels rise and endometrial growth stops.
    - With involution of the corpus luteum progesterone levels decline and menses ensues.
- Normal menstrual cycle
  - Requires maturation of the hypothalamic-pituitary-ovarian axis
    - Tends to be immature in first 2 years after menarche.
    - Immature pathway can lead to anovulatory cycles.
  - Normal cycle length is 21 to 35 days.
  - Menses typically lasts 3 to 7 days.
- Premenstrual syndrome
  - Timing
    - 1 to 2 weeks prior to menses
    - Resolves with menses

TABLE 15-2. CONTRACEPTIVE OPTIONS

Contraceptive	Number of Pregnancies Expected (per 100 women)	Dosing	Advantages	Disadvantages	Contraindications
Combined OCPs	5	Daily	Lighter periods, improves dysmenorrhea, decreases ovarian cysts, decreases ovarian cancer risk	Compliance, DVT risk: 15–20/100,000	Pregnancy, undiagnosed abnormal bleeding, liver disease, thromboembolic disease, HTN, lupus, breast cancer, migraine with aura, older than 35 years of age and smoker
OCP extended/continuous use	5	Daily	Same as OCPs above, fewer periods	Same as OCPs above, higher breakthrough bleeding rate	Same as OCPs above
Transdermal contraceptive patch	5	Weekly	Same as OCPs, improved compliance, bypass first-pass metabolism	Allergic skin reaction, same as OCPs	Same as OCPs, not well studied in patients weighing more than 90.7 kg (200 lb)
Vaginal ring	5	Every 3 weeks	Same as OCP, improved compliance, bypass first-pass metabolism	Vaginal irritation, same as OCPs; patient must insert and remove	Same as OCPs
Progestin-only pills	5	Daily	Approved with breastfeeding	Compliance	Pregnancy, breast cancer, active DVT, acute liver disease
Medroxyprogesterone acetate Injection	1	Every 3 months	Decreases incidence of sickle cell crisis, 50% have amenorrhea by fourth injection	Clinic appointment for injection, irregular bleeding, weight gain, delayed return of fertility, bone loss, depression	Pregnancy, breast cancer, active DVT, acute liver disease

(continued on next page)

TABLE 15-2. CONTRACEPTIVE OPTIONS (Continued)

Contraceptive	Number of Pregnancies Expected (per 100 women)	Dosing	Advantages	Disadvantages	Contraindications
Implantable rod	1	Every 3 years	Compliance	Must be placed by trained professional, irregular bleeding, acne	Pregnancy, breast cancer, active DVT, acute liver disease
Copper IUD	1	Every 10 years	Compliance	Insertion by trained professional, risk of uterine perforation, menses may be heavier with more cramping, PID	Distorted uterine cavity (large fibroid)
Progesterone IUD	1	Every 5 years (smaller version every 3 years)	Compliance, decreased menstrual flow	Insertion by trained professional, risk of uterine perforation, irregular bleeding in first 3 months, PID	Distorted uterine cavity (large fibroid)
Male condom	11–16	With intercourse	Prevention of STIs, over the counter	Compliance	Allergic reaction
Diaphragm with spermicide	15	With intercourse	Inexpensive, no hormones	Requires fitting in clinic, must leave in place 6–8 hours after intercourse	Allergic reaction, frequent bladder infections
Female sterilization	1	One-time procedure	One-time procedure	Requires referral to gynecology	Surgical procedure, regret
Emergency contraceptive[a]	15	Must use within 120 hours of unprotected intercourse		Requires prescription if younger than 17 years of age	Known pregnancy

DVT, deep vein thrombosis; HTN, hypertension; IUD, intrauterine contraceptive device; OCP, oral contraceptive pill; PID, pelvic inflammatory disease; STI, sexually transmitted infection.
[a]Not intended as regular form of birth control.

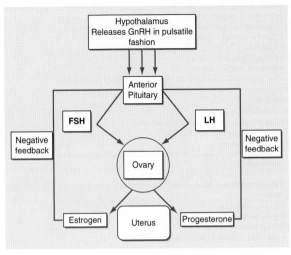

Figure 15-2   Hypothalamic-pituitary-ovarian axis. FSH, follicle-stimulating hormone; GnRH, gonadotropin-releasing hormone; LH, luteinizing hormone.

- Symptoms
  - Irritability
  - Mood swings
  - Trouble sleeping
  - Anxiety
  - Depression
  - Diarrhea
  - Constipation
- Treatment
  - Exercise
  - Healthy diet
  - Oral contraceptive pills (OCPs)
- Premenstrual dysphoric disorder: severe form of premenstrual syndrome that can be disabling
  - Treatment
    - Selective serotonin reuptake inhibitors
    - Drospirenone-ethinyl estradiol (Yaz) (only OCP with FDA approval for premenstrual dysphoric disorder)

ABNORMAL UTERINE BLEEDING

- Definitions
  - Oligomenorrhea: more than 35 days between menses
  - Amenorrhea: absence of menses for 6 months or more
  - Menorrhagia: menstrual flow more than 80 cc or lasting longer than 7 days
  - Metrorrhagia: intermenstrual bleeding
  - Dysfunctional uterine bleeding: used to describe abnormal bleeding in which no underlying cause is identified and usually implies anovulation (diagnosis of exclusion)
- Etiology
  - Anovulation

- Failure of rising estrogen levels to cause a decline in FSH and ultimately resulting in no decline in estrogen levels.
- Unopposed estrogen then leads to endometrial proliferation.
  - First 2 years after menarche.
  - Anorexia.
  - Excessive physical exercise.
  - Polycystic ovarian syndrome.
  - See below for endocrine dysfunctions that can lead to anovulation.
- Pregnancy
- Hematologic
  - Von Willebrand disease
  - Idiopathic thrombocytopenia purpura
- Endocrine and systemic dysfunctions
  - Thyroid dysfunction
    - Hypothyroidism is associated with increased peripheral conversion of testosterone to estradiol.
      - Menorrhagia occurs in 20% of patients.
    - Hyperthyroidism is associated with amenorrhea.
  - Diabetes
    - Insulin resistance
    - Anovulatory cycles
  - Liver disease
    - Impaired metabolism of estrogen
    - Decreased production of coagulation factors
  - Renal disease
    - May develop hyperprolactinemia leading to amenorrhea
- Infectious
  - Chlamydia
  - Gonorrhea
  - Trichomoniasis
  - Pelvic inflammatory disease
- Anatomic
  - Müllerian anomaly
    - Vaginal septum
    - Uterine didelphys
  - Uterine leiomyomas
  - Endometrial polyp
  - Endocervical polyp
  - Adenomyosis
    - Endometrial stoma within the myometrium
    - Symptoms include menorrhagia, dysmenorrhea and dyspareunia
    - Sometimes identified on ultrasound
- Exogenous hormones
  - Oral contraceptive pills: breakthrough bleeding seen 30% of the time in first three cycles.
  - Depot medroxyprogesterone acetate (DMPA) can be associated with irregular bleeding especially in the first year.
- Neoplasia
  - Cervical cancer
  - Endometrial hyperplasia or cancer
- Evaluation
  - Adolescent
    - Limited examination may be appropriate if not sexually active.
    - Consider testing for gonorrhea and chlamydia.
      - Cervical culture for DNA probe
      - Urine (must be dirty catch)

- Pregnancy test.
- Consider complete blood count (CBC) or von Willebrand testing if menorrhagia.
- Pelvic ultrasound (not always needed):
  - Transabdominal only if not sexually active
  - Helpful when müllerian anomaly suspected
- Reproductive age
  - CBC if patient reports heavy bleeding.
  - Pregnancy test.
  - TSH.
  - Pelvic ultrasound.
  - Endometrial biopsy if patient is 35 years of age or older:
    - Endometrial hyperplasia: referral to gynecology
    - Endometrial cancer: referral to gynecologic oncology
  - Pelvic examination.
  - Make sure Papanicolaou test is current.
- Postmenopausal bleeding (often spotting or light bleeding)
  - Pelvic examination
    - Look for other causes of bleeding:
      - Vaginal atrophy
      - hemorrhoids
  - Make sure Papanicolaou tests is current.
  - Pelvic ultrasound.
  - Endometrial biopsy:
    - If a transvaginal ultrasound shows an endometrial stripe measurement of 4 mm or less then unlikely to be hyperplasia or uterine malignancy (option to not perform biopsy)
- Management
  - Adolescent
    - Nonsteroidal antiinflammatory agents have been shown to decrease menstrual flow.
    - Combination oral contraceptive pill:
      - Confirm no contraindications to estrogen.
      - Consider a continuous OCP if patient desires to avoid menses.
    - DMPA:
      - Injection given every 3 months
      - Associated with more weight gain
  - Reproductive age
    - Nonsteroidal antiinflammatory drugs
    - OCPs
    - Progesterone therapy
    - DMPA
    - Cyclic medroxyprogesterone acetate (Provera)
      - 10 mg medroxyprogesterone acetate orally for 10 to 12 days each month
      - Will have withdrawal bleed within 1 week of stopping the medication
    - Continuous medroxyprogesterone acetate
    - Levonorgestrel-releasing intrauterine device (Mirena IUD)
      - Decreases menstrual blood loss by 80% to 90%
    - Surgical therapy
      - Hysteroscopy with removal of intrauterine pathology such as polyp or submucosal fibroid (if identified on ultrasound)
      - Endometrial ablation is an outpatient procedure resulting in destruction (ablation) of endometrial lining
      - Hysterectomy
        - Failed medical therapy
        - Large fibroids preventing less invasive surgery
        - Other additional diagnosis such as pelvic pain

- Postmenopausal
  - If endometrial hyperplasia and cancer are ruled out, then expectant management is appropriate (most bleeding light).
  - Hysteroscopy and polypectomy if endometrial polyp suspected.
  - Referral to gynecologic oncology if endometrial cancer.
- Emergency management of acute bleeding (adolescent and reproductive age)
  - Will need full evaluation as above.
  - Conjugated estrogen 2.5 mg orally every 6 hours followed by initiation of a combination OCP when bleeding improves (make sure no contraindications to estrogen).
  - If bleeding does not improve, then consider dilation and curettage.

VULVOVAGINAL DISORDERS

- Pertinent history
  - Symptoms
    - Itching
    - Vaginal discharge
    - Pain
    - Rash or lesions
    - Timing
  - Environmental
    - Changes in soaps or detergents
    - New medications (antibiotics)
    - New sexual partners
- Physical examination
  - Vulva
    - Erythema
    - Rash, lesions, skin changes
  - Vagina
    - Atrophy
    - Discharge (color, consistency, odor)
    - Lesions
    - Appearance of the cervix
- Diagnostic tests
  - Wet mount
    - Swab of vaginal side walls.
    - Place on glass slide.
    - Apply potassium hydroxide stain to one side.
      - Evaluate for pseudohyphae.
    - Apply saline to the other
      - Evaluate for clue cells: superficial epithelial cells with adherent bacteria.
      - Evaluate for *Trichomonas*.
  - PH swab
    - Normal vaginal pH: less than 4.5
    - Bacterial vaginosis: pH 4.7 to 5.7
    - Candidiasis: pH less than 4.5
    - Trichomoniasis: pH more than 5.0
  - Culture
    - Gonorrhea and chlamydia polymerase chain reaction (PCR) probe
    - Yeast culture
      - Consider if not responding to therapy.
      - Most medication treat *Candida albicans* but may not treat *Candida glabrata* or *Candida tropicalis*.
      - Herpes simplex virus (HSV): PCR of vulvar lesion if herpes suspected.
  - Biopsy

TABLE 15-3. MEDICATION OPTIONS FOR TREATMENT OF VAGINITIS[a]

Vaginitis	Treatment Medication	Dosing
Bacterial vaginitis	Metronidazole	500 mg PO BID × 7 days
	Metronidazole gel	0.75% gel, 1 applicator QHS × 5 days
	Clindamycin	300 mg PO BID ×7 days
Vulvovaginal candidiasis	Miconazole	100 mg vaginal suppository QHS × 7 days (OTC)
	Fluconazole	150 mg PO × 1
	Terconazole	1 applicator 0.4% cream QHS × 7 days
Trichomoniasis	Metronidazole	500 mg PO BID × 7 days or 2 g PO × 1
Atrophic vaginitis	Estrogen vaginal cream	½ applicator PV QHS × 2 weeks followed by 2 times a week for maintenance
	Estradiol vaginal tab	10 mcg PV QHS × 2 weeks followed by 2 times a week for maintenance

BID, twice daily; OTC, over the counter; PO, orally; PV, intravaginally; QHS, at bedtime.
[a]Does not include all treatment options available.

- Vaginal disorders (Table 15-3)
  - Bacterial vaginitis
    - Decrease in lactobacilli and increase in anaerobes
    - Gray discharge with odor
  - Vulvovaginal candidiasis
    - Thick, white vaginal discharge
    - Itching
  - Trichomonas vaginitis
    - Profuse, frothy vaginal discharge
    - Strawberry cervix
    - Sexually transmitted infection (partner needs treatment)
  - Atrophic vaginitis
    - Associated with menopause or sometimes seen in postpartum women who are breastfeeding.
    - May be associated with dyspareunia.
    - Loss of vaginal rugae; mucosa may be friable.
  - Cervicitis (see Sexually Transmitted Infections)
- Vulvar disorders
  - Contact dermatitis
    - Identify and remove source
    - Can treat with topical steroid cream
  - Folliculitis
    - Often the result of shaving
    - Can treat with antibiotic like cephalexin (Keflex)
  - Bartholin gland cyst or abscess
    - Cyst
      - 1 to 3 cm
      - Often asymptomatic
      - Does not require treatment
    - Abscess
      - Severe pain

- Treat with incision and drainage
- Biopsy as well if patient older than 40 years of age
- Lichen sclerosis
  - Smooth, white plaques (parchment paper)
  - Atrophy of labia
  - Obliteration of clitoris
  - Usually in postmenopausal women
  - Diagnosis through vulvar biopsy
  - Treatment with high-potency topical steroid
  - Associated with an increased chance of developing squamous cell carcinoma of vulva so monitor with clinical examinations
- Herpes (see Sexually Transmitted Infections)
- Molluscum contagiosum
  - Poxvirus
  - Transmitted through direct contact (children)
  - Transmitted through sexual contact (adults)
  - Pearly, dome-shaped papules with umbilicated center
  - Core contains intracytoplasmic virus
  - May resolve spontaneously
  - Can treat with physical or chemical destruction
- Condyloma
  - Papillomavirus, low-oncogenic type 6, 11
  - Sexually transmitted
  - Painless
  - Verrucous lesions, usually multifocal
  - Affects vulva, perineum, vagina, or cervix
  - HPV replicates in squamous cells
  - Most transient and clear in 2 years
  - Treatment
    - Chemical destruction
      - Podophyllin
      - Trichloroacetic acid
    - Physical destruction with cryotherapy
    - Immunological therapy with imiquimod 5% cream
    - Surgical removal (gynecology referral)
- Vulvar intraepithelial neoplasia (VIN)
  - White or pigmented lesion.
  - Diagnosis through biopsy.
  - VIN grade 1: follow with examinations every 4 to 6 months and repeat biopsy if concern.
  - VIN grade 2 or 3: treatment with wide local excision or laser therapy.
- Vulvar cancer: gynecologic oncology referral

SEXUALLY TRANSMITTED INFECTIONS (TABLE 15-4)

- Chlamydia
  - Caused by bacteria *Chlamydia trachomatis*
  - Screening should be offered to all women annually who are 25 years and younger.
  - Symptoms range from none to pelvic pain, vaginal discharge, and dysuria.
  - Diagnosis: urine or endocervical DNA probe.
- Gonorrhea
  - Caused by bacteria *Neisseria gonorrhoeae*.
  - Symptoms range from none to dysuria, vaginal discharge, and intermenstrual bleeding.
  - Diagnosis: urine or endocervical DNA probe.
- Herpes
  - Caused by HSV type 1 or type 2.

TABLE 15-4. RECOMMENDED TREATMENT FOR SEXUALLY TRANSMITTED INFECTIONS

Disease	Recommended Treatment (nonpregnant female)[a]
Chlamydia	Azithromycin 1 g PO × 1 OR
	Doxycycline 100 mg PO BID × 7 days
Gonorrhea	Ceftriaxone 250 mg IM × 1 OR
	Ciprofloxacin 500 mg PO × 1[b]
Herpes	Primary outbreak: acyclovir 400 mg PO TID × 7–10 days OR valacyclovir 1 g PO BID × 7–10 days
	Recurrent therapy: acyclovir 400 mg PO TID × 5 days OR valacyclovir 500 mg PO BID × 3–5 days
	Suppressive therapy: acyclovir 400 mg PO BID OR valacyclovir 500 mg-1 g PO daily
Pelvic inflammatory disease	Ceftriaxone 250 mg IM × 1 PLUS
	Azithromycin 1 gram po × 1 OR doxycycline 100 mg po bid × 7 days
	(if allergy to cephalosporins then use azithromycin 2 grams po × 1 as single agent therapy)
Syphilis	
Primary and secondary	Benzathine penicillin G 2.4 million units IM × 1
Latent and tertiary	Benzathine penicillin G 2.4 million units IM weekly × 3
CSF-proven neurosyphilis	Requires IV penicillin therapy
Pediculosis pubis	Permethrin 1% cream to affected area and rinse in 10 minutes
Scabies	Permethrin 5% cream to body and rinse in 8 hours OR ivermectin 0.2 mg/kg PO and repeat in 14 days

BID, twice daily; CDC, Centers for Disease Control and Prevention; CSF, cerebral spinal fluid; IM, intramuscularly; IV, intravenous; PO, orally, TID, 3 times daily.
[a]Not all options listed, see CDC website for full listing.
[b]Not as effective is some areas of United States.

- Symptoms range from no symptoms (many) to cyclic genital ulcerations, vaginal and vulvar pain, dysuria and dyspareunia.
- Diagnosis: culture of lesion for herpes PCR, serum for HSV-1 and HSV-2 immunoglobulin M (IgM) and IgG.
  - If serum returns positive for HSV-1, then could be caused by oral herpes or genital herpes.
  - HSV-1 causes 30% of genital herpes today.
- HPV (see Papanicolaou Test Screening and Management)
- Pelvic inflammatory disease
  - Definition: infection of upper genital tract (uterus and fallopian tubes)
  - Caused by multiple organisms including gonorrhea and chlamydia
  - Symptoms: lower abdominal pain, fever, vaginal discharge, dyspareunia, dysuria, irregular bleeding, right upper quadrant pain
  - Diagnosis: clinical findings, CBC to evaluate white blood cell count; send gonorrhea and chlamydia culture; order pelvic sonogram to look for a tuboovarian abscess
  - Inpatient treatment recommended when
    - Ill appearing (high fever, nausea)
    - Pregnant
    - Intravenous antibiotics needed
    - Tuboovarian abscess
  - Complications: pelvic adhesions, chronic pelvic pain, ectopic pregnancy, infertility (10%–15%)

- Syphilis
  - Caused by bacterium *Treponema pallidum*
  - Symptoms
    - Primary
      - Painless chancre lasting 3 to 6 weeks
    - Secondary
      - Rough, erythematous rash on palms of hands and soles of feet
      - Fever
      - Sore throat
      - Muscle aches
      - Fatigue
    - Latent
      - Often no symptoms
    - Tertiary
      - Seen in 15% of people not treated
      - 10 to 20 years after infected
      - Difficulty with movement
      - Paralysis
      - Blindness
      - Dementia
  - Diagnosis
    - Nontreponemal test such as rapid plasma reagin or VDRL
    - Confirmatory treponemal test such as *T. pallidum* particle agglutination
- Pediculosis pubis
  - Caused by crab louse *Phthirus pubis*
  - Symptoms: itching
  - Diagnosis: clinical examination for nits or adult lice; can remove and identify under the microscope
- Scabies
  - Caused by parasite *Sarcoptes scabiei*
  - Symptoms: itching and rash
  - Diagnosis: clinically based on papular rash and identification of burrows (often in webbing of fingers or skin folds); can perform scraping of burrow site for identification of mites or mite eggs under microscope
- Trichomoniasis (see Vulvovaginal Disorders)
- Hepatitis (not discussed here)
- Human immunodeficiency virus (not discussed here)

PELVIC PAIN

- Acute: less than 6 months in duration
  - Differential diagnosis
    - Pregnancy (including ectopic)
    - Pelvic inflammatory disease
    - Endometritis
    - Ovarian neoplasm
    - Ovarian cyst
    - Ovarian torsion
    - Endometriosis
    - Nongynecologic source: gastrointestinal, urologic, musculoskeletal
  - Evaluation
    - Pelvic examination
    - Pregnancy test
    - Urinalysis
    - CBC

TABLE 15-5. DIFFERENTIATING SYMPTOMS OF STRESS AND URGE INCONTINENCE

Symptom	Stress Incontinence	Urge Incontinence
Leakage with activity	Yes	No
Urge with leakage on route to restroom	No	Yes
Nocturia	No	Yes
Strong and sudden desire to void	Infrequent	Frequent

- Gonorrhea and chlamydia cultures
- Pelvic ultrasound
- Chronic: more than 6 months in duration. Consider referral to gynecology.

URINARY INCONTINENCE (TABLE 15-5)

- Diagnosis
  - Clinical diagnosis based on history
  - Urinalysis to rule out infection
  - Consider referral to gynecology, urogynecology, or urology for complete urodynamic testing
- Treatment options
  - Lifestyle modifications
    - Weight loss.
    - Avoid caffeinated and alcoholic beverages.
  - Physical therapy referral
  - Anticholinergic medication: most effective for urge incontinence
  - Pessary: requires fitting by gynecologist but may be effective with stress incontinence
  - Referral to gynecology, urogynecology or urology to discuss surgical options

MENOPAUSE

- Definition
  - Natural
    - Average age of menopause is 51.4 years.
    - Cessation of menses for 1 year.
    - Often preceded by irregular menses.
    - Loss of ovarian function and production of estrogen.
  - Surgical
    - Bilateral oophorectomy (often in conjunction with a hysterectomy)
    - Often more severe and sudden
  - Medical
    - Induced by chemotherapy
    - Induced by radiation
- Physiology
  - Menopause occurs secondary to a genetically programmed loss of ovarian follicles.
  - Variation in menstrual cycle prior to cessation of menses.
  - Elevated FSH serum level.
  - Preceded by perimenopause.
    - Variable cycle length (more than 7-day variation from 21 to 35 days)
    - Prolonged menstrual interval (>60 days)
- Perimenopause
  - Precedes menopause

- Average age 47.5
- Duration approximately 4 years
- Waxing and waning ovarian function
- Unpredictable bleeding
  - Amenorrhea
  - Heavy bleeding
- Varying vasomotor symptoms present
- Symptoms
- Hot flashes
  - Vasomotor instability
- Night sweats
  - Sleep disturbance
- Vaginal dryness
  - Dyspareunia
- Treatment
- Hormone therapy
  - Cyclic
    - Estrogen days 1 to 25
    - Progesterone days 16 to 25
  - Continuous
    - Combined estrogen and progesterone daily
  - Routes of administration
    - Oral
    - Transdermal
    - Vaginal creams
    - Vaginal rings
  - Benefits
    - Alleviate vasomotor symptoms
    - Treatment of vaginal atrophy
    - Prevention of osteoporosis
  - Risk
    - Increased for cardiovascular disease
    - Increased breast cancer
    - Increased thromboembolic events
- Estrogen therapy alone
  - Only for women with hysterectomy
  - Same as above applies
- Nonhormonal
  - Herbal treatments
    - Black cohosh
    - Soy supplements
    - St. John's Wort
  - Dietary supplements
    - Isoflavones
    - Vitamin E

CHAPTER 16

Perioperative Care of the Surgical Patient

Ronald S. Chamberlain, Vijayashree Murthy, Lauren S. Sparber, and Prasanna Sridharan

PERIOPERATIVE MEDICINE AND CLEARANCE OF THE SURGICAL PATIENTS

Evidence-based and patient-centered care paradigms have vastly changed the whole notion of caring for patients in the perioperative period. In the not-too-distant past, the primary role of internists or family practice physicians was centered on cardiac and pulmonary risk assessment and providing information to the referring surgeon as to whether the patient was low risk, moderate risk, high risk, or at too much risk for the planned elective procedure. Very little time, if any, was spent counseling the patient about modifiable risk factors, let alone intervening to improve many well-modifiable risk factors that could result in decreased surgical morbidity and mortality. After receipt of the "clearance letter," the surgeon would take the patient to the operating room, and the internist or hospitalist would make daily "social" rounds. As absurd as this process sounds, this scenario has been the status quo for the perioperative care of the surgical patient for more than a century. Table 16-1 outlines the old medical clearance approach and suggests a more modern approach to caring for the perioperative patient, which is patient centered and recognizes that there are inherent risks for the patient in each stage of the surgical continuum.

PREOPERATIVE RISK ASSESSMENT

Preoperative Cardiac Evaluation

Background

- Approximately 53.3 million patients undergo surgery in the United States each year, of which 1% to 6% will suffer a major cardiac event in the perioperative period.[1]
- Most life threatening among these events is postoperative myocardial infarction (MI), among which 15% to 25% will suffer in-hospital mortality.
- The primary purpose of the perioperative cardiac evaluation is to identify those patients at greatest risk of postoperative coronary event and to correct or modify those risks prior to surgical intervention.
- Although the primary cause of postoperative MI is because of coronary occlusion, stenosis, or plaque rupture, uncontrolled hypertension, preexisting untreated arrhythmias, and myocardial supply and demand mismatch play an undetermined but significant role.

History and Physical Examination

- Although diagnostic tests such as electrocardiograms (ECGs), echocardiograms, and stress tests play an important role in cardiac risk assessment, they are often over- or underused, that is ordered universally for all patients (unnecessarily increasing health care costs and patient risks), or not ordered when appropriate and necessary.
- Perhaps the best assessment of a patient's cardiac risk is an assessment of his or her functional status regarding the patient's ability to complete activities of daily living.
  - More specifically, questions should center on what specific activities a patient is able to perform and at what level of effort.
  - Poor-risk patients have been defined as those unable to perform activity requiring at least 4 metabolic equivalents of activity.
  - Examples of such activities are:
    - Able to climb one or more flights of stairs without severe fatigue
    - Able to walk a block at a brisk pace (>4 mph)
    - Able to run for a short distance
    - Able to perform heavy work around the home (mow the lawn, scrub the floors, etc.)
    - Able to participate in sporting activities[1]

TABLE 16-1. CURRENT AND FUTURE VISION OF THE MEDICAL CLEARANCE VISIT

Current Preoperative Clearance		
Preoperative	**Operative Course**	**Postoperative**
• Cardiac workup • ECG • Echocardiogram or stress test • Pulmonary workup • PFTs • ABGs • Letter detailing risk assessment	• Operation chosen was physician specific • Antibiotic choice and duration was anecdotal and surgeon driven • Anesthesia choice was general anesthesia • Rare consideration of postoperative pain control issues • DVT prophylaxis was mechanical only • Invasive monitoring was deemed safer for the patient • No nutritional concerns considered; postoperative TPN the norm	• Daily hospital visit by PMD or hospitalist was primarily social in nature • Appropriate follow-up

New Paradigm for Preoperative Clearance		
Preoperative Counseling	**Patient-Specific Operative Choice**	**Postoperative Plan**
• Weight reduction • Smoking cessation • Diabetic management • Nutritional counseling • Postoperative expectations for recovery • Family discussion to maximize postoperative recovery • Discuss need for rehab or subacute care postoperatively Cardiac Evaluation • ECG, echocardiogram, stress test • Coronary interventions to optimize cardiac status • Anticoagulant recommendations: ASA, warfarin (Coumadin), clopidogrel (Plavix), others Pulmonary Evaluation • ABG, PFTs • Counseling on spirometry and early ambulation postoperatively • Treatment of reversible deficits preoperatively with reassessment ID evaluation • MRSA testing and clearance • Antibiotic history to assess risk of MDR infection	• Preoperative counseling for expectations and recovery • Evidence-based perioperative antibiotic selection • Anesthesia choice: general, regional, local • Postoperative pain control: epidural, block, PCA • Appropriate DVT prophylaxis perioperatively • Avoid unnecessary tubes and lines early • Consider enteral feeding tube • Enteral nutrition over TPN • Single dose or ≤24 hr antibiotic duration	• Assess pain often • Ambulate early • Remove lines and tubes • Early feeding • Spirometry • PT and OT assessment • Discharge plan POD 1 • Family counseling • Appropriate follow-up

ABG, arterial blood gas test; ASA, aspirin; DVT, deep vein thrombosis; ECG, electrocardiogram; ID, infectious disease; MDR, multidrug resistant; MRSA, methicillin-susceptible *Staphylococcus aureus*; OT, occupational therapy; PCA, patient-controlled anesthesia; PFT, pulmonary function test; PMD, private medical doctor; POD, postoperative day; PT, physical therapy; TPN, total parenteral nutrition.

TABLE 16-2. PUBLISHED EXAMPLES OF SCORES AND SCALES PROVIDING PERIOPERATIVE RISK STRATIFICATION[2–4]

ACC/AHA Cardiac Risk Guidelines[2]

Major Risk Factors

• Unstable coronary syndromes	• Diabetes mellitus (needing insulin)
• Decompensated congestive heart failure (CHF)	• Severe/high-grade valvular lesions
• History of ventricular ectopy requiring therapy	• Age >70 years
• Uncontrolled/stable arrhythmias	

Intermediate Risk Factors

• Mild/stable angina	• Diabetes mellitus
• Prior myocardial infarction	• Renal insufficiency
• Compensated CHF	

Low Risk Factors

• Advanced age	• Poor functional capacity
• Abnormal electrocardiogram (ECG)	• Prior cerebrovascular accident (CVA)
• Stable nonsinus rhythm	• Poorly controlled hypertension

Eagle Criteria[3]

• Age >70 years	• History of angina
• Q wave on ECG	• Diabetes mellitus
• Ventricular ectopy	

Revised Cardiac Risk Index[4]

Risk Variables for Cardiac Event:

• High-risk surgery	• Renal insufficiency
• Ischemic heart disease	• Diabetes mellitus (needing insulin)
• History of CHF	• History of cerebrovascular disease

[a]Unclear utility outside of vascular surgery.

SPECIAL POPULATIONS

- A variety of risk-stratification tools based on information derived through a careful history has also been developed to better assess a specific patient's preoperative cardiac risks, such as the American College of Cardiology (ACC)/American Heart Association (AHA) Modifiable Risk Scale, the Revised Cardiac Risk Index, and the Eagle Criteria (primarily designed for patients undergoing vascular surgery[2–4]; Table 16-2.)
- Of note, it is not just patient health status that comes into play in determining surgical risks, but also the type of operation that is to be performed.
- Table 16-3 outlines the ACC/AHA criteria for high-, moderate-, and low-risk procedures.[3]
- A detailed physical examination is vital to a careful comprehensive assessment of cardiac risk.
  - Vitals signs, which are often glossed over as normal or stable, provide important clues to preexisting cardiac pathology.
  - Most importantly, the physical examination can reveal conditions that require treatment preoperatively to limit postoperative cardiac morbidity.
  - These conditions include:
    - (CHF) or pulmonary hypertension
    - Jugular venous distention
    - Pulmonary findings: crackles, wheezing, and so forth
    - S₃ gallop, distant heart sounds
      - Uncontrolled or untreated hypertension (systolic blood pressure [SBP] >180 mm Hg, diastolic blood pressure >100 mm Hg)

TABLE 16-3. RISK STRATIFICATION BASED ON TYPE OF SURGERY[2]

High Risk (Cardiac risk >5%):

- Major vascular surgery
- Prolonged surgery with marked volume shifts
- Emergency surgery

Moderate Risk (Cardiac risk >1% and <5%):

- Carotid endarterectomy
- Intraperitoneal/intrathoracic surgery
- Most orthopedic surgery
- Head and neck surgery

Low Risk (Cardiac risk <1%):

- Superficial and endoscopic procedures
- Cataract surgery
- Breast surgery

- Arrhythmia or tachycardia (eg, atrial fibrillation, reentrant pathways)
- Preexisting murmurs that can indicate significant valvular disease (eg, severe mitral regurgitation, aortic insufficiency, aortic stenosis)

Diagnostic Testing

- 12-Lead electrocardiogram
  - This is the most commonly used diagnostic test to evaluate a patient's cardiac risk.
  - ECGs can identify arrhythmias, reentrant pathways, cardiac blocks, prolonged intervals, prior myocardial injury, and current ischemia. That said, ECGs are not necessary for the majority of asymptomatic young patents undergoing moderate- to low-risk procedures.
  - ECGs are currently recommended for all males 40 years of age or older, and all females 50 years of age or older, patients of any age with high-risk comorbidities such as diabetes, CHF, angina, and so forth, or for those undergoing moderate- to high-risk surgical procedures.[2]
- Routine echocardiograms are not indicated in the medical evaluation of most surgical patients.
  - Echocardiogram is indicated when history or physical examination reveal significant reason to suspect valvular disease or significant myocardial dysfunction.
- Exercise or nuclear stress testing
  - There is no such thing as routine stress testing for older patients, nor prior to "big operations."
  - The decision to order an exercise or nuclear stress test should be undertaken after appropriate risk stratification (see Table 16-2), and the identification of high-risk patients.
  - Exercise stress testing is indicated for all patients able to exercise at 85% of their predicted maximal heart rate; patients who are unable to meet this goal should undergo either vasodilator-nuclear perfusion studies or dobutamine-echocardiography.
  - The benefits, contraindications, and limitations of these various modalities are beyond the scope of this chapter.
- Revascularization (who and when?)
  - Which patients require preoperative revascularization is ill defined and controversial.
  - However, truly high-risk patients such as those with left main coronary artery disease, severe left ventricular dysfunction, and severe aortic stenosis may have survival advantage from a revascularization procedure.
  - Elective surgery following a revascularization procedure (angioplasty and/or coronary artery bypass grafting) requires a minimum of 2 to preferably 6 weeks delay.[5]

Perioperative Treatment of Modifiable Risk Factors in Patients at Significant Risk of Cardiac Morbidity

- Behavioral Risk Factors
  - The role of the physician providing perioperative cardiac assessment is not limited to risk assessment, but rather must include treatment of modifiable risk factors and appropriate patient counseling.
  - Although nearly all physicians will treat a SBP higher than 180 mm Hg, all too few engage in counseling regarding smoking cessation and nutritional or diet counseling, which can play a pivotal role in the patient's perioperative outcome, and long-term outlook.
- Smoking Cessation
  - The toxic effects of smoking are mainly related to carbon monoxide and nicotine injury on the endothelial cells and the increased levels of oxidized low-density lipoprotein cholesterol.
  - Active as well as passive smoking and cigar smoke have all been linked to coronary artery disease.
  - Smoking cessation clearly has long-term benefits for improved pulmonary function, decreased cancer risk, and an overall improvement in health.
  - However, even short-term smoking cessation for weeks to months in the preoperative period that include, but are not limited to, the perioperative period is beneficial.
  - This modifiable risk factor management is most predictive of future need for coronary revascularization.
  - Prevention includes smoking cessation and training in proper breathing (incentive spirometry), which have the following advantages[6,7]:
    - Improved ciliary and small airway function
    - Decreased sputum production
    - Decreased risk of surgical site infection
    - Decreased overall postoperative complication rate
  - Counseling on smoking cessation is often ineffective on its own, and often times, adjunct therapies such as nicotine replacement therapies, bupropion, and varenicline can be used to improve the success rate.
- Nutrition and dietary counseling
  - Dietary habits, specific food consumption, or even certain micronutrients consumption, seem to play an important role in the development of coronary artery disease.
  - Evidence suggests that stress influences changes in food choice and appetite, promoting unhealthy dietary choices and mainly increasing consumption of sweet, fatty food.
  - Irregular meal patterns have been associated with increased energy intake, lower insulin sensitivity, and higher cholesterol levels, all known risk factors for coronary artery disease.
  - To promote cardiovascular health, diets should provide very low intake (ie, <1%) of trans fatty acids (hydrogenated fats).
  - Current evidence suggests that an intake of no more than 70 mmol or 1.7 g of sodium per day is beneficial in reducing blood pressure.[8]
  - Regular consumption of whole-grain cereals, legumes, fruits, and vegetables have potential health benefits, in particular for preventing obesity, diabetes, cardiovascular diseases, and various cancers.
- Hypertension
  - Preoperative blood control
    - It is imperative to control blood pressure (BP) prior to both elective and emergent surgical procedures, as conditions that ensue as a result of surgical therapy, such as pain, fluid shifts, blood loss, corticosteroid response, and catecholamine release, can result in wide fluctuations of BP postoperatively.
    - Preoperative BP higher than 180/110 mmm Hg can lead to an increased rate of intraoperative cardiac events or intraoperative fluctuations in BP.
    - It is routine to ask patients to continue current antihypertensive regimens up to the morning of surgery with the exception of diuretics that are often withheld in operations expected to result in significant blood loss or fluid shifts.

- This is particularly important in gastrointestinal (GI) tract surgery in which a preoperative bowel preparation may be administered and intravascular depletion may coexist as result.
- Acute beta-blocker or α_2-agonist (clonidine) withdrawals are most important to consider as this may result in rebound tachycardia or hypertension.
- In suspected pheochromocytoma, further investigations need to be done and surgery delayed.

- Postoperative BP control
  - The causes of postoperative hypertension are multifactorial, and unless life threatening should not be immediately treated with antihypertensive medications until all other factors are adequately controlled.
  - Most notably among these factors are the assurance of adequate postoperative pain control, the control of postoperative anxiety or agitation (which can result from hypoxia, hypercapnia, medications and their interactions, restraint, inadequate sedation), treatment of nausea and vomiting, and gastric or urinary bladder among others.
  - Treatment of postoperative hypertension is no different than the treatment of hypertension in other setting, except that diuretics are generally avoided until the patient is stable and intravenous fluids and nutrition has been discontinued.
  - A variety of parenteral, oral, and transdermal agents (clonidine) are available. (See the section Hypertension.)

- Perioperative beta-blocker use
  - Several landmark studies have documented the efficacy of preoperative β_1-selective blockers administered preoperatively to patients undergoing noncardiac surgery to decrease postoperative cardiac events.
  - The two largest studies evaluated the efficacy of beta-blockers in high-risk noncardiac surgery patients, and in vascular patients.[9,10]
  - In both studies, the goal of preoperative treatment was to achieve a heart rate of less than 65 beats per minute if SBP remained above 100 mm Hg; if this was not possible, a pulse of less than 80 beats per minute was targeted.
  - There is currently no data support the use of β_1-selective blockers in low-risk nonvascular surgery patients undergoing low-risk surgical procedure.
  - Information about whether intermediate-risk cardiac patients, or low-cardiac-risk patients undergoing intermediate- to high-risk surgical procedures is insufficient, and it should be considered on an individual case basis.

- Hypercholesterolemia
  - Hypercholesterolemia represents a significant risk factor for myocardial damage and coronary artery disease, with more than 40 million Americans having total cholesterol levels above 220 mg/dL.
  - Statin therapy has been a mainstay of treatment for this condition for more than a decade, and may be uniquely indicated for patients with other coexisting conditions such as diabetes or hypertension.
  - Whether statins should be continued or withheld in the perioperative period remains uncertain.
  - Initial concerns that statins may increase the risk of postoperative rhabdomyolysis have been subsequently refuted in a prospective study.[11,12]
  - Diabetics and patients undergoing vascular surgery may be ideal candidates for statin therapy to lower the occurrence of perioperative stroke, MI, or unstable angina.
  - Until such times as additional data is available, specific recommendations on what to do with statins cannot be made and should be individualized.

- Arrhythmia
  - Treatment and remediation of all preexisting arrhythmias (from underlying coronary artery disease, congestive cardiac failure or metabolic abnormalities like hypomagnesaemia or hypokalemia) is critical to ensure a smooth perioperative and anesthetic course.
  - The only exception to preoperative correction of arrhythmias is the asymptomatic ventricular premature beats.
  - Ideal management of specific arrhythmias, their potential interaction with anesthetic agents, and impact fluid shift and electrolyte abnormalities common to surgical patients may have on these is beyond the scope of this chapter (see the section Cardiac Disease).

TABLE 16-4. GUIDELINES FOR PREOPERATIVE CARDIAC RISK
ASSESSMENT IN PATIENTS WITH VALVULAR HEART
DISEASE AND PERIOPERATIVE CARDIAC MANAGEMENT
IN NONCARDIAC SURGERY[13]

Valvular Disease	Physical Findings and Cardiac Risk	Recommendations for Emergent Surgery	Recommendations for Elective Surgery
Aortic stenosis	Valve area <1 cm^2 class I recommendation	General anesthesia under hemodynamic monitoring.	Aortic valve replacement or balloon aortic valvuloplasty or transcatheter valve implantation prior to elective surgery
Mitral stenosis	Valve area <1.5 cm^2 and systolic pulmonary artery pressure <50 mmHg. Class I recommendation	Control of heart rate to avoid tachycardia and pulmonary edema. Strict control of fluid overload. Anticoagulation.	Percutaneous mitral commissurotomy (or open surgical repair) prior to high-risk cases. Rest same as emergent surgery
Mitral regurgitation	LV ejection fraction <30% Class I recommendation	Optimization of pharmacologic therapy to produce maximal hemodynamic stabilization before high-risk surgery	Perform elective surgery only if necessary
Aortic regurgitation	LV ejection fraction <30% Class I recommendation	Optimization of pharmacologic therapy to produce maximal hemodynamic stabilization before high-risk surgery	Perform elective surgery only if necessary

LV, left ventricular.

- Valvular Disease
  - The prevalence of valvular heart disease is approximately 2.5% and increases further in the patient group aged older than 75 years of age.
  - As life expectancy increases, the number of patients requiring surgical therapy who will have underlying valvular disease will increase exponentially in the next few decades.
  - Knowledge of the hemodynamic alterations and compensation mechanisms that accompany diseases of the valve apparatus is essential for a suitable treatment of patients with such preexisting diseases.
  - The most common valvular heart diseases lead to volume (mitral valve insufficiency) or pressure load (aortic stenosis) of the left ventricle and in the case of mitral stenosis to a pressure load on the left atrium.
  - Identification, optimization, or surgical correction of certain high-risk valvular conditions that pose significant surgical risk is critical.
  - Table 16-4 lists those valvular conditions most common among surgical patients with their associated risk, and treatment recommendation.
  - Depending on the underlying disease and the type of surgery planned a corresponding choice of anesthesia procedure and medication must be made.
  - In general, elective surgery should be delayed until correction of the valvular disease, particularly for stenotic lesions.

SPECIAL POPULATIONS

- Regurgitative valvular disease may also be severe and require surgical correction preoperatively, however, patients can often times be optimized medically there by permitting time-dependent surgical therapy to proceed (eg, cancer surgery).
- Perioperative prophylactic antibiotics should be administered to patients with congenital or valvular heart disease, prosthetic valves, mitral valve prolapse, or other cardiac abnormalities in accordance with ACC/AHA practice guidelines.

Preoperative Pulmonary Evaluation

Background

- Pulmonary complications contribute significantly to overall perioperative morbidity with frequency rates from 5% to 70% and account for approximately 25% of deaths occurring within 6 days of surgery. This wide range is caused by variations among studies in the definition of postoperative pulmonary complications, as well as variability in patient- and procedure-related factors.
- Postoperative pulmonary complication is defined as an abnormality that produces identifiable disease or dysfunction, is clinically significant, and adversely affects the clinical course and includes fever (because of microatelectasis), cough, dyspnea, bronchospasm, hypoxemia, atelectasis, hypercapnia, adverse reaction to a pulmonary medication, pleural effusion, pneumonia, pneumothorax, and ventilatory failure.
- Pulmonary complications occur much more often than cardiac complications in patients undergoing elective surgery to the thorax and upper abdomen complications prolong the hospital stay by an average of 1 to 2 weeks.
- The goal of perioperative pulmonary management is to identify patients at high risk of significant postoperative pulmonary complications (patients with preexisting lung disease, medical comorbidities, poor nutritional status, overall poor health, and smokers), so that appropriate interventions can be provided to minimize that risk.
- In most cases, even in high-risk patients, the procedure can be performed safely as planned, but occasionally postponement, modification, or cancellation are warranted.

Patient-Related Risk Factors

- Age
  - Age appears to be an independent yet controversial risk factor for postoperative pulmonary complications as some studies have shown that age is not a predictor for postoperative pulmonary complications.
  - Acceptable operative mortality rates can be achieved in older patients. In a study of perioperative mortality of patients older than 70 years of age, the unadjusted postoperative pulmonary complication estimates ranged from 4% to 45%, with a median postoperative pulmonary complication rate of 15%.[14]
  - As age is obviously a nonmodifiable risk factor, and the potential risk of complications does not invariably translate into increased mortality, surgery should not be declined because of advanced age alone.
- Obesity
  - Obesity (ie, body mass index [BMI] of >25 kg/m^2) causes a reduction in lung volume, ventilation-perfusion mismatch, and relative hypoxemia, which are accentuated after surgery.
  - In severe cases, obesity is associated with pulmonary hypertension, cor pulmonale, and hypercapnic respiratory failure (Pickwickian syndrome).
  - Left ventricular hypertrophy resulting from increased blood volume and cardiac output demands by hemodynamic overload, secondary to increased BMI and hypertension, is a usual feature.
  - Decreased ejection fraction resulting from ventricular dilatation is an important risk factor, and a careful examination should exclude or indicate necessary treatment prior to surgery.
  - Although some studies suggest that obesity increases the risk of postoperative pulmonary complications, others suggest that obesity is not an independent risk factor. In a review article, the risk of postoperative pulmonary complications was not excessive in 7 studies of obese patients who underwent abdominal or peripheral procedures.[15]
- Smoking
  - Patients who currently smoke have a twofold increased risk of postoperative complications, even in the absence of chronic obstructive pulmonary disease (COPD).

- The risk is highest in patients who smoked within the last 2 months.
- Forced expiratory volume at 1 second (FEV_1) decreases by approximately 30 mL per year in nonsmokers and 45 mL per year in smokers.
- Occupational exposures, airway hyperreactivity, and air pollution may interact with tobacco use to affect the severity of preexisting lung disease.
- Patients who quit smoking for more than 6 months have a risk similar to those who do not smoke, although the risk of postoperative pneumonia appears to remain elevated up to 1 year after smoking cessation.
- Other patient related factors:
  - COPD
    - This condition is one of the most important risk factors for postoperative pulmonary complications.
    - Patients with severe COPD (FEV_1 <40% predicted) are 6 times more likely to have a major postoperative complication.
    - Similarly, an FEV_1 less than 60% predicted was found to be an independent predictor of increased mortality in patients undergoing coronary artery bypass graft (CABG) procedures.
    - However, despite the increased risk, a prohibitive level of pulmonary function for an absolute contraindication is not apparent. One multivariable study reported that abnormal findings on chest examination (defined as decreased breath sounds, prolonged expiration, rales, wheezes, or rhonchi) were the strongest predictor of postoperative pulmonary complication rates (odds ratio, 5.8 [confidence interval, 1.04 to 32.1]).[16]
    - The benefits of surgery must be weighed against these complications. A careful preoperative evaluation of patients with COPD should include identification of high-risk patients and aggressive treatment.
    - Elective surgery should be deferred in patients who are symptomatic, have poor exercise capacity, or have acute exacerbation.
  - Asthma
    - Asthma increases the risk of bronchospasm, hypoxemia, hypercapnia, inadequate cough, atelectasis, and pulmonary infection following surgery.
    - Inadequate control of asthma preoperatively may increase the risk of these complications.
    - Optimal asthma control is defined as the absence of symptoms and an FEV_1 of greater than 80% of predicted or personal best.
  - Sleep apnea
    - Patients with obstructive sleep apnea are at increased risk for airway management in the immediate postoperative period including deterioration of sleep-disordered breathing, severe hypoxemia, and hypercapnia.
    - Individuals with sleep apnea who are also obese may present difficulties with endotracheal intubation or early postoperative upper airway obstruction, requiring reintubation or other therapies. In such patients, intraoperative and postoperative use of sedatives and narcotics should be minimized.
    - Careful monitoring in the postoperative period is required for worsening of sleep apnea, development of airway obstruction, or carbon dioxide retention.
    - In patients with suspected sleep apnea, the diagnosis should be confirmed and the severity should be assessed preoperatively with a formal polysomnographic sleep study, apnea-hypopnea index and the lowest oxygen saturation value during sleep.
    - Preoperative management should include nasal continuous positive airway pressure therapy. Regional rather than general anesthesia is a better option for these patients.
  - Neurologic impairment
    - Impaired sensorium is defined as:
      - An acutely confused or delirious patient who can respond to verbal or mild tactile stimulation or both
      - A patient with mental status changes, delirium, or both in the context of current illness
    - This does not include patients with stable chronic mental illness or dementia.
    - Patients with impaired sensorium or residual deficits from a previous stroke have an increased risk of postoperative pneumonia and respiratory failure.[17]

- Immunosuppression
  - Chronic steroid use is associated with an increased risk of postoperative pneumonia.
  - Daily use of alcohol within 2 weeks of surgery is associated with an increased risk of postoperative pneumonia and respiratory failure.
  - Insulin-treated diabetes is associated with an increased risk of postoperative respiratory failure.

Procedure-Related Risk Factors

- Surgical site
  - The incidence of postoperative pulmonary complications is inversely related to the distance of the surgical incision from the diaphragm.
  - The complication rates for upper abdominal surgery range from 17% to 76%.
  - For lower abdominal surgery (hip surgery [5 studies] and gynecologic or urologic procedures) the rate is 0% to 5%.
  - For high-risk thoracic surgeries (esophagectomy and thoracoabdominal aortic surgeries), the rate is 19% to 59%.
  - Abdominal aortic aneurysm repair is associated with the highest risk of postoperative pulmonary complications.[17]
- Duration of surgery
  - Patients undergoing procedures lasting longer than 2.5 to 4 hours have a higher incidence rate of pulmonary complications (40%) compared with those undergoing surgeries lasting shorter than 2 hours (8%).
- Type of anesthesia
  - Data are inconsistent about whether the pulmonary complication rate is lower with spinal or epidural anesthesia compared with general anesthesia.
  - Spinal or epidural anesthesia, in conjunction with general anesthesia, may be associated with a lower risk of postoperative pneumonia, venous thromboembolic disease, MI, renal failure, and respiratory depression.
  - Evidence suggests that the addition of neuraxial anesthesia, rather than avoidance of general anesthesia, may be the key to reducing pulmonary complications.
- Minimally invasive surgery
  - Laparoscopic abdominal surgery, particularly cholecystectomy, is associated with fewer postoperative pulmonary abnormalities and a shorter hospital stay. These techniques use small incisions, and the reduced manipulation of visceral organs minimizes the adverse effects on respiratory muscles.
  - Laparoscopic surgery leads to a 23% decrease in forced vital capacity (FVC) and a 16% decrease in FEV_1, and it is associated with a lower incidence of complications compared with laparotomy; therefore, even patients with severe COPD can tolerate surgery.
  - Video-assisted thoracoscopic surgery uses much smaller incisions without separation of the ribs; resulting in less postoperative pain, early ambulation and reduced pulmonary complications consequently, the hospitalization time is substantially reduced.

Preoperative History and Physical

- Obtain a complete history and perform a complete physical examination to help identify risk factors for pulmonary complications. Seek any current history of upper respiratory infections, smoking, exercise intolerance, unexplained dyspnea, sputum production, hemoptysis, or increased cough.
- Physical findings including increased chest circumference, presence of adventitious breath sounds such as wheezing, rales, rhonchi, accessory muscles of respiration, clubbing should be evaluated for preexisting pulmonary disease.
- Maximum laryngeal height of less than 4 cm has been observed with pulmonary complications.

Preoperative Testing and Laboratory Evaluation

- Pulmonary function tests
  - Routine performance of pulmonary function tests in the setting of nonpulmonary surgery has not been found to be useful, as pulmonary function tests result in only a marginal benefit in predicting postoperative complications. Rather, testing should be restricted to those patients with unexplained dyspnea or exercise intolerance.

- Preoperative identification of patients with asthma or COPD is important, to direct specific preoperative interventions, however, the degree of physiologic impairment (FEV_1 or FVC) does not correlate with the risk of postoperative pulmonary complications.
- Arterial blood gas tests
  - Although hypercapnia has been associated with an increased risk of postoperative pulmonary complications, routine testing of arterial blood gases is not recommended for preoperative pulmonary evaluation.
- Chest radiography
  - Clinicians frequently order chest radiography as part of a routine preoperative evaluation. This practice is often because of local institutional guidelines requiring chest radiography for all patients older than a particular age. However, chest x-ray studies add little to the clinical evaluation in healthy patients. Only 2 univariate studies stratified postoperative pulmonary complication rates on the basis of the finding of a normal or abnormal preoperative chest radiograph.[18,19] In their small, pooled patient sample ($N = 150$), 46% of patients with an abnormal preoperative chest radiograph had a postoperative pulmonary complication, and the rate for patients with a normal preoperative study was 25%.
  - Routine chest x-rays should not be performed routinely for preoperative evaluation in patients without risk factors.
- Renal function
  - Blood urea nitrogen level of 7.5 mmol/L or greater (>21 mg/dL) and serum creatinine level greater than 133 mmol/L (>1.5 mg/ dL) have been recognized as significant predictors for postoperative pulmonary complications. The risk has been observed to increase with increasing BUN levels.[17,20]
- Serum albumin
  - A low serum albumin level was also the most important predictor of 30-day perioperative morbidity and mortality.[21]

Risk Indices

- Although a number of scoring systems have been devised to predict an individual patient's risk of postoperative pulmonary complications, many of these systems have potential limitations.
  - Postoperative pneumonia and respiratory failure risk indices[17]
    - Described by Arozullah et al, the risk index incorporates the following procedure and patient factors:
      - Procedure: type of surgery (abdominal aortic aneurysm, thoracic, neurosurgery, upper abdominal, or peripheral vascular, neck), emergency surgery, general anesthesia
      - General health: age (<70 years), partially or fully dependent functional status, serum albumin (<30 g/L), weight loss
      - Immunosuppression: chronic steroid use, alcohol use, insulin-treated diabetes
      - Lung disease: COPD, smoking, preoperative pneumonia, dyspnea
      - Neurologic impairment
      - Fluid status: CHF, renal failure, BUN, preoperative transfusion
    - Points are assigned based on the relative risk of postoperative pulmonary complications associated with each factor. The points are totaled and the patient is assigned to a risk class (1 through 5, with points <10 to >40).
    - The risk of postoperative pneumonia and respiratory failure are less than 1% for patients in risk class 1, whereas patients in risk class 5 have a 15% risk of postoperative pneumonia and 30% risk of respiratory failure.
    - Cardiopulmonary and pulmonary risk indices
    - A combined cardiopulmonary risk index is proposed for risk stratification of pulmonary complications. Pulmonary risk factors have been added to the Goldman Cardiac Risk Index;[22] patients with a combined score of greater than 4 points (of a total of 10) are 17 times more likely to develop complications. These pulmonary risk factors include the following:
      - Obesity (ie, BMI >27 kg/m^2)
      - Cigarette smoking within 8 weeks of surgery
      - Productive cough within 5 days of surgery

- Diffuse wheezing within 5 days of surgery
- FEV_1/FVC ratio less than 70% and partial pressure of carbon dioxide ($PaCO_2$) more than 45 mm Hg
- American Society of Anesthesiologists (ASA) physical status classification system
  - This score is based on simple clinical criteria and is easy to quantify. Although subjective, assignment to physical status 1 through 5 indicates an increased level of severity and increased postoperative morbidity. The ASA classification, along with examples of each class, is described below:
    - ASA physical status 1: A normal, healthy patient without organic, physiologic, or psychiatric disturbance (eg, healthy with good exercise tolerance)
    - ASA physical status 2: A patient with controlled medical conditions without significant systemic effects (eg, controlled hypertension or controlled diabetes without systemic effects, cigarette smoking without COPD, anemia, mild obesity, age younger than 1 year or older than 70 years, pregnancy)
    - ASA physical status 3: A patient with medical conditions with significant systemic effects, intermittently with significant functional compromise (eg, controlled CHF, stable angina, old MI, poorly controlled hypertension, morbid obesity, bronchospastic disease with intermittent symptoms, chronic renal failure)
    - ASA physical status 4: A patient with a medical condition that is poorly controlled, associated with significant dysfunction and is a potential threat to life (eg, unstable angina, symptomatic COPD, symptomatic CHF, hepatorenal failure)
    - ASA physical status 5: A patient with a critical medical condition that is associated with little chance of survival with or without the surgical procedure (eg, multiorgan failure, sepsis syndrome with hemodynamic instability, hypothermia, poorly controlled coagulopathy)
    - ASA physical status 6: A patient who is brain dead and undergoing anesthesia care for the purposes of organ donation

Preoperative Treatment Measures

- The following preoperative measures help minimize pulmonary complications in at-risk patients:
- Cessation of smoking: at least 8 weeks prior to surgery.
- Training in proper breathing (incentive spirometry): Educate patients on lung expansion maneuvers. Consider inspiratory muscle training or pulmonary rehabilitation in high-risk patients.
- Inhalation bronchodilator therapy: Optimize COPD and asthma treatment regimens. Consider a course of systemic steroids if suboptimal control
- Control of infection and secretion for acute bronchitis.
- Weight reduction, when appropriate.

Perioperative Management of Diabetes

Background

- 8.3% of the U.S. population (25.8 million people) suffers from diabetes. It is estimated that 7 million diabetics in the United States (nearly one-quarter) are undiagnosed.[23]
- Mortality rates in diabetics are up to 5 times as high as in nondiabetics, ostensibly because of end-organ damage. Up to 25% of diabetic patients will undergo surgery during their lifetimes.
- Wound infection is the most common postoperative complication in diabetics (representing 66% of all postoperative complications in this group), and it accounts for nearly a quarter of perioperative mortalities.[24-27]
- Hospitalized patients suffering from poor glucose control and hyperglycemia are at greater risk for worse surgical outcomes and postoperative complications.[28,29]
- Tight glucose control (80–110 mg/dL) in postoperative critical care patients has been correlated with decreased morbidity and mortality.[30] Current guidelines suggest maintenance of blood glucose levels at 80 to 150 mg/dL.[24-27]
- There is no proven correlation between tight glucose control and decreased mortality in the nonintensive care unit setting, but given the established link between hyperglycemia and poor medical outcomes in an inpatient setting, maintaining glucose levels within strict limits is recommended.

- Diabetes increases the risk of cardiovascular and renal disease. Preoperative assessment of these patients should include cardiac risk stratification and evaluation of renal function.

Preoperative History and Physical

- Symptoms: polyuria, polydipsia, polyphagia, visual disturbances, neurologic changes in the lower extremity (numbness, tingling, pain), orthostatic hypotension (representative of autonomic dysfunction)
- Modifiable and behavioral risk factors: diet and nutrition, exercise history, weight gain or loss, smoking, alcohol consumption, illicit drug use
- Current therapy: diet, exercise, medication (oral, insulin, other medications that may affect blood glucose), monitoring, history of complications (hypoglycemia, ketoacidosis)
- Medical history: obesity, hypertension, visual disturbances, cerebrovascular accident (CVA), MI, heart failure, renal dysfunction, infections, foot ulceration, bowel and bladder dysfunction, erectile dysfunction, endocrine dysfunction, eating disorders
- Family history: diabetes, hypertension, hyperlipidemia, obesity, CVA, MI, peripheral vascular disease, endocrinopathies
- Physical examination: BMI, blood pressure (normal and orthostatic), pulses, funduscopy, foot examination, neurologic examination, airway evaluation

Preoperative Testing and Laboratory Evaluation

- Plasma glucose level: fasting plasma glucose 126 mg/dL or higher, 2-hour plasma glucose during 75 g oral glucose tolerance test 200 mg/dL or higher, or random plasma glucose 200 mg/dL or higher (with symptoms) are indicative of a diagnosis of diabetes.
- Hemoglobin A_{1c}: Glycated hemoglobin represents a 90-day index of glycemic control. HbA_{1c} 6.5% or higher is indicative of a diagnosis of diabetes.
- Cardiac function: lipid profile, ECG, exercise and nuclear stress test, echocardiogram (based on cardiac assessment and risk stratification)
- Renal function: metabolic panel, electrolytes, estimated glomerular filtration rate, urine microalbumin, urine glucose

Surgery in Diabetics: Other Implications and Considerations

- Approximately 7 million diabetics (one-quarter of all diabetics in the United States) are undiagnosed.[23] Diabetes should always be a consideration in preoperative patient evaluation.
- Diabetic patients with autonomic neurologic compromise may experience "silent ischemia" (myocardial ischemia without accompanying angina pectoris). Diabetics should be screened aggressively for cardiovascular risk factors prior to surgical interventions. Screening may include exercise and nuclear stress testing demonstrating ECG changes, or echocardiographic studies evaluating for cardiac wall motion abnormalities.
- Elective surgery should not be attempted in diabetic patients until adequate glycemic control is achieved. If current therapy is inadequate, it may be supplemented with "sliding scale" insulin or basal insulin prior to surgery. If a hyperglycemic patient requires emergency surgery, use intravenous (IV) regular insulin to rapidly correct hyperglycemia (supplementing potassium where necessary) while ensuring adequate fluid resuscitation.
- Fasting prior to surgery results in starvation, which forces the body into a catabolic state. Diabetic patients undergoing surgery should be scheduled for morning surgery, as early as possible, to minimize fasting.
- Surgery, anesthesia and pain result in metabolic stress, resulting in elevation of catabolic hormones (epinephrine, cortisol, glucagon, growth hormone) and cytokines, and inhibition of insulin.
- Postoperative pain, inflammation, fluid imbalance, and changes in tissue perfusion may necessitate diabetes treatment modification, especially in the use of subcutaneous insulin injection (because of inconsistency in absorption).
- Short procedures, or those performed under local anesthesia may only require observation. Longer procedures may require frequent periodic glycemic monitoring and insulin infusion.
- General anesthesia results in greater catecholamine release than spinal and epidural anesthesia, potentially resulting in a more prominent hyperglycemia.[31]

Perioperative Treatment of Diabetes

- For short and/or simple procedures, preoperative glucose management protocols may be continued.
- For long and/or complex procedures, IV regular insulin infusion is the recommended choice. A 7-minute half-life and 1-hour duration of effect make IV regular insulin the ideal candidate for basic intraoperative adjustment and control of rapid changes in blood glucose level.[32]
- Type 1 diabetes
  - Patients cannot produce endogenous insulin. Insulin supplementation is required at all times.
  - The normal schedule of basal (long-acting) insulin should be continued both on the night before and on the day of surgery.
  - Hypoglycemia can be prevented or controlled through infusion of any 5% dextrose solution (D_5 in water, D_5 in normal saline, D_5 in lactated Ringer) while patient is on nothing by mouth (NPO), until tolerance and resumption of normal diet postoperatively.
  - Lengthy and complex procedures may necessitate continuous glucose monitoring and IV insulin infusion.
- Type 2 diabetes managed by dietary restriction
  - Patients typically do not require insulin.
  - Blood glucose should be regularly checked, and hyperglycemia may be treated with short-acting insulin doses.
- Type 2 diabetes managed by oral medication
  - Most patients can be managed without the use of insulin.
  - No oral medications should be given on the day of surgery.
  - Short-acting sulfonylureas (ie, tolbutamide) and meglitinides (ie, repaglinide, nateglinide) may be given on the day prior to surgery. Long-acting sulfonylureas (ie, chlorpropamide, glipizide, glimepiride) should be discontinued 24 to 48 hours prior to surgery. Sulfonylureas and meglitinides may cause hypoglycemia in patients who are NPO, and should be held until oral (PO) intake is resumed postoperatively.
  - Biguanides (ie, metformin) should be discontinued 24 to 48 hours prior to surgery, and is contraindicated in patients with hepatic or renal failure. Metformin can cause lactic acidosis in patients with decreased renal function, and should especially be withheld in patients who will receive IV contrast during the procedure, and in patients undergoing procedures that may adversely affect hemodynamic stability or renal perfusion. If emergency surgery is required and the patient has received metformin, adequate estimated glomerular filtration rate should be maintained via fluid infusion to clear the drug. Metformin should also be held for 48 hours postoperatively, or until renal function is stable.
  - Thiazolidinediones (ie, rosiglitazone, pioglitazone, troglitazone) can result in fluid retention, which may complicate the postoperative course. They should be held several days prior to surgery, and should be held until PO intake is resumed postoperatively.
  - Incretin mimetics or glucagonlike peptide-1 (GLP-1) agonists (ie, exenatide, liraglutide) can slow GI tract motility, which may result in delayed recovery. They should be held the day of surgery, and should be held until PO intake is resumed postoperatively.
  - Incretin enhancers or dipeptidyl peptidase-4 (DPP4) inhibitors (ie, sitagliptin, saxagliptin, linagliptin) have few side effects, and may be continued. Because their mechanism of action is glucose-dependent in nature, they do not cause perioperative hypoglycemia, but because they act to reduces postprandial blood glucose, they are not likely to be of help in an NPO patient.
  - α-Glucosidase inhibitors (ie, miglitol, acarbose, voglibose) act to retard the digestion of starch in the intestine, and are only effective in the setting of PO intake. They should be held until normal diet is resumed postoperatively.
  - Blood glucose should be regularly checked, and hyperglycemia may be treated with short-acting insulin doses.
- Type 2 diabetes managed by insulin
  - If the patient is anticipated to resume a normal diet postoperatively, basal insulin should be administered the day of surgery. Long-acting insulin (ie, glargine, detemir) can be given at half dose or normal dose. Intermediate-acting insulin (ie, neutral protamine Hagedorn) can be given at a half to two-thirds dose.

- Intraoperatively, IV regular insulin drip is recommended. Glucose and potassium can be supplemented to prevent hypoglycemia and hypokalemia, respectively. Potassium supplementation may be contraindicated in patients with renal dysfunction.
- Hypoglycemia can be prevented or controlled using any 5% dextrose (D_5) solution.
- The patient's original insulin regimen and schedule may be resumed once the patient has resumed normal diet.

Postoperative Treatment of Insulin-Dependent Diabetes Mellitus Patients

- Basal insulin should be restarted 12 to 24 hours prior to discontinuation of IV regular insulin infusion. Dosing is 50% to 80% of total daily IV regular insulin dose, given either once daily, or split in half and given twice daily.
- If the patient is receiving total parenteral nutrition (TPN), give 1 unit of normal insulin (added to the bag) per 10 to 15 g of dextrose in the TPN solution.
- If the patient is receiving enteral nutrition, give 1 unit of insulin subcutaneously for each 10 to 15 g of carbohydrates, once every 4 hours if using a fast-acting insulin analog, or once every 6 hours if using regular insulin. For bolus feeding, give the dose as a bolus 15 to 20 minutes prior to the feed, based on the carbohydrate content.
- If the patient is tolerating PO intake, use 1 unit of fast-acting insulin analog or regular insulin for each 10 to 15 g of carbohydrates prior to each meal.
- If the patient is being fed enterally or parenterally, fingerstick glucose testing should be performed once every 4 to 6 hours if the patient is on fast-acting insulin analog, or once every 6 hours if the patient is on normal insulin. If the patient is tolerating PO intake, fingerstick glucose testing should be performed once before each meal and once immediately prior to bedtime.[32]
- As per the American College of Endocrinology, a target glucose of less than 110 mg/dL is recommended in critical care patients, and a target glucose of less than 180 mg/dL is recommended for all other inpatients.[33]

Perioperative Nutritional Management

Background

- Malnutrition is a medical condition defined as a nutrient imbalance (lack, excess, or incorrect proportion), secondary to insufficient or inappropriate diet. Causes include inadequate ingestion of protein and calories (protein-energy malnutrition), surplus caloric intake (overnutrition), nutrient loss (ie, chronic diarrhea, malabsorption), and additional energy expenditure (secondary malnutrition).
- Malnutrition is known to result in reduced wound-healing capacity, immunocompromise, and decreased cardiac and muscle function.
- Poor preoperative nutritional status has been correlated with higher rates of postoperative morbidity and mortality.[34]
- Perioperative restoration of nutritional status in malnourished patients is performed to:
  - Reduce the risk of intraoperative and/or postoperative complications
  - Support the patient during the catabolic stage precipitated by surgical intervention
  - Optimize the postoperative healing process
  - Restore normal GI tract function, such that the patient may promptly resume PO intake

Assessing the Need for Nutritional Support

- Preoperative nutritional support should be provided to patients with severe malnourishment, to patients having a procedure in which nutritional support has been proven to improve outcomes (ie, major abdominal surgery), and to patients in whom surgery can be safely delayed for 7 to 10 days (the timeframe for preoperative nutritional support).
- Postoperative nutritional support should be provided to mildly malnourished patients who cannot tolerate PO intake 7 to 10 days after surgery, and to severely malnourished patients who cannot tolerate PO intake 5 to 7 days after surgery. Postoperative nutrition should be started promptly if it is anticipated that a patient will be unable to tolerate PO intake 7 to 10 days after surgery.
- Enteral nutrition is always preferable to parenteral nutrition, as it is safer, more cost-effective, and is associated with better outcomes.[35–41]

- Nutritional support should only be provided in the setting of malnutrition. One study established that patients with borderline or mild malnutrition given TPN experienced a greater number of infectious complications, demonstrating that well-nourished patients may actually suffer worse outcomes with TPN.[42]
- The European Society for Clinical Nutrition and Metabolism guidelines recommend that patients with severe nutritional risk should receive nutritional support 10 to 14 days before major surgical intervention, even if surgery must be delayed.[43]

Assessing for Malnutrition

- Nutrition must be assessed comprehensively prior to planning surgical intervention, as it may help to evaluate intraoperative and perioperative risk, and whether or not nutritional support is appropriate. In the setting of malnourishment, nutritional assessment can reveal the degree of malnutrition.
- Numerous indexes and scoring systems exist for the assessment of malnutrition. Metrics used include serum albumin, serum transferrin, triceps skinfold thickness, delayed type hypersensitivity of skin, muscle wasting, weight loss, and percentage of ideal height and body weight.
- The prognostic nutrition index (PNI) can be used to predict the percentage risk of postoperative complication based on an equation using nutritional metrics exclusively.[44]

$$PNI\% = 158 - 16.6(Alb) - 0.78(TSF) - 0.20(TFN) - 5.8(DH),$$

where PNI% represents the percentage risk of postoperative complications; Alb represents serum albumin concentration (g/dL); TSF represents triceps skinfold thickness (mm); TFN represents serum transferrin concentration (g/dL); and DH represents delayed-type hypersensitivity reaction (DH = 0 if no reaction, 1 if induration <5 mm, 2 if induration >5 mm).

- Serum albumin measurements are a simple means by which to assess nutritional status. Low albumin levels correlate with increased morbidity and mortality in surgical patients.[45–47] Several studies recommend surgery should be postponed and nutritional support should be prioritized in patients with a serum albumin less than 3.25 g/dL.[48,49]

Calculating Appropriate Nutritional Support

- Caloric supplementation: 25 to 35 kcal/kg/day, or 1.5 to 1.75 times the basal energy expenditure[50]
  - Basal energy expenditure (Harris-Benedict equation)

$$In \ men, \ 66.47 + 13.75W + 5H - 6.76A$$
$$In \ women, \ 655.1 + 9.56W + 1.85H - 4.68A,$$

where W is weight (kg); H is height (cm); and A is age (years).

- Carbohydrate supplementation: 3 to 6 mg/kg/min (approximately 200–300 g/day)[51]
- Protein supplementation: 1.5 to 2 g/kg/day[50,51]
- Lipid supplementation: 10% to 25% of total calories[51]
- Overfeeding (supplementing >35 kcal/kg/day) is associated with increased rates of sepsis and metabolic complications.[52]
- Daily measurements of body weight, urine output, blood glucose, and electrolytes, and fluid intake should be considered when making modifications to a patient's nutritional therapy regimen.

Immunonutrition

- Immunological supplementation uses specific nutrients (arginine, glutamine, omega-3 fatty acids) to boost immune function in patients experiencing systemic stress.
- Although a relatively novel and controversial area of research, preliminary results have been resoundingly positive.
- Immune-system-enhancing formulas have been shown to reduce postoperative infectious and wound complications, as well as total hospital length of stay (LOS).[53–56] Studies focusing specifically on the immunonutrients arginine[57–59] and glutamine[60,61] have shown that supplementation may reduce infection and complication rates, as well as shorten total LOS.

Enhanced Recovery of Patients after Surgery (ERAS)

- ERAS, or the "fast track protocols"[62] represent a movement toward rapid perioperative restoration of metabolic and nutritional function.

- Key aspects of ERAS include the avoidance of prolonged preoperative fasting, resumption of PO intake soon after surgery, nutritional support with specialized nutrient supplementation, reduction of systemic stressors that stimulate catabolism, and early mobilization.[43,63,64]
- Possible benefits of ERAS include shorter LOS, rapid return of bowel function, prompt patient mobilization, decreased postoperative complication rates, patient ability to tolerate PO intake sooner, and lower 30-day readmission rates.[63]

Evidence for Nutritional Support

- The role of perioperative parenteral nutrition in malnourished surgical patients is highly controversial, with various studies presenting conflicting results. Preoperative TPN has not been conclusively shown to reduce intraoperative and postoperative mortality, although it may reduce postoperative complication rates.[42,65–67] Likewise, postoperative TPN has also failed to unequivocally demonstrate reductions in postoperative complication rates or postoperative survival.[66–71]
- The role of enteral nutrition in malnourished surgical patients has not been strongly established, but shows promise. The results of several studies on preoperative enteral nutrition have been hopeful.[72–75] Similarly, studies pertaining to postoperative enteral nutrition have presented positive results.[37,38,76–82]
- The role of enteral immunonutrition (immunological supplementation) in malnourished surgical patients has also shown hope. Supplementation of arginine, glutamine, and omega-3 fatty acids may reduce rates of postoperative complications and total hospital LOS.[55,57,60,83–85]

Other Considerations

- Refeeding syndrome may occur in patients with prolonged severe malnutrition who are provided nutritional support. Refeeding syndrome can manifest with:
  - Fluid imbalance: Insulin-induced sodium and water reabsorption (paired with nutritional support containing water, sodium and glucose) can result in fluid overload and CHF.
  - Electrolyte imbalance: Hypokalemia, hypomagnesemia, and hypophosphatemia can occur because of rapid cellular electrolyte intake triggered by the presence of insulin. Failure to replete can result in mortality.
  - Hyperglycemia: Prolonged malnutrition can result in insulin resistance. Large carbohydrate or glucose loads can precipitate hyperglycemia, dehydration, and hyperosmolar nonketotic coma. Carbohydrate loads in thiamine-deficient patients can precipitate Wernicke encephalopathy.
  - Heart arrhythmias: Severely malnourished patients may exhibit bradycardia, with rapid refeeding potentially resulting in rebound ventricular tachyarrhythmias or a prolonged QT interval. Arrhythmias may also be caused by electrolyte imbalance.

Perioperative Transfusion Medicine

Background

- Anemia is a widespread issue in the critically ill, with some institutions reporting up to 67% of critical care patients requiring blood transfusions during hospital admission.[86]
- Blood transfusion refers to the IV administration of blood (autologous blood, whole blood) and/or blood products (packed red blood cells, platelets, fresh frozen plasma [FFP], and cryoprecipitate).
- Other therapies, medications, and techniques may be used to reduce blood loss and obviate the need for transfusion.

Preoperative History and Physical

- Symptoms: fatigue, malaise, dyspnea, tachycardia, palpitations, angina, claudication, pallor, koilonychia, jaundice, bleeding diathesis, petechiae, purpura, ecchymoses, epistaxis, gingival bleeding, hematochezia
- Current therapy: medication (nonsteroidal antiinflammatory drugs [NSAIDs], salicylates, aspirin, warfarin, clopidogrel, fondaparinux, other anticoagulants), herbal medications and supplements (may affect coagulability), transfusions, iron and vitamin supplements, erythropoietin
- Medical history: anemias, thrombocytopenias, hemoglobinopathies, bleeding diathesis, hereditary blood dyscrasias (sickle cell anemia, hereditary spherocytosis, von Willebrand

disease, hemophilia, congenital afibrinogenemia, Bernard-Soulier syndrome, Glanzmann thrombasthenia, etc.), factor deficiencies, past transfusions, hypertension, cardiovascular disease, liver dysfunction, renal dysfunction, nutritional status, allergies
- Family history: anemias, thrombocytopenias, hemoglobinopathies, hereditary blood dyscrasias, hypertension, cardiovascular disease
- Physical examination: blood pressure, pulses, volume status, funduscopy, skin examination, joint examination

Preoperative Testing and Laboratory Evaluation

- Hematological evaluation: complete blood count (CBC), reticulocyte count, iron, total iron-binding capacity, ferritin levels, vitamin B_{12} levels, folate levels, peripheral blood smear, type and screen (recipient ABO and Rh blood group antigens), cross-matching (blood types, factors and antibodies of donor and recipient blood)
- Coagulation: activated partial thromboplastin time (aPTT), prothrombin time (PT) and international normalized ratio (INR), factor levels, fibrinogen level, platelet function tests
- Cardiac function: lipid profile, ECG, exercise and nuclear stress test, echocardiogram (based on cardiac assessment and risk stratification)
  - Patients with cardiovascular risk factors (at high risk of myocardial ischemia) are subject to different laboratory value criteria for transfusion eligibility

Preoperative Preparation for Surgery

- Modification or discontinuation of anticoagulant therapy: Oral anticoagulants are typically discontinued several days or weeks prior to surgery, and patients are bridged with unfractionated heparin (UFH) or low-molecular-weight heparin (LMWH) to prevent intractable intraoperative hemorrhage. In some cases, surgery may be delayed until the residual effects of anticoagulants have diminished. (See the section Perioperative Management of Anticoagulation.)
- Blood loss prophylaxis: Preoperative administration of aprotinin, ε-aminocaproic and tranexamic acid have been proposed for reducing intraoperative blood loss (and decreasing the likelihood of transfusion) in patients at high risk for excessive bleeding, with current literature supporting their use.[87-89]
- Allogeneic transfusion prevention and reduction: Preoperative administration of erythropoietin and vitamin K may reduce transfusion requirements in select populations. Preoperative blood collection (for intraoperative transfusion of autologous blood) can also reduce the need for allogeneic transfusion, although autologous blood transfusion is not recommended in patients with hemoglobin level greater than 10 g/dL.[90]

Intraoperative and Postoperative Management of Blood Loss

- Monitoring blood loss: Visual assessment of the operative field, paired with empirical measurement (suction canisters, laparotomy pads, drains).
- Monitoring oxygenation and perfusion: Vital signs, O_2 saturation, urine output, ECG, and in special cases, echocardiography and arterial blood gases.
- Monitoring for transfusion eligibility: Hemoglobin and hematocrit levels should be measured at the first sign of severe blood loss or organ and tissue ischemia. Indications for allogeneic and autologous red blood cell (RBC) transfusion:
- Hemoglobin level less than 6 to 7 g/dL
- Acute blood volume loss greater than 15%
- More than 20% decrease in blood volume, or systolic blood pressure less than 100 mm Hg secondary to blood loss
- Hemoglobin level less than 10 g/dL accompanied by symptoms (eg, chest pain, fatigue, dyspnea, light-headedness, orthostatic hypotension) or in the presence of significant cardiac disease
- Hemoglobin level less than 11 g/dL in patients at risk for multiple organ dysfunction syndrome[91]
- Other transfusion considerations: Blood pressure and intravascular volume should be adequately maintained through administration of colloids and crystalloids until indications for RBC transfusion are met. The main goal of transfusion is maintenance of organ perfusion. Intraoperative and postoperative RBC recovery (ie, cell salvage), deliberate hypotension and acute euvolemic hemodilution may also be considered.[90] Transfusion is not recommended in hemoglobin levels higher than 10 g/dL..

In patients with hemoglobin levels of 6 to 10 g/dL, transfusion is dictated by clinical circumstance (active bleeding, organ/tissue ischemia, etc.).[91]

- Other RBC transfusion products:
  - Specialized RBCs: Rare donor phenotypes, used in patients with unusual antibodies, rare blood types, and immunoglobulin A (IgA) deficiency.
  - Washed RBCs: Used to prevent febrile transfusion reactions and allergic transfusion reactions
  - Leukoreduced and leukofiltered blood: Used to prevent febrile transfusion reactions; favored in chronically transfused patients, organ transplant recipients, cancer patients, and cytomegalovirus (CMV)-seronegative patients.
  - Irradiated blood: Used to prevent graft versus host disease in at-risk patients.
  - CMV-safe blood: Used in CMV-negative infants, CMV-negative bone marrow and solid organ transplant recipients, and immunodeficient patients
  - Autologous cell salvage: May be acceptable to Jehovah's Witness patients.[92–97]
- Blood substitutes: Blood substitutes aim to mimic physiologic oxygen-carrying capacity and volume expansion without adverse effects. Two currently proposed strategies are perflurocarbon emulsions and hemoglobin-based RBC substitutes. Results from studies on blood substitutes have been largely conflicting, with many studies establishing unacceptable toxicities and adverse effects. Substitutes are not currently recommended for use.[91]

Intraoperative and Postoperative Management of Coagulopathy

- Visual assessment of coagulopathy: Visual inspection of the patient for signs of coagulopathy (microvascular blood loss) or major blood loss (suction canisters, laparotomy pads, drains).
- Laboratory assessment of coagulopathy: aPTT, PT/INR, platelet count, fibrinogen level, D-dimer, platelet function tests, thromboelastogram, thrombin time.
- Platelet transfusion: Platelet count should be obtained prior to platelet transfusion, and platelet function tests should be obtained if there is suspicion of drug-induced platelet dysfunction (ie, clopidogrel). Indications for platelet transfusion:
  - Platelet count less than 10×10^9/L
  - Platelet count less than 10 to 20×10^9/L with active bleeding
  - Platelet count less than 50×10^9/L after severe trauma
  - Bleeding time longer than 15 minutes
  - Platelet function tests show evidence of platelet dysfunction (ie, antiplatelet agents)[91]
- FFP transfusion: aPTT and PT/INR should be obtained prior to FFP transfusion. Indications for FFP transfusion:
  - PT longer than 17 seconds (INR >2.0), or aPTT more than 2 times normal
  - Clotting factor deficiency (<25% of normal value)
  - Massive transfusion (1 unit per 5 units of packed RBCs) or if clinically bleeding
  - Severe traumatic brain injury
  - Urgent reversal of warfarin therapy[91]
- Cryoprecipitate transfusion: Fibrinogen concentration should be obtained prior to cryoprecipitate transfusion in a bleeding patient. Indications for cryoprecipitate transfusion:
  - Fibrinogen less than 100 mg/dL
  - Hemophilia A
  - von Willebrand disease
  - Severe traumatic brain injury[91]
- Other transfusion considerations: Platelets transfusion is not indicated in heparin-induced thrombocytopenia (HIT), idiopathic thrombocytopenic purpura, or thrombotic thrombocytopenic purpura. FFP transfusion is not indicated if aPTT and PT/INR are normal. Cryoprecipitate transfusion is not indicated if fibrinogen concentration is higher than 150 mg/dL.
- Agents for treating excessive bleeding: Desmopressin (0.3 mcg/kg, intranasal or IV), fibrin glue and thrombin gel should be considered in the event of excessive bleeding.
- Recombinant activated factor VII (rFVIIa): When all other treatment modalities for microvascular bleeding (coagulopathy) have been exhausted, consider using rFVIIa.[90]

- Perioperative disseminated intravascular coagulopathy (DIC): Practitioners must maintain a high index of suspicion in patients at risk for DIC. The development of massive transfusion protocols allows for practitioner preparedness in the event that a patient develops DIC.

Risks and Adverse Effects of Transfusion

- Bacterial contamination of blood products: Bacterial contamination most commonly occurs in platelet transfusions and is the most common cause of transfusion-related mortality. Development of fever within 6 hours of transfusion may indicate sepsis.
- Transfusion-related acute lung injury (TRALI): Symptoms of noncardiogenic pulmonary edema (dyspnea, fever) occurring within 1 to 2 hours of transfusion may indicate incidence of TRALI. TRALI is the result of immune reactivity of leukocyte antibodies in transfusion products, and is one of the top three causes of transfusion-related mortality. Increased peak airway pressure may suggest incidence of TRALI.
- Infectious diseases: Although hepatitis B virus (HBV), hepatitis C virus (HCV), and human immunodeficiency virus (HIV) transmission via transfusion products were of major concern in the past, blood products are now regularly screened for HBV, HCV, HIV, and West Nile virus. To date, there exists no screening for severe acute respiratory syndrome and variant Creutzfeldt-Jakob disease.
- Transfusion reactions: Hemolytic transfusion reactions may manifest as tachycardia, hypotension, coagulopathy, decreased urine output, and hemoglobinuria. Nonhemolytic transfusion reactions may manifest as fever, chills, and urticaria, although these symptoms may be masked by anesthesia.[90]

Perioperative Anticoagulation

Background

- In patients undergoing anticoagulation therapy, the prospect of surgical intervention presents the potential risk of increased intraoperative hemorrhage. However, this must be balanced with the risk of precipitating thromboembolic phenomena through discontinuation of anticoagulant therapy.
- Evaluation of anticoagulant management in surgical patients, especially in patients on long-term anticoagulation (ie, warfarin and other vitamin K antagonist therapies), requires careful risk-to-benefit analysis. Although the question of whether or not to discontinue anticoagulant agents in the event of emergency surgery may not present a difficult decision, discontinuation prior to elective and nonurgent procedures requires a more complex discussion and decision-making process.
- Although minor surgical procedures may not necessitate discontinuation of warfarin, major surgeries typically require warfarin therapy. Patients at high risk for thromboembolic events may require "bridging therapy," to provide anticoagulation after discontinuation and before reinstatement of long-term warfarin therapy.

Surgery Not Requiring Warfarin Discontinuation

- Ophthalmic surgery: cataract extraction, trabeculectomy[98,99]
- GI tract endoscopy: upper endoscopy, colonoscopy, flexible sigmoidoscopy, endoscopic retrograde cholangiopancreatography, and biliary stenting without sphincterotomy, endosonography with fine-needle aspiration, capsule endoscopy, push enteroscopy[100]
  - Sphincterotomy, polypectomy, laser ablation and coagulation, pneumatic dilation, percutaneous endoscopic gastrostomy tube placement, and treatment of esophageal varices present a high risk of bleeding, and require discontinuation of anticoagulant therapy.[100]
- Dental procedures: uncomplicated extractions, endodontics, prosthetics, dental hygiene, restoration, periodontal therapy[101,102]
  - Complicated extractions, gingival, alveolar, and maxillofacial surgery require discontinuation of anticoagulant therapy.
- Dermatological procedures: Mohs micrographic surgery, simple excisions and repairs[103]
  - Rhytidectomy (face lift), blepharoplasty, hair transplantation, and other cosmetic and plastic surgical procedures require discontinuation of anticoagulant therapy.
- Other: joint and soft tissue aspiration and injection, minor podiatric procedures (nail avulsion, phenol matrixectomy)[104,105]

Preoperative History and Physical

- Current therapy: Medication (NSAIDs, salicylates, aspirin, warfarin, clopidogrel, fondaparinux, other anticoagulants), herbal medications and supplements (may affect coagulability), transfusions
- Medical and surgical history: arterial thromboembolism (ATE), venous thromboembolism (VTE), protein C and protein S deficiencies, antithrombin III deficiency, factor V Leiden mutation, antiphospholipid antibody syndrome, past transfusions, hypertension, hyperlipidemia, MI, CVA, rheumatic heart disease, atrial fibrillation (AFib), valve replacement, cancer
- Family history: ATE, VTE, protein C and protein S deficiencies, antithrombin III deficiency, factor V Leiden mutation, antiphospholipid antibody syndrome, hypertension, hyperlipidemia
- Physical examination: blood pressure, pulses, volume status

Preoperative Testing and Laboratory Evaluation

- Hematological evaluation: CBC (hemoglobin, hematocrit, platelet count), reticulocyte count, peripheral blood smear, type and screen (recipient ABO and Rh blood group antigens), cross-matching (blood types, factors and antibodies of donor and recipient blood)
- Coagulation: aPTT, PT/INR, factor levels, fibrinogen level, platelet function tests

Preoperative Warfarin Discontinuation

- Surgery is considered safe in patients with an INR less than 1.5.[106]
- In patients with an INR of 2.0 to 3.0, warfarin should be held for 5 days prior to surgery.
- In patients with an INR more than 3.0, warfarin may need to be held for a longer period of time (6 or more days).
- Major neurosurgical and noncardiac procedures may warrant waiting for INR less than 1.2.
- Coagulation studies (PT/INR) should be performed prior to surgery to ensure adequate reversal of anticoagulant therapy.

Emergency Warfarin Reversal

- FFP: Administration results in immediate reversal of warfarin anticoagulation. Risks include adverse effects of transfusion. INR should be checked periodically.
- Vitamin K: Vitamin K can be used in a semiurgent situation. Large doses (5–10 mg) may result in postoperative warfarin resistance.[107] A smaller dose (1.0–2.5 mg) is recommended. INR will typically normalize within 1 day of IV vitamin K administration.
- rFVIIa: rFVIIa administration is indicated in hemophiliacs who have factor VIII and factor IX inhibitors.[108]

Thromboembolic Risk Stratification and Bridging Recommendations

- High thromboembolic risk (1-year ATE risk >10% and 1-year VTE risk >10% while off warfarin; bridging therapy recommended)
  - Documented hypercoagulability secondary to protein C and protein S deficiencies, antithrombin III deficiency, factor V Leiden mutation, antiphospholipid antibody syndrome
  - Documented hypercoagulability, as evidenced by recurrent (two or more) episodes of ATE/VTE (not including atherosclerotic events such as MI, CVA)
  - ATE/VTE within the last 3 months
  - Rheumatic heart disease plus AFib
  - Mechanical heart valve plus AFib
  - Old model (single-disk, ball-in-cage) mechanical mitral valve replacement
  - Mechanical valve replacement within the last 3 months
  - AFib plus cardioembolism[108]
- Intermediate thromboembolic risk (1-year ATE risk 5%-10% and 1-month VTE risk 2%–10% while off warfarin; need for bridging therapy evaluated on an individual case basis)
  - Cerebrovascular disease with 2 or more CVAs or transient ischemic attacks, in the absence of cardioembolic risk factors
  - New model (ie, St. Jude) mechanical mitral valve replacement
  - Old model mechanical aortic valve replacement
  - AFib without cardioembolism, but with cardioembolic risk factors (ie, diabetes, hypertension, ejection fraction <40%, nonrheumatic heart valve disease, transmural MI within the last 1 month)
  - VTE occurring more than 3 to 6 months ago[108]

- Low thromboembolic risk (1-year ATE risk <5% and 1-month VTE risk <2% while off warfarin; bridging therapy not recommended)
  - Remote VTE (>6 months ago)
  - Stable cerebrovascular disease (without CVA or transient ischemic attack)
  - AFib without cardioembolic risk factors
  - New model mechanical aortic valve replacement[108]

Low-Molecular-Weight Heparin Bridging Criteria

- Inclusion criteria:
  - Patient age older than 18 years
  - Meets bridging recommendations (see above)
  - Medically and hemodynamically stable
  - Patient undergoing elective surgery or procedure[108]
- Exclusion criteria:
  - UFH/LMWH allergy
  - Patient weight more than 150 kg (330.7 lb)
  - Pregnancy plus mechanical heart valve
  - Bleeding disorder history
  - Intracranial bleeding history
  - Creatinine clearance less than 30 mL/min
  - GI tract bleeding within last 10 days
  - CVA or major trauma within last 14 days
  - HIT or severe thrombocytopenia history
  - Severe liver disease
  - Socioeconomic and domestic issues (potential noncompliance, language barrier, home environment unsuitable to therapy)[108]

Perioperative Low-Molecular-Weight Heparin Administration Protocol

- Preoperative LMWH protocol
  - If preoperative INR 2.0 to 3.0, discontinue warfarin 5 days prior to surgery
  - If preoperative INR 3.0 to 4.5, discontinue warfarin 6 days prior to surgery
  - Start LMWH 36 hours after patient received final warfarin dose
    - Enoxaparin 1 mg/kg subcutaneously every 12 hours
    - Enoxaparin 1.5 mg/kg subcutaneously every 24 hours
    - Dalteparin 120 units/kg subcutaneously every 12 hours
    - Dalteparin 200 units/kg subcutaneously every 24 hours
    - Tinzaparin 175 units/kg subcutaneously every 24 hours
  - Give last dose of LMWH 24 hours prior to surgery
  - Check INR prior to surgery[108]
- Postoperative LMWH protocol
  - Resume LMWH 24 hours after surgery (if adequate hemostasis is achieved)
  - Restart warfarin (at preoperative dose) on postoperative day 1
  - Daily PT/INR until hospital discharge
  - Periodic PT/INR until therapeutic INR range reached
  - CBC (with platelet count) on postoperative days 1,3, and 7 (to assess for HIT)
  - Discontinue LMWH once therapeutic INR range reached[108]

Risks and Considerations of Bridging Therapy

- Bleeding: 0.5% to 5.0% risk of bleeding associated with UFH or LMWH[108]
- HIT is said to occur in 3% of patients receiving UFH, and in 1% of patients receiving LMWH.[109] HIT may occur within 1 day of initiating bridging therapy. Close monitoring of platelet count is encouraged.
- Epidural hematoma: Insertion or removal of epidural catheters while on bridging therapy can result in the formation of epidural hematomas. Lumbar puncture or epidural catheter removal should only be performed 12 hours after last thromboprophylactic LMWH dose, or 24 hours after last treatment LMWH dose. LMWH should be given at least 2 hours after an epidural catheter has been removed.

- LMWH is not recommended in pregnant women with mechanical heart valves.[108]
- Routine antifactor Xa levels may be used to monitor the effects of LMWH anticoagulation.

Antiplatelet Agents

- Aspirin and clopidogrel should be discontinued 7 to 10 days prior to surgery.
- Aspirin and clopidogrel may be resumed 24 hours after surgery (if adequate hemostasis is achieved).
- Patients undergoing noncardiac surgery who are at high risk for cardiac events, patients undergoing CABG, and patients undergoing percutaneous coronary intervention (PCI) should be continued on aspirin up to and after surgery.
  - If aspirin is interrupted prior to CABG, it may be resumed 6 to 48 hours after CABG.
- Patients undergoing noncardiac surgery who are at high risk for cardiac events, and patients undergoing CABG should have clopidogrel discontinued 5 to 10 days prior to surgery.
  - If clopidogrel is interrupted prior to PCI, it may be resumed after PCI with a 300- to 600-mg loading dose.
- Patients undergoing surgery within 6 weeks of bare metal coronary stent placement should be continued on aspirin and clopidogrel perioperatively.
- Patients undergoing surgery within 12 months of drug-eluting coronary stent placement should be continued on aspirin and clopidogrel perioperatively.
- In coronary stent patients, if antiplatelet therapy has been interrupted prior to surgery, the patient should receive bridging therapy with UFH, LMWH, direct thrombin inhibitors (ie, hirudin, bivalirudin, lepirudin, desirudin, argatroban, melagatran, dabigatran), or glycoprotein IIb/IIIa inhibitors (ie, abciximab, eptifibatide, tirofiban).[110]

Management of Preexisting Liver Disease in the Surgical Patient

Background

- Assessing the risk of surgery and anesthesia in patients with hepatic dysfunction is challenging because of the numerous functions of the liver, as any or all functions can be impaired.[111]
- Liver disease comprises a large spectrum of hepatic dysfunction including asymptomatic transaminitis, cirrhosis, and end-stage liver disease.
- The most common causes of advanced liver disease are chronic viral infections (HCV and HBV), alcohol abuse, nonalcoholic fatty liver disease, nonalcoholic steatohepatitis (NASH), autoimmune disease, drugs or toxins, metabolic disorders (α_1-antitrypsin deficiency, hemochromatosis, and Wilson disease), and biliary tract diseases.
- Surgical patients with liver disease are at an increased risk of complications and morbid outcomes, but the extent of that risk depends on certain factors including type and severity of hepatic dysfunction, the surgical procedure, type of anesthesia along with certain perioperative events such as hypotension, sepsis, and hepatotoxic drugs.[112,113]
- Most published data regarding surgical risk in the patient with liver disease has come from studies specifically from patients with cirrhosis, but less information is available on patients with milder disease.[114,115]
- It has been estimated that many patients with end-stage liver disease will undergo surgery in the last 2 years of their lives.[115,116]

Preoperative History and Physical

- Assess for risk factors such as prior blood transfusions, tattoos, illicit drug use, sexual promiscuity, family history of jaundice or liver disease, history of jaundice or fever following anesthesia, alcohol use (current and prior use along with quantity), and a complete review of current medications.
- Physical examination findings suggestive of liver disease include: increased abdominal girth, fatigue, jaundice, palmar erythema, pruritus, splenomegaly and spider telangiectasias. In men, gynecomastia and testicular atrophy should also be assessed.

Preoperative Testing and Laboratory Evaluation

- Should include laboratory tests to assess blood counts, coagulopathy, electrolyte abnormalities, and markers of hepatic synthetic function.

Estimating Surgical Risk

- Assessing surgical risk in the patient with hepatic dysfunction, several factors must be evaluated including severity of hepatic dysfunction, the urgency of surgery or an alternative to surgery, along with coexisting medical conditions.
- In urgent situations, risk assessment is less important. In most cases, there is adequate time for proper risk assessment, optimization of the patient, and discussion of alternatives to surgery.
- Risk factors associated with morbidity and mortality in patients with cirrhosis[111]
  - Type of surgery: abdominal (especially cholecystectomy, gastric resection or colectomy), cardiac, emergency, hepatic resection
  - Patient condition: anemia, ascites, Child-Turcotte-Pugh class (C > B), encephalopathy, hypoalbuminemia, hypoxemia, infection, jaundice, malnutrition, portal hypertension, and prolonged PT (>2.5 seconds above the control that does not correct with vitamin K)
- Contraindications to surgery in patients with liver disease:[111]
  - Acute alcoholic hepatitis, acute viral hepatitis, Child-Turcotte-Pugh class C cirrhosis, fulminant hepatic failure, severe chronic hepatitis, severe coagulopathy (PT greater than 3 seconds despite vitamin K administration, platelet count <50,000 mm³), and severe extrahepatic complications (acute renal failure [ARF], cardiomyopathy, heart failure, hypoxemia).
- The primary predictor of operative risk in a patient with cirrhosis has been the Child-Turcotte-Pugh classification for the past 30 years, but more recently studies have shown that the Model for End-Stage Liver Disease (MELD) score may be superior.[117]
  - Child-Turcotte-Pugh Classification (Table 16-5)
    - The most recent study in 2011 of 138 patients undergoing abdominal surgery showed mortality rates of 10%, 17%, and 63% for patients with Child-Turcotte-Pugh class A, B, and C, respectively.[118]
    - Patients with Child-Turcotte-Pugh class A cirrhosis and portal hypertension are at increased risk of postoperative jaundice, ascites, and encephalopathy.[119]
  - MELD Score: a statistical model predicting survival in patients with cirrhosis.
    - It is typically used to select patients for liver transplant, but more recently has shown promising results as a predictor of surgical risk in patients with cirrhosis.[120]
    - It has been suggested that a patient with a MELD score below 10 can undergo elective surgery, whereas a score of 10 to 15 indicates that surgery should proceed with caution; if a patient has a MELD score higher than 15, the patient should not undergo surgery.[121]
    - The calculation is based the patient's serum bilirubin, creatinine, and INR for PT:

$$= (3.8 \times ln \text{ bilirubin value}) + (11.2 \times ln \text{ INR}) + (9.6 \times ln \text{ creatinine value}),$$

where bilirubin and creatinine values are in milligrams per deciliter (mg/dL) and *ln* represents natural logarithm.

TABLE 16-5. CHILD-TURCOTTE-PUGH CLASSIFICATION

Parameters	1 Point	2 Points	3 Points
Encephalopathy	None	Minimal	Advanced (Coma)
Ascites	Absent	Controlled	Refractory
Bilirubin (mg/dL)	<2	2–3	>3
Albumin (g/L)	>35	28–35	<28
INR	<1.7	1.7–2.3	>2.3
Prothrombin (seconds over control)	<4	4–6	>6

INR, international normalized ratio.

- Patients with mild to moderate liver disease without cirrhosis usually tolerate surgery, but should be optimized prior to surgery.

Preoperative Treatment of Liver Disease

- Assess for jaundice, coagulopathy, ascites, electrolyte abnormalities, renal dysfunction, and encephalopathy.
  - Coagulopathy should be corrected with vitamin K if the PT is elevated. FFP and diamino-8-D-arginine vasopressin (dDAVP) may also be required.
  - Thrombocytopenia should be corrected if the platelet count is below 50,000 mm^3.
  - Optimal surgical technique and maintenance of low central venous pressure may help decrease blood loss.[122]
- Renal function should be evaluated with creatinine and BUN levels.
- Volume status must be assessed and corrected.
- Nephrotoxic substances, such as NSAIDs and aminoglycosides should be avoided.
- Electrolyte abnormalities: hypokalemia and metabolic alkalosis should be corrected to reduce the likelihood of encephalopathy and cardiac arrhythmias.
- Ascites should be treated with diuretics prior to surgery and possibly paracentesis, if there is not enough time ascites can be drained at the time of surgery.
- Gastroesophageal varices should be treated prophylactically.
- Encephalopathy should be treated with lactulose and protein restriction, and avoid sedatives and narcotics in these patients.
- Perioperative nutritional support can reduce the frequency of postoperative complications and short-term mortality.[123]

Postoperative Treatment of Liver Disease

- Observe closely for hepatic decompensation, which often presents with worsening jaundice, encephalopathy, and ascites.
- Monitor liver function with PT and serum bilirubin concentration. However, the serum bilirubin concentration usually rises, particularly after complicated surgery, multiple blood transfusions, excessive bleeding, hemodynamic instability, or systemic infection.
- Renal function, serum electrolytes, and glucose should also be monitored carefully.

Management of Preexisting Renal Disease in the Surgical Patient

Chronic Renal Insufficiency and End-Stage Renal Disease

Background

- Patients with chronic kidney disease not currently on dialysis and patients with end-stage renal disease (ESRD) frequently need surgical interventions.[124]
- All patients with renal disease need appropriate cardiac risk stratification because of the fact that chronic renal insufficiency (CRI) is an independent risk factor for perioperative cardiac complications.[125]
- Impairment of kidney function results in both excretory and synthetic dysfunction leading to elevated levels of BUN, creatinine, various protein metabolites as well as decreased levels of erythropoietin, active vitamin D_3, acid, potassium, sodium, and water excretion leading to excess surgical morbidity.
- Careful evaluation perioperatively by a nephrologist is warranted to reduce complications including ARF, hyperkalemia, volume overload, and infections.
- A significant mortality risk of 1% to 4% exists in patients with ESRD undergoing surgery.[124,126]

Preoperative Risk Assessment

- A thorough cardiovascular risk assessment is warranted in patients with CRI or ESRD because of an increased perioperative morbidity risk.
- Please refer to the section Preoperative Cardiac Evaluation to review predictors of preoperative cardiovascular risk.
- Patients with chronic kidney disease can be divided into 4 categories:[124,127]
  - Chronic renal failure but not on dialysis
  - ARF with or without dialysis
  - Stable renal failure undergoing hemodialysis or peritoneal dialysis
  - Kidney transplant patients with impaired renal function

- Evaluate patients with CRI being treated conservatively.
  - Establish duration of CRI and level of impairment.
  - Is the elevated BUN and creatinine levels prerenal, intrarenal, postrenal, or a combination including CRI?
  - Euvolemic patients that are responsive to diuretics and have no significant electrolyte or bleeding abnormalities usually do not require dialysis prior to surgery.
  - Patients with edema, CHF, or pulmonary congestion and are responsive to diuretics require further cardiovascular evaluation and if optimal, fluid overload may be the cause. Combination diuretic therapy may be warranted preoperatively.
  - Diabetic patients tend to have cardiovascular disease or be volume overloaded. Preoperative dialysis may be necessary.
- Avoid potential nephrotoxic agents in patients with renal impairment.
  - Antibiotics (aminoglycosides)
  - Antifungals (amphotericin)
  - Antivirals (acyclovir)
  - Sedatives
  - Muscle relaxants
  - NSAIDs
  - Radiocontrast material including iodinated and gadolinium
    - Acetylcysteine or sodium bicarbonate along with hydration may reduce the risk of ARF if iodinated contrast cannot be avoided.[128]
  - Demerol (meperidine) for postoperative pain caused by seizures because of the accumulation of normeperidine in CRI patients.
- Electrolyte abnormalities must by assessed and corrected perioperatively.
- Renal transplant and dialysis patients
  - Evaluate patient to see if adequately dialyzed and determine preoperative and postoperative dialysis requirements and timing.
  - Patients currently on hemodialysis usually require preoperative dialysis within 24 hours of the surgical procedure to avoid volume overload, excessive bleeding, and hyperkalemia.
  - Peritoneal dialysis patients undergoing abdominal surgery should be switched to hemodialysis until wound healing is complete.
  - Peritoneal dialysis can continue in patients undergoing nonabdominal surgery.
  - Evaluate medications and dosage requirements for transplant patients because the immunosuppressive drugs affect the cytochrome P450 system and can precipitate nephrotoxicity or rejection.

Perioperative Treatment of Kidney Disease

- Volume status
  - Euvolemia should be attained preoperatively to minimize complications.[129]
  - Volume contraction can be caused by third-space fluid loss, diarrhea, vomiting, and nasogastric suctioning.
- Electrolyte abnormalities
  - Hyperkalemia may be caused by acidosis, transfusions, tissue breakdown, angiotensin-converting enzyme inhibitors, beta-blockers, heparin, rhabdomyolysis, and the use of Ringer lactate as a replacement fluid, which contains potassium.
    - Preoperative dialysis should be performed for patients on dialysis.
    - Patients with CRI, not on dialysis will need an alternative form or potassium excretion.
  - Hypokalemia can be caused by third-space fluid loss, diarrhea, vomiting, and nasogastric suctioning.
  - Hypomagnesemia can happen concurrently with hypokalemia.
  - Chronic acidosis is common in patients with chronic kidney disease and may be worsened by surgery, which puts the patient at increased risk of hyperkalemia, myocardial depression, and cardiac arrhythmia.
  - Hypocalcemia and hyperphosphatemia may be caused by rhabdomyolysis.
  - Hyponatremia can be caused by use of hypotonic fluids or the inappropriate secretion of antidiuretic hormone.

- Coagulopathy
  - Platelet dysfunction is associated with uremia.
    - Dialysis for ESRD patients
    - Desmopressin (0.3 mcg/kg IV or intranasally) may be used.
    - Cryoprecipitate (10 units over 30 minutes).
    - RBC transfusions for patients with coexisting anemia.
    - Preoperative desmopressin for patients with a history of prior uremic bleeding.
  - Heparin-free dialysis should be used to decrease bleeding risk.
- Antibiotic prophylaxis
  - Renal dosing may be necessary.

Acute Renal Failure

Background

- Surgery has been associated with an increased risk of ARF.[129]
- Patients with chronic renal insufficiency (CRI) are at increased risk of ARF.
- The approach to ARF in the perioperative setting is not substantially different from the nonoperative setting.
- Certain factors to be considered include
  - Intraoperative hemodynamic changes, especially hypotension.
  - Certain procedures have an adverse effect on renal function.
  - Possibility of bleeding.

Specific Issues

Corticosteroids

- Corticosteroids are clearly savior medications in the right clinical setting, however, for the most part they are viewed as negatively affecting wound healing, and increasing patient infection risk if they are continued through the perioperative period.
- Historically, a nonevidence-based approach in which surgeons gave a "100, a 100, and a 100 mg of [hydrocortisone sodium succinate] Solu-Cortef," to almost any patient on corticosteroid supplementation was the standard, however, recent data has permitted a more evidence-based approach to perioperative corticosteroid administration to limit their deleterious effects.
- It has now become quite clear that "stress dose" steroids are only indicated when the hypothalamic-pituitary-adrenal axis (HPAA) is suppressed.
- The corticosteroid dose below which HPAA suppression is difficult to predict. Many patients take supraphysiologic doses of prednisone (5 mg/day long term, 7.5–10 mg/day for 1 month, more than 20 mg/day for 1 week, or high doses of other inhaled corticosteroids) for a variety of conditions and may show evidence of HPAA suppression.
- The time to recovery of normal adrenal function after stopping corticosteroids varies from a few days to several months. The best plan is to assume that patients receiving corticosteroids within 3 months of surgery have some degree of HPAA suppression and should receive perioperative supplementation.
- When using perioperative corticosteroid supplementation, doses should parallel the physiologic response of the normal adrenal gland to surgical stress, providing only very short-term supplementation.
- Depending on the dose the patient is taking prior to surgery and the type of operative procedure, the following schedule can be used:
  - In the case of a minor surgery, in a patient on more than 10 mg/day of prednisone (or equivalent), 25 to 100 mg of hydrocortisone at induction is sufficient. Postoperatively, patients resume the usual dose of corticosteroid the next day.
  - In the case of a major operation, 100 mg of hydrocortisone every 8 hours for 24 hours should be used, on the day of surgery, then the dose of prednisone should be decreased rapidly (ie, 50% per day, down to the usual steroid dose). Oral corticosteroid therapy should be resumed when GI tract function returns.
  - In the case of ambulatory procedures, administer hydrocortisone (100 mg IV/IM) at discharge, along with a prescription for a rapid taper of prednisone or resumption of the previous steroid dose. A patient taking a high dose of steroids for immunosuppression should be maintained during the perioperative period. For example, for a patient taking

TABLE 16-6. RISK FACTORS FOR POSTOPERATIVE NAUSEA AND VOMITING IN ADULTS[130]

Patient-specific risk factors	Female patients
	Nonsmokers
	Previous history of PONV and motion sickness
Anesthetic risk factors	Volatile anesthetics
	Nitrous oxide
	Use of intraoperative or postoperative opioid
Surgery-related risk factors	Type of surgery (laparoscopy, ear-nose-throat, neurosurgery, breast, strabismus, laparotomy, plastic surgery)
	Duration of surgery (each 30-minute increase in duration increases PONV risk by 60%, so that a baseline risk of 10% is increased by 16% after 30 minutes)

60 mg of prednisone per day, hydrocortisone at 250 to 300 mg/day parenterally is recommended until the patient can resume the normal oral dose.
- Remember that when calculating the hydrocortisone dose, prednisone is 4 times stronger.

Postoperative Nausea and Vomiting (PONV) (Table 16-6)
- Nausea and vomiting are important in the perioperative period as they may interrupt the procedure when a patient is under regional anesthesia or limit discharge following surgery.
- Management:
  - Not all surgical patients will benefit from antiemetic prophylaxis; thus, identification of patients who are at increased risk is imperative. The first step in reducing PONV risk is to reduce baseline risk factors among patients at risk (which includes use of regional anesthesia, use of propofol for induction and maintenance of anesthesia, use of intraoperative supplemental oxygen, use of hydration, avoidance of nitrous oxide, avoidance of volatile anesthetics, minimization of intraoperative and postoperative opioid, and minimization of neostigmine)
  - Specific Measures (Table 16-7)
  - If PONV occurs within 6 hours after surgery, patients should not receive a repeat dose of the prophylactic antiemetic. An emetic episode more than 6 hours after surgery can be treated with any of the drugs used for prophylaxis except dexamethasone and transdermal scopolamine.

TABLE 16-7. MANAGEMENT OF POSTOPERATIVE NAUSEA AND VOMITING

No prophylaxis or dexamethasone
5-HT$_3$ antagonist[a] plus second agent
Triple therapy with 5-HT$_3$ antagonist[a] plus 2 other agents[b] when PONV occurs <6 hours after surgery
Triple therapy with 5-HT$_3$ antagonist[a] plus 2 other agents[b] when PONV occurs >6 hours after surgery

5-HT$_3$, serotonin.
[a]Small-dose 5-HT antagonist dosing: ondansetron 1.0 mg, dolasetron 12.5 mg, granisetron 0.1 mg, and tropisetron 0.5 mg.
[b]Alternative therapies for rescue: droperidol 0.625 mg IV, dexamethasone (2–4 mg IV), and promethazine 12.5 mg IV.

Perioperative Management of the Trauma Patient

- Trauma remains the third most common cause of death for all individuals regardless of age.
  - Initial management of seriously injured patients includes performance of the primary survey (the ABCs—*a*irway with cervical spine protection, *b*reathing, and *c*irculation).
  - Shock caused by hemorrhagic, cardiogenic, neurogenic, or septic pathophysiology requires prompt intervention. In patients without clear operative indications and persistent hypotension, one should systematically evaluate the five potential sources of blood loss: scalp, chest, abdomen, pelvis, and extremities. The preoperative SBP target for patients with torso arterial injuries is higher than 90 mm Hg. Conversely, optimal management of traumatic brain injury includes maintaining the SBP at higher than 90 mm Hg.
  - All patients with blunt injury should be assumed to have unstable cervical spine injuries until proven otherwise; one must maintain cervical spine precautions and inline stabilization. Thoracoabdominal trauma should be evaluated with a combination of chest radiograph, focused assessment with sonography for trauma, and pelvic radiograph. Extremity examination and radiographs should be used to search for associated fractures.
  - Immediate operative intervention for penetrating abdominal injury should include maintenance of hemodynamic stability and significant external arterial hemorrhage; and specific treatment based on the presenting symptoms and anatomic location of injury. If a weapon is still in place, it should be removed in the operating room, because it could be tamponading a lacerated blood vessel.
  - Management of blunt abdominal injuries should include physical examination and ultrasound to rapidly identify patients requiring emergent laparotomy. Computed tomographic scanning is the mainstay of evaluation in the remaining patients to more precisely identify the site and magnitude of injury.
  - Antibiotics: All injured patients undergoing an operation should receive preoperative antibiotics. The type of antibiotic is determined by the anticipated source of contamination in the abdomen or other operative region; additional doses should be administered during the procedure based on blood loss and the half-life of the antibiotic. Extended postoperative antibiotic therapy is administered only for open fractures or significant intraabdominal contamination. Tetanus prophylaxis is administered to all patients according to published guidelines.
  - Prophylaxis for thromboembolism: Patients at higher risk for venous thromboembolism example those with multiple fractures of the pelvis and lower extremities, those with coma or spinal cord injury, those requiring ligation of large veins in the abdomen and lower extremities, and morbidly obese patients should receive LMWH prophylaxis.
  - Thermal protection: Hemorrhagic shock impairs perfusion and metabolic activity throughout the body, with resultant hypothermia that may result in coagulopathy and myocardial irritability in the operating room. Management should include comfortable ambient temperature, covering stabilized patients with warm blankets, administering warmed IV fluids and blood products and heated inhalation through the ventilatory circuit.
  - Treatment of specific intracranial, head and neck, thoracic, abdominal, and extremity injuries is beyond the scope of this chapter. Pregnant and geriatric patients pose a special challenge in this scenario.
- Perioperative management of trauma patients:[131]
  - Initial resuscitation involves initial volume loading to attain adequate preload (10 L during the initial 6–12 hours), followed by judicious use of inotropic agents or vasopressors.
  - During shock resuscitation a hemoglobin level of more than 10 g/dL is generally accepted to optimize oxygen delivery. After the first 24 hours of resuscitation, a more judicious transfusion of a hemoglobin level of less than 7 g/dL in the euvolemic patient limits the adverse inflammatory effects of stored RBCs.
  - Invasive monitoring with pulmonary artery catheters is controversial but may be a critical adjunct in patients with multiple injuries who require advanced inotropic

support. This information on the patient's volume status, cardiac function, peripheral vascular tone, response to vasoactive agents, and metabolic response to injury permits appropriate therapeutic intervention. Although norepinephrine is the agent of choice for patients with low systemic vascular resistance who are unable to maintain a mean arterial pressure of more than 60 mmHg, patients may have an element of myocardial dysfunction requiring inotropic support. The role of relative adrenal insufficiency is another controversial area.

Perioperative Management of the Burn Patient

- With advances in fluid resuscitation, improvements in critical care, and the advent of early excision of the burn wound, survival has become an expectation even for patients with severe burns.
- American Burn Association recommendations for referral to specialized burn centers include:
  - Partial-thickness burns greater than 10% total body surface area
  - Burns involving the face, hands, feet, genitalia, perineum, or major joints
  - Third-degree burns in any age group
  - Electrical burns, including lightning injury
  - Chemical burns
  - Inhalation injury
  - Burn injury in patients with complicated preexisting medical disorders
  - Patients with burns and concomitant trauma in which the burn is the greatest risk. If the trauma is the greater immediate risk, the patient may be stabilized in a trauma center before transfer to a burn center.
  - Burned children in hospitals without qualified personnel for the care of children
  - Burn injury in patients who will require special social, emotional, or rehabilitative intervention.
- Management guidelines[132] (Table 16-8):
  - Patients with upper airway injury, partial pressure of arterial oxygen: fraction of inspired oxygen ratio less than 200 mm Hg or carbon monoxide toxicity should be intubated for inhalation injury.
  - IV fluid resuscitation for patients with burns greater than 20% total body surface area (children with >15% total body surface area) should be titrated to mean arterial pressure greater than 60 mm Hg and urine output greater than 30 mL/hour.
  - Never administer prophylactic antibiotics other than tetanus vaccination.
  - Early excision and grafting of full thickness and deep partial thickness burns improves outcomes.
  - Appropriate management of decreased urine output, increased ventilator airway pressures, and hypotension.
- The details of management of burn wound, nutrition, and complications of burn injuries are beyond the scope of this chapter.

TABLE 16-8. PARKLAND FORMULA

Initial 24 hours: Adults	Initial 24 hours: Children
Lactated Ringer solution 2–4 mL/kg/% burn over 24 hours—given in the first 8 hours postinjury. Additional fluid required for inhalation injury. Urine output of 30 mL/h.	Lactated Ringer solution at 5000 mL/m² body surface area burn/24 hr plus 2000 mL/m² body surface area burn/24 hr given in the first 8 hours postinjury. Urine output of 1 mL/kg/h.
Subsequent 24 hours: Adults	*Subsequent 24 hours: Children*
1 mL/kg/% body surface area burn/day	3750 mL/m² body surface area burn/day plus 1500 mL/m² total body surface area/day

Perioperative Management of the Bariatric Patient

- Obesity is defined as BMI more than 30 kg/m².
- More than 33 % of adults in the United States (approximately 72 million people) are obese.[133]
- Success of a bariatric surgery depends on a series of factors and requires a multidisciplinary team with complete dedication and a comprehensive understanding of how to manage obese patients.[134]
- The clinical and surgical team should consider morbid obesity as a disease and must be prepared to care for critically ill bariatric surgical patients with cardiopulmonary failure, serious wound problems, and ventilatory and nutritional support.[134]
- Comorbid diseases associated with obesity include but are not limited to:
  - Cardiovascular diseases (hypertension, hypercholesterolemia, dyslipidemia, diabetes mellitus type 2)
  - Hematologic abnormalities (prophylactic treatment for deep venous thrombosis and pulmonary embolism)
  - Pulmonary diseases (preoperatively assess for obstructive sleep apnea COPD and risk for developing pneumonia, atelectasis, and respiratory failure postoperatively; chest physiotherapy instruction)
  - Renal dysfunction (renal insufficiency is not a contraindication for surgery)
  - GI tract diseases (gastroesophageal reflux disease), peptic ulcer disease, *Helicobacter pylori*, gastric ulcers, and cholelithiasis
  - Hepatic abnormalities (NASH)
    - Patients with metabolic syndrome, and diagnosed with NASH should have a liver biopsy during surgery to observe fibrosis or the evolution to cirrhosis.[135]
  - Endocrine dysfunction (hypothyroidism, hyperthyroidism, Cushing disease)
  - Diabetes mellitus (strict glucose control is necessary)
  - Psychological issues
- All comorbid conditions must be documented and controlled to decrease the risk of the procedure.
- Careful evaluation perioperatively is imperative in the successful outcome of the bariatric patient.
- For specifics of bariatric surgery, see the section Perioperative Management of the Bariatric Patient.

Perioperative Management of the Cancer Patient

- No guidelines for anesthesia procedures in cancer patients have been developed.
- Competent immune cells particularly CD4+ T-helper 1 type cells, CD8+ cytotoxic T cells, and natural killer (NK) cells may be suppressed by surgical inflammation, some anesthetics, and inadvertent anesthesia management, which may render cancer patients susceptible to tumor recurrence and metastasis after surgery.[136]
- Hypotension, hypovolemia, and hypoxia
  - Cancer patients are frequently at risk of intraoperative hypotension owing to preoperative malnutrition, dehydration and intraoperative hypovolemia by hemorrhage.
  - Hypoxia is strongly associated with tumor progression and metastasis, and the number of hypotensive episodes during a surgery has been deemed to be the single most significant risk factor associated with a shorter disease-free interval.[137]
- Blood transfusion
  - Allogeneic blood transfusion is recognized to have diverse immunomodulatory effects and this immunosuppression may increase the risk of cancer recurrence.
- β-Adrenergic antagonists
  - Mobilization of antitumor CD8+ T cells and NK cells into circulation from the marginal pool is promoted by endogenous catecholamines.
  - β-adrenergic antagonists reduce vascular endothelial growth factor secretion from malignant human cells and provide a novel clinically effective therapeutic strategy for several cancer types.

- Opioids
  - Morphine causes immunosuppression and also increases migration of cancer cells. Methylnaltrexone and fentanyl a peripheral μ-opioid receptor antagonist have been approved for palliative care.
- Volatile anesthetics, anesthetic induction drugs, and cyclooxygenase inhibitors
  - Volatile anesthetics such as halothane, isoflurane and sevoflurane suppress NK cell activity and suppress lymphocyte functions.
  - Propofol has only minor effects on NK cells and lymphocytes. Propofol also has cyclooxygenase-2 inhibiting activity and thus prevents tumor progression, vascular endothelial growth factor production and NK cell inhibition.
  - Regional anesthesia including peripheral nerve blockades, epidural and spinal anesthesia not only provide pain relief by acting at the origin of pain impulses they also block surgery-induced perioperative immunosuppression.
- Perioperative nutrition
  - Cancer patients present with preoperative malnutrition that engenders immunosuppression.
  - Oral and/or enteral perioperative immunonutrition with arginine and omega-3 fatty acids can enhance NK cell activity and improve outcomes in cancer patients.

REFERENCES

1. Kullen KA, Hall MJ, Golosinskiy A. Ambulatory surgery in the United States, 2006. *Natl Health Stat Report*. 2009;11:1-28.

2. Eagle KA, Berger PB, Calkins H, et al. American College of Cardiology. American Heart Association. ACC/AHA guideline update for perioperative cardiovascular evaluation of non cardiac surgery—executive summary: a report of the American College of Cardiology/American Heart Association Task Force on Practice Guidelines (Committee to update the 1996 Guidelines on Perioperative Cardiovascular Evaluation for Noncardiac Surgery). *J Am Coll Cardiol*. 2002;39:542-553.

3. Eagle KA, Coley CM, Newell JB, et al. Combining clinical and thallium data optimizes preoperative assessment of cardiac risk before major vascular surgery. *Ann Intern Med*. 1989;110:859-866.

4. Lee TH, Marcantonio ER, Manione CM, et al. Derivation and prospective validation of a simple index for prediction of cardiac risk of major noncardiac surgery. *Circulation*. 1999;100:1043-1049.

5. Brilakis ES, Orford JL, Fasseas P, et al. Outcome of patients undergoing balloon angioplasty in the two months prior to noncardiac surgery. *Am J Cardiol*. 2005;96: 512-514.

6. Hermanson B, et al. Beneficial six year outcome of smoking cessation in older men and women with coronary heart disease: results from the CASS registry. *N Engl J Med*. 1988;319:1365.

7. Cameron A, Davis K, Rogers W. Recurrence of angina after coronary artery bypass surgery: predictors and prognosis (CASS Registry). *J Am Coll Cardiol*. 1995;26:895.

8. Diet, Nutrition and the Prevention of Chronic Diseases. Report of a Joint WHO/FAO Expert Consultation. WHO Technical Report Series No. 916. Geneva: World Health Organization, 2003.

9. Mangano DT, Layug EL, Wallace A, et al. Effect of atenolol on mortality and cardiovascular morbidity after noncardiac surgery. *N Engl J Med*. 1996;335:1713-1720.

10. Poldermans D, Boersma E, Bax JJ, et al. The effect of bisoprolol on perioperative mortality and myocardial infarction in high risk patients undergoing vascular surgery. *N Engl J Med*. 1999;341:1789-1794.

11. Poldermans D, Bax JJ, Kertai MD, et al. Statins are associated with a reduced incidence of perioperative mortality in patients undergoing major noncardiac vascular surgery. *Circulation*. 2003;107:1848-1851.

12. Lindenauer PK, Pekow P, Wang K, et al. Lipid lowering therapy and in hospital; mortality following major non cardiac surgery. *JAMA*. 2004;291:2092-2099.

13. Poldermans D, Bax JJ, Boersma E, et al. Guidelines for preoperative cardiac risk assessment and perioperative cardiac management in non-cardiac surgery: the Task Force for Preoperative Cardiac Risk Assessment and Perioperative Cardiac

Management in Noncardiac Surgery of the European Society of Cardiology (ESC) and endorsed by the European Society of Anaesthesiology (ESA). *Eur J Anaesthesiol.* 2010;27(2):92-137.

14. Hall JC, Tarala RA, Hall JL, Mander J. A multivariate analysis of the risk of pulmonary complications after laparotomy. *Chest.* 1991;99:923-927.

15. Blouw EL, Rudolph AD, Narr BJ, Sarr MG. The frequency of respiratory failure in patients with morbid obesity undergoing gastric bypass. *AANA J.* 2003;71:45-50.

16. Lawrence VA, Dhanda R, Hilsenbeck SG, Page CP. Risk of pulmonary complications after elective abdominal surgery. *Chest.* 1996;110:744-750.

17. Arozullah AM, Daley J, Henderson WG, Khuri SF. Multifactorial risk index for predicting postoperative respiratory failure in men after major noncardiac surgery. The National Veterans Administration Surgical Quality Improvement Program. *Ann Surg.* 2000;232:242-253.

18. Fogh J, Willie-J rgensen P, Brynjolf I, et al. The predictive value of preoperative perfusion/ventilation scintigraphy, spirometry and x-ray of the lungs on postoperative pulmonary complications. A prospective study. *Acta Anaesthesiol Scand.* 1987;31: 717-721.

19. Cooper MH, Primrose JN. The value of postoperative chest radiology after major abdominal surgery. *Anaesthesia.* 1989;44:306-309.

20. Arozullah AM, Khuri SF, Henderson WG, Daley J. Development and validation of a multifactorial risk index for predicting postoperative pneumonia after major noncardiac surgery. *Ann Intern Med.* 2001;135:847-857.

21. Gibbs J, Cull W, Henderson W, Daley J, Hur K, Khuri SF. Preoperative serum albumin level as a predictor of operative mortality and morbidity: results from the National VA Surgical Risk Study. *Arch Surg.* 1999;134:36-42.

22. Goldman L, Caldera DL, Nussbaum SR, et al. Multifactorial index of cardiac risk in noncardiac surgical procedures. *N Engl J Med.* 1977;297:845-850.

23. Centers for Disease Control and Prevention. National diabetes fact sheet: national estimates and general information on diabetes and prediabetes in the United States, 2011. Available at http://www.cdc.gov/diabetes/pubs/pdf/ndfs_2011.pdf. Issued 2011. Accessed May 1,2012.

24. Hall GM, Page SR. Diabetes and surgery. *Emergency and Hospital Management.* London, UK: BMJ Publishing; 1999.

25. Hirsch IB, McGill JB, Cryer PE, et al. Perioperative management of surgical patients with diabetes mellitus. *Anesthesiology.* 1991;74(2):346-359.

26. Alberti KG, Thomas DJ. The management of diabetes during surgery. *Br J Anaesth.* 1979;51(7):693-710.

27. Gavin LA. Perioperative management of the diabetic patient. *Endocrinol Metab Clin North Am.* 1992;21(2):457-475.

28. Umpierrez GE, Isaacs SD, Bazargan N, et al. Hyperglycemia: an independent marker of in-hospital mortality in patients with undiagnosed diabetes. *J Clin Endocrinol Metab.* 2002;87:978-982.

29. Pomposelli JJ, Baxter JK 3rd, Babineau TJ, et al. Early postoperative glucose control predicts nosocomial infection rate in diabetic patients. *J Parenter Enteral Nutr.* 1998;22:77-81.

30. van den Berghe G, Wouters P, Weekers F, et al. Intensive insulin therapy in the critically ill patients. *N Engl J Med.* 2001;345:1359-1367.

31. Grigoleit HG. Anesthesia and blood glucose. *Acta Diabetologica.* 1973;10:569-574.

32. Meneghini LF. Perioperative management of diabetes: translating evidence into practice. *Cleve Clin J Med.* 2009;76(suppl 4):S53-59.

33. Garber AJ, Moghissi ES, Bransome ED, et al. American College of Endocrinology position statement on inpatient diabetes and metabolic control. *Endocr Pract.* 2004;10:77-82.

34. Studley HO. Percentage of weight loss: a basic indicator of surgical risk in patients with chronic peptic ulcer. *JAMA.* 1936;106:458-460.

35. Lim STK, Choa RG, Lam KM, et al. Total parenteral nutrition versus gastrostomy in the preoperative preparation of patients with carcinoma of the esophagus. *Br J Surg.* 1981;68:69-72.

36. Sako K, Lore JM, Kaufman S, et al. Parenteral hyperalimentation in surgical patients with head and neck cancer: a randomized study. *J Surg Oncol.* 1981;16:391-402.

37. Kudsk KA, Croce MA, Fabian TC, et al. Enteral versus parenteral feeding: effects on septic morbidity after blunt and penetrating abdominal trauma. *Ann Surg.* 1992;215:503-515.

38. Moore EE, Jones TN. Benefits of immediate jejunostomy feeding after major abdominal trauma: a prospective, randomized trial. *J Trauma.* 1986;26:874-881.

39. Campos ACL, Meguid M. A critical appraisal of the usefulness of perioperative nutritional support. *Am J Clin Nutr.* 1992;55:117-130.

40. Reilly JJ, Hull SF, Albert N, et al. Economic impact of malnutrition: a model system for hospitalized patients. *J Parenter Enteral Nutr.* 1988;12:371-376.

41. Pacelli F, Bossola M, Papa V, et al. Enteral vs. parenteral nutrition after major abdominal surgery: an even match. *Arch Surg.* 2001;136:933-936.

42. Veterans Affairs Total Parenteral Nutrition Cooperative Group. Perioperative total parenteral nutrition in surgical patients. *N Engl J Med.* 1991;325:525-532.

43. Weimann A, Braga M, Harsanyi L, et al. ESPEN guidelines on enteral nutrition: surgery including organ transplant. *Clin Nutr.* 2006;25:224-244.

44. Dempsey DT, Buzby GP, Mullen JL. Nutritional assessment in the seriously ill patient. *J Am Coll Nutr.* 1983;2:15-22.

45. Reinhardt GF, Myscofski JW, Wilkens DB, et al. Incidence and mortality of hypoalbuminemic patients in hospitalized veterans. *J Parenter Enteral Nutr.* 1980;4: 357-359.

46. Yamanaka H, Nishi M, Kanemaki T, et al. Preoperative nutritional assessment to predict postoperative complications in gastric cancer. *J Parenter Enteral Nutr.* 1989;13:286-291.

47. Gibbs J, Call W, Henderson W, et al. Preoperative serum albumin level as a predictor of operative mortality and morbidity. Results from the national VA Surgical Risk Study. *Arch Surg.* 1999;134:36-42.

48. Kudsk KA, Tolley EA, DeWitt RC, et al. Preoperative albumin and surgical site identify surgical risk for major postoperative complications. *J Parenter Enteral Nutr.* 2003;27:1-9.

49. Daley J, Khuri SF, Henderson W, et al. Risk adjustment of the postoperative morbidity rate for the comparative assessment of the quality of surgical care: results of the National Veterans Affairs Surgical Risk Study. *J Am Coll Surg.* 1997;185:328-340.

50. Salvino RM, Dechicco RS, Seidner DL. Perioperative nutrition support: who and how. *Cleve Clin J Med.* 2004;71(4):345-351.

51. Jacobs DG, Jacobs DO, Kudsk KA, et al. Practice management guidelines for the nutritional support of the trauma patient. *J Trauma.* 2004;57:660-678.

52. Torosian MH. Perioperative nutrition support for patients undergoing gastrointestinal surgery: critical analysis and recommendations. *World J Surg.* 1999;23:565-569.

53. Daly J, Lieberman M, Goldfine J, et al. Enteral nutrition with supplemental arginine, RNA, and omega-3 fatty acids in patients after operation: immunologic, metabolic, and clinical outcome. *Surgery.* 1992;112:56-67.

54. Braga M, Gianotti L, Vignali A, et al. Artificial nutrition after major abdominal surgery: impact of route of administration and composition of the diet. *Crit Care Med.* 1998;26:24-30.

55. Heyland DK, Novak F, Drover JW, et al. Should immunonutrition become routine in critically ill patients? A systematic review of the evidence. *JAMA.* 2001;286:944-953.

56. Braga M, Gianotti L, Nespoli L, et al. Nutritional approach in malnourished surgical patients: a prospective randomized study. *Arch Surg.* 2002;137:174-180.

57. Garth AK, Newsome CM, Simmance N, et al. Nutritional status, nutrition practices and postoperative complications in patients with gastrointestinal cancer. *J Hum Nutr Diet.* 2010;23:393-401.

58. Marik PE, Zaloga GP. Immunonutrition in high-risk surgical patients: a systemic review and analysis of the literature. *J Parenter Enteral Nutr.* 2010;34:378-386.

59. Drover JW, Dhaliwal R, Weitzel L, et al. Perioperative use of arginine-supplemented diets: a systemic review of the evidence. *J Am Coll Surg.* 2011;212(3):385-399.

60. Novak F, Heyland DK, Avenell A, et al. Glutamine supplementation in serious illness: a systemic review of the evidence. *Crit Care Med.* 2002;30:2022-2029.

61. Loi C, Zazzo JF, Delpierre E, et al. Increasing plasma glutamine in postoperative patients fed an arginine rich immune-enhancing diet—a pharmacokinetic randomized controlled study. *Crit Care Med.* 2009;37:501-509.

62. Drover JW, Cahill NE, Kutsogiannis J, et al. Nutrition therapy for the critically ill surgery patient: we need to do better! *J Parenter Enteral Nutr.* 2010;34:644-652.

63. Waters JM. Postoperative nutrition: past, present, and future. *Support Line.* 2011;32(5):2-7.

64. Bozzetti F, Gianotti L, Braga M, et al. Postoperative complications in gastrointestinal cancer patients: the joint role of the nutritional status and the nutritional support. *Clin Nutr.* 2007;26:698-709.

65. Heyland DK, Montalvo M, MacDonald S, et al. Total parenteral nutrition in the surgical patient: a meta-analysis. *Can J Surg.* 2001;44:102-111.

66. Klein S, Kinney J, Jeejeebhoy K, et al. Nutrition support in clinical practice: review of published data and recommendations for future research directions. *J Parenter Enteral Nutr.* 1997;21:133-156.

67. Torosian MH. Perioperative nutrition support for patients undergoing gastrointestinal surgery: critical analysis and recommendations. *World J Surg.* 1999;23:565-569.

68. Collins JP, Oxby CB, Hill GL. Intravenous amino acids and intravenous hyperalimentation as protein-sparing therapy after major surgery. A controlled clinical trial. *Lancet.* 1978;1:788-791.

69. Preshaw RM, Attisha RP, Hollingsworth WJ, et al. Randomized sequential trial of parenteral nutrition in healing of colonic anastomoses in man. *Can J Surg.* 1979;22:437-439.

70. Woolfson AMJ, Smith JAR. Elective nutritional support after major surgery: a prospective randomized trial. *Clin Nutr.* 1989;8:15-21.

71. Sandstrom R, Drott C, Hyltander A, et al. The effect of postoperative intravenous feeding (TPN) on outcome following major surgery evaluated in a randomized study. *Ann Surg.* 1993;217:185-195.

72. Flynn MB, Leightty FF. Preoperative outpatient nutritional support of patients with squamous cancer of the upper aerodigestive tract. *Am J Surg.* 1987;154(4):359-362.

73. Foschi D, Cavagna G, Callioni F, et al. Hyperalimentation of jaundiced patients on percutaneous transhepatic biliary drainage. *Br J Surg.* 1986;73(9):716-719.

74. Shukla HS, Rao RR, Banu N, et al. Enteral hyperalimentation in malnourished surgical patients. *Indian J Med Res.* 1984;80:339-346.

75. von Meyenfeldt MF, Meijerink WJHJ, Rouflart MMJ, et al. Perioperative nutritional support: a randomized clinical trial. *Clin Nutr.* 1992;11:180-186.

76. Graham TW, Zadrozny DB, Harrington T. The benefits of early jejunal hyperalimentation in the head-injured patient. *Neurosurgery.* 1989;25:729-735.

77. Dominioni L, Trocki O, Mochizuki H, et al. Prevention of severe postburn hypermetabolism and catabolism by immediate intragastric feeding. *J Burn Care Rehabil.* 1984;5:106-112.

78. Jensen GL, Sporay G, Whitmire S, et al. Intraoperative placement of the nasoenteric feeding tube: a practical alternative? *J Parenter Enteral Nutr.* 1995;19:244-247.

79. Schroeder D, Gillanders L, Mahr K, et al. Effects of immediate postoperative enteral nutrition on body composition, muscle function, and wound healing. *J Parenter Enteral Nutr.* 1991;15:376-383.

80. Bastow MD, Rawlings J, Allison SP. Benefits of supplementary tube feeding after fractured neck of femur: a randomized controlled trial. *Br Med J.* 1983;287(6405):1589-1592.

81. Beattie AH, Prach AT, Baxter JP, et al. A randomized controlled trial evaluating the use of enteral nutritional supplements postoperatively in malnourished surgical patients. *Gut.* 2000;46(6):813-818.

82. Delmi M, Rapin CH, Bengoa JM, et al. Dietary supplementation in elderly patients with fractured neck of femur. *Lancet.* 1990;335(8696):1013-1016.

83. Gianotti L, Braga M, Vignali A, et al. Effects of route of delivery and formulation of postoperative nutritional support in patients undergoing major operations for malignant neoplasms. *Arch Surg.* 1997;132(11):1222-1229.

SPECIAL POPULATIONS

84. Heys SD, Walker LG, Smith I, et al. Enteral nutritional supplementation with key nutrients in patients with critical illness and cancer. A meta-analysis of randomized controlled clinical trials. *Ann Surg.* 1999;229(4):467-77

85. Senkal M, Mumme A, Eickhoff U, et al. Early postoperative enteral immunonutrition: clinical outcome and cost-comparison analysis in surgical patients. *Crit Care Med.* 1997;25:1489-96

86. Zilberberg MD, Stern LS, Wiederkehr DP, et al. Anemia, transfusions and hospital outcomes among critically ill patients on prolonged acute mechanical ventilation: a retrospective cohort study. *Crit Care.* 2008;12:R60.

87. Ma HP, Keyoumu N, Chen L, et al. A meta-analysis on efficacy of antifibrinolytic agents during perioperative period in patients undergoing coronary artery bypass grafting treated with antiplatelet agents. *Zhonghua Xin Xue Guan Bing Za Zhi.* 2011;39(8):759-763.

88. Sniecinski RM, Karkouti K, Levy JH. Managing clotting: a North American perspective. *Curr Opin Anaesthesiol.* 2012;25(1):74-79.

89. Henry DA, Carless PA, Moxey AJ, et al. Anti-fibrinolytic use for minimising perioperative allogeneic blood transfusion. *Cochrane Database Syst Rev.* 2011;(3):CD001886.

90. American Society of Anesthesiologists Task Force on Perioperative Blood Transfusion and Adjuvant Therapies. Practice guidelines for perioperative blood transfusion and adjuvant therapies: an updated report by the American Society of Anesthesiologists Task Force on Perioperative Blood Transfusion and Adjuvant Therapies. *Anesthesiology.* 2006;105(1):198-208.

91. Townsend CM, Beauchamp DR, Evers MB, et al. *Sabiston Textbook of Surgery.* 19th ed. Philadelphia: Saunders, 2012. Chapter 11. Principles of preoperative and operative surgery. 223-225.

92. Blajchman MA. The clinical benefits of the leukoreduction of blood products. *J Trauma.* 2006;60(suppl 6):S83-90.

93. Nichols WG, Price TH, Gooley T, et al. Transfusion-transmitted cytomegalovirus infection after receipt of leukoreduced blood products. *Blood.* 2003;101: 4195-4200.

94. Schroeder ML. Transfusion-associated graft-versus-host disease. *Br J Haematol.* 2002;117:275-287.

95. Popovsky MA. Frozen and washed red blood cells: new approaches and applications. *Transfus Apher Sci.* 2001;25:193-194.

96. Fasano R, Luban NL. Blood component therapy. *Pediatr Clin North Am.* 2008;55: 421-445.

97. Hillyer CD, Shaz BH, Zimring JC, et al. *Transfusion Medicine and Hemostasis: Clinical and Laboratory Aspects.* Philadelphia: Elsevier; 2009. Chapter 48. Management of patients who refuse blood transfusion. 279-282.

98. Dunn AS, Turpie AG. Perioperative management of patients receiving oral anticoagulants: a systematic review. *Arch Intern Med.* 2003;163:901-908.

99. Konstantatos A. Anticoagulation and cataract surgery: a review of the current literature. *Anaesth Intensive Care.* 2001;29:11-18.

100. Eisen GM, Baron TH, Dominitz JA, et al. Guideline on the management of anticoagulation and antiplatelet therapy for endoscopic procedures. *Gastrointest Endosc.* 2002;55:775-779.

101. Wahl MJ. Dental surgery in anticoagulated patients. *Arch Intern Med.* 1998;158:1610-1616.

102. Weibert RT, Le DT, Kayser SR, Rapaport SI. Correction of excessive anticoagulation with low-dose oral vitamin K1. *Ann Intern Med.* 1997;126:959-962.

103. Billingsley EM. Intraoperative and postoperative bleeding problems in patients taking warfarin, aspirin, and nonsteroidal anti-inflammatory agents. A prospective study. *Dermatol Surg.* 1997;23:381-383.

104. Thumboo J, O'Duffy JD. A prospective study of the safety of joint and soft tissue aspirations and injections in patients taking warfarin sodium. *Arthritis Rheum.* 1998;41:736-739.

105. Lanzat M, Danna AT, Jacobson DS. New protocols for perioperative management of podiatric patients taking oral anticoagulants. *J Foot Ankle Surg.* 1994;33:16-20.

106. White RH, McKittrick T, Hutchinson R, Twitchell J. Temporary discontinuation of warfarin therapy: changes in the international normalized ratio. *Ann Intern Med.* 1995;122:40-42.

107. Crowther MA, Donovan D, Harrison L, McGinnis J, Ginsberg J. Low-dose oral vitamin K reliably reverses over-anticoagulation due to warfarin. *Thromb Haemost.* 1998;79:1116-1118.

108. Jaffer AK, Brotman DJ, Chukwumerije N. When patients on warfarin need surgery. *Cleve Clin J Med.* 2003;70(11):973-984.

109. Warkentin TE, Levine MN, Hirsh J, et al. Heparin-induced thrombocytopenia in patients treated with low-molecular-weight heparin or unfractionated heparin. *N Engl J Med.* 1995;332:1330-1335.

110. Douketis JD, Berger PB, Dunn AS, et al. The perioperative management of antithrombotic therapy: American College of Chest Physicians Evidence-Based Clinical Practice Guidelines (8th ed.). *Chest.* 2008;133(6 suppl):299S-339S.

111. Friedman LS. The risk of surgery in patients with liver disease. *Hepatology* 1999;29(6):1617-1623.

112. O'Leary JG, Yachimski PS, Friedman LS. Surgery in the patient with liver disease. *Clin Liver Dis* 2009;13(2):211-231.

113. Patel T. Surgery in the patient with liver disease. *Mayo Clin Proc.* 1999;74(6):593-599.

114. Ziser A, Plevak DJ, Wiesner RH, et al. Morbidity and mortality in cirrhotic patients undergoing anesthesia and surgery. *Anesthesiology.* 1999;90(1):42-53.

115. Garrison RN, Cryer HM, Howard DA, Polk HC Jr. Clarification of risk factors for abdominal operations in patients with hepatic cirrhosis. *Ann Surg.* 1984;199(6):648-655.

116. Keegan MT, Plevak DJ. Preoperative assessment of the patient with liver disease. *Am J Gastroenterol.* 2005;100(9):2116-2127.

117. O'Leary JG, Friedman LS. Predicting surgical risk in patients with cirrhosis: from art to science. *Gastroenterology.* 2007;132(4):1609-1611.

118. Neeff H, Mariaskin D, Spangenberg HC, et al. Perioperative mortality after non-hepatic general surgery in patients with liver cirrhosis: an analysis of 138 operations in the 2000s using Child and MELD scores. *J Gastrointest Surg.* 2011;15:1.

119. Bruix J. Treatment of hepatocellular carcinoma. *Hepatology.* 1997;25:259.

120. Teh SH, Nagorney DM, Stevens SR, et al. Risk factors for mortality after surgery in patients with cirrhosis. *Gastroenterology.* 2007;132:1261.

121. Hanje AJ, Patel T. Preoperative evaluation of patients with liver disease. *Nat Clin Pract Gastroenterol Hepatol.* 2007;4(5):266-276.

122. Alkozai EM, Lisman T, Porte RJ. Bleeding in liver surgery: prevention and treatment. *Clin Liver Dis.* 2009;13:145.

123. Nompleggi DJ, Bonkovsky HL. Nutritional supplementation in chronic liver disease: an analytical review. *Hepatology.* 1994;19:518.

124. Krishnan M. Preoperative care of patients with kidney disease. *Am Fam Physician.* 2002;66(8):1471-1476.

125. Lee TH, Mangione CM, et al. Derivation and prospective validation of a simple index for prediction of cardiac risk of major noncardiac surgery. *Circulation.* 1999;110:859-866.

126. Kellerman PS. Perioperative care of the renal patient. *Arch Intern Med.* 1994;154: 1674-1688.

127. Tilney NL, Lazarus JM. Surgical care of the patient with renal failure. Philadelphia: Saunders; 1982:22.

128. Recio-Mayoral A, Chaparro M, Prado B, et al. The reno-protective effect of hydration with sodium bicarbonate plus N-acetylcysteine in patients undergoing emergency percutaneous coronary intervention: the RENO Study. *J Am Coll Cardiol.* 2007;49 (12):1283-1288.

129. Joseph AJ, Cohn SL. Perioperative care of the patient with renal failure. *Med Clin North Am.* 2003;87:193-210.

130. Gan TJ, Meyer T, Apfel CC, et al. Consensus guidelines for managing postoperative nausea and vomiting. *Anesth Analg.* 2003;97(1):62-71.

131. West MA, Shapiro MB, Nathens AB, et al: Inflammation and the host response to injury, a large-scale collaborative project: Patient-oriented research core-standard operating procedures for clinical care. IV. Guidelines for transfusion in the trauma patient. *J Trauma* 2006;61:436-439.

132. Alvarado R, Chung KK, Cancio L, et al. Burn resuscitation. *Burns.* 2009;35:4-14.

133. Flegal KM, Carroll MD, Ogden CL, Johnson CL. Prevalence and trends in obesity among U.S. adults, 1999-2000. *JAMA.* 2002;288:1723.

134. Tambascia, M. Chapter 7. Preoperative evaluation of patients. In: Pitombo C, Jones K, Higa K, Pareja JC, eds. *Obesity Surgery: Principles and Practice.* New York: McGraw-Hill; 2007. 61-66, http://www.accesssurgery.com/content.aspx?aID=147165. Accessed February 19, 2013.

135. Dixon JB, Bhathal PS, O'Brich PE: Nonalcoholic fatty liver disease: Predictors of nonalcoholic steatohepatitis and liver fibrosis in the severely obese. *Gastroenterology.* 2001;121:91-100.

136. Kurosawa S. Anesthesia in patients with cancer disorders. *Curr Opin Anaesthesiol.* 2012 Mar 23; Epub ahead of print: PMID: 22450698.

137. Younes RN, Rogartko A, Brennan MF. The influence of hypotension and perioperative blood transfusion on disease free survival in patients with complete resection of colorectal liver metastases. *Ann Surg.* 1991;214:107-113.

CHAPTER 17

Common Psychiatric Emergencies

Nina Khachiyants

GENERAL APPROACHES TO EMERGENCY PSYCHIATRIC EVALUATION

In 2002, the American Psychiatric Association defined psychiatric or behavioral emergency as "an acute disturbance of thought, mood, behavior, or social relationships that requires an immediate intervention defined by the patient, family or the community."

Safety

- Safety is the first priority.
- Always evaluate the patient for imminent danger to self or others.
- General precautions:
  - Defer the interview if safety is not assured.
  - Order pharmacologic or physical restraints or seclusion if patient shows signs of agitation, aggressiveness, or potential violence toward self or others.
  - Call security for backup.
  - Interview the patient with police if you feel unsafe.
  - Order as-needed medications or physical restraints over the phone before seeing the patient, if necessary.
  - Order one-to-one observation.
  - Maintain a safe distance from the patient (at least 1 arm's length).
  - Always have an escape route (do not let patient block the exit; open a door behind you).

Agitation and Violence

Major factors associated with patient violence:

- Acute illness
- Psychosis
- Substance abuse
- History of violence

Identify early signs of anger:

- Muscular tension: clenched fists; "ready to jump" position
- Face expression: furled brows, flashed face, clenched teeth, clenched jaw
- Voice: raised or lowered

Identify signs of anger escalation:

- Verbal or physical threats
- Restlessness, pacing
- Throwing objects
- Acts of violence

Treatment

Deescalation of Agitation

Anger management and behavioral intervention:

- Remain calm.
- Help patient recognize and accept angry feelings.
- Empathize, but do not touch an angry patient.
- Speak in short command sentences, for example, "Mr. Smith, calm down."
- Do not argue with an angry patient.
- Ask for assistance from other staff.

- Restraints and/or seclusion as needed (last resort).
- Use as needed medications (always offer voluntarily first).

Pharmacotherapy for Acute Agitation and Psychosis

- Haloperidol: 0.5–10 mg orally (PO) every 1 to 4 hours as needed; maximum dose 100 mg/day
  - 10 mg PO dose equivalent to 5 mg intramuscularly or intravenously (IM/IV)
  - 5 mg PO dose equivalent to 2.5 mg IM/IV
  - 2 mg PO dose equivalent to 2 mg IM/IV
- Lorazepam:
  - Best choice for agitation caused by acute alcohol or benzodiazepine withdrawal.
  - Parameters for use: agitation, tremor, sweating, blood pressure (BP) greater than 160/100 mm Hg; heart rate (HR) faster than 100 beats per minute (bpm); temperature higher than 37.8°C (100°F). Hold if BP is less than 90/55 mm Hg; HR is less than 60 beats per minute; respiratory rate less than 12 breaths per minute.
  - Use 2 to 6 mg PO/IM/IV; divide twice daily (BID), 3 times daily (TID). Maximum 10 mg/day. Use 1 to 2 mg/day PO/IM/IV in elderly patients.
  - Reassess need for treatment.
  - Taper dose gradually (15%–20% dose reduction daily).
  - Watch for paradoxical agitation in elderly patients.
  - Advantages: relatively short half-life (10–20 hours), lack of active metabolites.
- Diazepam:
  - Best choice for agitation caused by acute alcohol or benzodiazepine withdrawal.
  - Parameters for use: agitation, tremor, sweating, BP higher than 160/100 mm Hg; HR higher than 100 bpm; temperature higher than 37.8°C (100°F).
  - Hold if BP less than 90/55 mm Hg; HR less than 60 bpm; respiratory rate less than 12 breaths per hour. Use 20 mg PO every 2 hours until sedated.
  - Contraindications: age older than 65 years, chronic obstructive pulmonary disease, sleep apnea, liver diseases.
  - Not reliably absorbed when used IM.
  - Reassess need for treatment.
  - Taper dose gradually (15%–20% dose reduction daily).
  - Avoid use in elderly patients because of increased risk of respiratory depression, oversedation, disinhibition, paradoxical agitation.
- Olanzapine:
  - 10 mg PO/IM, can repeat in 2 hours and 6 hours as needed; maximum dose 30 mg/24h
  - Also works effectively in case of alcohol and benzodiazepine withdrawal agitation; also effective in small doses: 2.5 to 5 mg PO for psychosis and agitation in elderly patients.
  - Watch for postural hypotension, bradycardia after IM injection.
  - Simultaneous use of olanzapine and benzodiazepines is not recommended because of additive sedating and cardiovascular toxic effect.
  - Available in oral rapid disintegrating preparation.
- Ziprasidone:
  - 10 mg IM every 2 hours or 20 mg IM every 4 hours; maximum dose 40 mg/24h.
  - Contraindicated in patients with known history of QT prolongation (including congenital QT prolongation), recent acute myocardial infarction, or uncompensated heart failure.
- Aripiprazole:
  - Use 9.5 mg/1.3 mL IM or 7.5 mg/mL IM; can repeat every 2 hours as needed. Use 5.25 mg/0.7 mL IM in elderly patients; maximum dose 30 mg/day.
  - Less sedating than olanzapine or quetiapine.
  - Watch for orthostatic hypotension after IM injection.
  - Simultaneous use of aripiprazole and benzodiazepines is not recommended because of additive sedating and cardiovascular toxic effect.
  - Available in liquid and oral rapid disintegrating preparations.
- Quetiapine:
  - Start 25 mg PO BID, then increase by 50 to 150 mg/day up to 300 to 400 mg/day; divide BID, TID; maximum 800 mg/day

- Loxapine:
  - 2.5 to 10 mg daily/TID for elderly demented patients
- **Combination of haloperidol (Haldol) 5 mg and lorazepam 2 mg IM:** for severe agitation.
- **Combination of trazodone 25 to 50 mg BID and olanzapine 2.5 mg/day:** for violent behavior or agitation in elderly demented patients.

SELECTED PSYCHIATRIC EMERGENCIES

Delirium

Definition

Fluctuating disturbance because of direct physiologic consequences of a general medical condition, medication side-effects, or substance intoxication or withdrawal that develops over a short period of time (usually hours to days) and manifested as problems with:

- **Consciousness** (reduced ability to focus, sustain, or shift **attention**)
- **Cognition** (memory, orientation, language deficit)
- **Thought process and content** (tangentiality, incoherence, paranoid, and other delusions)
- **Perception** (illusions, hallucinations)
- **Affect** (dysphoria, lability, anxiety)
- **Behavior** (agitation, lethargy)

Delirium Subtypes

- Hyperactive (agitated, hyperalert), recognized more often.
- Hypoactive (lethargic, hypoalert), underrecognized, especially in people older than 65 years of age.
- Mixed (includes alternating features of both)

Diagnosis

Rule of thumb: Any sudden changes in consciousness, cognition, or behavior in an elderly person should be considered delirium, until proven otherwise, and possible etiologies should be promptly and thoroughly investigated.

Selective Mental Status Examination Findings

- A fluctuating level of consciousness
- Confusion
- Disorientation
- Psychomotor activation (agitation, combativeness) or retardation
- Picking at clothes or sheets
- Falling asleep during the interview
- Mumbling or shouting speech
- Incoherent, illogical, or disorganized thought process
- Paranoid or other delusional thoughts
- Perceptual abnormalities (illusions, visual, auditory, tactile, gustatory, olfactory hallucinations)
- Irritability
- Anxiety
- Depression
- Euphoria
- Sundowning in elderly demented patients (cognitive, behavioral, emotional disturbances occurring in the late afternoon, evening, or at night)

Etiologies

- Intracranial
  - Epilepsy, head trauma, meningitis, encephalitis, neoplasm, vascular disorders
- Extracranial
  - Endocrine: hypoglycemia, hyperglycemia, pituitary, pancreatic, adrenal, parathyroid, thyroid hypofunction or hyperfunction
  - Pulmonary: hypoxia, pneumonia
  - Cardiovascular: hypotension, hypertension, cardiac failure, arrhythmias

- Liver: hepatic encephalopathy
- Kidney: uremic encephalopathy, urinary retention or urinary tract infection
- Vitamin deficiency: thiamine, nicotinic acid, vitamin B_{12}, folate
- Dehydration (inadequate fluid intake, diuretics use, sweating)
- Major electrolyte disturbances of any cause
- Systemic infections, intoxications, fever, sepsis
- Constipation or fecal impaction
- Pain, thirst, and hunger
- Alcohol withdrawal and intoxication syndrome
- Sensory impairments
- Polypharmacy (and drug interactions), including over-the-counter medications
- Drug reaction or intoxication: anticholinergic agents, sedative-hypnotic, alcohol, benzodiazepines, opioids, anticonvulsants, antihypertensive agents, antiparkinsonian agents, antipsychotic drugs, cardiac glycosides, cimetidine, ranitidine, clonidine, insulin, disulfiram, steroids, phenytoin, salicylates, phencyclidine

Risk Factors for Delirium

- Preexisting cognitive impairment and dementia
- Depression
- Psychosis
- Catatonia
- Hyponatremia, hypernatremia
- Visual impairment, hearing impairment, and other sensory deprivation
- Use of indwelling catheter
- Use of physical restraints
- Multiple medication use
- Return from hospitalization

Risk Factors for Developing Postsurgical Delirium

- General anesthesia.
- Exposure to meperidine.
- Exposure to benzodiazepines (benzodiazepines with longer half-life are more strongly associated with delirium than short-acting preparations).
- A previous history of delirium.
- Alcohol-related medical problems.
- Preoperative use of narcotic analgesics.
- Admission to neurosurgery.
- In elderly hospitalized patients, the risk of delirium decreased significantly after day 9.
- In elderly post-hip-surgery patients, most cases of delirium occurred during postoperative days 2 to 5.

Clinical Manifestations

- **Core features:** altered (decreased) level of consciousness, diminished ability to focus, sustain, or shift attention, cognitive impairment, disorientation in time and place, relatively rapid onset (hours to days), relatively brief duration (days to weeks), fluctuations in intensity of the symptoms during the day.
- **Associated symptoms:** thought process disorganization, perceptual disturbances (illusions, hallucinations), psychomotor retardation or hyperactivity, sleep-wake cycle disruption, emotional liability, behavioral disturbances (agitation, disorganization), autonomic hyperactivity, myoclonus, dysarthria.

Clinical Evaluation

- Vital signs (temperature, pulse, respiration rate, oxygen saturation, BP including orthostatic)
- Mental status examination (arousal, attention, orientation)
- Neurologic examination (evidence of head trauma, nuchal rigidity, papilledema, reflexes, motor or sensory deficit, focal neurologic signs, seizures)
- Chest: heart (arrhythmia, murmurs, cardiomegaly); lungs (excursion, auscultation, cough)
- Abdomen (liver enlargement, bladder or urinary retention, palpable fecal impaction)
- Skin (lesions, signs of dehydration, inflammation)

Diagnostic Studies

- Laboratory tests
  - Full blood examination (complete blood count [CBC], creatinine, electrolytes, glucose, calcium, liver function tests)
  - Urinalysis; midstream urine specimen (if urinalysis abnormal)
  - Prothrombin time, partial thromboplastin time (if indicated)
- Urine toxicology screen
- Chest x-ray
- Cardiac enzymes
- Electrocardiogram (ECG)
- Blood, sputum, urine cultures, and sensitivity (if fever present, cough and/or abnormal chest radiograph, urinary urgency, abnormal urinalysis)
- Arterial blood gases (if shortness of breath, cough present, or abnormal chest radiograph)
- Thyroid function tests
- Vitamin B_{12} and folate serum levels
- VDRL, human immunodeficiency virus (HIV) test
- Computed tomography (CT) of the brain (if history of falls, patient on anticoagulant therapy, or focal neurologic signs present)
- Lumbar puncture (if headache, fever, and meningeal symptoms present)
- Electroencephalogram (EEG) (may assist in determining etiology: epileptic or nonepileptic seizure activity)
  - Characteristic EEG findings in delirium: diffuse slowing of background activity; delirium because of alcohol or sedative-hypnotic withdrawal: low-voltage fast activity.

Differential Diagnosis

It is important to differentiate delirium from other conditions because delirium may be life-threatening and should be approached as an emergency.

- Dementia
  - A gradually progressing course.
  - Lack of fluctuation in and out of a confusional state (except for Lewy body dementia).
  - Much less major attentional deficit and fewer sleep disturbances.
  - Differentiation is less straightforward as dementia progresses and alertness and attention are impaired.
- Depression
  - May present with a reduced level of alertness, emotional lability, and appearing withdrawn
  - Can be distinguished on the basis of an EEG (lack of diffuse slowing of background activity)
- Schizophrenia and psychosis
  - Hallucinations and delusions are better organized and more constant than in delirium.
  - Usually no changes in level of consciousness or orientation.
- Factitious disorder
  - Reveal factitious nature of symptoms by greater inconsistencies on mental status examination.
  - Can be distinguished on the basis of an EEG (lack of diffuse slowing of background activity).

Treatment

- Identify promptly the cause of delirium where possible.
- Address the possible cause and any precipitating factors for delirium.
- Start with nonpharmacologic interventions: provide psychological, physical, sensory, and environmental support; one-to-one nursing observation for safety reasons (if agitated or restless); allowing family members or regular sitter to stay with the patient; frequent assurance and reorientation to person, place, and time (familiar pictures, calendars, clocks); keep light on, avoid eye patches; relaxation strategies to assist with sleep.

Pharmacologic Interventions

- **Antipsychotic medications** are indicated to treat cognitive impairment, behavioral and severe emotional disturbances (severe anxiety, hallucinations, fear, delusions) when these symptoms cannot be controlled by nonpharmacologic methods, and it is causing significant distress to the patients and placing them or others at risk.
- **Haloperidol:** (First-line treatment, although not U.S. Food and Drug Administration approved for IV use, or for the treatment of delirium). Start 0.5 mg PO BID and titrate upward if necessary (in elderly patients). Usual dose 2 mg PO every 4 hours as needed. May use 2 to 10 mg PO, IM or IV depending on patient's age, weight, physical condition, or severity of psychosis.
- **Caution:** IV haloperidol may be complicated by torsades de pointes (cardiac arrhythmia with QT prolongation), which is an uncommon but life-threatening complication.
- Low doses of **risperidone** (0.25–2 mg/day), **olanzapine** (2.5–10 mg/day), and **quetiapine** (12.5–50 mg/day) may be used to treat delirium.
- **Lorazepam:** 0.5 to 2 mg every 4 hours as needed for agitation in delirium, although its use is mostly justified in combination with antipsychotic medications, or in cases of delirium that are induced by drug (benzodiazepines) or alcohol withdrawal. High risk of "paradoxical agitation" after benzodiazepine administration in elderly patients. Always try to obtain informed consent from patient (if possible), or from family and caregivers.

Neuroleptic Malignant Syndrome (Table 17-1)

Definition: Neuroleptic malignant syndrome (NMS) is a life-threatening medical emergency that can occur anytime during treatment with neuroleptic medications and is characterized by a distinctive clinical syndrome that includes mental status changes, rigidity, fever, and autonomic dysfunction.

Incidence rate: 0.2% to 2%; mortality: 10% to 20%

Causative Agents

- **First-generation antipsychotics more than second-generation antipsychotics**
- **High-potency antipsychotics more than low-potency antipsychotics**
- **Typical antipsychotics (first-generation antipsychotics):** haloperidol, fluphenazine, chlorpromazine, thioridazine, mesoridazine, perphenazine, loxapine, trifluoperazine, thiothixene
- **Atypical antipsychotics (second-generation antipsychotics):** risperidone, paliperidone, ziprasidone, quetiapine, olanzapine, aripiprazole, olanzapine, clozapine
- **Antiemetic drugs** (metoclopramide, promethazine)
- **Antiparkinson medication withdrawal** (L-dopa or dopamine agonist withdrawal, as well as dose reductions and a switch from one agent to another)
  - Risk factors: male gender, young age (20–40 years), acute agitation, preexisting medical, neurologic or psychiatric conditions, infection, recent surgery, acute catatonia, dehydration, recent or rapid dose escalation, a switch from one agent to another, high-potency agents, IM administration, depot form.
  - Associated risk factors: Concomitant use of lithium or other psychotropic drugs, antihistamines (prochlorperazine), comorbid substance abuse (have not been substantiated in case-control studies).
  - Pathogenesis: The exact cause of NMS is unknown; possibly secondary to dopaminergic receptor blockade in nigrostriatal dopamine pathways (producing rigidity, fever, and autonomic instability), or because of direct toxic effect of neuroleptics on skeletal muscles.

Diagnosis

The diagnosis should be suspected when any two of the four cardinal clinical features—mental status change, rigidity, fever, or dysautonomia—appear in the setting of neuroleptic use or dopamine withdrawal.

Remember the acronym: FARGO

- **F**ever
- **A**utonomic instability (hypotension, tachycardia, urinary incontinence, diaphoresis)
- **R**igidity ("lead-pipe")
- **G**ranulocytosis (eg, leukocytosis, as well as other laboratory result **abnormalities:** increased lactic dehydrogenase, liver function tests abnormalities, laboratory evidence of muscle injury [eg, elevated creatinine phosphokinase, myoglobinuria])
- **O**rientation changes (confusion, coma, mutism, other mental status changes)

Clinical Manifestations

Typical Symptoms

The tetrad of NMS symptoms are:

- **Mental status changes** in the form of an agitated delirium with confusion rather than psychosis, catatonic signs and mutism; may progress to profound encephalopathy with stupor and eventual coma.
- **Muscular rigidity** is generalized; "lead pipe rigidity" or resistance through all ranges of movement, tremor, cogwheel rigidity, dystonia, opisthotonus, trismus, chorea, and other dyskinesias. Also sialorrhea, dysarthria, and dysphagia.
- **Hyperthermia** (38°C–40°C [100.4°F–104°F]).
- **Autonomic instability** (tachycardia, labile or high BP, tachypnea, dysrhythmias, profuse diaphoresis).

Atypical Symptoms

A mild or absent rigidity; temperature is absent. From a practical clinical point of view, it seems reasonable to consider the diagnosis of NMS when any two of the tetrad of symptoms are present in the setting of an offending agent.

Differential Diagnosis

- **Serotonin syndrome:** The most common differential diagnosis; usually caused by use of selective serotonin reuptake inhibitors (SSRIs) and has a presentation similar to NMS, although NMS patients lack shivering, hyperreflexia, myoclonus, and ataxia. Nausea, vomiting, and diarrhea are also a common part of the prodrome in serotonin syndrome and are rarely described in NMS. Rigidity and hyperthermia are less severe than in patients with NMS.
- **Malignant hyperthermia:** A rare genetic condition; occurring with use of potent halogenated inhalational anesthetic agents and succinylcholine. May present with hyperthermia, muscle rigidity, autonomic instability, although often more fulminant.
- **Malignant catatonia:** The most difficult to differentiate from NMS; however, in this syndrome, there is usually a behavioral prodrome of some days or weeks that is characterized by psychosis, agitation, and catatonic excitement. The motor symptoms are more in the form of dystonic or bizarre posturing, waxy flexibility, and stereotyped repetitive movements. Laboratory values are typically normal. The two conditions may overlap.
- **Central anticholinergic syndrome:** Associated with therapeutic (in elderly patients), or toxic doses of drugs with anticholinergic activity; present with encephalopathy and elevated body temperatures that are usually not as severe as in NMS. Other symptoms of NMS (diaphoresis, rigidity, and elevated creatine kinase [CK] levels) are absent in this condition, although flushing, mydriasis, and bladder distension are common features.
- **Clozapine-induced "benign" fever** and **creatinine phosphokinase elevation:** Absence of other symptoms of NMS
- **Acute intoxication with cocaine, amphetamines, phencyclidine, and ecstasy:** Manifest as psychomotor agitation, delirium, and psychosis. Hyperthermia and rhabdomyolysis can develop, usually in association with increased physical exertion and environmental high temperature conditions. Rigidity is not prominent.
- **Withdrawal of intrathecal baclofen therapy:** Although NMS-like symptoms (dysautonomia, altered mental status, fever, and elevated creatine kinase [CK] level) may occur in this condition, the increased muscle tone is often in a form of rebound spasticity rather than rigidity. Reduced γ-aminobutyric acid (GABA) activity is thought to be the pathophysiologic cause. The symptoms reversal with reinstitution of therapy, and benzodiazepines administration.
- **Other disorders:** meningitis, encephalitis, systemic infections (eg, pneumonia, sepsis) seizures, acute hydrocephalus, acute spinal cord injury, heat stroke (neuroleptics predispose to heat stroke by impairing thermoregulation), acute dystonia, tetanus, acute porphyria, thyrotoxicosis, central nervous system vasculitis

Laboratory Test Abnormalities

- **Elevated serum CK:** In NMS, CK is typically more than 1000 IU/L and can be as high as 100,000 IU/L (the degree of CK elevation correlates with disease severity and prognosis, and usually normalizes after an NMS resolution). Normal CK can be seen early in the onset of NMS, or if rigidity is not well developed. CK elevation is not specific for NMS and

SPECIAL POPULATIONS

may be seen in combative, agitated, or psychotic patients, also caused by intramuscular injections, physical restraints, and without any specific explanation.

- **Leukocytosis** is a consistent laboratory finding with a white blood cell count typically 10,000 to 40,000/mm^3 (left shift may be present).
- **Mild elevations of lactate dehydrogenase, alkaline phosphatase, and liver transaminases** (aspartate aminotransferase, alanine aminotransferase) are common but not specific.
- **Electrolyte abnormalities, such as** hypocalcemia, hypomagnesemia, hypo- and hypernatremia, hyperkalemia, and metabolic acidosis are frequently observed.
- **Myoglobinuria** and acute renal failure can result from rhabdomyolysis.
- **Low serum iron concentration** (mean 5.71 µmol/L; normal 11 to 32 µmol/L) is commonly observed in NMS patients and is a sensitive (92%–100%) but not specific marker for NMS among acutely ill psychiatric patients.

Additional Tests

- **Head magnetic resonance imaging (MRI) and CT** (to exclude structural brain diseases and infections) are typically normal in NMS, but diffuse cerebral edema has been reported in the setting of severe metabolic derangements.
- **Cerebral spinal fluid (CSF)** is usually normal, although a nonspecific protein elevation has been reported.
- **EEG** to rule out nonconvulsive status epilepticus. In NMS patients, generalized slow wave activity is seen.

Treatment

- **Aggressive and supportive care in NMS is essential to reduce mortality.**
- **Immediate discontinuation of causative agent is the single most important treatment in NMS.**
- **Discontinue other potential contributing psychotropic agents:** lithium, serotonergic agents, anticholinergic drugs.
- **Admission to the medical intensive care unit is required** for close inpatient monitoring of clinical signs and laboratory values.
- **Correct cardiac and respiratory instability:** mechanical ventilation, antiarrhythmic agents, or emergent pacemaker placement may be required in severe cases.
- **Correct dehydration caused by fever and diaphoresis** by maintaining euvolemic state. Use intravenous fluids. If CK is significantly elevated, use high-volume intravenous fluids with urine alkalinization to prevent renal failure from rhabdomyolysis.
- **Reduce fever** using cooling blankets; ice water gastric lavage or ice packs in the axilla may be used if required. Role of acetaminophen or aspirin to lower temperature in NMS is not established.
- **Decrease BP** if markedly elevated. Clonidine is effective in NMS-related hypertension. Nitroprusside may have advantages by also facilitating cooling through cutaneous vasodilatation.
- **Use heparin or low-molecular-weight heparin** to prevent deep venous thrombosis.
- **Use low doses of benzodiazepines** (lorazepam 1–2 mg PO every 4 hours as needed or IM if nausea and vomiting; maximum dose 10 mg/day. Clonazepam 0.5–2 mg PO TID; maximum dose 20 mg/day) to control severe agitation, if indicated.

Dantrolene, bromocriptine, amantadine: frequently used, although the efficacy of any of these medications is controversial.

- **Dantrolene** (direct-acting skeletal muscle relaxant): 0.25 mg/kg to 2 mg/kg IV every 6 to 12 hours. Typical daily doses are 3 to 5 mg/kg; max: 10 mg/kg/day; effective for treatment of malignant hyperthermia, as well as rigidity; effective within minutes after administration. Avoid use in abnormal liver function tests (hepatotoxic). Suggested treatment: 3 to 10 days.
- **Bromocriptine** (dopamine agonist; restores lost dopaminergic tone): 2.5 mg (through nasogastric tube) every 6 to 8 hours; titrated up to a maximum dose of 40 mg/day for 10 days after NMS is controlled and then tapered slowly.
- **Amantadine** (has dopaminergic and anticholinergic effects): start 100 mg orally or via gastric tube and then titrate upward as needed to a maximum dose of 200 mg every 12 hours.
- **Electroconvulsive therapy** is indicated if (a) the patient is not responding to medical therapy in the first week; (b) residual catatonia persists after other symptoms of NMS have resolved; and (c) malignant catatonia is suspected as an alternative or concomitant disorder.

Electroconvulsive therapy complications: General anesthesia-related complications, cardiovascular complications (ventricular fibrillation and cardiac arrest), status epilepticus, uncontrolled spontaneous seizures, and aspiration pneumonia, anoxic brain injury. Nondepolarizing agents are not recommended because of induced hyperkalemia and cardiac arrhythmias in patients with rhabdomyolysis and autonomic dysfunction.

Common complications: Dehydration, electrolyte imbalance, acute renal failure associated with rhabdomyolysis, cardiac arrhythmias including torsades de pointes and cardiac arrest, myocardial infarction, cardiomyopathy, respiratory failure from chest wall rigidity, aspiration pneumonia, pulmonary embolism, deep venous thrombophlebitis or thrombosis, thrombocytopenia, disseminated intravascular coagulation, seizures from hyperthermia and metabolic derangements, hepatic failure.

Prognosis

Most episodes resolve within 2 weeks (mean recovery times are 7 to 11 days). NMS symptoms persisting for 6 months with residual catatonia are reported. Most patients recover without neurologic sequelae except for those with severe hypoxia or significantly elevated temperatures for a long duration.

Restarting Neuroleptics

Patients restarted on neuroleptic agents may or may not have a recurrent NMS episode. If neuroleptic medication is required, risk may be minimized by the following measures: Wait at least 2 weeks before restarting therapy, even longer if any clinical residual symptoms of NMS exist; use lower rather than higher potency neuroleptic agents; start with low doses and titrate upward slowly; avoid concomitant lithium; avoid dehydration; carefully monitor for possible NMS reemergence.

Serotonin Syndrome (Table 17-1)

Definition: Serotonin syndrome is a potentially life-threatening condition caused by excess serotonin (serotonin toxicity) in the central nervous system because of a combination of drugs that increase serotonergic transmission.

Causative Agents

- **SSRIs:** fluoxetine, fluvoxamine, paroxetine, sertraline, citalopram, escitalopram
- **Selective serotonin-norepinephrine reuptake inhibitors:** venlafaxine, duloxetine
- **Tricyclic antidepressants:** clomipramine, imipramine, amitriptyline, nortriptyline, desipramine, doxepin, amoxapine, trimipramine, protriptyline
- **Other antidepressants:** mirtazapine
- **Monoamine oxydase inhibitors (MAOIs):** classical, irreversible and nonselective— phenelzine, tranylcypromine, isocarboxazid
- **Reversible monoamine oxydase type A (MAO-A) inhibitors:** moclobemide
- **Selective monoamine oxydase type B (MAO-B) inhibitors:** selegiline (Eldepryl)
- **Other MAOI:** linezolid
- **Opioid analgesics:** tramadol, fentanyl, dextromethorphan, pethidine
- **Serotonin-releasing agents:** fenfluramine, amphetamines, methylenedioxymethamphetamine (MDMA, Ecstasy)
- **Miscellaneous:** Lithium, tryptophan, St. John's wort

Diagnosis

- Hunter Serotonin Toxicity Criteria (the most sensitive and specific in diagnosing serotonin syndrome):
- Requires at least 1 of the following characteristic symptoms:
  - Spontaneous clonus
  - Inducible clonus with agitation or diaphoresis
  - Ocular clonus with agitation or diaphoresis
  - Tremor and hyperreflexia, or hypertonia
  - Temperature above 100.4°F (38°C), and ocular or inducible clonus

Clinical Manifestations

- **Mental status changes:** confusion, delirium, disorientation
- **Neuromuscular excitation:** tremor, clonus, hyperreflexia, myoclonus, rigidity
- **Autonomic instability:** hypertension, hypotension, hyperthermia, shivering and chills tachycardia, tachypnea, diaphoresis, tremor, flushing, sialorrhea, mydriasis

- **Gastrointestinal disturbances:** nausea, vomiting, diarrhea, abdominal cramps
- **Neurologic changes:** coma, lethargy, seizures, insomnia, dizziness, ataxia and incoordination, nystagmus, Babinski sign
- **Cognitive-behavioral disturbances:** agitation, irritability, anxiety, hallucinations

Severity of Serotonin Syndrome

- **Mild serotoninergic features:** Nausea, diarrhea, anorexia, insomnia, irritability, anxiety, decreased libido. May occur with therapeutic use of many serotonergic drugs; self-limited and often resolves after discontinuation or dose reduction of offending agent.
- **Moderate toxicity:** Symptoms cause the patient marked distress and require supportive measures and symptomatic treatment.
- **Severe serotonin toxicity or serotonin crisis:** Medical emergency; rapidly elevating temperature, muscle rigidity, severe autonomic instability, which may progress to multiorgan failure if not treated promptly within hours. Most often caused by combinations of MAOI and SSRI.

Etiology

Most commonly occurs with combinations of drugs acting at different receptor sites, most commonly including a MAOI and a SSRI. Less commonly occurs with other combinations of serotonergic drugs, overdoses, and even single-drug therapy in susceptible individuals.

TABLE 17-1. DIFFERENTIAL DIAGNOSIS BETWEEN SEROTONIN SYNDROME AND NEUROLEPTIC MALIGNANT SYNDROME

Feature	Serotonin syndrome	Neuroleptic Malignant Syndrome
Mechanism	Serotonin excess	Dopamine antagonism
Symptom onset	Minutes to hours	Days to weeks
Symptom duration	Less than 24 hours	5–14 days
Neuromuscular	Myoclonus, hyperreflexia	Bradykinesia, "lead pipe" rigidity, extra-pyramidal side-effects (EPS), hyperkinesias
Gastrointestinal tract	Nausea, vomiting, diarrhea, abdominal cramps	Absent
Rhabdomyolysis, myoglobinuria	Rare	Common
Metabolic acidosis	Rare	Common
Elevated transaminases	Uncommon	Common
Low serum iron	Absent	Common
Leukocytosis	Uncommon	Common
CPK	Uncommon	Common

CPK, creatinine phosphokinase; NMS, neuroleptic malignant syndrome.

Other Differential Diagnoses

- Nonconvulsive seizures (toxic ictal delirium): mostly because of encephalopathy, various drugs overdose (most commonly phenothiazines) or withdrawal (most commonly alcohol or benzodiazepines). EEG is usually diagnostic; treatment with benzodiazepines decreases seizure activity, and clinically differentiates nonconvulsive seizures from serotonin toxicity.
- Acute baclofen withdrawal (typically caused by intrathecal pump failure): difficult to distinguish from serotonin toxicity, need only be considered in a few patients, rapid improvement with reinstitution of baclofen.

- Central nervous system infections (encephalitis, meningitis): absence of neuromuscular excitation, characteristic CSF findings, absence of isolated neck rigidity or other meningeal signs, absence of increased intracranial pressure signs (bradycardia in association with hypertension).
- Anticholinergic delirium: associated with therapeutic (in elderly patients), or toxic doses of drugs with anticholinergic activity; absence of neuromuscular excitation, bowel sounds absent, constipation, urinary retention, decreased salivation, decreased sweating (dry skin).
- Sympathomimetic toxicity: absence of neuromuscular excitation.
- Malignant hyperthermia: exposure to anesthetic agents and absence of neuromuscular excitation, more fulminant.

Treatment

- **Immediate discontinuation of causative agent** is the single most important treatment in serotonin syndrome (resolution of symptoms within 24 hours after the withdrawal of the offending medication[s] in most patients). Serotonin toxicity may worsen progressively over a several hours after ingestion of offending agent or drug combination. At least 6 hours of observation is required for patients with moderate serotonin toxicity (12 hours of observation for serotonergic drugs with long half-life such as fluoxetine, or a slow-release formulations such as venlafaxine).
- **Severe serotonin toxicity requires admission to the medical intensive care unit** (with focus on airways, breathing and circulation, as well as prevention of rhabdomyolysis, renal failure, and disseminated intravascular dissemination caused by hyperthermia and muscle damage).
- **Treatment for all forms of serotonin toxicity includes supportive care and symptomatic treatment:**
  - **Hyperthermia:** antipyretics, aggressive external cooling measures (cooling blankets, ice, mist, fans)
  - **Renal failure prevention:** IV hydration
  - **Hypertension:** nifedipine 30 to 60 mg ER PO daily; maximum 120 mg/day; propranolol (β_1- and β_2-nonselective blocker) 20 to 40 mg PO BID
  - **Sympathetic overstimulation:** propranolol (β_1- and β_2-nonselective blocker) 20 to 40 mg PO BID
  - **Nausea and vomiting:** antiemetics: promethazine (H_1 block) 12.5 to 25 mg PO/IM/IV every 4 to 6 hours as needed; maximum dose 50 mg/dose PO/IM; 25 mg/dose IV); promethazine should be used with extreme caution only in mild serotonin toxicity, and contraindicated in moderate or severe serotonin toxicity because of such side effects as respiratory depression, seizures, urinary retention. Metoclopramide (D_2 central and peripheral receptor block) 5 mg PO TID or 5 to 10 mg PO every 4 hours as needed; metoclopramide should be used with extreme caution only in mild serotonin toxicity, and contraindicated in moderate or severe serotonin toxicity because of such side effects as renal impairment and hypertension.
  - **Rigidity, seizures, and agitation:** benzodiazepines (lorazepam 1–2 mg PO every 4 hours as needed or IM if nausea and vomiting; maximum 10 mg/day. Clonazepam 0.5–2 mg PO TID; maximum 20 mg/day).
  - **Extreme agitation, psychosis:** chlorpromazine (D_2-receptor antagonist) 10 to 25 mg PO TID; maximum 100 mg/day. Chlorpromazine is a preferable agent for sedation in serotonin toxicity; monitor for hypotension (patients should receive sufficient volume load).
  - **Moderate and severe serotonin toxicity:** cyproheptadine (a $5\text{-}HT_2$ antagonist) 4 to 8 mg PO every 1 to 4 hours (maximum 32 mg/day) or 0.25 mg/kg/day divided every 1 to 4 hours in children (available in 4-mg tablets and a syrup 2 mg/5 mL; no parenteral formulation is available).
  - **Overdose of serotonergic agents:** activated charcoal (warranted only if administered within 1 hour after ingestion)

SUBSTANCE-INDUCED ACUTE PSYCHIATRIC EMERGENCIES (TABLE 17-2)

Other Intoxications

- **Carbon monoxide:** depression, lethargy, confusion, delirium, hallucinations, nausea and vomiting, headache, flulike symptoms, hypotension, tachycardia, arrhythmias, respiratory arrest.
- **Treatment:** stop exposure to carbon monoxide, 100% oxygen via nonrebreather mask, hyperbaric oxygen.

SPECIAL POPULATIONS

TABLE 17-2.   CLINICAL MANIFESTATIONS AND TREATMENT OF SUBSTANCE-RELATED DISORDERS

Substance	Symptoms of Intoxication	Treatment of Intoxication	Symptoms of Withdrawal	Treatment of Withdrawal
Alcohol	Aggressive or inappropriate sexual behavior, mood lability, impaired judgment, attention, or memory, slurred speech, incoordination, unsteady gait, stupor, or coma	No specific treatment. Supportive: IV fluids, B-complex vitamins, thiamine (100 mg PO TID for 1–2 weeks for Wernicke encephalopathy, and for 3–12 months for Korsakoff syndrome), magnesium. Mechanical ventilation in respiratory depression.	Tremor, anxiety, autonomic hyperactivity (hypertension, tachycardia, sweating), insomnia, nausea and vomiting, visual and tactile hallucinations-formications (sense of bugs crawling under the skin leading to injurious self-picking behavior) seizures, delirium tremens	Lorazepam[a] Chlordiazepoxide[b] Correct fluid and electrolyte imbalance Thiamine, magnesium, calcium, potassium supplementation if needed
Amphetamines, cocaine; dopaminergic	Euphoria, auditory hallucinations, tactile hallucinations-formications (sense of bugs crawling under the skin leading to injurious self-picking behavior), paranoid delusions, hypervigilance, ideas of reference, psychomotor agitation, aggression, mydriasis, hypertension, tachycardia, arrhythmia, nausea and vomiting	Symptom resolution within 24–48 hours. Consider short-term use of antipsychotics, benzodiazepines, beta-blockers, urine acidification (vitamin C, cranberry juice) to promote renal excretion	Anxiety, tremor, depression (increased risk of suicide), increased appetite, headache	Antidepressants, benzodiazepines
Cannabis: cannabinoid receptors	Impaired motor coordination, euphoria, anxiety, sensation of slowed time, impaired judgment, social withdrawal, increased appetite, conjunctival injection, dry mouth, tachycardia	None	None	None

Opiates: μ-receptor agonists	Initial euphoria followed by apathy, dysphoria, psychomotor agitation or retardation, drowsiness or coma, slurred speech, impairment in attention or memory, pupillary constriction	Naloxone- 1 mg IV every 3 min until improvement Max: 10 mg	Dysphoria, nausea and vomiting, fever, chills, lacrimation, runny nose, abdominal cramps, diarrhea, muscle spasms, insomnia, yawning, pupillary dilatation, piloerection, sweating	Clonidine, methadone
PCP (phencyclidine): NMDA receptor agonist	Hallucinations, delusions, bizarre, or catatonic behavior, violence toward self and others, belligerence, agitation, hypertension, tachycardia, nystagmus, ataxia, dysarthria, tremor, increased muscle tone/rigidity, seizures, diaphoresis, lacrimation, hypersalivation, numbness or diminished sensitivity to pain, hyperacusis	Benzodiazepines, antipsychotics	None	Urine acidification (vitamin C, cranberry juice) to promote renal excretion
MDMA (Ecstasy)- 3,4-Methylenedioxy-methamphetamine (club drug): serotonergic and dopaminergic	Visual and auditory hallucinations, delusions, depersonalization, derealization, depersonalization, increased emotional closeness to others and social relatedness, muscle tension, autonomic instability, teeth clenching, seizures, hyperthermia, hepatic and renal failure	No specific treatment	Anxiety, panic attacks, insomnia, depersonalization, depression, psychosis	Antidepressants, benzodiazepines, antipsychotics

(continued on next page)

SPECIAL POPULATIONS

TABLE 17-2. CLINICAL MANIFESTATIONS AND TREATMENT OF SUBSTANCE-RELATED DISORDERS (Continued)

Substance	Symptoms of Intoxication	Treatment of Intoxication	Symptoms of Withdrawal	Treatment of Withdrawal
Other hallucinogens: serotonergic (agonist/antagonist)	Anxiety, depression, ideas of reference, fear of losing one's mind, paranoid ideations, impaired judgment, derealization, depersonalization, illusions, hallucinations, pupillary dilatation, tremor, incoordination, tachycardia, sweating	Talking down, antipsychotics, benzodiazepines	None	None
Inhalants: GABA receptor enhancer	Belligerence, apathy or euphoria, assaultiveness, impaired judgment, blurred vision or diplopia, stupor or coma, dizziness, nystagmus, incoordination, slurred speech, unsteady gait, lethargy, depressed reflexes, generalized muscle weakness	Antipsychotics if delirious or agitated	None	None
Benzodiazepines: GABA receptor agonists	Inappropriate sexual or aggressive behavior, impairment in memory, attention, concentration, confusion, respiratory depression	Flumazenil	Autonomic hyperactivity (hypertension, tachycardia, diaphoresis), insomnia, anxiety, hallucinations, agitation, tremor, seizures	Benzodiazepines

GABA, γ-aminobutyric acid; IV, intravenously; Max, maximum; NMDA, N-methyl-D-aspartate; PO, orally; TID, 3 times daily.
[a]Lorazepam 1–2 mg PO every 2–4 hours for the first 24 hours. Use lorazepam 1 mg PO every 2 hours as needed for breakthrough symptoms, then taper over the next 7–10 days.
[b]Chlordiazepoxide protocol:
    Chlordiazepoxide 50 mg PO every 6 hours × 4 doses.
    Chlordiazepoxide 25 mg PO every 6 hours × 4 doses.
    Chlordiazepoxide 10 mg PO every 6 hours × 4 doses.
    Chlordiazepoxide 10 mg PO every 12 hours × 2 doses, then stop.
    Use chlordiazepoxide 25 mg or 50 mg PO every 6 hours as needed for breakthrough symptoms.

- **Anticholinergic intoxication:** delirium, agitation, aggression, confusion, visual hallucinations, pupillary dilatation, hot and dry skin, dry mouth, tachycardia, hypertension, urinary retention, constipation. **Treatment:** discontinue anticholinergic agent, gastric lavage and activated charcoal in severe overdose, physostigmine salicylate, benzodiazepines for seizures and agitation. *(Do not use phenothiazine antipsychotics because of their anticholinergic properties.)*
- **Anabolic steroids (abused by bodybuilders):** psychosis, aggression, violent and assaultive behavior. **Treatment:** discontinue offending drug, antipsychotics or benzodiazepines for psychosis, agitation.

SELECTED MOST COMMON PSYCHIATRIC EMERGENCIES CAUSED BY ACUTE MEDICAL AND NEUROLOGIC CONDITIONS AND DRUG SIDE-EFFECTS (TABLE 17-3)

SELECTED MOST COMMON PSYCHIATRIC EMERGENCES CAUSED BY MEDICALLY UNEXPLAINED SYMPTOMS

Conversion Disorder

Definition: Impairment of function of some part of the nervous system that cannot be explained by organic pathology (anatomical or physiologic) of the central or peripheral nervous system. It typically occurs as a result of stress and causes significant dysfunction.

Etiologies

- **Primary gain:** Repression of unconscious intrapsychic conflict and conversion of mental symptom (severe anxiety or unacceptable thought) into physical symptom. Symptoms are produced unconsciously.
- **Secondary gain:** May be classically conditioned learned behavior that serves as a nonverbal means to gain, to cope, to control, to manipulate, or to avoid.

Diagnosis

Based on the apparent absence of organic pathology and the following features:

- Abrupt occurrence of the symptom or deficit, which follows an acute stress or conflict.
- The disorder is usually manifested first during adolescence or in the patient's twenties.
- Patient is predisposed to having histrionic, dependent, or antisocial personality traits or disorder.
- Past history of conversion symptoms.
- Patient tends to have lower intelligence, limited insight, and frequently from lower socioeconomic class.
- *La belle indifférence*—indifference to having the symptom or deficit, which would be frightening or anxiety-provoking in unafflicted person.
- Comorbid depressive or anxiety disorder.

Clinical Manifestations

Most common conversion symptoms are paralysis, blindness, and mutism.

- **Motor symptoms:** paresis, paralysis, aphonia, mutism, tics, blepharospasm, torticollis, opisthotonus, abnormal movements, gait disturbances, falling, astasia-abasia, urinary incontinence
- **Sensory symptoms:** paresthesia, anesthesia (stocking-and-glove, hemianesthesia), blindness, tunnel vision, deafness, anosmia
- **Seizure symptoms:** pseudoseizures—difficult to differentiate from actual seizures—tongue biting, urinary incontinence, injuries after falling are not common in pseudoseizures.
- **Visceral symptoms:** globus hystericus, psychogenic vomiting, pseudocyesis (false pregnancy), syncope, urinary retention
- **Mixed presentation**

Clinical Evaluation

A comprehensive and thorough physical and neurologic evaluation and laboratory investigations are warranted to rule out medical disorders.

TABLE 17-3.   PSYCHIATRIC MANIFESTATIONS OF SELECTED MEDICAL CONDITIONS

	Medical Condition	Characteristic Medical Symptoms and Signs	Acute Confusional State Delirium	Psychosis/ Agitation	Mania	Depression	Anxiety	Diagnostic Tests
Metabolic/Endocrine disorders	Hypoglycemia	Generalized weakness, tremor, dizziness, nausea, hunger, insomnia, seizures, low serum glucose	++	+		+	++	Serum glucose, electrolytes
	Hyperglycemia	Nausea, vomiting, drowsiness, seizures, high serum glucose	+	+		++		Serum glucose, electrolytes (sodium), urine for glucose and ketones
	Hyponatremia	Headache, confusion, nausea and vomiting, anorexia, muscle spasms and weakness, cerebral edema, seizures, coma, low serum sodium	++				+	Serum and urine sodium and osmolality
	Hypernatremia	Lethargy, generalized edema, thirst, respiratory paralysis, seizures, coma, high serum sodium	++					Serum and urine sodium and osmolality
	Hypothyroidism (myxedema madness)	Cold intolerance, weight gain, dry skin, coarse hair, face edema	++	+		+++		TSH, T_4, T_3, thyroid-stimulation test Thyroid imaging studies

	Clinical features						Laboratory tests
Hyperthyroidism	Heat intolerance, weight loss, warm moist skin, hair loss, tremor, palpitations		+	++	+	+	TSH, T₄, T₃, thyroid-stimulation test Thyroid imaging studies
Hypocalcemia	Perioral paraesthesia, muscle spasms, Trousseau sign (carpal spasm induced by blood pressure cuff inflation), Chvostek sign (facial spasm induced by tapping of inferior zygoma), laryngospasm, cardiac arrhythmias	+	+		+	+	Serum calcium PTH ECG (QT and ST prolongation)
Hypercalcemia	Generalized weakness, anorexia, constipation, nausea and vomiting, polyuria, dyspepsia, bone pain, renal stones, soft tissue calcification	+	++		++	++	Serum calcium PTH ECG (short QT and wide T wave)
Hypoparathyroidism	Dry skin, diarrhea, muscle spasms, numbness, paraesthesias, CHF, tremor, rigidity, low serum calcium		+		+	+	Serum calcium, phosphorus, PTH
Hyperparathyroidism	Constipation, dyspepsia, weight loss, renal stones, bone pain, proximal muscle weakness, high serum calcium	+	+		+	+	Serum calcium, phosphorus, PTH, bone x-ray

(continued on next page)

SPECIAL POPULATIONS

TABLE 17-3. PSYCHIATRIC MANIFESTATIONS OF SELECTED MEDICAL CONDITIONS (*Continued*)

Medical Condition	Characteristic Medical Symptoms and Signs	Acute Confusional State Delirium	Psychosis/ Agitation	Mania	Depression	Anxiety	Diagnostic Tests
Hypercortisolism (Cushing syndrome)	Weakness, truncal obesity, buffalo hump, hirsutism, skin stretch marks, moon face, acne, hypertension, impaired glucose tolerance, osteoporosis, high serum and urine cortisol level, high serum sodium, low serum potassium	+	+	++	++	++	Serum, urine cortisol, dexamethasone suppression test, serum sodium, potassium, imaging studies (head, adrenals)
Adrenocortical insufficiency (Addison disease/crisis)	Hypotension, orthostasis, joint and muscle pain and weakness, dizziness, anorexia, nausea and vomiting, hyperpigmentation, sweating, loss of consciousness, fever, low serum sodium, and glucose, high serum potassium and calcium	+			++	++	Serum and urine cortisol, serum aldosterone, renin, serum sodium, potassium, imaging studies (abdominal CT)
Pheochromocytoma	Headache, sweating, flashing, palpitations, paroxysmal hypertension, tachycardia				+	+++	24-hour urine assay for catecholamines, metanephrines, vanillylmandelic acid
Hepatic encephalopathy	Asterixis, ataxia, seizures, fetor hepaticus, abnormal liver function tests, high ammonia level	++	+	+	+		CBC, PT/PTT, liver function tests, serum ammonia level

	Symptoms						Diagnostic evaluation
Acute/chronic renal failure	Oliguria, nausea and vomiting, anorexia, muscle cramps, arrhythmias, dehydration or generalized edema, itching, dizziness, high serum creatinine, potassium phosphate	+		+		+	CBC, serum electrolytes and creatinine, urinalysis, renal imaging
Acute intermittent porphyria	Abdominal pain, nausea and vomiting, constipation, hypertension, tachycardia, seizures, peripheral neuropathy	++		++	+	++	Urine porphyrins, Watson–Schwartz test/ Hoesch test
Structural Brain Diseases — Stroke	Focal motor or sensory deficit, other neurologic symptoms	+	+	+	+	+	Neurologic examination, head CT or MRI
Seizure disorder	Tonic-clonic muscle contractions, aura, episodic staring, automatism	+	++			+	Neurologic examination, comprehensive medical evaluation, head CT or MRI, EEG
Subdural hematoma	Headache, focal neurologic deficit	+				+	Head CT or MRI neurologic examination
Intracranial tumor	Headache, nausea and vomiting, focal motor or sensory deficit, optic nerve edema	+	+	+	+	+	LP (opening pressure is increased), only after head CT or MRI

(continued on next page)

TABLE 17-3. PSYCHIATRIC MANIFESTATIONS OF SELECTED MEDICAL CONDITIONS (Continued)

Medical Condition	Characteristic Medical Symptoms and Signs	Acute Confusional State Delirium	Psychosis/ Agitation	Mania	Depression	Anxiety	Diagnostic Tests
Normal pressure hydrocephalus	Gait abnormality, urinary incontinence	++			+		LP (opening pressure is normal), head CT or MRI
Hypoxic brain injury	Evidence of cardiac or respiratory failure, myocardial infarction, severe congestive heart failure, respiratory paralysis, shock, asphyxia, or carbon monoxide poisoning	++	+			+	Chest x-ray, ECG, arterial blood gases, pulmonary function tests
Neurosyphilis	Headache, nausea and vomiting, nuchal rigidity, vertigo, hyperreflexia, cranial nerve palsies, Argyll-Robertson pupils, gait abnormalities, seizures, mental status changes, stroke	+	+	+	+	+	VDRL, FTA-ABS, enzyme immunoassay test
Bacterial meningitis	Fever, headache, nuchal rigidity, Brudzinski or Kernig signs, nausea and vomiting, photophobia, petechial rash, mental status changes	++	+			+	LP for opening pressure (after head CT or MRI), CSF assay for cells, glucose, protein, CSF culture

Infections

	Clinical features					Workup
Tuberculous meningitis	Headache, fever, weight loss, meningeal signs, SIADH	++		+		LP for opening pressure (after head CT or MRI), CSF assay for cells, glucose, protein, acid-fast bacteria; CSF culture
Cryptococcal meningitis		++		‡	‡	LP for opening pressure (after head CT or MRI), CSF assay for cells, glucose, protein, CSF and serum cryptococcal antigen, head CT or MRI
Viral meningitis	Fever, headache, nuchal rigidity, Brudzinski and Kernig signs—all mild (less prominent than in bacterial meningitis)—nausea and vomiting, photophobia, mental status changes, seizures, zoster eruption in VZV, maculopapular rash in measles, vesicular rash in herpes simplex meningitis, lymphadenopathy and splenomegaly in Epstein-Barr infection	‡		+		LP for opening pressure (after CT or MRI), CSF assay for cells, glucose, protein, CSF for latex antigen test to differentiate from other etiologies

(continued on next page)

TABLE 17-3. PSYCHIATRIC MANIFESTATIONS OF SELECTED MEDICAL CONDITIONS (Continued)

Medical Condition	Characteristic Medical Symptoms and Signs	Acute Confusional State Delirium	Psychosis/ Agitation	Mania	Depression	Anxiety	Diagnostic Tests
AIDS	Fever, weight loss, lymphadenopathy, neurologic changes	+	+	+	++	+	HIV serology and Western blot; CSF testing of HIV PCR for AIDS-dementia complex
Thiamine deficiency	Wernicke encephalopathy (acute and completely reversible with treatment): ataxia, mental status changes/confusion, ophthalmoplegia (horizontal nystagmus, lateral orbital palsy, gaze paralysis. See treatment in Table 17-1. Korsakoff syndrome (chronic and irreversible in more than 80% of cases, even with treatment): anterograde amnesia, impaired recent memory, confabulations. Dry beriberi: peripheral neuropathy, impairment of sensory, motor, and reflex functions. Wet beriberi: mental status changes, confusion, tachycardia, cardiomegaly, CHF, edema in addition to peripheral neuropathy.	+	+		+		Thiamine level

VITAMIN DEFICIENCY

	Condition	Clinical features						Diagnostic tests
Other	Vitamin B$_{12}$ deficiency	Ataxia, peripheral neuropathy (paresthesias, impaired senses of tough, vibration, pressure, proprioception, decreased deep tendon reflexes), GI tract symptoms, memory loss, megaloblastic anemia; common causes: pernicious anemia, achlorhydria, Crohn disease/short bowel syndrome, metformin use	+		+	+	+	+	Serum vitamin B$_{12}$ and folate levels, homocysteine level, CBC with red cell indices, methylmalonic acid level, Schilling test
	Niacin deficiency (pellagra)	Skin lesions—bilateral, symmetric, at pressure points or sun-exposed areas—stomatitis, glossitis, nausea and vomiting, constipation, diarrhea, abdominal distention, dementia	+		+	+	+	+	Mostly clinical diagnosis; urine N-methylnicotinamide (NMN) level
	Systemic lupus erythematosus	Arthritis, myalgias, malaise, fatigue, malar rash (butterfly rash), photosensitivity, oral and vaginal ulcers, fatigue, weight loss, alopecia, lymphadenopathy	+		++	++	+	+	Antinuclear antibodies (ANA) and anti-DNA antibody tests

AIDS, acquired immunodeficiency syndrome; CBC, complete blood count; CHF, congestive heart failure; CSF, cerebral spinal fluid; CT, computed tomography; ECG, electrocardiogram; EEG, electroencephalogram; FTA-ABS, fluorescent treponemal antibody absorption; GI, gastrointestinal; HIV, human immunodeficiency virus; LP, lumbar puncture; MRI, magnetic resonance imaging; PCR, polymerase chain reaction; PT, prothrombin time; PTH, parathyroid hormone; PTT, partial thromboplastin time; SIADH, syndrome of inappropriate secretion of antidiuretic hormone; T$_3$, triiodothyronine; T$_4$, thyroxine; TSH, thyroid-stimulating hormone; VZV, varicella-zoster virus; + mild symptoms; ++ moderate symptoms; +++ severe symptoms.

Diagnostic Studies

• Conversion disorder is a diagnosis of exclusion.
• As many as 25% to 50% of patients with conversion disorder have associated organic pathology.

Laboratory

• Full blood examination (CBC, creatinine, electrolytes, glucose, calcium, liver function tests)
• Urinalysis (if urinalysis abnormal)
• CT brain (to exclude stroke, tumor, infection)
• Lumbar puncture (if headache, fever and meningeal symptoms present),
• EEG (may assist in determining etiology: epileptic or nonepileptic seizure activity)
• Prothrombin time (PT), partial thromboplastin time (PTT) (if indicated)
• Urine toxicology screen
• Chest x-ray
• Cardiac enzymes
• ECG
• Thyroid function tests
• Vitamin B_{12} and folate serum levels
• VDRL and HIV tests

Differential Diagnosis

• **Paresis, paralysis:** Attempts to drop paralyzed hand onto face results in failure of hand to drop onto face, but next to face.
• **Anesthesia:** Sensory deficit does not conforms dermatomal distribution; exact half-body split in hemianesthesia.
• **Blindness:** No relative afferent pupillary defect, swinging hand in front of "blind eye" causes tracking eye movements.
• **Aphonia:** normal coughing (inability to cough because of vocal cord paralysis in true aphonia).
• **Pseudoseizures:** Gag reflexes and papillary reflexes are preserved in pseudoseizures; no postictal prolactin elevation, video-monitoring EEG does not confirm true seizure activity.
• **Astasia-abasia:** Patients rarely fall, are rarely injured, unable to walk, but able to dance with suggestion.
• **Parenteral lorazepam** is indicated in selected cases to obtain additional historical information.

Prognosis

• Favorable, with resolution of symptoms in 90% to 100% within several days or weeks after initial presentation.
• Good prognostic factors: sudden onset, identifiable stressor, good premorbid functioning.

Treatment

• Reassurance
• Behavioral therapy
• Insight-oriented supportive psychotherapy
• Psychodynamic or psychoanalytic interventions
• Relaxation exercises

Factitious Disorder

Definition: Intentional production or falsification of the symptoms or signs of medical or mental disorders in order to assume the sick role.

  Diagnosis based on the following criteria (*Diagnostic and Statistical Manual of Mental Disorders IV-TR*):

• Intentional production or feigning of physical or psychological signs or symptoms.
• The motivation for the behavior is to assume the sick role.
• External incentives for the behavior (economic gain, avoiding legal responsibilities, or improving physical well-being, as in malingering) are absent.

Types

- With predominantly psychological signs and symptoms
- With predominantly physical signs and symptoms—Munchausen syndrome (polysurgical or hospital addiction): severe form of factitious disorder in which a patient presents with very elaborate medical or surgical histories in order to be repeatedly admitted to the hospital, and even to be intentionally exposed to painful and risky tests, procedures, or surgeries.
- With combined psychological and physical signs and symptoms.
- Pseudologia fantastica is a form of factitious disorder in which the patient presents factual material that is intermixed with extensive, dramatic, colorful, and conflicting fantasies.

Etiologies

- **Psychologic factors:** poorly consolidated sense of self, difficulties in reality testing and regarding emotional experiences as real. Assuming the sick role may serve to stabilize impaired sense of self, and evoke responsiveness of caregiver in a safe and structured context.
- **Biologic factors:** nonspecific brain dysfunction, including impairment of information processing.

Clinical Manifestations

Suspect factitious disorder if patient has the following features:

- History of multiple hospitalizations to different medical facilities, malpractice and insurance claims.
- Very elaborate, dramatic, colorful medical and personal history presentation.
- Patient is insisting, evasive, argumentative.
- Patient may be in the professional health care or medical field, or related to health care field.

Factitious Disorder with Predominantly Psychological Signs and Symptoms

- Depression
- Amnesia
- Psychosis (hallucinations, delusions)
- Bipolar disorder type I
- Dissociative identity disorder
- Pain disorder
- Bereavement
- Posttraumatic stress disorder
- Hypersomnia
- Eating disorders
- Transsexualism
- Substance-related disorders

Factitious Disorder with Predominantly Physical Signs and Symptoms (Munchausen Syndrome)

- **Abdominal pain:** Look for numerous surgical scars ("railroad abdomen").
- **Bleeding:** Look for intentional intake of anticoagulant medications, or contamination of laboratory samples (urine) with blood.
- **Heart rhythm disorders:** Look for intentional intake of stimulants or amphetamine to induce tachycardia, beta-blockers to induce bradycardia, or digitalis to induce arrhythmia.
- **Fever:** Look for possible manipulation with thermometer.
- Sepsis: Look for possible contamination of IV lines with urine, feces, or dirt to induce septicemia.
- **Hypoglycemia:** Look for intentional intake of hypoglycemic medications or insulin injections.
- **Skin lesions:** Look for linear pattern in skin areas the patient is able to reach.

Clinical Evaluation

Thorough medical and neurologic workup, as well as laboratory investigations are warranted to rule out medical and neurologic disorders.

Diagnostic Studies

- **Laboratory:** There is no specific laboratory test for factitious disorder.
- **Psychological testing**

Differential Diagnosis

- **Somatization disorder:** Onset before age 30 years, involvement of multiple organs or systems (at least 4 pain symptoms, 2 gastrointestinal symptoms, 1 sexual symptom, and 1 pseudoneurologic symptom) versus onset at any age and voluntary production of factitious symptoms and signs, and willingness to undergo multiple painful, and invasive procedures and surgeries in factitious patient.
- **Conversion disorders:** Lack of knowledge of medical terminology, hospital rules, lack of temporal connection between the symptom or deficit and severe stress or conflict.
- **Hypochondriasis:** No intentional symptom production, lack of willingness to undergo multiple painful, and invasive procedures and surgeries in contrast with factitious patient.
- **Antisocial personality disorder:** Antisocial persons do not demonstrate willingness to undergo multiple painful, and invasive procedures and surgeries in contrast with factitious patient, although both conditions have common features (pathologic lying, manipulative behavior, substance abuse, lack of close relationships).
- **Borderline personality disorder:** Difficult to differentiate, as borderline persons often demonstrate self-mutilating acts, identity crisis, attention-seeking and manipulative behavior, although they are lacking multiple hospitalizations and surgeries and do not demonstrate willingness to undergo multiple painful and invasive procedures and surgeries in contrast to the factitious patient.
- **Schizophrenia:** Presence of positive symptoms (bizarre delusions, auditory hallucinations, disorganized speech and behavior) and negative symptoms (social withdrawal, flat affect, amotivation, abulia); only a few patients with factitious disorders present with frank psychotic symptoms.

Prognosis

In most cases prognosis is poor, especially in cases of multiple prolonged hospitalizations and disability caused by multiple surgeries that are incompatible with normal social, occupational, and personal life.

Treatment

- Early diagnosis is crucial in order to avoid unnecessary hospitalizations and dangerous invasive procedures.
- Educate hospital staff to establish rapport with the patient.
- Offer supportive individual psychotherapy with close countertransference monitoring.

Malingering

Definition: Intentional production, falsification, or exaggeration of physical or psychological symptoms that motivate person to seek hospitalization for some obvious external incentives such as obtaining financial compensation, free hospital bed for night, getting drugs, avoiding military duty, work, difficult or dangerous situations, evading police, court appointments, or criminal prosecution.

Diagnosis

Suspect malingering if a person has the following features:

- Significant discrepancy between the person's vague, ill-defined complains, or disability and the objective findings.
- Clinical findings appear compatible with self-inflicting injuries.
- Uncooperative and evasive behavior during clinical assessment and treatment.
- Nonadherence with recommended treatment regimen.
- Avoidance of diagnostic tests and medical procedures to establish diagnosis.
- Giving up initially presented symptoms on exposure to tests and procedures.
- Requesting discharge from hospital against medical advice.
- Claiming physical disability or requesting disability benefits for condition that lacks objective findings.
- Presence of homeless person in psychiatric emergency room during cold, winter season with suicidal threats and requesting admission.
- Antisocial personality traits or disorder and substance abuse are common concomitant conditions.

- Attorney referral for clinical evaluation or other medicolegal context of presentation (prisoner presents with foreign body ingestion to get out of prison).
- Evidence of several episodes of injury or undiagnosed diseases in past medical records.

Etiologies

- Malingering is not medical or psychiatric diagnosis, but a condition that may be a focus of clinical attention.
- The presence of obvious, definable goal and external motivation is the main feature of this condition.

Clinical Manifestations

- Vague, ill-defined, subjective symptoms that are difficult to refute
- Physical symptoms: headache, nausea, dizziness, vertigo, back and neck pain, chest pain, abdominal pain, blurred vision, hearing loss, paresis or paralysis, seizures
- Psychological symptoms: anxiety, panic attacks, depression, amnesia, psychosis
- Symptoms that are nor congruent with recognized medical or psychiatric conditions
- Preoccupation with compensation rather than with treatment
- Knowledge of the legal-medical precedents and law, and claim procedures

Clinical Evaluation

Thorough medical and neurologic workup, as well as laboratory investigations are warranted to rule out medical and neurologic disorders.

Diagnostic studies (to sort out auditory, ophthalmologic, labyrinthine, neurologic, and other medical conditions)

- Audiometry
- Brainstem audiometry
- Ophthalmoscopy
- Visual- and auditory-evoked potentials
- Galvanic skin response
- Electromyography, nerve conduction study
- EEG

Differential Diagnosis

- **Factitious disorder:** External incentives are absent; psychological need to obtain and to maintain sick role.
- **Conversion disorder and other somatoform disorder:** External incentives are absent; suggestion or hypnosis is not effective for symptom resolution.
- **Other specific features that differentiate malingering from genuine diseases** (see the section Diagnosis)

Treatment

- Clinician should never assume malingering before thorough objective clinical, radiological, and laboratory evaluation.
- Clinician should never demonstrate any suspicion or become angry while dealing with a person suspected of malingering.
- Establish rapport with a person, which is essential for correct diagnosis.
- Use an intensive treatment approach including inpatient and outpatient observation to reveal symptoms that could be consistently present only when a person is under close observation.
- Encourage and reassure a person to give up his or her symptoms without losing face.

SUGGESTED READING

1. Glick RL, Berlin JS, Fishkind AB, Zeller SL. *Emergency Psychiatry: Principles and Practice.* Philadelphia: Lippincott Williams & Wilkins; 2008; 117-123; 125-131; 213-221; 227-281.
2. Hall RCW, Gardner ER, Ropkin MD, et al. Unrecognized physical illness prompting psychiatric admission: a prospective study. *Am J Psychiatry.* 1981;25:1315-1320.
3. Blumenfield M, Tiamson-Kassab M. *Psychosomatic Medicine. A Practical Guide.* 2nd ed. Philadelphia: Lippincott Williams & Wilkins; 2009; 123-127; 156-160; 163-166.

4. Bernstain CA, IsHak WW, Weiner ED, Ladds BJ. *On Call Psychiatry*. 2nd ed. Philadelphia: Saunders; 2001; 17-39; 125-134; 135-148.

5. Tomb D. *Psychiatry*. 6th ed. Philadelphia: Lippincott Williams & Wilkins; 1999; 56-61; 105-114; 132-136.

6. Davis S. Violence in psychiatric patients: a review. *Hosp Community Psychiatry*. 1991;42:585-590.

7. Pedersen DD. *Psych Notes. Clinical Pocket Guide*. 2nd ed. Philadelphia: F.A. Davis; 2008: 163-164.

8. Sadock BJ, Sadock VA. *Synopsis of Psychiatry*. Philadelphia: Lippincott Williams & Wilkins; 2003; 323-329; 668-675; 903-905; 993-994; 998.

9. Tropea J, Slee JA, Brand CA, Gray L, Snell T. Clinical practice guidelines for the management of delirium in older people in Australia. *Australas J Ageing*. 2008;27:150-156.

10. McIntyre JS, Charles SC. *Quick Reference to the American Psychiatric Association Practice Guidelines for the Treatment of Psychiatric Disorders*. Arlington, VA: Compendium; 2006.

11. Strawn, JR, Keck, PE Jr, Caroff, SN. Neuroleptic malignant syndrome. *Am J Psychiatry*. 2007;164:870.

12. Wijdicks E. *Neuroleptic malignant syndrome*. Last updated May 6, 2010. http://www.uptodate.com/home/content/topic.do?topicKey=medneuro/5946.

13. Shalev A, Hermesh H, Munitz H. Mortality from neuroleptic malignant syndrome. *J Clin Psychiatry*. 1989;50:18.

14. Levenson JL. Neuroleptic malignant syndrome. *Am J Psychiatry*. 1985;142:1137.

15. Velamoor VR. Neuroleptic malignant syndrome. Recognition, prevention and management. *Drug Saf*. 1998;19:73.

16. Keck PE Jr, Pope HG Jr, Cohen BM, et al. Risk factors for neuroleptic malignant syndrome. A case-control study. *Arch Gen Psychiatry*. 1989;46:914.

17. Hermesh H, Aizenberg D, Weizman A, et al. Risk for definite neuroleptic malignant syndrome. A prospective study in 223 consecutive in-patients. *Br J Psychiatry*. 1992;161:254.

18. Berardi D, Amore M, Keck PE Jr, et al. Clinical and pharmacologic risk factors for neuroleptic malignant syndrome: a case-control study. *Biol Psychiatry*. 1998;44:748.

19. Koch M, Chandragiri S, Rizvi S, et al. Catatonic signs in neuroleptic malignant syndrome. *Compr Psychiatry*. 2000;41:73.

20. Adnet P, Lestavel P, Krivosic-Horber R. Neuroleptic malignant syndrome. *Br J Anaesth*. 2000;85:129.

21. Brent J. Monoamine Oxidase Inhibitors and the Serotonin Syndrome. In: Haddad LM, Shannon MW, Winchester JF, eds. Clinical Management of Poisoning and Drug Overdose. 3rd ed. Philadelphia, PA: W.B. Saunders Company; 1998:459-463.

22. Burkhalter A, Julius DJ, Katzung BG. Histamine, serotonin, & the ergot alkaloids. In: Katzung BG, ed. *Basic and Clinical Pharmacology*. 7th ed. Stamford, CT: Appleton and Lange; 1998:273-277.

23. Mills KC. Serotonin syndrome. A clinical update. *Crit Care Clin*. 1997;13:763-783.

24. Isbister GK, Buckley NA, Whyte IM. Serotonin toxicity: a practical approach to diagnosis and treatment. *Med J Aust*. 2007;187:361-365.

25. Dunkley EJ, Isbister GK, Sibbritt D, et al. The Hunter Serotonin Toxicity Criteria: simple and accurate diagnostic decision rules for serotonin toxicity. *QJM*. 2003;96: 635-642.

26. Isbister GK, Bowe SJ, Dawson A, Whyte IM. Relative toxicity of selective serotonin reuptake inhibitors (SSRIs) in overdose. *J Toxicol Clin Toxicol*. 2004;42:277-285.

27. Sternbach H. The serotonin syndrome. *Am J Psychiatry*. 1991;148:705-713.

28. Whyte IM. Serotonin toxicity/syndrome. In: *Medical Toxicology*. 3rd ed. Philadelphia: Lippincott Williams & Wilkins; 2004:103-106.

29. Shelton RC. The nature of the discontinuation syndrome associated with antidepressant drugs. *J Clin Psychiatry*. 2006;67(suppl 4):3-7.

30. Van Sweden B, Mellerio F. Toxic ictal delirium. *Biol Psychiatry*. 1989;25:449-458.

31. Mohammed I, Hussain A. Intrathecal baclofen withdrawal syndrome—a life-threatening complication of baclofen pump: a case report. *BMC Clin Pharmacol*. 2004;4:6.

32. Radomski JW, Dursun SM, Reveley MA, Kutcher SP. An exploratory approach to the serotonin syndrome: an update of clinical phenomenology and revised diagnostic criteria. *Med Hypotheses.* 1999;55:218-224.

33. Graudins A, Stearman A, Chan B. Treatment of the serotonin syndrome with cyproheptadine. *J Emerg Med.* 1998;16:615-619.

34. Gillman PK. The serotonin syndrome and its treatment. *J Psychopharmacol.* 1999;13: 100-109.

35. Utah Poison Control Center. Serotonin syndrome. *Utox Update.* 2002;4(4). http://uuhsc.utah.edu/poison/healthpros/utox/Vol4_No4.pdf

36. Lipowski ZJ. Delirium in the Elderly Patient. New England Journal of Medicine. 1989;320:578-582.

Appendix

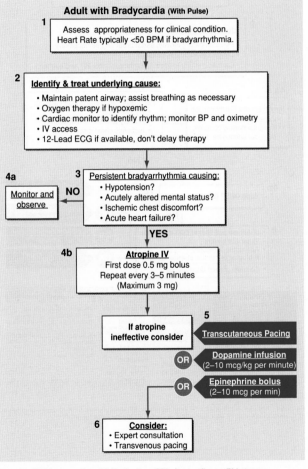

Figure A-1 BPM, beats per minute; BP, blood pressure; ECG, electrocardiogram; IV, intravenous.

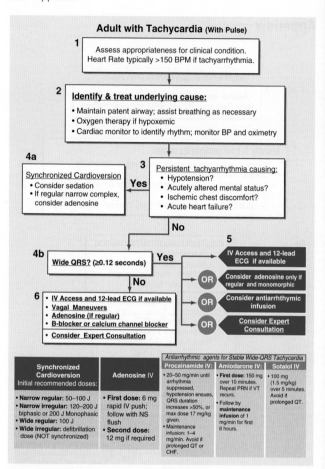

Figure A-2 B-blocker, beta-blocker; BPM, beats per minute; BP, blood pressure; CHF, congestive heart failure; ECG, electrocardiogram; IV, intravenous; PRN, as needed; VT, ventricular tachycardia.

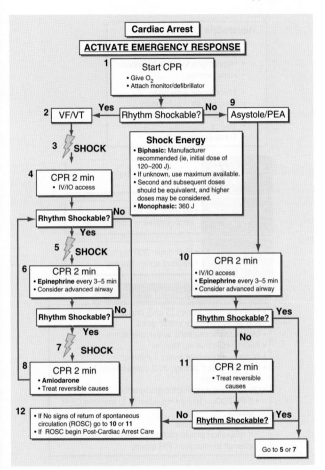

Figure A-3 CPR, cardiopulmonary resuscitation; IO, intraosseous infusion; IV, intravenous; PEA, pulseless electrical activity; ROSC, return of spontaneous circulation; VF, ventricular fibrillation; VT, ventricular tachycardia.

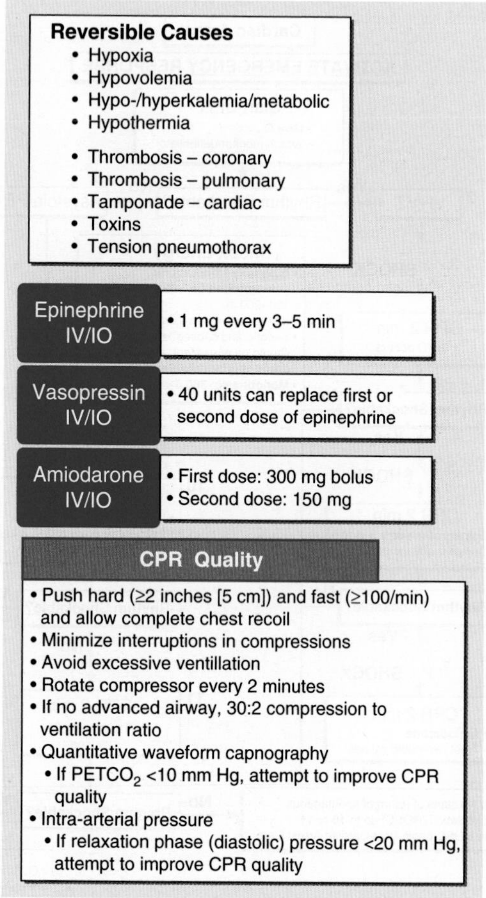

Reversible Causes
- Hypoxia
- Hypovolemia
- Hypo-/hyperkalemia/metabolic
- Hypothermia

- Thrombosis – coronary
- Thrombosis – pulmonary
- Tamponade – cardiac
- Toxins
- Tension pneumothorax

Epinephrine IV/IO	• 1 mg every 3–5 min
Vasopressin IV/IO	• 40 units can replace first or second dose of epinephrine
Amiodarone IV/IO	• First dose: 300 mg bolus • Second dose: 150 mg

CPR Quality
- Push hard (≥2 inches [5 cm]) and fast (≥100/min) and allow complete chest recoil
- Minimize interruptions in compressions
- Avoid excessive ventilation
- Rotate compressor every 2 minutes
- If no advanced airway, 30:2 compression to ventilation ratio
- Quantitative waveform capnography
  - If $PETCO_2$ <10 mm Hg, attempt to improve CPR quality
- Intra-arterial pressure
  - If relaxation phase (diastolic) pressure <20 mm Hg, attempt to improve CPR quality

Figure A-4   CPR, cardiopulmonary resuscitation; IO, intraosseous infusion; IV, intravenous; $PETCO_2$, partial pressure of end-tidal carbon dioxide.

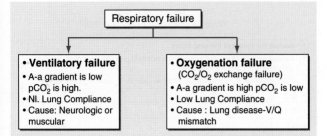

Figure A-5 A-a, alveolar-arterial; Nl, normal limits; pCO₂, partial pressure of carbon dioxide; V/Q, ventilation perfusion scan.

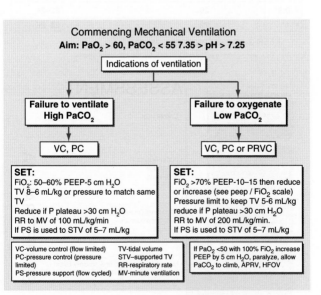

Figure A-6 APRV, airway pressure release ventilation; FiO₂, fraction of inspired oxygen; HFOV, high-frequency oscillatory ventilation; PaCO₂, arterial partial pressure of carbon dioxide; PaO₂, arterial oxygen partial pressure; PEEP, positive end-expiratory pressure; PRVC, pressure-regulated volume control.

| Target PaO$_2$ >60 |
| What FiO required to achieve this? |

- **Assess the extent of the lung injury**
- **Assess patient' chest wall compliance NORMAL** or **LOW I.e.** obesity, edema, abdominal compartment syndrome

FiO$_2$	Normal C$_w$ Compliance PEEP in cmH$_2$O	Low C$_w$ Compliance
0.3	5	10
0.4	8	12
0.5	10	14
0.6*	12	16
0.7*	14	18
0.75*	16	20
0.8*	18	22
0.9*	20	22–24
1*	22	24–26

PEEP-positive end expiratory pressure

Figure A-7   PaO$_2$, arterial oxygen partial pressure; FiO$_2$, fraction of inspired oxygen.

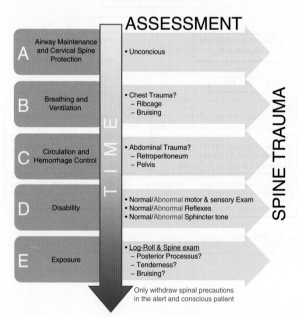

Figure A-8

ATLS Hemorrhage Classification

Estimated Blood Loss Based on Patient's Initial Presentation*

	Class I	Class II	Class III	Class IV
Blood loss (mL) and percent loss	Up to 750 up to 15%	750–1500 15–30%	1500–2000 30–40%	>2000 >40%
Pulse Rate (bpm)	<100	100–120	120–140	>140
Blood Pressure	Normal	Normal	Decreased	Decreased
Pulse Pressure (mm Hg)	Normal or ↑	↓	↓	↓
Respiratory Rate (breaths/min)	14–20	20–30	30–40	>35
Urine Output (mL/hr)	>30	20–30	5–15	Negligible
CNS/Mental status	Slightly anxious	Mildly anxious	Anxious, confused	Confused, lethargic
Fluid replacement	Crystalloid	Crystalloid	Crystalloid and blood	Crystalloid and blood

(*Based on 70 kg male)

Figure A-9   CNS, central nervous system.

Glasgow Coma Score		Score
Eye opening	Spontaneous	4
	To speech	3
	To pain	2
	None	1
Best **Verbal** response	Oriented	5
	Confused	4
	Innapropriate words	3
	Incomprehensible sounds	2
	None	1
Best **Motor** response	Obeys	6
	Localizes	5
	Withdraws	4
	Abnormal flexion to pain	3
	Extensor response to pain	2
	None	1

Figure A-10

Index

Note: Page number followed by *f* and *t* indicates figure and table respectively.

Color Insert

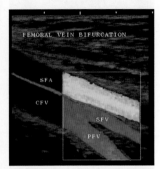

Figure 1-2 Ultrasound anatomy of the superficial femoral artery and the bifurcation of the common femoral vein. Note colored Doppler direction. BART, blue away from, red toward (the transducer).

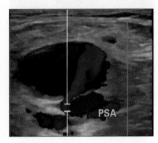

Figure 4-20 Two-dimensional arterial ultrasound and colored Doppler of the patient with femoral artery pseudoaneurysm. PSA, posterior spinal artery. (Image recreated by Maria Levitov.)

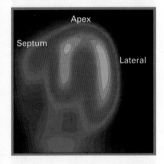

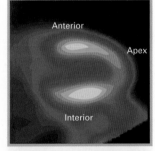

Figure 4-17 Correlation of coronary anatomy and imaging segments (positron emission tomography, single-photon emission computed tomography, etc). (Images recreated by Maria Levitov.)

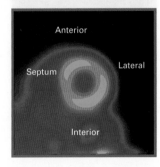

1

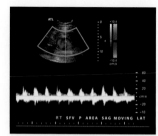

Figure 4-21 Two-dimensional arterial ultrasound continuous wave and colored Doppler of the patient with femoral artery arteriovenous fistula.

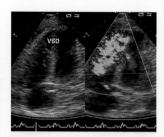

Figure 4-24 Echocardiogram in apical 4-chamber view of the acquired ventricular septal defect (VSD) complicating septal (left anterior descending artery distribution) ST-segment elevation myocardial infarction.

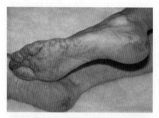

Figure 4-22 Livedo reticularis in patient with atheroemboli.

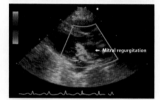

Figure 4-28 Echocardiogram in parasternal long axis view of a patient with acquired mitral valve regurgitation and inferior wall myocardial infarction (right coronary artery distribution).

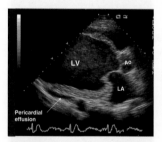

Figure 4-23 Echocardiogram in parasternal long axis view of the patient with severe dilative cardiomyopathy. Ao, aorta; LA, left atrium; LV, left ventricle.

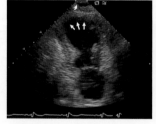

Figure 4-34 Takotsubo dilated cardiomyopathy ("broken heart syndrome"). Note disproportional apical involvement (ballooning [white arrows]).

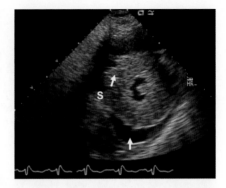

Figure 4-36 Echocardiogram in parasternal short axis view of a patient with restrictive cardiomyopathy (cardiac amyloidosis). Notice symmetrical nature of the left ventricle wall thickening, small pericardial effusion, and speckled (S) myocardial pattern.

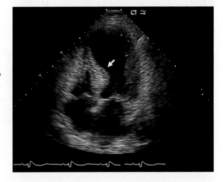

Figure 4-38 Echocardiogram (echo) in apical 4-chamber view of a patient with hypertrophic cardiomyopathy (HCMP). Note intraventricular septal thickness greatly exceeds free wall thickness. Two-dimensional echo differential diagnosis between acquired and congenital HCMP is difficult.

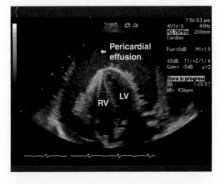

Figure 4-44 Echocardiogram in subcostal view a patient with pericardial effusion and cardiac (pericardial) tamponade. LV, left ventricle; RV, right ventricle.

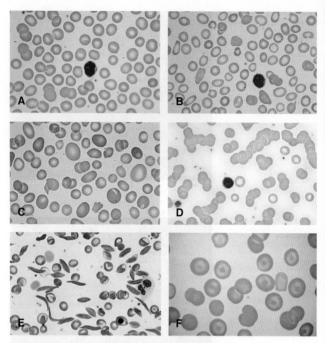

Figure 7-1   Peripheral blood smears. **A.** Normal peripheral blood smear. Small lymphocyte in center of field.
Note that the diameter of the red blood cell is similar to the diameter of the small lymphocyte nucleus.
B. Hypochromic microcytic anemia of iron deficiency. Small lymphocyte in field helps assess the red blood
cell size. **C.** Macrocytosis. These cells are both larger than normal (mean corpuscular volume >100 femtoliters)
and somewhat oval in shape. Some morphologists call these cells *macroovalocytes.* **D.** Rouleaux formation. Small
lymphocyte in center of field. These red cells align themselves in stacks and are related to increased serum
protein levels. **E.** Sickle cells. Homozygous sickle cell disease. A nucleated red cell and neutrophil are also in
the field. **F.** Target cells. Target cells are recognized by the bull's-eye appearance of the cell. Small numbers of
target cells are seen with liver disease and thalassemia. Larger numbers are typical of hemoglobin C disease.

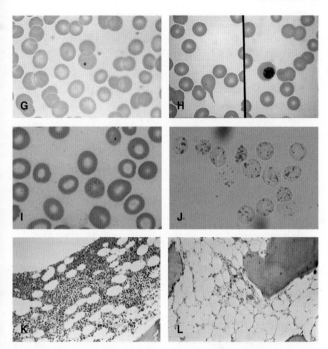

G. Howell-Jolly bodies. Howell-Jolly bodies are tiny nuclear remnants that normally are removed by the spleen. They appear in the blood after splenectomy (defect in removal) and with maturation and dysplastic disorders (excess production). **H.** Teardrop cells and nucleated red blood cells characteristic of myelofibrosis. A teardrop-shaped red blood cell (*left panel*) and a nucleated red blood cell (*right panel*) as typically seen with myelofibrosis and extramedullary hematopoiesis. **I.** Stippled red cell in lead poisoning. Mild hypochromia. Coarsely stippled red cell. **J.** Heinz bodies. Blood mixed with hypotonic solution of crystal violet. The stained material is precipitates of denatured hemoglobin within cells. **K.** Normal bone marrow. Low-power view of normal adult marrow (H and E stain), showing a mix of fat cells (clear areas) and hematopoietic cells. The percentage of the space that consists of hematopoietic cells is referred to as *marrow cellularity*. In adults, normal marrow cellularity is 35% to 40%. If demands for increased marrow production occur, cellularity may increase to meet the demand. As people age, the marrow cellularity decreases and the marrow fat increases. Patients older than 70 years of age may have a 20% to 30% marrow cellularity. **L.** Aplastic anemia bone marrow. Normal hematopoietic precursor cells are virtually absent, leaving behind fat cells, reticuloendothelial cells, and the underlying sinusoidal structure. (From Longo DL, et al., eds. *Harrison's Principles of Internal Medicine.* 18th ed. New York: McGraw-Hill; 2011.)

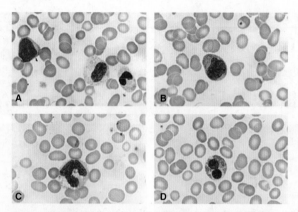

Figure 7-3   Myelodysplastic syndrome (oligoplastic myelogenous leukemia). **A.** Blood film. Blast, monocyte, and pseudo-Pelger-Huët cell. **B.** Blood film. Monocyte. **C.** Blood film. Monocyte. **D.** Blood film. Dysmorphic eosinophil with very small granules. (From Lichtman MA, et al. *Lichtman's Atlas of Hematology.* New York: McGraw-Hill; © 2007 by The McGraw-Hill Companies, Inc. All rights reserved.)

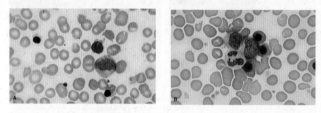

Figure 7-4   **A.** Blood film. Two nucleated red cells and a promyelocyte and a lymphocyte. The red cells show occasional but increased poikilocytosis. The patient had metastatic renal carcinoma to several sites including marrow. **B.** Blood film. White cell concentrate (buffy coat). Three nucleated red cells, 2 myelocytes, and a segmented neutrophil are evident. Another nucleated red cell can be partially visualized at right margin of field. In this case the blood film did not have evidence of a leukoerythroblastic reaction, but evidence was found in a film of the white cell concentrate. Because the white cell concentrate is the layer between the red cells and plasma in centrifuged blood, the red cells aspirated with the white cells are usually of lower density than average and reticulocyte rich, as evident here. Red cell morphology is not representative of the direct blood film. Patient had carcinoma of the lung metastatic to marrow. In leukoerythroblastic reactions, the red cell precursors that escape the marrow are usually orthochromatic erythroblasts, although occasionally earlier precursors may be seen. (From Lichtman MA, et al. *Lichtman's Atlas of Hematology.* New York: McGraw-Hill; © 2007 by The McGraw-Hill Companies, Inc. All rights reserved.)

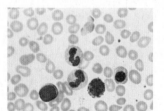

Figure 7-5   Teardrop-shaped red blood cells indicative of membrane damage from passage through the spleen, a nucleated red blood cell, and immature myeloid cells indicative of extramedullary hematopoiesis are noted. This peripheral blood smear is related to any cause of extramedullary hematopoiesis. (From Longo DL, et al., eds. *Harrison's Principles of Internal Medicine.* 18th ed. New York: McGraw-Hill; 2011.)